VIDEO CONTENT AND RESOURCES FROM DR. TEBBETTS

DVD 1

■ **Breast Augmentation: A Masterclass Curriculum**

1.1 Introduction – Redefining Patient Outcomes
1.2 Requirements for Optimal Patient Outcomes
1.3 Evolution of Tissue-based Implant Selection Systems
1.4 Five Critical Decisions and Measurements
1.5 Clinical Application of the High Five™ Systems
1.6 Implant Selection Principles and Processes
1.7 Preoperative Marking
1.8 Premedications and Anesthesia
1.9 Surgical Processes and Techniques
1.10 Prospective Hemostasis Principles
1.11 Pocket Dissection Sequence
1.12 Incision and Pocket Access
1.13 Inferiomedial (Zone 2) Pocket Dissection
1.14 Transition to the Lateral Pocket Dissection (Zone 3 and 4)
1.15 Medial Pocket (Zone 5) Dissection
1.16 Implant Insertion and Positioning
1.17 Incision Closure
1.18 Postoperative Adjuncts
1.19 Recovery and PACU Care
1.20 Postoperative Care for the 24-hour Recovery
1.21 Redefining the Patient Experience

Running time = 97 minutes

DVD 2 INCLUDING RESOURCES FOLDER

■ **Instrumentation, Anesthesia, and Postoperative Care**

2.1 Surgical Instrumentation for Augmentation
2.2 Anesthesia for Augmentation
2.3 IMF Augmentation in Real Time
2.4 PACU Management Post Augmentation
2.5 Patient in Step Down Immediately Pre Discharge
2.6 Instructions to Patient Caregiver
2.7 Phone Call to Patient Afternoon of Surgery

Running time = 142 minutes

RESOURCES FOLDER

The Resources Folder located on Disk 2 is only acc_____ on standard DVD players. To access the Resources folder on a co_____ "Open" (Windows and Macintosh).

00. **Accessing Materials in the R_____**

01. **Tebbetts Published Pape_____**

    1.01 What is Adequa_____ (June, 1996)
    1.02 Patient Acceptanc_____ed Implants (July, 2000)
    1.03 Greatest Myths in Brea_____ation (June, 2001)
    1.04 Informed Consent Article (Sep__ 2002)
    1.05 TEPID System Implant Selection by Tissues (April, 2002)
    1.06 High Five™ Augmentation Decision System (Dec, 2005)
    1.07 24-hour Augmentation Recovery Part 1 (Jan, 2002)
    1.08 24-hour Augmentation Recovery Part 2 (Jan, 2002)
    1.09 Dual Plane Augmentation (April, 2001)
    1.10 Out Points Criteria for Breast Implant Removal (Oct, 2004)
    1.11 BASPI Decision and Management Algorithms (Oct, 2004)
    1.12 Wishes and Tissues - Concerns about Dimensional Systems (Jan, 2006)
    1.13 Axillary Endoscopic Breast Augmentation - a 28-year Experience (Dec, 2006)
    1.14 Zero Percent Reoperation rate at 3 years (Nov, 2006)

02. **Tebbetts Informed Consent Materials**

    2.1 Patient Education and Informed Consent
    2.2 Common Questions and Answers
    2.3 Patient Images Analysis with Surgeon Dialogue

03. **Patient Images Analysis and Surgeon Dialogue**

    3.1 Patient Images Analysis with Surgeon Dialogue
    3.2 Patient Images Analysis without Surgeon Dialogue

04. **High Five™ System Form and Clinical Evaluation Sheet**

    4.1 High Five™ System Measurements Techniques Illustrated
    4.2 Five Critical Decisions in Breast Augmentation
    4.3 High Five™ Comprehensive Clinical Evaluation Sheet

05. **Surgical Scripts for Inframammary and Axillary Breast Augmentation**

    5.1 Axillary Breast Augmentation Script
    5.2 Inframammary Breast Augmentation Script

06. **Requirements for Out-to-Dinner Augmentation and 24-hour Recovery**

07. **Dr. Tebbetts' Course Handout - Processes that Redefine a Practice**

08. **Integrated Anesthesia PACU and Stepdown Protocol**

09. **Augmentation Instruments and Equipment**

10. **Post-op Instructions – Dr. Tebbetts' Recipe for Augmentation Recovery**

11. **FDA PMA Studies and Tebbetts Published Data Comparison Table**

Please see inside back cover for DVDs 3 & 4.

AUGMENTATION
MAMMAPLASTY

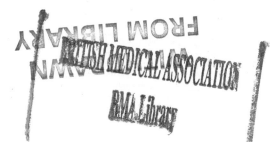

AUGMENTATION
MAMMAPLASTY

REDEFINING THE PATIENT AND SURGEON EXPERIENCE

JOHN B. TEBBETTS, M.D.

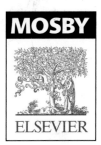

MOSBY
ELSEVIER

MOSBY

ELSEVIER

MOSBY an imprint of Elsevier Inc.

ISBN: 978-0-323-04112-6

British Library Cataloguing in Publication Data
A catalogue record for this book is available from the British Library

Library of Congress Cataloging in Publication Data
A catalog record for this book is available from the Library of Congress

Notice
Medical knowledge is constantly changing. Standard safety precautions must be followed, but as new research and clinical experience broaden our knowledge, changes in treatment and drug therapy may become necessary or appropriate. Readers are advised to check the most current product information provided by the manufacturer of each drug to be administered to verify the recommended dose, the method and duration of administration, and contraindications. It is the responsibility of the practitioner, relying on experience and knowledge of the patient, to determine dosages and the best treatment for each individual patient. Neither the Publisher nor the author assumes any liability for any injury and/or damage to persons or property arising from this publication.

The Publisher

Commissioning Editor: **Sue Hodgson**
Development Editor: **Ben Davie**
Project Manager: **Rory MacDonald**
Designer: **Charlotte Murray/Kirsteen Wright**
Illustrator: **Christy Krames**
Marketing Manager (UK/USA): **Radha Mawrie**

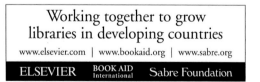

ELSEVIER   **your source for books,**
journals and multimedia
in the health sciences
www.elsevierhealth.com

The publisher's policy is to use **paper manufactured from sustainable forests**

Working together to grow
libraries in developing countries

www.elsevier.com | www.bookaid.org | www.sabre.org

ELSEVIER   BOOK AID International   Sabre Foundation

Printed in China
Last digit is the print number: 9 8 7 6 5 4 3 2 1

CONTENTS

ACKNOWLEDGEMENTS

Terrye and Kas for their love, support, patience, and sacrifice of family time that allowed me to pursue this project. Special thanks to Terrye for her unique perspectives, solutions, and constant work that have made our clinical practice enjoyable, productive, and rewarding, and for her insights and encouragement to prioritize our patients and redefine their experience.

Don and Shirley McGhan for demonstrating more than two decades ago that breast implant manufacturer commitment and support of surgeon education can be real, and for providing opportunities and friendship that encouraged my development of implants and clinical systems that have redefined the breast augmentation experience for our patients.

Dan Carlisle for his friendship, support, and help in developing anatomic, form stable, gel and saline implants.

Bill Adams, M.D., Steve Teitelbaum, M.D. and other emerging surgeons who have stimulated my thinking, challenged my thoughts, contributed ideas, and implemented proved processes that offer a bright future and a redefined experience for our augmentation patients.

Christy Krames for her illustration skills, commitment, and patience throughout the project.

Sue Hodgson, Rory MacDonald, Ben Davie, Charlotte Murray, and their team at Elsevier for their patience, persistence, and help as we worked to "get it right".

DEDICATION

To Terrye and Kas.

INTRODUCTION

The patient experience in breast augmentation has been redefined during the past decade. Advances in every aspect of breast augmentation currently enable a majority of patients to be out to dinner the evening of their augmentation surgery, and enable up to 95% to return to full normal activities within 24 hours following surgery. Patients can expect this level of recovery with any type of currently available breast implant, and they can expect equal recovery with any currently described implant pocket location and with inframammary, periareolar, and axillary incision approaches.

Less than a decade ago, patients required some or all of the following after a breast augmentation procedure: compressive bandages, special straps or bras, drains, intercostal blocks, pain pumps, nerve stimulation devices, narcotic strength pain medications, muscle relaxants, motion exercises, restricted normal activities, and 1 to 2 weeks to return to full, normal activities. Today, improvements in every process in breast augmentation have made all of these postoperative measures completely unnecessary, allowing patients to experience dramatically different recovery.

Refinements in processes that have redefined patient recovery have also redefined patients' longer term outcomes and have reduced reoperation rates. Less than a decade ago, 15–20 percent reoperation rates within just 3 years following breast augmentation were documented in Food and Drug Administration (FDA) premarket approval application (PMA) studies. Currently, in large peer reviewed and published studies with up to 7 year followup, refined processes resulted in a 3% reoperation rate, and one 50 consecutive cases series in a recent PMA study documented a zero percent reoperation rate at 3 years.

These dramatic improvements for patients did not evolve from solution based thinking and designing new surgical techniques. The redefined patient experience resulted from process based thinking, reexamining all of the major process categories in breast augmentation, including patient education, informed consent, clinical evaluation, operative planning and implant selection, anesthetic techniques, surgical techniques, and postoperative care. Basic principles of process engineering and motion and time study, implemented by all of the world's most successful businesses, were invaluable as a framework to examine and improve processes in breast augmentation.

The processes described in this book have been refined over more than a decade and a half. Each process has been documented, implemented, and tested, collecting data that have been peer reviewed and published in *Plastic and Reconstructive Surgery*, the most respected professional journal in plastic surgery. This approach to process analysis, with outcomes confirmed by peer review, has produced an entirely different patient experience and redefined outcomes for breast augmentation patients.

The extent to which patients can benefit from these dramatic improvements depends on surgeon implementation of proved processes. The goal of this book is to provide surgeons a framework of proved processes to deliver a new level of patient experience and outcome in breast augmentation.

The history of breast augmentation is interesting. For more than four decades, many surgeons have considered breast augmentation a simple operation, basing clinical evaluation, implant selection, and surgical technique selections entirely on subjective parameters and surgeon preference of incision location, pocket location, and implant type. As recently as 2002, this type of approach produced up to 20% reoperation rates within 3 years following augmentation in FDA PMA studies. For more than three decades, the patient experience in augmentation remained largely unchanged. Implant options for patients declined when the "breast implant crisis" of the early 1990s prompted the FDA in the United States to remove silicone gel filled implants from the market, while a greater range of implant products remained available to patients in other parts of the world. Despite additional research supporting the safety and efficacy of silicone gel filled implants, FDA concerns regarding several additional issues including excessively high reoperation rates have delayed FDA approval of conventional and new designs of silicone gel filled devices. A majority of surgeons in the United States currently recommend and use round, smooth shell, saline filled implant devices, a design that was developed more than three decades ago.

While other medical technology fields have continually progressed with device and application innovations, breast augmentation has in some ways gone full circle in reverse.

New implant designs have not changed appreciably since 1994. Fewer implant alternatives are available to patients in the United States today compared to the 1980s. The obvious question is, "Why?"

Surgeons learn by apprenticeship. An apprenticeship educational model encourages solution based thinking. Solution based thinking is linear and algorithmic, defining a specific set of solution alternatives to address a surgical objective or problem. Solution based thinking compares one solution or technique to another, and potentially limits advancement by encouraging choices from currently available alternatives and channeling thought into a debate mode (one technique or solution versus another) instead of a continuous improvement mode (how do we improve processes to better apply every technique or implant solution).

Process based thinking, in contrast to solution based thinking, focuses on the processes and subprocesses that ultimately determine actions and outcomes. Instead of encouraging debate and choices between currently available solution alternatives (technique or implant), process based thinking encourages continuous improvement in the processes that determine optimal use of all solution alternatives. Instead of focusing on which technique or implant is currently "best", process based thinking encourages more optimal use of every available alternative by improving the processes of patient education, clinical evaluation, decision making, surgical execution, and postoperative management.

Process oriented thinking encourages surgeons to question every detail of every process, analyzing and seeking improvements in the details of each subprocess. More detailed analysis of processes stimulates lateral thinking that often sparks innovation. Analyzing the details of one process can stimulate surgeons to recognize seemingly small actions that, alone or in combination, may dramatically affect outcomes and results. For example, analyzing steps and movements in an augmentation operation using motion and time study principles (analyzing the steps in the operation process) to shorten operative and anesthesia times revealed surgical technical maneuvers that were inadvertently and unnecessarily increasing tissue trauma and bleeding. Optimizing one set of processes (eliminating unnecessary steps or movements during the operation) resulted in refinements and outcome improvements in another set of processes (surgical techniques).

Many businesses spend considerable resources to acquire and implement "best practices" (proved processes) that were developed by other companies and acquired through highly paid consultants. These companies then carefully and precisely implement the "best practices" and gather data to determine the effectiveness of each process before making any changes to the best practices "recipe". Plastic surgeons often learn of new or improved processes in professional education venues or by reading professional journals. Instead of implementing the process exactly as described, plastic surgeons often only partially implement the processes as described, or make changes to the process based on personal preference or subjective opinion before gathering data on which to base changes in the process. The surgeon tendency to modify a proved recipe (best practice, proved process) before exactly implementing the proved process can dramatically slow improvements in the patient experience and outcomes.

Surgeon educational methods and venues have also remained largely unchanged for three decades. Highly effective education models developed and used by the world's most successful businesses require staged, repetitive educational encounters, assess the effectiveness of the education process by verification and testing, and base employee incentives and rewards on testing performance. In plastic surgery, education methods and venues seldom utilize staged, repetitive learning encounters. Testing to evaluate the effectiveness of education methods and information transfer is rare. Attendee opinions gleaned from educational venue evaluation forms often determines content and curriculum of future education venues and methods. Absent objective performance evaluations, surgeon incentives to change are limited, and limit progress for the patient and the patient's experience.

Surgeons rarely read any book cover to cover. Instead, surgeons usually access printed information when they need information about an operation that they are planning to perform in the near future. The primary limitation of all printed information for surgeons is the inability to assure transmission of essential information when the surgeon accesses only a single chapter or index reference. The only method to credibly address surgeons' needs is purposeful redundancy in a book, reiterating critical information in multiple locations to assure that the critical information is available to surgeon readers when they access limited content in a book.

This book focuses on proved processes that have a 15 year track record of delivering a redefined patient experience, improved outcomes, and lower reoperation rates in breast augmentation. Our responsibility as plastic surgeons is to our patients—to predictably deliver a continually improving level of patient experience and outcome. We have an opportunity to advance our patients' experience and outcome by applying process based thinking and best practices principles to our education methods and venues and our surgical practices. To the extent that this book can contribute to that effort, it will meet its objectives.

A Personal Historical Perspective

Historical perspectives of breast augmentation reflect surgeons' priorities and focus on the evolution of breast implant devices and surgical techniques. Throughout the history of breast augmentation, surgeons have prioritized and focused on implants and techniques. This focus is ingrained in decades of surgeons by surgical training, a preceptorship learning process that teaches linear thinking based on a problem–solution model. Given a problem—in this case inadequate breast volume—surgeons choose their preferences of implant device and surgical techniques to address the problem. The patient experience, including education, informed consent, recovery, outcomes, and reoperation rates, has largely evolved secondarily and passively as the result of surgeons' decision processes and choices of devices and techniques. The author's historical perspective was initially device and technique oriented, but has evolved to become more patient oriented. History suggests that optimal outcomes, safety and efficacy in augmentation prioritize the patient experience and decision processes that determine outcomes. Breast implant devices do not impact patient outcomes as much as surgeon and patient decisions and surgeon execution.

Viewing history from the perspective of the patient points out surgeon inadequacies and shortcomings that prompt the question, "Why didn't I recognize this earlier in my career?" In the end (and supposedly from the beginning), the patient is why surgeons exist, and surgeons' primary responsibility is the ultimate safety and outcome for patients. Surgeons focus on devices and techniques that are less important to patient outcomes compared to decisions and decision processes. Surgical techniques and implants are important, but the best of both do not deliver optimal outcomes if patient education and decision making processes are not optimal.

> Throughout the history of breast augmentation, surgeons have prioritized and focused on implants and techniques
>
> The patient experience, including education, informed consent, recovery, outcomes, and reoperation rates, has largely evolved secondarily and passively as the result of surgeons' decision processes and choices of devices and techniques

Decision processes based on scientifically valid data are essential to optimize patient outcomes in breast augmentation

When surgeons and patients base decisions and choices on *opinion and preferences* instead of *scientifically valid data*, history reflects the impact of opinion over science on the patient experience, recovery, outcomes, and reoperation rates

The scientific method is the foundation of evidence based medicine and essential to generate scientifically valid data. Decision processes based on scientifically valid data are essential to optimize patient outcomes in breast augmentation. Surgeons' and breast implant manufacturers' application of the scientific method to implant device design, clinical testing, and surgeons' evolution of surgical techniques have profoundly affected the history of breast augmentation and the patient experience over the past four decades. Surgeons' preferences of device and technique affect surgeon and patient decisions that, in turn, define safety, efficacy, and outcomes. When surgeons and patients base decisions and choices on *opinion and preferences* instead of *scientifically valid data*, history reflects the impact of opinion over science on the patient experience, recovery, outcomes, and reoperation rates. The continuing prevalence of decisions based on suboptimal knowledge and opinions instead of science is the reason that a majority of patients continue to experience 10 days or longer to recover and continue to endure reoperation rates of up to 20% in just 3 years following augmentation according to United States Food and Drug Administration (FDA) premarket approval (PMA) data.

This historical perspective derives from a patient's viewpoint, not a device and technique viewpoint. Events that are unquestionably positive for surgeons and patients validate the premise that prioritizing the patient and the patient experience and outcome over devices and techniques optimizes the patient experience.

■ THREE PHASES OVER FOUR DECADES OF BREAST AUGMENTATION

In the United States, the history of breast augmentation can be viewed in three phases or periods: (1) a phase of device and procedure oriented evolution, (2) a period of device and technique validation, and (3) a phase of redefining the patient experience, outcomes, and reoperation rates

In the United States, the history of breast augmentation can be viewed in three phases or periods: (1) a phase of device and procedure oriented evolution, (2) a period of device and technique validation, and (3) a phase of redefining the patient experience, outcomes, and reoperation rates. While some overlap of these periods exists, these three phases have largely occurred sequentially. Table 1-1 diagrams these three periods and key events that define each phase.

The following historical perspective is not intended as a comprehensive historical document of breast augmentation or breast implants. The objective of this perspective is to provide insight into the author's observations, thought processes, and events that influenced the content of this book. A detailed and well documented history of the evolution of breast implant designs is available for interested readers in the Institute of Medicine's book entitled *Safety of Silicone Breast Implants*, published in 1999.[1] Several

Table 1-1. Historical timeline of breast augmentation.

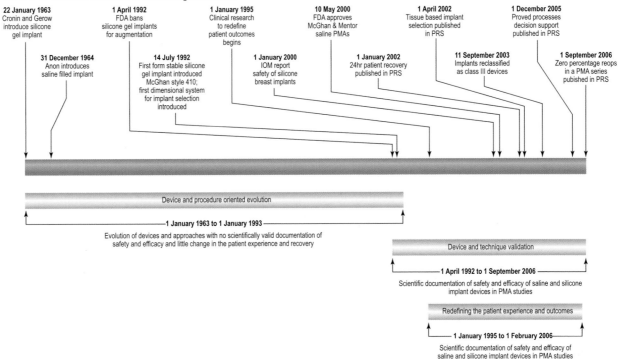

authors have attempted to classify breast implant types into specific "generations" of implants. These classifications are arbitrary and non-scientific with respect to outcomes because they classify devices according to device characteristics instead of classifying specific devices according to patient outcomes. Patient outcomes and reoperation rates have varied significantly within certain classes of devices, so global characterization of outcomes by implant class (e.g. textured shell implants or smooth shell implants, generation 1–5, etc.) without specifying the specific product manufacturer, style, and code of device is scientifically meaningless.

1963–1993: Device and Procedure Oriented Evolution

The silicone gel filled breast implant was introduced in 1963 by Drs Cronin and Gerow.[2] The author's perspective based on personal clinical experience with breast augmentation began in 1977 as a plastic surgery resident. At that time, a majority of surgeons performed breast augmentation through an inframammary incision, placing smooth shell, silicone gel filled implants in a submammary pocket location. Capsular contracture rates were high (in the range of 10–15% or more in most practices), but were accepted by most surgeons and patients as an acceptable tradeoff of breast augmentation. Periareolar and axillary approaches to augmentation had been reported, but a majority of United States surgeons used the inframammary incision approach.

Cronin implants produced by Dow Corning Corporation in the 1960s were filled with a firm silicone gel. By the mid 1970s, the gel filler was changed to be much softer and more compliant, with a less highly cross-linked silicone gel. Shells were made thinner on most implants to decrease shell palpability for increased "naturalness". Device failures were usually diagnosed at surgery to address grade 3 or 4 capsular contracture, because breast imaging with mammography was less common and less accurate, and an intact or disrupted implant was often impossible to differentiate on physical examination. At operation for failed devices, surgeons encountered a capsular space containing a very fluid silicone gel material, and surgeons sometimes concluded that the shell had disintegrated because it was very thin and sometimes exceedingly difficult to identify within the silicone gel filler as it was removed from the pocket.

Implant designs in the 1970s included round and shaped implants. Shaped implant designs were limited, and all shaped implants had smooth shells filled with very non-cohesive silicone gel. Shaped implants and some round implants were designed with patches of various materials on the posterior surface of the implant to encourage adherence of the posterior surface of the implant to the pectoralis major muscle or the chest wall, ostensibly to prevent future ptosis. Unfortunately, descent of the breast parenchyma and soft tissues while the fixed implant remained in place superiorly produced aesthetic compromises that resulted in fixation patches being removed from most implant designs by the mid 1970s.

Double lumen implants, with an inner lumen containing silicone gel and an outer lumen to accept relatively small volumes of saline, were also available during the 1970s and 1980s. To attempt to reduce rates of capsular contracture, some surgeons placed steroids in a small volume of saline in the outer lumens of double lumen implants. While steroids placed in the periprosthetic pocket prior to incision closure predictably resulted in significant soft tissue thinning in the inferior pole of the breasts and a high incidence of implant extrusions, steroids in moderate concentrations (e.g. 20 mg of methylprednisolone in 20 cc of saline) placed in the outer lumen of double lumen implants did not produce significant tissue thinning and may have been partially effective at reducing capsular contracture.

In 1981, a fluorosilicone barrier layer was added to the interior walls of implant shells filled with silicone gel in an attempt to limit diffusion of low molecular weight silicone through the implant shell (silicone bleed). This barrier layer, the Intrasheil® barrier, was developed by McGhan Corporation and subsequently licensed to Mentor Corporation for use in their implants. During the 1980s, both McGhan and Mentor Corporations modified shell designs by making shells thicker in an attempt to increase shell longevity.

Other implant designs were introduced in the 1980s, including polyurethane covered silicone gel filled implants (Vogue, Meme, and Replicon). All polyurethane covered implant devices were subsequently withdrawn from the United States market due to questions about the possible carcinogenicity of breakdown products of the polyurethane and a high failure rate of the devices due to thin shells and underfill relative to mandrel volume. Misti Gold breast implants (Bioplasty, St Paul, Minn.) filled with polyvinylpyrrolidone (PVP) hydrogel were introduced in the late 1990, but were subsequently withdrawn from the United States and British markets when osmotic effects of the hydrogel resulted in marked volume increases in the device post implantation.

The 1976 Medical Device Amendments to the Federal Food, Drug, and Cosmetic Act required manufacturers of medical devices to demonstrate a reasonable assurance of safety and efficacy for certain medical devices, and gave the FDA authority over those devices. Breast implants, however, were "grandfathered" into the regulatory process at that time, and manufacturers of implants were not required to provide the FDA with scientific evidence of product safety unless issues and questions arose about previously marketed devices. In 1991, prompted largely by questions about possible effects of silicone, the FDA published a new regulation that required breast implant manufacturers to submit premarket approval applications (PMAs).

In 1991, the FDA asked manufacturers to submit PMA data on their silicone gel implants. After examining the data, the FDA Advisory Panel concluded that insufficient scientific evidence existed to verify the safety and efficacy of silicone gel filled implants, but recommended the devices remain available to augmentation and reconstruction patients while studies accumulated more data. The FDA commissioner at the time, David Kessler, M.D., a pediatrician by training, overruled the panel and in April, 1992 called for a "voluntary moratorium" on all silicone gel implants from the United States market for primary breast augmentation. He allowed gel implants to remain available under adjunct study criteria for some reoperation patients and for reconstruction patients. No scientific data basis existed then or exists today to logically support the validity of that decision.

Several common themes exist in the history of the period from 1963 to 1993. Breast implant designs were largely derived from intuitive perceptions of individual surgeons or breast manufacturer personnel including bioengineers and, in many instances, marketing personnel. Most devices were used under Investigational Device Exemptions (IDEs) or 510k rules that allowed a new device to be classified as roughly equivalent to an existing device. These two sets of FDA rules were very lenient with respect to requiring substantive scientific data in large amounts under clinical review organization (CRO) supervision. As a result, surgeons and manufacturers became extremely complacent during this period and failed to accumulate enough valid scientific data with adequate followup to satisfy the requirements for an FDA PMA study which is the type of study required by the FDA to approve Class III devices such as breast implants.

Anecdotal reports about implant types and surgical techniques being published in the plastic surgery literature prior to 1992 did not fulfill the requirements for valid scientific studies according to FDA criteria, and when these data were submitted to the FDA, the FDA ruled that they were inadequate to establish safety and efficacy. Even in PMA studies structured by breast implant manufacturers, followup percentage was low, reoperation rates were extremely high within just 3 years following augmentation, documentation of study cases was poor, and CRO supervision pointed out discrepancies relative to the protocols.

The result was the commissioner's "voluntary moratorium" on silicone gel breast implants for primary breast augmentation in the United States in 1992. Technically, the commissioner did not ban the devices, but asked for a voluntary moratorium on the use of silicone gel implants for primary breast augmentation. Right or wrong, silicone gel implants were no longer an available option for women desiring augmentation. Why and how did that occur?

The moratorium on gel implants for primary augmentation in 1992 resulted from three decades of complacency and business as usual by surgeons and breast implant manufacturers, not recognizing and prioritizing the importance of proactively designing and performing well structured scientific protocols with CRO supervision to assure collection of valid scientific data to address key questions of safety and efficacy. Instead of focusing on this priority, all existing companies during those three decades focused on marketing and remarketing similar implant designs under slightly different forms, calling them "new" products to make them attractive to the surgeon market (a practice that

> The moratorium on gel implants for primary augmentation in 1992 resulted from three decades of complacency and business as usual by surgeons and breast implant manufacturers, not recognizing and prioritizing the importance of proactively designing and performing well structured scientific protocols with CRO supervision to assure collection of valid scientific data to address key questions of safety and efficacy

continues today). Not a single breast implant in the period from 1963 to 1991 was subjected to rigorous PMA testing to gather long-term data *before* the product was released and used in large numbers of patients. The results of this approach were: (a) many products had serious design flaws or high shell failure rates that became apparent after many devices had been implanted in patients (Vogue, Meme, Replicon, Misti Gold, Inamed Style 153, Mentor Siltex salines, PIP prefilled salines, peanut oil filled implants, and others), and (b) negative media and medicolegal consequences arose from untoward outcomes and the result of inadequate testing before bringing products to market. Patient advocate groups, patients, and the FDA became aware of this history and a pattern of introducing devices that had not been adequately investigated prior to market introduction. This awareness has prompted the FDA to be much more stringent with FDA PMA study requirements and require much more data, and longer term data before approving these devices. Although history was clear with respect to evolving concerns about implants prior to 1991, surgeons, surgeon professional organizations, and implant manufacturers did not proactively respond in an effective manner to establish scientifically valid safety and efficacy data for the devices that would satisfy public and FDA concerns about the devices. Had such data been available, the moratorium of 1992 and its effects on options for patients might well have been avoided.

1993–2006: Device and Technique Validation

The FDA commissioner's "voluntary" ban of silicone breast implants for primary augmentation in 1991, overruling his own Advisory Panel's recommendations, was a wakeup call for plastic surgeons and breast implant manufacturers. Surgeon professional organizations and their respective research entities responded by encouraging and funding more scientifically designed protocols to document improvement in quality of life following breast augmentation and verify critical issues of safety and efficacy of the devices. Surgeons and breast implant manufacturers immediately shifted focus from silicone gel to saline filled devices. Implant manufacturers instituted PMA studies for saline and silicone gel filled implants that embodied much more rigorous testing and better, more scientific study design with stricter monitoring by CROs.

Breast implant manufacturers' augmentation product line offerings to surgeons decreased dramatically with the ban of silicone gel implants. In negotiations with the FDA, manufacturers successfully negotiated the initiation of adjunct studies that enabled surgeons to continue to use silicone gel implants for primary and revision augmentation for indications listed in Table 1-2.

> The FDA commissioner's "voluntary" ban of silicone breast implants for primary augmentation in 1991, overruling his own Advisory Panel's recommendations, was a wakeup call for plastic surgeons and breast implant manufacturers

Table 1-2. **Silicone gel adjunct study indications for primary and reoperation augmentation**
A. Congenital and developmental deformities
• Scoliosis, isolated rib deformities
• Thoracic hypoplasia
• Tuberous breast deformity (constricted lower pole deformities)
• Pectus excavatum and pectus carinatum
• Poland's syndrome
• Congenital absence of the breast
B. Acquired deformities
• Ptosis requiring mastopexy
• Grade III or IV capsular contracture
C. Augmentation revision
• Implant rupture following breast augmentation
D. Saline implants deemed unsuitable for medical reasons
• Thin (inadequate) soft tissue thickness or coverage
• Severe skin wrinkling

Criteria for participation in adjunct studies were designed and intended to allow continued use of older design silicone gel implants for the specific indications listed in Table 1-2. These criteria were flexible enough, however, to enable "creative" surgeons to continue to use older generation silicone gel implants for primary augmentation. Instead of rigidly adhering to the letter of the FDA's intent with regard to these criteria, some surgeons continued to use silicone gel implants for primary augmentation by "creatively" performing minor ancillary procedures such as a crescent excision of a small amount of areolar skin (calling it a mastopexy), diagnosing minor chest wall abnormalities that exist in a majority percentage of patients as "thoracic hypoplasia" or "congenital chest wall deformities", or by deeming skin and subcutaneous tissue coverage as too thin for placement of a saline implant. Breast implant manufacturers and their CROs have had little or no effect on policing strict indications in adjunct studies, and surgeon professional organizations have no policing powers over their members, hence surgeon compliance with indications in adjunct studies remains a matter of personal professional ethics. Unfortunately, surgeons who are willing to be "creative" with inclusion criteria establish a track record with the FDA and patient advocate groups that negatively impacts the reputation of credible surgeons, and has enabled special interest groups to point out blatant diversions from adjunct study indications that negatively impact the FDA and further complicate bringing state-of-the-art implant products to patients.

The ban on silicone gel stimulated the introduction of implants with alternative filler materials, but none of the alternative filler devices measured up to their marketing claims

Breast implant manufacturers and their CROs have had little or no effect on policing strict indications in adjunct studies, and surgeon professional organizations have no policing powers over their members, hence surgeon compliance with indications in adjunct studies remains a matter of personal professional ethics

The ban on silicone gel stimulated the introduction of implants with alternative filler materials, but none of the alternative filler devices measured up to their marketing claims during the 1990s during the 1990s. In 1991, the Bioplasty Corporation introduced the Misti Gold implant, filled with polyvinylpyrrolidone hydrogel, marketed to be more radiolucent than silicone gel. The PIP Corporation in France introduced an implant filled with a hydrated polysaccharide gel marketed as hydrogel that claimed similar superiorities to silicone gel. Subsequent reports of volume increases in these devices after implantation due to an osmotic pressure gradient prompted the British Medical Devices Agency to issue an alert in December 2000, citing a lack of studies validating safety and efficacy of the devices. Both types of implant were withdrawn from the United States market. In 1994, the Trilucent implant, filled with soybean oil, was introduced by the Lipomatrix Corporation in the United States. The radiolucency of the Trilucent implant and its more natural feel compared to saline were primary marketing points, but subsequent problems with oil bleed, tissue irritation, and a foul odor post implantation resulted in withdrawal of the product from the United States market in 1999. In each of these cases, more scientifically conducted studies with optimal CRO supervision and longer followup would likely have demonstrated the inherent design problems with the devices before premature marketing, and implantation in larger numbers of patients subsequently resulted in reoperations for removal or replacement of these poorly designed and inadequately tested implants.

Interestingly, today's most state-of-the-art form stable cohesive silicone gel device, the Allergan/Inamed Style 410, was already designed at the time of the 1991 ban of silicone gel. McGhan Medical (acquired by Inamed and subsequently by Allergan) proceeded with introduction of these devices in Europe in 1993, accompanied by a comprehensive educational initiative that introduced the first dimensional system that supported the implant selection decision process. The widespread use of the Style 410 in Europe and other countries internationally began in 1993, and combined with a more objective, dimensional approach to implant selection, advanced the state-of-the-art in breast augmentation outside the United States. For the first time in the history of breast augmentation, options for surgeons and patients in the United States were limited to older devices and saline devices with known higher shell failure rates compared to surgeons and patients in other parts of the world. Patients seeking more implant options began having augmentation outside the United States, often in surroundings that were suboptimal and by surgeons with suboptimal training and experience.

From a more positive perspective, beginning in 1992 plastic surgeons and other investigators compiled a large amount of more valid scientific data supporting the safety and efficacy of breast implants. Perhaps the most compelling compilation of information that reviews all existing literature is the Institute of Medicine's report in book form

In each of these cases, more scientifically conducted studies with optimal CRO supervision and longer followup would likely have demonstrated the inherent design problems with the devices before premature marketing, and implantation in larger numbers of patients subsequently resulted in reoperations for removal or replacement of these poorly designed and inadequately tested implant

Perhaps the most compelling compilation of information that reviews all existing literature is the Institute of Medicine's report in book form entitled *Safety of Silicone Breast Implants* published in 1999[1]

entitled *Safety of Silicone Breast Implants* published in 1999.[1] This comprehensive work resulted from an exhaustive review and evaluation of existing literature by non-plastic surgeon experts from many fields of medicine, and represents the most unbiased, scientific review of available information to date. To address concerns of links between silicone gel implants and risks of connective tissue diseases and symptoms, a meta analysis of over 87 000 women published in the *New England Journal of Medicine* found no association between silicone gel implants and incidence of connective tissue diseases.[3]

In December of 2001, Inamed Corporation resubmitted their PMA application for silicone gel implants. This PMA was reviewed in October 2003 by an FDA Advisory Panel when the FDA was required by law to review the PMA within a specified time frame, but despite a panel recommendation for approval, the FDA determined that the PMA was not approvable, meaning that the implants were not approved for marketing pending additional studies and information. With submission of additional information, both Inamed (now Allergan) and Mentor Corporations have received FDA approval for their older generation, conventional silicone gel filled implants, now marketed under new names.

In August 1999, the FDA issued a regulation that required all saline filled breast implants to be PMA approved prior to sale in the United States market. Companies that had preamendments or 510k cleared saline devices were allowed to continue to sell these devices until the FDA ruled on the PMAs. On May 10, 2000, the FDA approved Inamed and Mentor Corporations' PMAs for saline filled breast implants. All other saline breast implants of other manufacturers continued as investigational devices because they were not PMA approved. In order for patients to have devices other than the Inamed and Mentor saline devices, the patients were required to enroll in Investigational Device Exemption (IDE) studies in augmentation, reoperation, and reconstruction cohorts. Safety and efficacy data from IDE studies are used to support future PMA submissions by the respective manufacturers of investigational devices.

> Historically, breast implant manufacturers and surgeons have tended to lump different styles or designs of devices together to facilitate regulatory and marketing considerations, and to control testing and regulatory costs

Historically, breast implant manufacturers and surgeons have tended to lump different styles or designs of devices together to facilitate regulatory and marketing considerations, and to control testing and regulatory costs. For example, all smooth shell, saline devices have been lumped together for FDA approval, while significant differences in shell technology can exist within the group. Textured surfaces on implants are often considered as a group by regulatory bodies and even by surgeons, when substantial differences exist that affect shell longevity of different textured devices and that affect implant–soft tissue dynamics post implantation. Not reporting outcomes data by specific implant device or product code, while satisfying marketing and cost concerns, tends to benefit the poorest performing devices at the expense of the better performing devices with respect to device longevity, clinical efficacy, and patient outcomes. The FDA does not require breast implant manufacturers to disclose adverse events by individual device style codes, only by broader categories. As a result, specific devices with higher device failure rates remain on the market longer than optimal because their higher failure rates are hidden in failure rate data for broader categories of products. Most recent examples include the Mentor Siltex saline filled implant that has a substantially higher shell failure rate compared to other Mentor products (yet remains available), and the Allergan/Inamed Style 153 double lumen implant that was withdrawn from the United States PMA study in 2005.

While the FDA approved Inamed and Mentor saline devices in 2000, the PMA submissions for these devices and issues that arose during subsequent FDA Advisory Panel hearings further challenged plastic surgeons. An average 17% reoperation rate within just 3 years following augmentation in the saline PMAs and even higher reoperation rates in the older generation silicone gel PMAs prompted serious concerns among FDA Advisory Panel members. Additional concerns expressed by Advisory Panel members during these hearings and subsequent hearings for the silicone gel PMAs in October of 2003 included: (1) level, depth, and methods of patient education and informed consent, (2) modes, frequency, and management of silicone gel implant device failures, including management of "silent ruptures", and (3) methods of monitoring and managing symptoms or symptom complexes that may or may not be associated with connective tissue disease or other undefined symptom complexes.[4–6]

Regardless of progress documenting safety and efficacy of both saline and silicone gel filled implants, three categories of substantive issues became apparent to the author beginning in 1993:

1. Reoperation rates for breast augmentation patients were unacceptably high, despite rationalizations by plastic surgeons and plastic surgeon professional organizations

2. Significant concerns exist among non-plastic surgeon scientists, patients, patient advocate groups, and the FDA regarding the issues listed previously and the fact that there seemed to be no defined management algorithms to address these concerns, and

3. For more than three decades, the routine patient experience, recovery and reoperation rates had not changed significantly for breast augmentation patients.

Not reporting outcomes data by specific implant device or product code, while satisfying marketing and cost concerns tend to benefit the poorest performing devices at the expense of the better performing devices with respect to device longevity, clinical efficacy, and patient outcomes

An average 17% reoperation rate within just 3 years following augmentation in the saline PMAs and even higher reoperation rates in the older generation silicone gel PMAs prompted serious concerns among FDA Advisory Panel members

While patients and surgeons need more accurate reporting of device performance by specific implant type or style code by manufacturers, many other issues that affect patient outcomes are not device dependent. Significant issues that had persisted for more than three decades are more surgeon and patient related compared to implant device related. Significantly more reoperations are performed for surgeon and patient related issues compared to device failures. Definitive answers for management of areas of patient and FDA concern come from surgeons, not from implants or implant manufacturers. Surgeons, not breast implant devices, most impact each patient's experience, recovery, reoperation rates, and complication rates. While discomforting from a surgeon perspective, these realizations point out opportunities for improvement in surgical decision making processes and surgical practices and techniques that could substantially improve patient outcomes and the patient experience.

1995–2006: Redefining Patient Experience and Outcomes

The "voluntary moratorium" on silicone gel breast implants of 1992 is a turning point in the history of breast augmentation from two perspectives: (1) it dramatically changed the complacent, business as usual approach of surgeons and breast implant manufacturers to a more scientifically accountable and verifiable approach to safety and efficacy, and (2) it stimulated development of comprehensive, proved processes, peer reviewed and published in the most respected professional journal in plastic surgery, that have dramatically impacted the patient experience and outcomes.

The patient experience is the whole of the patient's experience with breast augmentation—patient education, informed consent, clinical evaluation, decisions and choices, operative planning and implant selection, the surgical procedure, recovery, and future reoperations. Prior to 1992, outcomes evaluation by plastic surgeons often consisted of showing selected before and after pictures in professional presentations and publications, judging decision processes and choices by whether "it's what the patient wants" (regardless of whether the patient really knows what she may be asking), and documenting "long term outcomes" at 1 or 2 years by personal recollections of reoperation rates and causes. Although some of these practices continue, many have changed dramatically. The most respected journal in plastic surgery has instituted a much more stringent review process for manuscript submissions, requiring reviewers to focus on the scientific validity of study design and data during the review process. Anecdotal reports are declining in favor of more objective, scientifically valid studies in which data support conclusions instead of conclusions being based on opinions. In professional

> The patient experience is the whole of the patient's experience with breast augmentation—patient education, informed consent, clinical evaluation, decisions and choices, operative planning and implant selection, the surgical procedure, recovery, and future reoperations

forums, surgeons are beginning to better focus on data instead of opinions, though substantial opportunities exist for further improvement. Recognizing and acknowledging that surgeon decisions and actions impact outcomes in breast augmentation far more than specific implant devices prompted a paradigm shift in the author's thinking post 1992 and stimulated a comprehensive reexamination of established surgical practices in every area of breast augmentation that impacts the patient experience and outcomes.

Beginning in 1994 with the author's introduction of the first dimensional system for breast implant selection,[7] surgeons began to recognize that specific, objective, quantifiable parameters could assist surgeons in selecting breast implants according to individual patient tissue characteristics and limitations. Although the first generation of these systems, the McGhan/Inamed BioDimensional™ System, allowed surgeons to pick implants to force tissues to a desired or requested result without specific, limiting parameters to protect patients' tissues, this two dimensional system represented a first step in changing the totally subjective system of implant selection to a more quantifiable and objective process. Subsequent process and outcomes based thinking evolved a more sophisticated three dimensional approach to basing implant selection on objective and quantifiable tissue parameters that included tissue stretch, the third dimension.[8] The most recent evolution of systems for defined, process based decision making, the High Five™ System,[9] prioritizes patient safety and tissue protection long-term by defining and prioritizing key decisions in breast augmentation while incorporating the previous objective measurement systems to individualize implant choices to individual patient tissue requirements and limitations.

A majority of uncorrectable deformities and tissue compromises following breast augmentation result from surgeon and patient decisions that fail to optimize long-term soft tissue coverage over implants and protect patient tissues long-term. This realization prompted evolution of evidence based (tissue measurements based) selection of implant pocket location and refined surgical techniques that allow surgeons to provide maximal, optimal, long-term soft tissue coverage and extremely rapid recovery while minimizing tradeoffs traditionally associated with submuscular implant placement.[10] Currently, instead of arbitrarily selecting implant pocket location based on perceived preferences and tradeoffs, surgeons and patients have evidenced based, objective criteria on which to base these critical decisions.

Recognizing that optimal patient decision processes require optimal patient education, informed consent, and accountability, a staged, repetitive process for patient education

---

Sidebar notes:

Beginning in 1994 with the author's introduction of the first dimensional system for breast implant selection,[7] surgeons began to recognize that specific, objective, quantifiable parameters could assist surgeons in selecting breast implants according to individual patient tissue characteristics and limitations

The most recent evolution of systems for defined, process based decision making, the High Five™ System,[9] prioritizes patient safety and tissue protection long-term by defining and prioritizing key decisions in breast augmentation while incorporating the previous objective measurement systems to individualize implant choices to individual patient tissue requirements and limitations

A majority of uncorrectable deformities and tissue compromises following breast augmentation result from surgeon and patient decisions that fail to optimize long-term soft tissue coverage over implants and protect patient tissues long-term

Using defined decision assist processes and extensive, integrated documents to verify patient accountability for specific requests and situations, the author's system of patient education and informed consent was the first such comprehensive system published in the plastic surgery literature

evolved to encourage patients to become more thoroughly informed and participate more actively in the decision making processes prior to breast augmentation.[11] Using defined decision assist processes and extensive, integrated documents to verify patient accountability for specific requests and situations, the author's system of patient education and informed consent was the first such comprehensive system published in the plastic surgery literature. Patients now can have an opportunity to more thoroughly understand their options and the potential consequences of their choices and requests, helping them understand why their tissues may realistically limit what is safely achievable in breast augmentation.

Acknowledging that FDA and patient concerns and questions must be addressed by expert surgeons with a wide range of backgrounds, experience, and expertise, a group of surgeons selected for their diversity, expertise, and commitment collaborated in a Breast Augmentation Surgeons for Patients Initiative (BASPI) to address FDA and patient concerns listed previously in this chapter. The goal of this collaboration was to deliver peer reviewed and published, specific answers to areas of patient and FDA concern by defining decision and management algorithms to address each of the following specific areas of concern: implant size exchange, capsular contracture grades 3–4, infection, stretch deformities (implant bottoming or displacement), silent rupture of gel implants, and patients presenting with undefined symptom complexes (connective tissue disease or other).[12]

While breast implant designs have changed substantially over more than three decades prior to 2000, no peer reviewed study specifically addressed processes that define and impact patient recovery

Patient recovery is also a parameter that undeniably distinguishes differences in surgical techniques that are virtually impossible to differentiate by other parameters

While breast implant designs have changed substantially over more than three decades prior to 2000, no peer reviewed study specifically addressed processes that define and impact patient recovery. Countless studies and anecdotal reports in the literature promote a particular incision approach, pocket location, or surgical technique, but no study over more than three decades correlated specific decisions, processes, and surgical techniques with dramatic improvements in patient recovery and reoperation rates. Patient recovery following breast augmentation correlates directly with quality of longer-term outcomes, because processes that determine the amount of bleeding and tissue trauma during augmentation also determine the degree of inflammation and intensity of wound healing processes that occur postoperatively and impact incidence of capsular contracture, hematoma, seroma, and infection. Patient recovery is also a parameter that undeniably distinguishes differences in surgical techniques that are virtually impossible to differentiate by other parameters. Using principles of motion and time study and other principles of process engineering to analyze surgical practices and techniques dramatically changed patient recovery. Regardless of incision location or pocket location, 96% of 627

Regardless of incision location or pocket location, 96% of 627 patients in our study were able to return to full normal activities within 24 hours, and a majority of those patients to be out to dinner the evening of their breast augmentation[13,14]

patients in our study were able to return to full normal activities within 24 hours, and a majority of those patients to be out to dinner the evening of their breast augmentation.[13,14] While addressing long-term issues of safety and efficacy of implant devices, identifying and defining proved processes that impact patient recovery provides surgeons tools to offer patients a totally redefined patient experience short-term that subsequently impacts long-term outcomes.

The integration of proved processes in clinical practice ultimately defines the potential of those processes to impact patient outcomes. Optimal validation of proved processes not only requires peer review and publication in the most respected journal in the specialty, but also requires that the processes stand up to the ultimate clinical scrutiny in plastic surgery—evaluation in a breast implant PMA study monitored by an independent clinical review organization and the FDA. Studies cited in this chapter enabled more than 1600 consecutive patients to experience a 3% overall reoperation rate with up to 7 year followup compared to a 17% average reoperation rate at just 3 years in Inamed and Mentor saline PMA studies.[10,13–15] More importantly, these same processes integrated in clinical practice dramatically improved reoperation and complication rates in a PMA study. For the first time in the history of breast augmentation, a peer reviewed and published study in the most respected journal in the specialty documented a zero percent reoperation rate at 3 year followup in a PMA study for breast implants[16]. This study was independently monitored by a CRO and is part of the Allergan/Inamed PMA study for the Style 410 form stable, cohesive gel implant that is currently under review by the FDA.

From a patient perspective, the progression of the history of breast augmentation in the United States is encouraging. After decades of status quo with respect to implant devices, today's implants are subjected to an unprecedented and improved level of scientific scrutiny to assure optimal patient safety and efficacy. After three decades of relatively small changes in patient recovery, the patient experience, and evidence based patient outcomes, defined processes now exist in the peer reviewed plastic surgery literature that provide surgeons with tools and templates for patient education, decision making, implant selection, and surgical techniques that enable patients to predictably expect a 24-hour return to normal activities following breast augmentation and a chance for minimal reoperation rates and complications long term. During the past decade, advancements in breast augmentation have eclipsed changes that occurred over more than three decades of previous history.

Studies cited in this chapter enabled more than 1600 consecutive patients to experience a 3% overall reoperation rate with up to 7 year followup compared to a 17% average reoperation rate at just 3 years in Inamed and Mentor saline PMA studies[10,13–15]

For the first time in the history of breast augmentation, a peer reviewed and published study in the most respected journal in the specialty documented a zero percent reoperation rate at 3 year followup in a PMA study for breast implants

After three decades of relatively small changes in patient recovery, the patient experience, and evidence based patient outcomes, defined processes now exist in the peer reviewed plastic surgery literature that provide surgeons tools and templates for patient education, decision making, implant selection, and surgical techniques that enable patients to predictably expect a 24-hour return to normal activities following breast augmentation and a chance for minimal reoperation rates and complications long-term

▓ REFERENCES

1. Institute of Medicine: *Safety of silicone breast implants*. Washington, D.C, National Academy Press, 1999.

2. Cronin TD, Gerow FJ: *Augmentation mammaplasty: a new "natural feel" prosthesis*. Transactions of the Third International Congress of Plastic Surgery, October 13–18, 1963. Amsterdam, The Netherlands. Excerpta Medica Foundation, 1963, pp 41–49.

3. Sanchez-Guerrero J, Colditz GA, Karison EW, Hunter DJ, Speizer FE, Liang MHY: Silicone breast implants and the risk of connective-tissue diseases and symptoms. *N Engl J Med* 332(25):1666–1670, 1995.

4. Food and Drug Administration. U.S. Food and Drug Administration. General and Plastic Surgery Devices Panel Meeting Transcript. Washington, D.C. February 18, 1992.

5. Food and Drug Administration. U.S. Food and Drug Administration. General and Plastic Surgery Devices Panel Meeting Transcript. Washington, D.C. March 1–3, 2000. Online. Available: http://www.fda.gov/cdrh/gpsdp.html#030100.

6. Food and Drug Administration. U.S. Food and Drug Administration. General and Plastic Surgery Devices Panel Meeting Transcript. Washington, D.C. October 14–15, 2003. Online. Available: http://www.fda.gov/ohrms/dockets/ac/03/transcripts/3989T1.htm.

7. Tebbetts JB: *Dimensional augmentation mammaplasty using the BioDimensional™ System*. Santa Barbara: McGhan Medical Corporation, 1994, pp 1–90.

8. Tebbetts JB: A system for breast implant selection based on patient tissue characteristics and implant–soft tissue dynamics. *Plast Reconstr Surg* 109(4):1396–1409, 2002.

9. Tebbetts JB, Adams WP: Five critical decisions in breast augmentation using 5 measurements in 5 minutes: the high five system. *Plast Reconstr Surg* 116(7):2005–2016, 2005.

10. Tebbetts JB: Dual plane (DP) breast augmentation: optimizing implant–soft tissue relationships in a wide range of breast types. *Plast Reconstr Surg* 107:1255, 2001.

11. Tebbetts JB: An approach that integrates patient education and informed consent in breast augmentation. *Plast Reconstr Surg* 110(3):971–978, 2002.

12. Adams WP, Bengtson BP, Glicksman CA, Gryskiewicz JM, Jewell ML, McGrath MH, Reisman NR, Teitelbaum SA, Tebbetts JB, Tebbetts T: Decision and management algorithms to address patient and Food and Drug Administration concerns regarding breast augmentation and implants. *Plast Reconstr Surg* 114(5):1252–1257, 2004.

13. Tebbetts JB: Achieving a predictable 24 hour return to normal activities after breast augmentation Part I: Refining practices using motion and time study principles. *Plast Reconstr Surg* 109:273–290, 2002.

14. Tebbetts JB: Achieving a predictable 24 hour return to normal activities after breast augmentation Part II: Patient preparation, refined surgical techniques and instrumentation. *Plast Reconstr Surg* 109:293–305, 2002.

15. Tebbetts JB: Patient acceptance of adequately filled breast implants using the tilt test. *Plast Reconstr Surg* 106(1):139–147, 2000.

16. Tebbetts JB: Achieving a zero percent reoperation rate at 3 years in a 50 consecutive case augmentation mammaplasty PMA study. *Plast Reconstr Surg* 118(6):1453–1457, 2006.

Ten Essentials

■ TEN ESSENTIALS TO OPTIMIZE PATIENT OUTCOMES

Proved processes currently enable surgeons to optimize breast augmentation outcomes according to principles of evidence based outcomes analysis.[1-11] Using principles of process engineering and quality control, surgeons can evaluate and apply 10 essentials derived from proved processes to redefine patient outcomes long-term. The processes that have produced a redefined level of patient experience and outcome in breast augmentation are detailed in the chapters of this book. Table 2-1 lists 10 essential processes that are required to predictably deliver an optimal patient experience, recovery, and outcome.

> Using principles of process engineering and quality control, surgeons can evaluate and apply 10 essentials derived from proved processes to redefine patient outcomes long-term

Table 2-1. Ten essential processes for optimal patient experience, recovery, and outcome

1. Prioritize evidence based outcomes analysis and surgeon accountability
2. Prioritize and optimize patient education, informed consent, and patient accountability
3. Optimize surgeon education and process implementation using proved educational models, modern technology, verifiability, and surgeon incentives
4. Prioritize and protect patients' tissues long-term by choosing implant pocket location to assure optimal long-term tissue coverage of the implant and by avoiding implant sizes or projection that are likely to cause excessive stretching, tissue thinning, and parenchymal atrophy
5. Implement objective, tissue based clinical evaluation, preoperative decisions, operative planning and implant selection
6. Prioritize and consider implant design, filler distribution dynamics, and implant–soft tissue dynamics during preoperative patient education, implant selection, and operative planning
7. Design and dissect the implant pocket to "fit" the implant selected
8. Minimize trauma and bleeding, eliminate blunt dissection, and apply prospective hemostasis principles
9. Optimize outcomes prospectively by managing factors that speed recovery
10. Manage untoward occurrences using defined processes; define end points for implant removal without replacement

An optimal outcome from breast augmentation is more than a "happy" patient and selected before and after results to support individual surgeons' presentations and publications

An optimal outcome from breast augmentation is more than a "happy" patient and selected before and after results to support individual surgeons' presentations and publications. Patient desires may include a larger breast and a desired cup size, but ultimately the quality of her outcome depends on more specific, objective, and scientifically verifiable criteria. For every patient, an optimal outcome is a result derived from knowledge-based decisions with accountability, an optimal surgical experience, rapid recovery and return to normal activities, and minimal complications and reoperations over her lifetime. A paradigm shift in evaluating breast augmentation outcomes is occurring in this decade—the result of Food and Drug Administration (FDA) and public demands that evidence based outcomes improve, combined with the development, peer review, and publication of proved processes and improved implant devices that enable surgeons to deliver a redefined level of outcomes.

A paradigm shift in evaluating breast augmentation outcomes is occurring in this decade—the result of Food and Drug Administration and public demands that evidence based outcomes improve, combined with the development, peer review, and publication of proved processes and improved implant devices that enable surgeons to deliver a redefined level of outcomes

The FDA, patients, and patient advocates evaluate optimal outcomes based on objective data from premarket approval (PMA) studies. PMA studies are the most scientifically constructed and stringently monitored studies on breast augmentation. For more than two decades, PMA data established an unenviable track record of 15–20% reoperation rates within 3 years of augmentation.[12–14] Fortunately, that track record is improving, and proved processes are available that enable surgeons to deliver a 3% reoperation rate with up to 7 year followup,[2,3,5,10] and a zero percent reoperation rate at 3 years in a PMA series of 50 consecutive patients.[11]

Ten essentials derived from these peer reviewed and published processes provide a framework for surgeons to integrate with personal practice preferences and provide optimal outcomes in augmentation based on verifiable data.

1. Prioritize evidence based outcomes analysis and surgeon and patient accountability

For the past two decades, most breast augmentation outcomes data in peer reviewed and published studies as well as anecdotal reports indicated a high level of patient satisfaction and low reoperation rates. Surgeons introduced and refined operative techniques including axillary and umbilical incision approaches and endoscopic pocket dissection. During these two decades, however, two things did not improve appreciably—patients' perioperative experience and recovery, and reoperation rates. Incredibly high reoperation rates within just 3 years of augmentation were exposed in data from FDA saline PMA studies.[12–14] FDA Advisory Panel members and patient advocate representatives strongly criticized these reoperation rates and suggested a need for more scientifically constructed studies, long-term followup, evidence based outcomes analysis, and patient and surgeon accountability including a data registry for augmentation.

Scientific examination of the root causes of high reoperation rates and prolonged patient morbidity in the early postoperative period requires *objective* data for analysis. *Subjective* data and terms established a two decade track record of high reoperation rates and little improvement in the patient experience. Truly scientific analysis of *objective* data, while uncomfortable or even threatening to some surgeons, is the best method to assure optimal patient outcomes and improvement in the patient experience in breast augmentation.

Patient outcomes begin with the surgeon. If the surgeon does not prioritize evidence based outcomes analysis of objective data, the track record suggests that the patient experience, outcomes, and reoperation rates are unlikely to improve. Tissue based clinical analysis and implant selection enable objective outcomes analysis, using *objective* rather than *subjective* assessment parameters. Many surgeons oppose data collection and reporting through an independently managed registry. If verifiably advancing patient outcomes and lowering reoperation rates is a priority, mandatory reporting of baseline preoperative objective tissue measurements, operative data, postoperative measurements, and detailed reporting of all reasons for reoperations is the best method to assure objective analysis of processes and outcomes.

2. Prioritize and optimize patient education, informed consent, and patient accountability

Suboptimal outcomes in augmentation frequently result from suboptimal preoperative decisions by the patient and the surgeon. Decisions affect outcomes. The quality of decisions relates directly to the knowledge base of the patient and surgeon and the processes by which they use this knowledge base to make decisions.

Informed consent law mandates that patients make choices and decisions about their care. Surgeons are responsible for providing information to patients about the potential benefits and risks of all available options for treatment. Current scope of patient education in augmentation is highly variable, and depends not only on the information provided to the patient, but whether the patient reads and uses the information, and specifically *how* the patient uses the information to make choices and decisions.

Patient outcomes begin with the surgeon. If the surgeon does not prioritize evidence based outcomes analysis of objective data, the track record suggests that the patient experience, outcomes, and reoperation rates are unlikely to improve. Tissue based clinical analysis and implant selection enables objective outcomes analysis, using *objective* rather than *subjective* assessment parameters

Decisions affect outcomes. The quality of decisions relates directly to the knowledge base of the patient and surgeon and the processes by which they use this knowledge base to make decisions

Most current patient education methods and materials provided by professional organizations and surgeons do not optimally address two specific areas that are critically important to optimizing patient education—*verifiability* or testing to assess whether patients have assimilated critical information, and *proved decision support processes* to assure decision making pathways that have been shown to optimize outcomes and minimize reoperation rates (Table 2-2). Regardless of the amount of information provided to patients, absent some form of testing or verification to assure their assimilation of the information, the patient never builds an optimal knowledge base. Absent specific guidance in decision processes using processes that have been shown to improve outcomes, patients are unlikely to make optimal choices that ensure optimal long-term outcomes.

Assuming that surgeons optimize all of the previously mentioned factors, patients may nevertheless make requests, choices, or decisions that may adversely affect their long-term outcomes. A common example is requesting an implant size or dimensions that exceed the base width of available soft tissue coverage, or that may excessively stretch or thin envelope tissues or cause parenchymal atrophy in the future. Surgeons cannot predict or control some of these factors. Patients must be accountable for their requests and choices, provided they have been given optimal education and decision support. Processes to assure this accountability are detailed in Chapter 4. A third critically

> Patients must be accountable for their requests and choices, provided they have been given optimal education and decision support

> A third critically deficient area in patient education and informed consent is documenting patient requests and decisions after optimal education

Table 2-2. Patient education basic processes and current deficiencies.

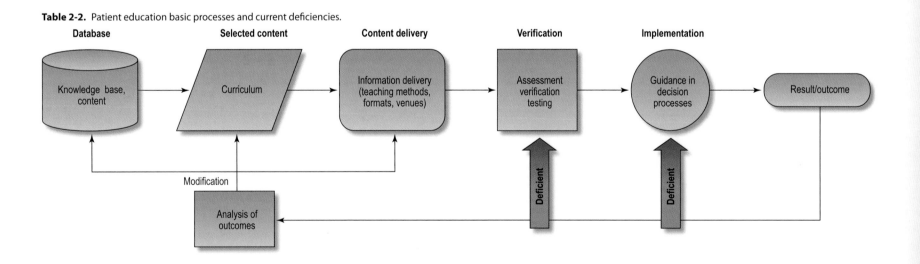

deficient area in patient education and informed consent is *documenting patient requests and decisions* after optimal education. This documentation can be integrated into the educational process in a staged, repetitive manner that provides information, decision support, and line item documentation of patient choices to assure patient and surgeon accountability.[7] All of the documents in this system are included in the Resources folder on the DVDs that accompany the book for surgeons to use or modify to suit individual practice preferences.

3. Optimize surgeon education and process implementation using proved educational models, modern technology, verifiability, and surgeon incentives

If optimizing patient outcomes and the patient experience is an objective, surgeons must access and implement proved processes that speed recovery, reduce complication and reoperation rates, and minimize negative effects of implants on patients' tissues over time.

The track record of 15–20% reoperation rates and two decades of minimal change in the patient's perioperative experience suggest a need for reexamination of surgeon education processes. Individual surgeon presenters, program chairs, and surgeon questionnaire suggestions currently determine content for most surgeon education venues, instead of defining content to include proved processes that have been shown to positively impact outcomes and reoperation rates in peer reviewed and published studies. Most current surgeon education programs prioritize individual surgeon techniques and preferences and encourage panel discussions or debates that are rarely based on verifiable data that validate proved processes. Professional organizations routinely rely on surgeon questionnaires from one educational venue to make decisions about content and format for subsequent venues, prompting the question of whether those who need to be educated are best qualified to determine content that might best change their two decade old track record.

Meaningful impact to improve outcomes for significant numbers of patients requires a comprehensive approach to surgeon education that integrates essential components of valid education models that have proved successful in industry and medicine. Three critical components are largely absent in current surgeon education and implementation of proved processes: (1) a defined curriculum derived from a knowledge base of reviewed and published processes that have been shown to impact outcomes, (2) verifiability

> If optimizing patient outcomes and the patient experience is an objective, surgeons must access and implement proved processes that speed recovery, reduce complication and reoperation rates, and minimize negative effects of implants on patients' tissues over time

Table 2-3. Deficiencies in surgeon education and implementation of proved processes.

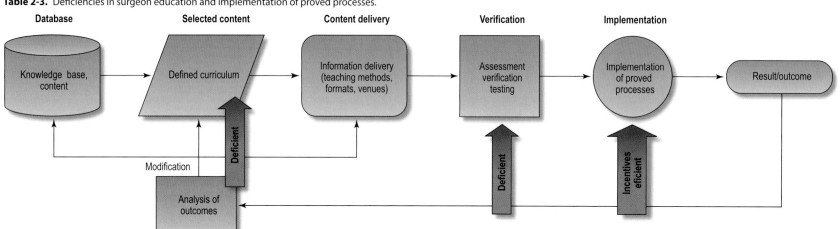

of information exchange by proved testing methodologies (in venues or online), and (3) incentives (positive or negative) to encourage surgeons to implement proved processes (Table 2-3).

The roles of professional organizations and implant manufacturers in surgeon education should be non-competitive and complementary, to most logically use resources for optimal effectiveness. While surgeon professional organizations state that they are most qualified to educate surgeons, critics may question their two decade old track record. Addressing the needs mentioned previously may improve that track record. Implant manufacturers have a fiduciary responsibility to their stockholders to promote their products; hence most of their surgeon education program content is product oriented and marketing directed.

Professional organizations and implant manufacturers might more effectively optimize patient outcomes by considering some or all of the following measures:

1. Commission a group of independent scientists working with plastic surgeon content experts to define a knowledge base of peer reviewed and published processes that have been shown to positively impact patient outcomes.

> The roles of professional organizations and implant manufacturers in surgeon education should be non-competitive and complementary, to most logically use resources for optimal effectiveness

2. Define a standardized, core curriculum that prioritizes proved processes shown to impact all impact products and all surgical procedures.

3. Define a decision process framework that comprehensively addresses variables critical to patient outcomes while providing flexibility for individual surgeon preferences and training.

4. Design educational venues and delivery methods according to established education model guidelines to include verifiability of information exchange.

5. Prioritize content, decision processes, and scientific assessment of objective data as a core curriculum in professional organization programs; then supplement the core curriculum with subjective and personal surgeon opinion content as time and resources allow.

6. Provide basic core content of proved processes that apply to all implant products in implant manufacturer education forums, while continuing to promote product oriented content.

7. Establish an online knowledge base accessible to all surgeons and patients that includes all information that will be used in any educational curriculum.

8. Expand online educational venues that meaningfully incorporate state-of-the-art education methodologies used by business and industry.

9. Establish an independently managed registry depository for breast augmentation and implant data that is transparent to patients and surgeons.

10. Jointly define incentives and disincentives to encourage better surgeon implementation of proved processes and compliance with reporting requirements.

4. Prioritize and protect patients' tissues long-term by choosing implant pocket location to assure optimal long-term tissue coverage of the implant and by avoiding implant sizes or projection that are likely to cause excessive stretching, tissue thinning, and parenchymal atrophy

These decision processes are detailed in Chapter 9.

Breast implants can have adverse effects on patients' tissues and increase risks of reoperations or uncorrectable deformities if surgeons and patients make suboptimal preoperative choices and decisions. Excessively large implants can cause excessive stretch or thinning of patient tissues that is irreversible. When combined with normal effects of aging, thinning of soft tissues can compromise skin quality and reduce the efficacy of

Breast implants can have adverse effects on patients' tissues and increase risks of reoperations or uncorrectable deformities if surgeons and patients make suboptimal preoperative choices and decisions

lifting procedures or other revisional procedures. Excessively projecting implants, especially when used in patients with tight envelopes (anterior pull skin stretch less than 2.5 cm), can cause atrophy of breast parenchyma that is irreversible and that compromises implant coverage and patients' ability to nurse. No surgical procedure can improve the quality of tissues that have been compromised by excessively large or excessively projecting breast implants.

To minimize risks of tissue compromise or uncorrectable loss of tissue coverage and uncorrectable deformities long-term, patients and surgeons must make optimal decisions preoperatively—carefully selecting breast implant size, dimensions, and projection to optimize long-term soft tissue coverage and minimize risks of excessive tissue stretch, thinning or atrophy. Making optimal decisions requires that surgeons objectively evaluate and consider individual patient tissue characteristics, avoiding arbitrary choices that attempt to drive tissues to a desired result.

> Select implant pocket location to maximize available soft tissue coverage over all areas of the implant for the patient's lifetime, regardless of perceived advantages of a pocket location that provides less soft tissue coverage

Essential principles to protect patients' tissues and minimize reoperations, negative tissue consequences, and uncorrectable deformities long-term include (Table 2-4):

1. Select implant pocket location to *maximize available soft tissue coverage over all areas of the implant for the patient's lifetime*, regardless of perceived advantages

Table 2-4. Essentials to protect patient tissues from irreversible compromises and uncorrectable deformities

Essential principle	Potential consequences if ignored
1. Select implant pocket location to *maximize available soft tissue coverage over all areas of the implant for the patient's lifetime*	Implant edge visibility, implant edge palpability, visible traction rippling
2. Select base width of implant equal to or less than base width of patient's parenchyma preop	Implant edge visibility, implant edge palpability, visible traction rippling
3. Avoid excessively projecting breast implants	Parenchymal atrophy, chest wall deformities, excessive skin stretch and thinning, subcutaneous tissue thinning
4. Avoid excessively large implants in all patients	Implant edge visibility, implant edge palpability, visible traction rippling, parenchymal atrophy, chest wall deformities, excessive skin stretch and thinning, subcutaneous tissue thinning

of a pocket location that provides less soft tissue coverage. For the vast majority of patients, this means selecting either a dual plane or partial retropectoral pocket location.

2. Select an implant with a base width equal to or less than the base width of the patient's existing breast parenchyma in order to assure optimal, long-term soft tissue coverage. The only exception to this principle is breast base width less than 10 cm in breasts such as tubular or severely constricted lower pole breasts. When surgeons attempt to honor patient requests to narrow the gap between the breasts (intermammary distance or IMD) by selecting implants with a base width wider than the patient's parenchyma, surgeon and patient risk edge visibility, palpability, traction rippling, and synmastia long-term. These are potentially uncorrectable deformities with irreversible tissue compromises. Subpectoral or dual plane placement, preserving all medial origins of the pectoralis major intact along the sternum to the level of the sixth rib, usually enables surgeons to safely narrow the intermammary distance to 3–4 cm. Surgeons should inform patients preoperatively and require patients to specifically acknowledge long-term risks of choosing implants with a base width greater than the base width of their existing breast parenchyma.

3. Avoid excessively projecting breast implants, especially when choosing an implant to purposefully increase projection in breasts with limited envelope compliance (anterior pull skin stretch less than 3 cm). While highly projecting implants may have limited indications in glandular ptotic breasts to fill a previously projecting lower envelope, highly projecting implants should never be selected to force tissues to a projection that the tissues have never previously been. Even when used in glandular ptotic breasts, highly projecting implants maximize weight for any given base width—perhaps improving aesthetics temporarily, but at the risk of adding maximal weight per base width in a breast whose tissues have already proved that they stretch excessively (glandular ptosis). Highly projecting implants should never be used to force a patient's tissues to a projection that the tissues have never previously experienced with pregnancy or nursing so as to avoid irreversible parenchymal atrophy, chest wall deformities, and loss of soft tissue coverage in order to protect patients' tissues and optimize long-term outcomes. Few, if any, indications exist in primary breast augmentation for high or extra high projection implants.

4. Avoid excessively large implants in all patients, but especially in patients whose tissues are thin by objective measurements (soft tissue pinch thickness, STPT, less

Avoid excessively projecting breast implants, especially when choosing an implant to purposefully increase projection in breasts with limited envelope compliance (anterior pull skin stretch less than 3 cm)

Avoid excessively large implants in all patients, but especially in patients whose tissues are thin by objective measurements

than 2 cm superior to breast parenchyma, or soft tissue pinch thickness less than 1 cm in any area of the breast). While the number of variables precludes identifying a specific volume or weight of implant that is excessively large, surgeons should carefully consider the size and weight of normal breasts that deteriorate in appearance over time and encourage patients to carefully consider all risks of uncorrectable deformities and irreversible tissue compromises that may occur with implants larger than 350 cc. Rarely, some patients experience irreversible tissue consequences with implants much smaller than 350 cc, and all patients should be informed and document their preoperative acceptance that surgeons cannot totally predict the soft tissue consequences of breast implants over time.

5. Implement objective, tissue based clinical evaluation, preoperative decisions, operative planning and implant selection

Base decisions on objective measurements and proved (peer reviewed and published) processes, limiting non-scientific subjective parameters, and avoiding opinions based on personal preference instead of data.

Two basic formulas are invaluable during preoperative planning. The first formula (Table 2-5) is:

Result = Envelope + Parenchyma + Implant

Table 2-5. Components that affect final breast volume.

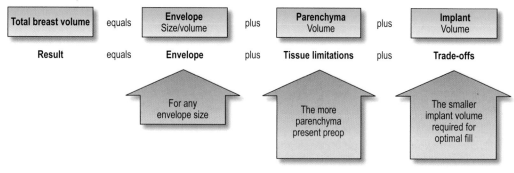

This formula reminds the surgeon that the final result following augmentation is determined by the characteristics of each patient's soft tissue envelope (volume and stretch), and by the amount of fill in the envelope, consisting of the patient's existing parenchyma and the volume and characteristics of the implant. When considering a desired result, patient and surgeon must be aware that forcing tissues to a desired result may have serious, irreversible consequences. The ideal volume for each patient's envelope is the *least* volume that will provide adequate fill of the envelope for optimal aesthetics and the desired result. Accurately estimating optimal volume for each patient's envelope requires the surgeon to consider not only what the patient *wants*, but the width and compliance of the existing envelope (measured by base width and anterior pull skin stretch) and the contribution of the patient's existing parenchyma to stretched envelope fill (PCSEF).[6,10] When a patient's envelope compliance measured by anterior pull skin stretch is less than 3 cm, and the patient's envelope is already filled by existing parenchyma (a breast with adequate upper pole fill preoperatively judged in oblique and lateral photographs), surgeon and patient should select less implant volume to avoid overstretching and thinning the envelope, exposing implant edges or creating visible traction rippling, or causing subsequent parenchymal atrophy.

A second formula (Table 2-6) is:

Result = Desired dimensions (volume) – Tissue limitations – Tradeoffs

> The ideal volume for each patient's envelope is the least volume that will provide adequate fill of the envelope for optimal aesthetics and the desired result

Table 2-6. Optimal result is limited by patient tissue characteristics and tradeoffs.

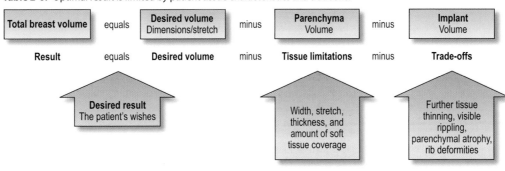

Tempering desires with reality reconciles wishes with tissues, reminding patient and surgeon that although one or both might wish for a specific volume breast, tissue limitations, tradeoffs, and risks might prompt both to consider what the tissues will safely accommodate with the least long-term tradeoffs and risks

This formula reminds the surgeon and patient that the desired result is limited by the amount and characteristics of the patient's existing tissues and the patient's and surgeon's willingness to accept responsibility and accountability for decisions that may exceed the capability of the tissues to safely accommodate a specific volume. Tempering desires with reality *reconciles wishes with tissues*, reminding patient and surgeon that although one or both might *wish* for a specific volume breast, tissue limitations, tradeoffs, and risks might prompt both to consider *what the tissues will safely accommodate with the least long-term tradeoffs and risks*.

Optimizing outcomes requires optimizing the parameters and processes that surgeons use to make preoperative decisions and select implants. Absent objective data and defined decision processes, individual surgeons continue to base decisions on subjective parameters and personal opinions—precisely the methods that established a two decade old track record of 15–20% reoperation rates.[12–14] Currently, in the most respected professional journals in plastic surgery, few published studies on breast augmentation outcomes derive conclusions from quantified, objective data.

Scientific analysis of outcomes requires objective data derived from quantifiable parameters used in preoperative evaluation, selection of implant pocket location, and selection of implant and surgical techniques

Scientific analysis of outcomes requires *objective data* derived from *quantifiable parameters* used in preoperative evaluation, selection of implant pocket location, and selection of implant and surgical techniques. Preoperative decision processes can dramatically impact long-term outcomes and tissue consequences. Optimizing decision processes according to process engineering principles requires *defining processes*, and *testing them* by consistent implementation and *monitoring*. Terms such as "thin", "thick", "stretchy", or "tight" are subjective and preclude scientifically valid analysis. Quantifying tissue parameters with objective measurements is rapid, effective, and allows objective analysis of results and outcomes data. Outcomes data analysis and process analysis are essential tenets of evidence based medical practices that are well established in many other medical disciplines, but are just evolving in plastic surgery.

To optimize outcomes, surgeons should follow basic principles of evidence based medicine, basing decisions on quantifiable parameters, recording objective data that can be analyzed scientifically, and refining and defining decision making processes according to established principles of process engineering.

Peer reviewed and published processes currently exist that use five simple measurements and prioritize five essential decisions in breast augmentation that surgeons can complete in 5 minutes or less—processes that have a documented 3% overall reoperation rate at

Peer reviewed and published processes currently exist that use five simple measurements and prioritize five essential decisions in breast augmentation that surgeons can complete in 5 minutes or less—processes that have a documented 3% overall reoperation rate at up to 7 year followup compared to previous 15–20% reoperation rates at just 3 years

up to 7 year followup[2,3,5,9,10] compared to previous 15–20% reoperation rates at just 3 years.[12–14] These methods also resulted in dramatically improved perioperative experience and 24 hour return to normal activities,[5] a 0.2% reoperation rate for implant size exchange[2,3,5] compared to an average 8.7% rate for size exchange in saline PMA studies,[12–14] and a zero incidence of uncorrectable tissue deformities at up to 7 year followup.[2,3,5] The five critical decisions that delivered these results are prioritized and described in detail in the paper entitled "Five critical decisions in breast augmentation using 5 measurements in 5 minutes: the high five system".[10] Chapter 7 details the High Five™ System.

By implementing published processes for quantitative tissue assessment and implant selection,[6,10] surgeons can totally eliminate the use of sizer implants for primary breast augmentation. Elimination of sizers in primary augmentation reduces tissue trauma and risk of pocket contamination by repeated introduction and removal of sizers, reduces costs, and reduces risks of contamination from reused sizers. Preoperatively selecting implants according to these established systems, and eliminating sizer use, avoids ordering multiple sizes of implants for straightforward primary cases, and substantially reduces operative times and resultant total perioperative narcotics doses, both of which directly impact the patient experience and outcome.[4,5]

6. Prioritize and consider implant design, filler distribution dynamics, and implant–soft tissue dynamics during preoperative patient education, implant selection, and operative planning

Chapter 6 comprehensively addresses each of these topics.

The previous discussion of item 4 identified specific implant factors that can have negative effects on patients' tissues over time. Item 5 referenced quantifiable tissue evaluation parameters and decision processes to improve outcomes. When selecting breast implants, surgeons should consider additional implant parameters based on peer reviewed and published or PMA data that have been shown to affect patient outcomes.[2,3,4,6,10,11]

Implant longevity is critically important to patients. Surgeons and patients should carefully evaluate all available data on implant failure rates. Patients should be aware preoperatively of the failure rates of available implant designs by specific product number, not by product category. Unfortunately, specific information that could impact

Implant longevity is critically important to patients. Surgeons and patients should carefully evaluate all available data on implant failure rates

surgeon and patient decisions is only partially available in current data from implant manufacturers. Manufacturers are currently required by the FDA to report device failure rates by broad categories of implant devices. For patients and surgeons to make optimal decisions, manufacturers should compile and disclose device failure rates by individual product number, style, or type—not by broad categories. Manufacturers currently have device failure data by product number or style, but have not made the data available. Data that are currently available even in manufacturer advertisements help distinguish products by device failure rates.

More than a decade of experience indicates that implants filled to a volume that minimizes shell collapse and folding reduces device failure rates.[2,3,5] Surgeons and patients sometimes overlook such data, preferring to select implants based on perceived, subjective palpability or "naturalness" considerations instead of selecting implant designs and filler volumes to maximize the life of the device. An interesting question for patients who request the ultimate in a "soft, natural" (translated, underfilled) implant is "How soft for how long is worth a reoperation?" Patients should be informed preoperatively of implant fill issues (manufacturer's recommended fill versus mandrel volume of the device) for inflatable and prefilled implants in order to make informed choices.

When considering implant design options, surgeons should recognize differences in implant designs and implant–soft tissue interactions that can affect reoperation rates and require more detailed preoperative planning considerations. For example, full height, form stable implants that do not experience upper pole collapse and shell folding when upright require a more accurate estimate of optimal volume for a patient's envelope and optimal position of the inframammary fold. With this type of device, excessive volume or an excessively short nipple to inframammary fold distance (failure to accurately reposition the inframammary fold when needed), results in excessive upper breast fullness. In contrast, reduced height, form stable implants, and all current round implants that experience upper pole collapse in the upright position may be more forgiving with respect to volume selection, but they may not control and maintain upper breast fullness as well, depending on tissue and surgeon variables.

Anatomic or shaped implants that are truly form stable (minimize upper pole collapse when upright) provide surgeons and patients with additional options. To control shape in a breast, a surgeon must be able to control distribution of fill within the breast. *To control distribution of fill in a breast, the surgeon must first be able to control distribution of fill within the implant.* With saline or non-cohesive fill implants, the only means of controlling distribution of fill within the implant is to add more filler compared to the original mandrel volume of the device, with a tradeoff of increased firmness that has been shown to not be a significant factor to patients who are informed of the tradeoffs preoperatively.[2] In contrast, form stable, highly cohesive silicone gel filled implants maintain their shape with a lower fill volume-to-mandrel volume ratio, enabling better control of distribution of fill with less firmness.

At least 31 clinical and tissue factors, and at least 22 surgeon variables[6] affect every breast augmentation result (Table 2-7). Establishing valid comparative cohorts with this many variables has limited surgeons' ability to publish scientifically valid studies that compare implant devices or surgical techniques. During operative planning and implant selection, the more variables the surgeon considers, and the more objective data the surgeon records, the more likely scientific analysis of outcomes data can lead to improved patient outcomes.

> At least 31 clinical and tissue factors, and at least 22 surgeon variables affect every breast augmentation result

7. Design and dissect the implant pocket to "fit" the implant selected

Chapters 13, 14, and 15 address principles, sequence, and details of pocket dissection through inframammary, axillary, and periareolar incision approaches.

Prior to the development of polyurethane covered and textured silicone shell implants, implant options were limited to smooth shell implants. In the United States, during the 1980s and prior to the FDA ban on silicone gel filled devices, most patients and surgeons preferred and used silicone gel filled devices. Gel filled devices during that period experienced significant gel bleed. Combined with more traumatic blunt dissection techniques prevalent during that period, capsular contracture rates were relatively high. To attempt to reduce those rates, surgeons dissected pockets that were much larger than the implant, and frequently recommended implant displacement exercises to keep the pocket open against the forces of wound contracture and healing. The obvious tradeoffs of these techniques were: (a) inability to optimally control the position of the device within the pocket and therefore inability to optimally control the shape of the breast, (b) patient compliance issues with displacement exercises, (c) persistent issues with capsular contracture despite all these efforts (traumatic blunt dissection with tissue trauma and bleeding persisted as a likely cause, as did all basic wound healing mechanisms), and (d) creation of larger internal wound surface areas relative to the size of the implant device.

Table 2-7. Surgeon and patient variables to control for valid scientific studies

Clinical and tissue factors	Surgeon factors
Genetic factors	Incision approach
Hormonal factors	Parenchymal dissection
Pregnancy history	Location Extent
Nursing history	Pocket dissection method
Age	Pocket dissection technique
Medications (especially birth control pills and hormones)	Degree of tissue trauma
Skin thickness	Bleeding intraoperatively
Skin compliance	Blood remaining in tissues Blood remaining in pocket
Breast parenchyma Amount	Pocket dimensions
Base width	Pocket dissection plane—submammary or subpectoral
Height Consistency	Division of pectoralis origins
Attachments to pectoralis	Location
Attachments to serratus	Extent
Attachments to deep subcutaneous fascia	Method of implant leak testing
	Method of implant fill
	Implant fill accuracy
Capsule Thickness	Implant insertion method
Compliance	Implant positioning method
Degree of contracture	Tissue closure method
Age of capsule	Postoperative bandaging methods
Attachments to pectoralis	Postoperative implant motion exercises
Attachments to serratus	Postoperative activity regimen
Pectoralis major muscle Thickness	Postoperative drug regimen
Compliance	
Degree of contraction	
Degree of passive tension	
Size of periprosthetic pocket	
Shape of periprosthetic pocket	
Patient arm position	
Patient degree of pectoralis contraction (passive or active)	
Implant fill volume	
Air in implant	

The development of form stable, anatomic or shaped implants in the early 1990s necessitated better control of the position of the implant in the pocket to minimize occurrence of implant malposition. With these devices, surgeons learned to adjust pocket dissection techniques to make the pocket "fit" the implant more precisely by slightly underdissecting the lateral portion of the pocket initially, then incrementally enlarging it to "fit" the base width footprint of the implant after the implant is in place.[3,5,15] Interestingly, mobile and supine views of these textured, form stable implants in place clearly demonstrate lateral shift and movement of the implant when patients lie supine, due to movement that occurs 3 or more months postoperatively at the interface between the capsule and the surrounding soft tissues. This degree of movement for naturalness, however, does not increase implant malposition rates with *anatomic* devices with Biocell[TM] texturing. In 1664 consecutive reported cases,[2,3,5] using optimal planning[6] and surgical[3,5] techniques, with up to 7 year followup, implant malposition with full height anatomic implants occurred in only 0.1 % of cases. During the same period, the implant malposition rate for round implants in saline PMA studies averaged 2%.

In ongoing PMA studies for conventional (non-form stable) gel filled implants, data suggest lower rates of capsular contracture compared to earlier generations of gel implants. In addition, electrocautery dissection techniques evolved to minimize bleeding and tissue trauma,[3,5] contributing to even lower rates of capsular contracture. As a result, surgeons no longer needed to dissect pockets that were much larger than the implant, even with smooth shell implants. With newer generation conventional round gel implants, and with all shaped, form stable gel implants, surgeons using optimal planning and dissection techniques can now dissect pockets that more nearly match the dimensions of implants, minimizing wound surface area, minimizing reoperations due to implant displacement or malposition, better controlling breast shape, and eliminating unproved and unnecessary patient displacement exercises.

With newer generation conventional round gel implants, and with all shaped, form stable gel implants, surgeons using optimal planning and dissection techniques can now dissect pockets that more nearly match the dimensions of implants

Shaped breast implants, and shaped, form stable implants in particular, are now available in various heights and widths. When using full height, form stable implants, surgeons must assure adequate superior pocket dimensions to accommodate the full height of the implant and avoid folding or compression of the upper pole of the device. With reduced height, shaped implants, surgeons must carefully assess the width of the device relative to its height, and avoid excessive upper pocket dissection that might encourage implant rotation with implants that are wider than they are tall (base width exceeds implant vertical height). Any qualified plastic surgeon can readily acquire the surgical skills to dissect and tailor optimal pocket sizes for various implant types, provided the surgeon plans optimally and executes pocket dissection techniques following published, proved techniques.[2,3,5,6,7,10]

8. Minimize trauma and bleeding, eliminate blunt dissection, and apply prospective hemostasis principles

These techniques are described in Chapters 10–13.

Surgical techniques are currently published that enable over 85% of patients to be out to dinner the evening of surgery and return to full normal activities within 24 hours.[5] These techniques address the most basic principles of surgery—minimizing tissue trauma and minimizing bleeding *prospectively* to minimize blood in tissues that creates inflammation, pain, and an excessive wound healing response. By preventing bleeding before it starts and by totally eliminating all blunt dissection during pocket development, these techniques allow surgeons to dramatically redefine the perioperative patient experience. By minimizing bleeding and trauma that incite a more aggressive wound healing response, the techniques help reduce risks of capsular contracture and infection compared to rates in comparable PMA studies.[12–14]

Peer reviewed and published data indicate that techniques of monopolar electrocautery forceps and needlepoint pocket dissection, and techniques of prospective hemostasis dramatically decrease patient recovery times.[5] Additionally, these simple techniques dramatically decrease morbidity and totally *eliminate any need* for all of the following adjuncts that detract from patient recovery: drains, intercostal blocks, invasive pain pumps, compression bandages, compression bras, compression or positioning straps, implant displacement exercises, narcotic strength pain medications, and limitation of normal activities such as lifting and driving. Patients can shower the afternoon of surgery without bandages, perform all normal activities including arm lifting above the head and lifting normal objects, and can go to dinner the evening of surgery.

Prospective hemostasis is a term that describes dissection techniques that prevent bleeding before it ever starts, reducing even small amounts of blood that soak into tissues and cause unnecessary, additional inflammation. These techniques are described in detail in a previous publication.[5] While electrocautery dissection techniques using a blade tip or needle tip electrocautery are far superior to any type of blunt dissection, dissection with *monopolar*, needlepoint electrocautery handswitching forceps is another quantum improvement. Using a single instrument for dissection and hemostasis enables the

Sidebar notes:

Surgical techniques are currently published that enable over 85% of patients to be out to dinner the evening of surgery and return to full normal activities within 24 hours

By preventing bleeding before it starts and by totally eliminating all blunt dissection during pocket development, these techniques allow surgeons to dramatically redefine the perioperative patient experience

Prospective hemostasis is a term that describes dissection techniques that prevent bleeding before it ever starts, reducing even small amounts of blood that soak into tissues and cause unnecessary, additional inflammation

surgeon to eliminate unnecessary instrument exchange to control a bleeder if it occurs, dramatically reducing the amount of blood that can soak into adjacent tissues while trying to control the bleeding vessel.

Blunt dissection for pocket development in breast augmentation, though still commonly practiced, is unnecessarily traumatic, uncontrolled, and causes more bleeding compared to state-of-the-art electrocautery dissection. By totally eliminating even the most limited blunt dissection, surgeons can reduce trauma and bleeding and deliver dramatically improved outcomes to patients. Direct vision during pocket dissection enables optimal control by the surgeon. Any incision approach or technique that does not require and provide *direct internal vision* (or endoscopic, direct internal vision) within the pocket as dissection proceeds, deprives the surgeon and patient of optimal control of tissue trauma, bleeding, and accuracy of pocket dissection, each of which can significantly impact outcomes.

> Blunt dissection for pocket development in breast augmentation, though still commonly practiced, is unnecessarily traumatic, uncontrolled, and causes more bleeding compared to state-of-the-art electrocautery dissection

9. Optimize outcomes prospectively by managing factors that speed recovery

Factors that speed recovery also improve outcomes by minimizing tissue trauma, minimizing bleeding, reducing operative times, reducing narcotics perioperatively and eliminating them postoperatively, and decreasing morbidity by providing patients a much more rapid return to normal activities and work.[5] Chapter 17 details the processes that enable patients to be out to dinner the evening of their breast augmentation and return to full normal activities within 24 hours.

Optimal outcomes are the result of patient education,[7] quantifiable clinical tissue assessment,[6,10] patient and surgeon decision making,[7] operative planning and perioperative protocols that reduce operative times and drug dosages,[5] surgical techniques that reduce tissue trauma and bleeding,[5] and postoperative management regimens that eliminate unnecessary adjuncts and support patients to early normal activity.[5] Proved, peer reviewed and published processes can help surgeons deliver a dramatically improved perioperative experience and improved outcomes to patients.[2-11]

> Proved, peer reviewed and published processes can help surgeons deliver a dramatically improved perioperative experience and improved outcomes to patients

Table 2-8 lists the processes that are essential to predictably deliver the most rapid recovery and lowest complication and reoperation rates.

Preoperative planning, perioperative anesthesia and stepdown protocols and surgical scripts[5] can avoid unnecessary prolongation of operative times and resultant total

Table 2-8 **Essential processes to deliver out to dinner and 24 hour recovery**
• Staged, repetitive patient education and documented informed consent
• Quantitative tissue assessment
• Tissue based implant selection
• Surgeon and patient decision making based on knowledge base
• Defined decision processes that are validated
• Preoperative planning to eliminate time waste
• Eliminate use of implant sizers and unnecessary postoperative adjuncts
• Techniques of prospective hemostasis
• No touch techniques for ribs and periosteum
• Precise pocket dissection to fit the implant
• Minimize narcotic medications
• Rapid mobilization
• Elimination of the following adjuncts: bandages, straps, drains, pain pumps, intercostal blocks, bupivacaine (Marcaine) in the pocket, narcotic strength pain medications, muscle relaxants, pulsed electromagnetic therapy, or other neurostimulation therapy

Reducing narcotic dosage is essential to delivering state-of-the-art results in breast augmentation, and reducing narcotic dosage begins with avoiding unnecessarily prolonged operative times due to inadequate planning, sizer use, implant selection, or suboptimal surgical techniques

perioperative narcotics dosage. A narcotized patient awakens slower, is more prone to nausea and vomiting, is unmotivated and often unable to resume normal activities within the first 8 hours postoperatively, is more prone to constipation, and with available narcotic medication is less motivated to resume normal activities. Reducing narcotic dosage is essential to delivering state-of-the-art results in breast augmentation, and reducing narcotic dosage begins with avoiding unnecessarily prolonged operative times due to inadequate planning, sizer use, implant selection, or suboptimal surgical techniques. Eliminating narcotics postoperatively with patients requiring only ibuprofen for discomfort dramatically redefines the postoperative patient recovery experience.[5]

Defining and practicing proved processes improves surgeon performance. Surgeons less than 5 years in practice now routinely deliver 24 hour return to normal activities by reading, practicing, and modifying published anesthesia protocols, surgical operative scripts, recovery and stepdown protocols, and postoperative patient management protocols.[10] Implementing proved processes before attempting to modify those proved processes minimizes surgeon time waste, frustration, and suboptimal results and outcomes.

Assuming optimal implementation of proved processes through recovery and stepdown, management of the patient in the first 8 hours postoperatively is key to optimal outcomes

Assuming optimal implementation of proved processes through recovery and stepdown, management of the patient in the first 8 hours postoperatively is key to optimal outcomes.[5,11] Early mobilization and activity conflict with patient and surgeon instincts. Early mobilization and activity require patient compliance derived from education and staff support to help overcome natural fears and apprehension. Altering surgeon instincts and habits is more difficult. Many surgeons including the author were taught that early mobilization increases risks of bleeding, a self-fulfilling prophecy using blunt dissection techniques popular at that time. Using refined dissection techniques, early mobilization does not increase risks of bleeding.[5,9,10] Eliminating unnecessary adjuncts that absolutely preclude state-of-the-art recovery is difficult for many surgeons. The fact that surgeons with very limited experience can deliver 24 hour recovery should help encourage surgeons to implement processes that deliver improved outcomes.

Postoperative management during the first 8 hours after augmentation is critically important to predictably enable patients to be out to dinner and resume full normal activities within 24 hours.[5] Before leaving the surgery facility, staff reviews complete postoperative instructions with patients and caregivers. Patients raise their fully extended arms in a "jumping jack" motion, touching the backs of their hands above their heads with five repetitions as the caregiver observes. The patient repeats these stretching exercises every hour until bedtime after returning home. Patients are instructed to take a 2 hour nap after returning home, and the caregiver is instructed to wake and get the patient out of bed immediately at the end of 2 hours. After a light snack to avoid medication on an empty stomach, the patient takes 800 mg ibuprofen, waits 20 minutes, and enters a hot shower where she is instructed to wash her hair and wash all markings off her breasts and chest. Out of the shower, the patient is instructed to blow dry her hair and repeat her hands over her head exercises, and not to return to bed under any circumstances, instead, engaging in normal activities and leaving the house to go shopping, to a movie, or out to dinner. When the patient returns home, before bedtime she is instructed to lie with full weight on her breasts for 15 minutes, repeated nightly for the first 4 weeks. Timed phone calls from staff to home and mobile phones at the end of the 2 hour nap period and before bedtime to provide support and assure compliance are absolutely critical to help patients and caregivers overcome apprehension and optimally comply with the postoperative regimen. Peer reviewed and published methods of delivering 24 hour recovery have been developed and refined over a decade, are currently being reproduced by other surgeons, and have redefined the patient experience in breast augmentation. The greatest impediments to success with this regimen are surgeon apprehension, failure to implement defined perioperative protocols, overmedication with narcotic strength pain medication, addition of other unnecessary

Peer reviewed and published methods of delivering 24 hour recovery have been developed and refined over a decade, are currently being reproduced by other surgeons, and have redefined the patient experience in breast augmentation

medications and adjuncts, and lack of disciplined, stringent compliance measures in the 8 hours immediately postoperatively.

10. Manage untoward occurrences using defined processes; define end points for implant removal without replacement

In addition to the above, the patient should be educated preoperatively about specific management, end point, and cost protocols should untoward events occur. Chapter 16 presents detailed, algorithmic approaches to managing common challenges in breast augmentation.

No surgeon or patient wants to deal with problems or reoperations postoperatively. Unfortunately, breast augmentation surgery involves factors that neither surgeons nor patients can control, and untoward outcomes and complications can occur that sometimes require reoperations. Problems are occasionally unavoidable, but when problems and eventualities are a surprise to a patient and the patient's family, the problem is compounded and can result in medicolegal action.

Avoiding surprise requires that surgeons provide patients specific information about problems and eventualities preoperatively, and assure patient understanding and acceptance of responsibility for the decision to have surgery using repetitive, detailed informed consent documents.[7] Integrated into the patient education and informed consent process, these documents provide the following specific information: nature of the problem, risk of occurrence, specific management measures, key events or conditions that will trigger specific measures, approximate success and failure rates of treatment of the problem, risks and possible eventualities if the problem is not correctable, approximate costs of treatment, who is responsible for each type and amount of cost of treatment, end points at which the surgeon will recommend implant removal without replacement, potential appearance of the breasts after implant removal, and whether additional surgical procedures may be necessary or whether they may improve the appearance of the breasts after implant removal. Although this information is comprehensive and requires surgeon commitment to integrate into patient education and informed consent, it is critically important.

Defined, peer reviewed and published decision and management algorithms derived from multiple surgeons' experience can be exceedingly helpful in managing untoward events and occurrences.[8] These algorithms are not intended to define a standard of practice.

Defined, peer reviewed and published decision and management algorithms derived from multiple surgeons' experience can be exceedingly helpful in managing untoward events and occurrences

Instead, they are designed as a framework and checklist for decisions and management alternatives, and to assist with informed consent and involving the patient in choosing alternatives during difficult periods. The Breast Augmentation Surgeons for Patients Initiative (BASPI) algorithms are a valuable reference and help in managing occurrences which happen rarely and therefore are not a routine part of every surgical practice.

Defining end points for implant removal without replacement is difficult, and must fit each individual surgeon's practice pattern and preferences.[9] When difficult circumstances occur, end points for removal without replacement that the surgeon has defined preoperatively and the patient has accepted in detailed, line item signed informed consent documents are invaluable. If the patient is not aware of these end points preoperatively, she and her family are much less likely to understand and accept them postoperatively if problems occur, persist, or recur. As difficult as implant removal without replacement is, surgeons and patients must remember that patient tissue is an irreplaceable commodity. Prolonged surgical efforts at implant salvage that prolong inflammation and repeated surgical trauma can produce irreversible damage to tissues and uncorrectable deformities that patients can avoid by timely implant removal without replacement. A smaller breast without significant, uncorrectable deformity is always preferable to a larger, deformed breast with irreversible tissue damage.

> When difficult circumstances occur, end points for removal without replacement that the surgeon has defined preoperatively and the patient has accepted in detailed, line item signed informed consent documents are invaluable

> Prolonged surgical efforts at implant salvage that prolong inflammation and repeated surgical trauma can produce irreversible damage to tissues and uncorrectable deformities that patients can avoid by timely implant removal without replacement

■ CONCLUSION

Ten essentials, implemented over a 30 year clinical experience in breast augmentation, predictably deliver rapid, out-to-dinner recovery and return to normal activities within 24 hours of breast augmentation.[5] In 1664 peer reviewed and published cases with up to 7 year followup, implementation of the processes referenced in this chapter resulted in a 3% overall reoperation rate, a 1.8% reoperation rate for implant size exchange, zero uncorrectable deformities following breast augmentation,[2,3,5] and a zero percent reoperation rate in a PMA series at 3 year followup.[11]

> Ten essentials, implemented over a 30 year clinical experience in breast augmentation, predictably deliver rapid, out-to-dinner recovery and return to normal activities within 24 hours of breast augmentation

■ REFERENCES

1. Tebbetts JB: What is adequate fill? Implications in breast implant surgery. *Plast Reconstr Surg* 97(7):1451–1454, 1996.

2. Tebbetts JB: Patient acceptance of adequately filled breast implants using the tilt test. *Plast Reconstr Surg* 106(1):139–147, 2000.

3. Tebbetts JB: Dual plane (DP) breast augmentation: optimizing implant–soft tissue relationships in a wide range of breast types. *Plast Reconstr Surg* 107:1255, 2001.

4. Tebbetts JB: Achieving a predictable 24 hour return to normal activities after breast augmentation Part I: Refining practices using motion and time study principles. *Plast Reconstr Surg* 109:273–290, 2002.

5. Tebbetts JB: Achieving a predictable 24 hour return to normal activities after breast augmentation Part II: Patient preparation, refined surgical techniques and instrumentation. *Plast Reconstr Surg* 109:293–305, 2002.

6. Tebbetts JB: A system for breast implant selection based on patient tissue characteristics and implant–soft tissue dynamics. *Plast Reconstr Surg* 109(4):1396–1409, 2002.

7. Tebbetts JB: An approach that integrates patient education and informed consent in breast augmentation. *Plast Reconstr Surg* 110(3):971–978, 2002.

8. Tebbetts JB: Decision and management algorithms to address patient and Food and Drug Administration concerns regarding breast augmentation and implants. *Plast Reconstr Surg* 114(5):1252–1257, 2004.

9. Tebbetts JB: Out points criteria for breast implant removal without replacement and criteria to minimize reoperations following breast augmentation. *Plast Reconstr Surg* 114(5):1258–1262, 2004.

10. Tebbetts JB, Adams WP: Five critical decisions in breast augmentation using 5 measurements in 5 minutes: the high five system. *Plast Reconstr Surg* 116(7):2005–2016, 2005.

11. Tebbetts JB: Achieving a zero percent reoperation rate at 3 years in a 50 consecutive case augmentation mammaplasty PMA study. *Plast Reconstr Surg* 118(6):1453–1457, 2006.

12. Food and Drug Administration. U.S. Food and Drug Administration. General and Plastic Surgery Devices Panel Meeting Transcript. Washington, D.C. October 14–15, 2003. Online. Available: http://www.fda.gov/ohrms/dockets/ac/03/transcripts/3989T1.htm.

13. Food and Drug Administration. U.S. Food and Drug Administration. General and Plastic Surgery Devices Panel Meeting Transcript. Washington, D.C. February 18, 1999.

14. Food and Drug Administration. U.S. Food and Drug Administration. General and Plastic Surgery Devices Panel Meeting Transcript. Washington, D.C. March 1–3, 2000. Online. Available: http://www.fda.gov/cdrh/gpsdp.html#030100.

15. Tebbetts JB: *Dimensional augmentation mammaplasty using the BioDimensional™ System*. Santa Barbara: McGhan Medical Corporation, 1994, pp 1–90.

Patient Education, Decisions, and Informed Consent

Decisions affect patient outcomes and the patient experience more than any surgical technique or implant device. A staged, repetitive system of patient education, integrated with detailed informed consent documents, best assures optimal patient education and informed consent.[1] Optimal decisions require knowledge applied through valid decision making processes. Few, if any, prospective breast augmentation patients begin the patient experience knowing what they need to know to make optimal decisions for an optimal outcome. Even fewer patients understand alternative decision processes and decision pathways that lead to predictably optimal outcomes in breast augmentation. Current reoperation rates in United States Food and Drug Administration (FDA) and Health Canada studies,[2-4] and the reasons for reoperations and suboptimal outcomes support the previous statements. Data in FDA premarket approval (PMA) studies and current rates of litigation suggest a need and opportunities for surgeons to provide patients better and more information and to improve patient education, decision making, and informed consent prior to breast augmentation.

While patient education is critically important to outcomes, reoperation rates and the patient experience, legally valid and properly documented informed consent prior to having a breast augmentation is equally important. Creating optimal content and decision pathways that satisfy proved educational models and simultaneously satisfying legal requirements for informed consent is demanding. To optimally accomplish these tasks, surgeons must commit time and resources to optimize all areas of patient education and informed consent.

> Decisions affect patient outcomes and the patient experience more than any surgical technique or implant device

▥ PATIENT EDUCATION AND INFORMED CONSENT: A PROCESS WITH REQUIREMENTS

Current law in the United States mandates that patients, not surgeons, make the ultimate decisions of the specific medical care the patient considers in her best interest

Informed consent in breast augmentation is a process, not a document or even a set of documents. Current law in the United States mandates that patients, not surgeons, make the ultimate decisions of the specific medical care the patient considers in her best interest. This does not mean that the patient cannot and should not seek information and decision support assistance from her surgeon. Law requires, however, that at the conclusion of the patient education process, the patient chooses treatment options.

To some surgeons, requirements of informed consent law may seem to conflict with surgical training and common processes in surgical practice. As a colleague once stated: "After all, the surgeon, not the patient, really knows best when making decisions regarding size, incision location, pocket location, and implant type and size." While this colleague's opinion may be shared by many surgeons, it does not satisfy the requirements of informed consent law.

Potential medicolegal problems arise when surgeons focus on the surgeon's preferences to the detriment or exclusion of providing comprehensive information to patients and allowing the patients to make informed decisions

Informed consent law requires that surgeons inform patients of all available treatment alternatives and provide information explaining the potential benefits and relative risks of each alternative. Surgeons' perceptions of potential benefits and relative risks are irrevocably linked to the surgical skill set derived from residency and postgraduate training, and from marketing and economic considerations that are a reality in any surgical practice. Potential medicolegal problems arise when surgeons focus on the surgeon's preferences to the detriment or exclusion of providing comprehensive information to patients and allowing the patients to make informed decisions. Surgeons are certainly free to have and express individual opinions regarding the benefits and risks of any choice. Difficulties can arise when a surgeon expresses personal opinions based on clinical experience and either fails to inform patients of other available alternatives, or manipulates peer reviewed and published information for marketing purposes or to mask a limited surgical skill set. To optimally address patients' educational needs and legal requirements for informed consent, surgeons should advise patients of all available alternatives, with all known (peer reviewed and published) potential benefits and risks, while honestly advising patients of the surgeon's personal clinical experience and preferences.

▥ VALID PATIENT EDUCATIONAL PROCESSES

Optimal outcomes require optimal processes

Optimal outcomes require optimal processes. The processes of patient education and informed consent should logically follow established models of proved educational

Figure 3-1. Basic education and training process.

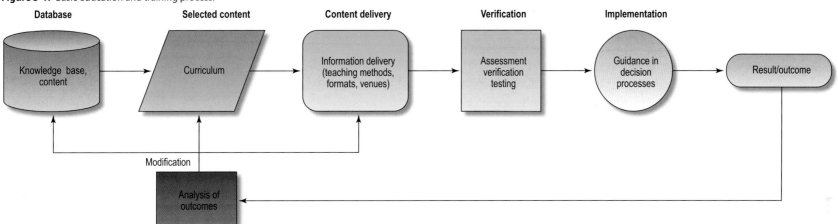

models and processes that meet legal requirements for informed consent. Figure 3-1 illustrates components that are essential to any valid educational model or process.

From a medicolegal perspective, patient education should be staged and repetitive, providing patients with information, allowing the patient time to digest the information, providing opportunities for the patient to ask questions and clarify the information, and repeating the steps before asking the patient to make definitive choices and decisions. Surgeons can best meet this requirement by providing patients extensive information in printed form prior to the first office visit, have a patient educator spend time with the patient to review the information and answer questions prior to the surgeon consultation, and carefully document each stage of the patient education and informed consent process.

Processes of patient education and informed consent must be comprehensive and carefully documented to assure optimal medicolegal compliance. These requirements can be accomplished while optimizing surgeon time use by implementing a system of information documents, patient choice documents, and informed consent documents that are integrated and used at sequential patient encounters. The system currently in use in the author's practice has evolved over a 26 year period, has been subjected to detailed legal scrutiny, and has been peer reviewed and published in the journal *Plastic and Reconstructive Surgery*.[1]

The primary source of content for our comprehensive patient education is our book entitled *The Best Breast*, first published in 1999, and now in its second edition. This book

> Processes of patient education and informed consent must be comprehensive and carefully documented to assure optimal medicolegal compliance

is the most comprehensive source of information about breast augmentation for patients, and the second edition is extensively referenced to provide scientific validity for the content based on our peer reviewed and published articles in *Plastic and Reconstructive Surgery.* The book is available at bookstores and through http://www.Amazon.com, or by calling our office at (+1)214-220-2712. The book website, http://www.thebestbreast. com, contains extensive content excerpts from the book and additional references and links for patients seeking information about breast augmentation.

In our initial telephone calls with patients, we request that each patient read *The Best Breast* before scheduling a patient educator consultation, because content from the book is much more extensive compared to any series of patient educator or surgeon visits. Content from the book forms an invaluable knowledge base for a patient that subsequently enables the patient to communicate much more effectively with a patient educator and the surgeon. Our comprehensive system then integrates content from *The Best Breast* with an extensive and constantly evolving system of informed consent documents, and the entire system is designed for surgeon efficiency. Optimally educated patients are capable of making over 90% of all decisions that relate to their breast augmentation before ever seeing a surgeon, enabling the surgeon to focus more precisely on key issues individual to the patient during the consultation and examination process.

To best understand how this comprehensive system actually applies in clinical practice, surgeons should *first read the original article from the journal* or online at the journal's website, http://www.plasreconsurg.com. *With the overview the article provides, the surgeon should then read in detail each of the individual documents that apply at each patient encounter in order, as a patient would read them.* Each of these documents is available in Adobe Acrobat™ pdf format in the Resources folder on the DVDs that accompany this book. Surgeons can use these resources for review or as templates to individualize similar documents.

Thoroughly understanding this system requires that surgeons read this chapter, and then read each of the informed consent documents in sequence, paying special attention to when and how the documents apply at each patient encounter

Table 3-1 lists each of the documents in the author's patient education in the order in which the documents are used at each patient encounter. Thoroughly understanding this system requires that surgeons read this chapter, and then read each of the informed consent documents in sequence, paying special attention to when and how the documents apply at each patient encounter. A summary of the patient education process will provide a basis for understanding how this document system can be comprehensive, staged, and repetitive, while maximizing surgeon efficiency.

Table 3-1. An overview of the informed consent process and documents

Patient encounter	Personnel	Document name and number
1. Initial patient call	Patient coordinator and/or patient educator	Surgeon's written information of choice, in the author's practice, the book entitled *The Best Breast* Professional societies' brochures of choice
2. Patient educator consult	Patient educator	1. Patient Educator Checklist 2. Patient Preferences for Augmentation 3. Augmentation Decisions Flowchart 4. How Did We Do Informing You? 5. Will Anyone Else Be Involved—Part 1 6. Will Anyone Else Be Involved—Part 2
3. Surgeon consultation	Surgeon	7. Clinical Evaluation Form 8. Surgeon Consultation Notes 9. Patient Images Analysis
4. Documents packet provided to patient when surgery scheduled	Surgery scheduling coordinator	10. General Disclosure and Consent for Augmentation 11. Verification of Informed Consent (*Applicable specialized informed consent documents #12–#20) 12. Informed Consent for Patients Desiring Augmentation Mammaplasty with a Round Breast Implant 13. Informed Consent for Patients Desiring Augmentation Mammaplasty with an Anatomic Breast Implant 14. Informed Consent for Patients Desiring Augmentation Mammaplasty and Who Have a Family History of Breast Cancer 15. Informed Consent for Patients Desiring Augmentation with a Large (>350 cc) Breast Implant 16. Informed Consent for Patients Desiring Augmentation with a Larger Implant than Dr. [Surgeon's Name] Feels is Optimal for the Patient's Tissues 17. Informed Consent for Patients Desiring Augmentation Mammaplasty Through a Belly Button (Umbilical) Incision 18. Informed Consent for Patients Desiring Endoscopic Axillary or Umbilical Augmentation 19. Request for Larger Implants 20. Request to Remove Implants 21. Request for Implant With Mastopexy 22. Disclosure and Consent for HIV Test 23. Anesthesia Important Information For You 24. Information on Financial Policies

*Specialized informed consent documents. One or more may be used depending on patient's specific choices, medical history, or tissue requirements. Each document listed in the right column is available in the Resources folder on the DVDs accompanying the book.

■ APPLYING EDUCATION AND INFORMED CONSENT SYSTEMS IN PRACTICE MANAGEMENT

Patient Encounters During a Staged, Repetitive Education and Informed Consent Process

In our practice, four patient encounters occur during the patient education and informed consent process (Table 3-1):

1. The initial telephone call to the office and followup with patient information (*The Best Breast*)
2. A patient educator consultation (including viewing a detailed consultation DVD with accompanying paper documentation of Choices and Preferences)
3. A surgeon consultation (tissue measurements, reconciling wishes with tissues, and imaging and photo analysis)
4. Finalization of informed consent documents, drawing blood for laboratory studies, and presurgical instructions and checklists.

A structured patient education curriculum, designed to present realistic alternatives and information, is staged and repeated to maximize opportunities for the patient to learn and make optimal decisions

Key patient education and informed consent events occur at each patient encounter. Most importantly, a structured patient education curriculum, designed to present realistic alternatives and information, is *staged and repeated* to maximize opportunities for the patient to learn and make optimal decisions. During this staged, repetitive process, specific decision support processes and documents aid the patient and our staff in helping make decisions that optimize the patient's experience and outcome, while minimizing short- and long-term risks and potential problems.

Initial Telephone Call and Information Provided to the Patient

Following the initial patient phone call to the office, the author provides each patient with a copy of his book entitled *The Best Breast* (available online, at most bookstores, or by contacting the author's office) and requires that the patient acknowledge having read the book prior to a patient educator consultation that precedes the surgeon consultation. If a patient is unwilling to attempt to read the materials provided, we usually suggest that the patient seek treatment elsewhere. If the patient makes an effort to read and digest the information, we are always willing to provide additional information and support to complement the initial information. While generic materials traditionally provided to patients by professional societies and other sources are helpful, none provides the depth of information that a surgeon can provide by committing time and resources to provide much more detailed information backed by peer reviewed and referenced data. More importantly, no generic materials to our knowledge provide meaningful decision support algorithms or processes, and none provides any significant level of testing or verification to assure a specific level of patient understanding and acceptance of responsibility for patient requests and choices.

Patient Educator Consultation

The patient educator consultation is usually scheduled on a separate day from the surgeon consultation to allow maximum flexibility of patient educator time with the patient while minimizing potential interference with optimal efficiency when the surgeon is seeing patients.

At the patient educator consultation, the patient views a DVD that reiterates information in *The Best Breast*, but in a structured manner that defines and clarifies alternatives in terms of what a surgeon can realistically deliver. A copy of the patient educator DVD from our practice is included in the set of DVDs with this book. Patients view this DVD at the time of their patient educator consultation in the office, or prior to the patient educator visit at home. The DVD is designed to be a stark, face-to-face discussion, devoid of entertaining but non-educational distractions, bells, and whistles. The content of the DVD is integrated with and complemented by additional content in a printed document that the patient refers to while watching the DVD in stages. This document, entitled "My Preferences and Information I Fully Understand and Accept", asks the patient to choose from specific options presented in stages following a discussion of each topic on the DVD.

The patient educator DVD content provides a framework for patient decision making that encourages the patient to choose from realistic alternatives that seek to minimize "gray areas" and present more "black and white" alternatives. The DVD also encourages the patient to list questions or topics for further discussion with the patient educator. While viewing the DVD in stages, the patient reads and signs, paragraph by paragraph, the detailed informed consent document entitled "My Preferences and Information I Fully Understand and Accept" that sequentially asks the patient to make choices after reading the book and hearing verbal presentations on the DVD. These choices and preferences are not final, but provide documentation that the patient has received and understands essential printed and visual information, and further documents the patient's decision processes. The Choices and Preferences document asks several key questions in two or

> The patient educator DVD content provides a framework for patient decision making that encourages the patient to choose from realistic alternatives that seek to minimize "gray areas" and present more "black and white" alternatives

> The Choices and Preferences document asks several key questions in two or three different ways, allowing the staff and surgeon to judge the consistency of a patient's answers and the knowledge level of the patient

three different ways, allowing the staff and surgeon to judge the consistency of a patient's answers and the knowledge level of the patient. Equally importantly, the answers in the document enable staff and surgeon to identify inconsistencies or hidden patient agendas that may or may not be realistic in the patient's individual clinical setting.

Thoroughly understanding the functionality of the patient education and informed consent system requires that surgeons assume the role of the patient, read all of the written materials and informed consent documents in the system, and watch the entire patient education DVD. Each component of the system has a specific function, and the components integrate to reinforce information and ask important questions repetitively in different ways to test the patient's understanding of the content and also test the consistency of the patient's answers.

The patient educator transfers the patient's preliminary choices to the Clinical Evaluation Form that the surgeon uses during the surgeon consultation, and asks the patient to initial her choices once again on the Clinical Evaluation Form to provide repetitive documentation of the patient's requests and choices.

The patient educator thoroughly reviews each of the topics in the Choices and Preferences document, answering all patient questions, and encouraging the patient to discuss any additional topics or concerns. A thorough discussion of any questions the patient has listed while watching the patient education DVD or during the patient educator review assures a documented opportunity for the patient to ask questions and have the questions answered to her satisfaction (another opportunity occurs at the surgeon consultation, and a third opportunity with the patient educator before signing operative consent forms). Each opportunity to ask questions and having those questions answered to the patient's satisfaction is documented repetitively on sequential informed consent documents used at each of the question encounters.

The Surgeon Consultation

Prior to the surgeon consultation, the patient has read an extensive amount of information, reviewed information in stages, viewed a patient education DVD, stated her preliminary preferences and choices on the Choices and Preferences document, and completed a patient educator consultation to review and clarify the information and answer questions. With this preparation, the surgeon consultation can focus on quantifying the patient's tissue characteristics and breast measurements, and answering the key question, "Knowing the patient's preferences stated on the Choices and Preferences document, and quantifying patient tissue characteristics, can the surgeon predictably deliver what the patient is requesting with optimal safety and efficacy long-term?" The patient education, decision making, and informed consent process helps the patient reconcile her *wishes* with the *realities of her tissues*. If any of her requests are suboptimal given her individual tissue characteristics, surgeon and patient reconcile potential compromises, and finalize choices during the surgeon consultation.

Before entering the consultation room, the surgeon reviews the patient's Choices and Preferences document, and assures consistency of the choices on that document with choices that the patient educator transferred to the Clinical Evaluation Form. This content is included in Adobe Acrobat™ pdf format in the Resources folder on the DVDs that accompany this book.

During the surgeon consultation, the surgeon completes five basic measurements and makes five critical decisions in less than 5 minutes using the High Five™ System. This system is discussed in detail in Chapter 4. Using this quantifiable, efficient system, the surgeon completes choices of pocket location (soft tissue coverage), implant volume, implant type, position of the inframammary fold to set intraoperatively, and incision location. The surgeon can ask the patient to initial these choices at the time of the surgeon consultation, assuring another level of documentation of the patient's choices.

The funnel analogy—understanding what is optimal fill for each individual patient

During the surgeon consultation, discussing a "funnel analogy" often helps the patient understand optimal fill for her individual breast dimensions. The following dialogue from the surgeon has been extremely useful in helping patients understand the concept of optimal fill based on individual tissue characteristics.

You must choose the appearance you prefer, choosing whether you prefer a more natural appearing breast, or a more rounded, basketball appearing upper breast [the surgeon can choose a personal descriptive analogy; the analogy should attempt to eliminate "grays" and ask for "black and white" choices]. Once we know your preferences, our measurement system provides a very accurate approximation of the amount of fill required to produce the look you desire, given the width of your breast and your individual amount of skin stretch.

The patient education, decision making, and informed consent process helps the patient reconcile her *wishes* with the *realities of her tissues*

During the surgeon consultation, discussing a "funnel analogy" often helps the patient understand optimal fill for her individual breast dimensions

The wider your breast, and the greater your skin stretch, the greater the amount of fill that we must place into your breast to fill it adequately for an optimal result. If we stop short of the optimal amount of fill, your upper breast will not be adequately filled, and your breast may have a "rock in a sock" appearance. In the opposite situation, if you have a narrow breast and minimal skin stretch, your breast does not require and will not accommodate as much fill. If we attempt to place excessive fill in your breast, you may have excessive upper breast fullness and bulging with a breast that appears more like a basketball compared to a natural breast.

In addition to trying to achieve the appearance you desire, you must remember that even without a breast augmentation, larger breasts tend to lose an optimal appearance and position sooner than more normal size breasts. Remember that your choices now are very likely to affect how your breasts look as you grow older, and the quality of your tissues that a surgeon may have to deal with in the future.

Imagine that we have a funnel in the top of your breast. As we pour fill into the funnel, the lower portion of your breast fills first until it reaches its limit of stretch. This may be a bit uncomfortable, but let's determine the maximum amount your skin will stretch forward by grasping the skin and pulling it until you feel discomfort and the skin stops (Figure 3-2, A, B). [During this maneuver, the surgeon grasps the areolar skin immediately beside the nipple and stretches it maximally forward, noting the location of maximal stretch with a fingernail (Figure 3-2, B), and then releases the skin. At this maximum stretch distance from the breast, the surgeon cups the hand around the lower pole of the breast at a distance approximately equal to the maximal skin stretch (Figure 3-2, C), and continues the dialog.]

If I cup my hand at an equal distance around your lower breast at this point of maximal stretch, if you will look down, you can visually get an idea of how full your lower breast will be at maximal skin stretch without overstretching or damaging the skin (Figure 3-2, C). From this point of maximal stretch, I will align my pen onto your upper chest (Figure 3-2, D), and you can get an idea of the area under the pen that will be filled in the upper breast.

While maximally stretching the skin and demonstrating maximal fill, the surgeon carefully watches the patient's expression as the surgeon demonstrates the amount of fill to assess a positive or negative response. The surgeon also asks: "How does that amount of fill look to you?" If the patient makes any type of excuse for not being able to judge adequacy of size using this technique, the surgeon should say: "There is no better way to accurately judge visually than by looking at your own tissues and how much they will stretch. Let's repeat this again until you feel comfortable judging and telling me whether this amount of fill and size is agreeable to you."

Figure 3-2, A-D. Maximally stretching the periareolar skin (*A*) defines anterior pull skin stretch and (*B*) demonstrates to the patient the maximal amount of stretch her skin will tolerate. By cupping the hand equidistant from the breast at this distance (*C*), the patient can visualize on her own breast the approximate amount of fullness that augmentation using the High Five™ system will create. By connecting the point of maximal stretch with the upper chest using a pen (*D*), the patient can visualize the amount of fullness that will be achieved in the upper breast.

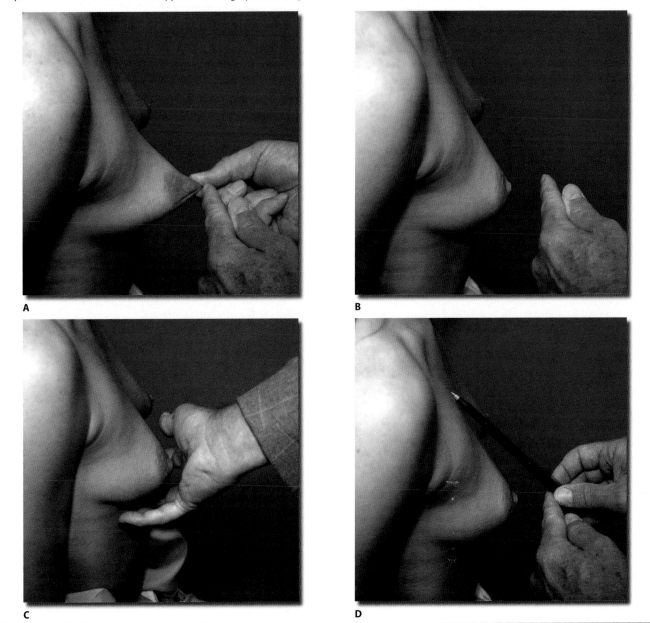

A

B

C

D

If the size appears too large to the patient, the surgeon responds:

As we add filler to our funnel, the lower breast will fill until it reaches its limit of stretch, and the lower breast must be full before we achieve fill in the middle and upper breast. We can certainly stop short of the maximal stretch size I showed you, but if we do, we risk your having an empty middle or upper breast. Which would you prefer, a smaller breast that is emptier in the middle and upper breast, or a slightly larger breast in the lower breast that allows us to fill the middle and upper breast?

When the lower pole of your breast fills to this point, if we continue adding filler, the middle of the breast will fill, and the last portion of the breast to fill will be the upper breast. Once the upper breast is appropriately full, allowing for stretch, to produce a natural appearing breast, if we continue to pour more filler into the funnel, your upper breast will continue to bulge more and more and look more and more unnatural. If you requested a breast that does not appear unnatural, at some point, depending on the width and skin stretch of your breast, we must stop pouring fluid into the funnel. At that point, we have put as much filler into your breast as your skin will accommodate, unless we sacrifice soft tissue coverage or unless we accept a much more unnatural appearing breast.

The most important thing for you to understand from our stretching and measuring your tissues is that each woman's breast, depending on the width and skin stretch, requires enough fill to fill the entire breast, not just the lower breast. When we have placed adequate fill to fill the lower, middle, and upper breast, if we add any more fill, the breast will appear unnaturally bulging in the upper breast. Therefore the amount required to adequately fill your breast is also the maximum amount we can safely place in the breast without producing an unnatural appearance.

The amount required to adequately fill your breast is also the maximum amount we can safely place in the breast without producing an unnatural appearance

In previous documents and on the Clinical Evaluation Form, the patient has expressed and initialed her desire for either a "natural appearing breast" or an "unnatural appearing breast". No other options are available. This allows the surgeon to better define exactly what the patient may be expecting, and forces the patient to make more definitive decisions that a surgeon can more likely deliver, compared to shades of gray that no surgeon can deliver.

Encouraging the patient to visualize her result using her own tissues on her own chest is much more accurate, truthful, realistic, and valid compared to having her visualize a result using pictures or test implants stuffed into a bra that has no correlation with the patient's own tissue stretch characteristics

Maximally stretching the patient's periareolar skin to the point of discomfort is a powerful tool to demonstrate that overstretching skin has consequences, and that the measurement system is built to maximally fill the envelope without overfilling or overstretching and damaging the skin. Encouraging the patient to visualize her result using her own tissues on her own chest is much more accurate, truthful, realistic, and valid compared to having her visualize a result using pictures or test implants stuffed into a bra that has no correlation with the patient's own tissue stretch characteristics.

If the patient has stated a specific *volume* she desires in her implant on the Choices and Preferences document, the surgeon completes the High Five™ System measurements and analysis, and then must reconcile the patient's volume request with the volume the system recommends. The High Five™ System Clinical Evaluation Form has a specific line on the form that allows the surgeon to factor in a specific number of cc's to accommodate "Patient requests" that do not coincide with the system's recommendations.

Preoperative photographic imaging and a critically important discussion

The author prefers capturing preoperative digital images personally, using the patient encounter to further assure documentation of what breast augmentation can do and what it cannot do. After capturing at least five standardized views using a digital capture system and database, the patient sits beside the surgeon and views her anteroposterior view image on the display. The surgeon then uses the Images Analysis Sheet (Table 3-2) from the documents set included in the Resources folder on the DVD that accompany this book, placing the document in front of the patient, and reviews the following with the patient and her husband or significant other.

This conversation with the patient is one of the most important of all patient encounters. This discussion combines the reality of the patient viewing her preoperative anatomy with a clear, powerful set of statements that define reality and define what a breast augmentation can and cannot deliver. While viewing the patient's preoperative anteroposterior chest view, the surgeon asks the patient to read and initial each of the following items after the surgeon clarifies each printed statement using statements similar to the statements below.

The text from the Patient Images Analysis document precedes the surgeon's comments for each topic enclosed in quotes.

1. L/R breast larger—YOUR BREASTS WILL NEVER MATCH, AND DIFFERENT SIZE OR FILL IMPLANTS WILL NOT MAKE THEM MATCH.

Table 3-2. **Images analysis document**

Patient Images Analysis
Factors Unlikely to Change and Things That Will Not Be Totally Corrected
after Your Breast Augmentation

Patient: _____

Date: _____

❏ L/R breast larger—YOUR BREASTS WILL NEVER MATCH, AND DIFFERENT SIZE OR FILL IMPLANTS WILL NOT MAKE THEM MATCH.

❏ L/R breast is higher on chest—BREAST LEVELS ON THE CHEST WILL NEVER MATCH ON THE TWO SIDES.

❏ L/R nipple–areola higher on chest—NIPPLE LEVELS WILL NEVER MATCH ON THE TWO SIDES.

❏ Nipple position on the breast mounds is different on the two sides—NIPPLE POSITION AND DIRECTION WILL NEVER MATCH ON THE TWO SIDES.

❏ L/R fold beneath breast higher on chest—LEVEL OF MY BREASTS ON THE CHEST WILL NOT MATCH ON THE TWO SIDES.

❏ The position of the entire breast on the chest wall will not change, and nipple position will not change. If one fold beneath the breast is lower than the other, it will also be lower after your augmentation.

❏ The gap between the breasts will be similar to what it is now in order to avoid risks of visible implant edges and traction rippling in the cleavage area, both of which can be uncorrectable.

❏ Chest wall differences exist on the two sides that cannot be corrected and will affect breast shape.

❏ The basic shape and configuration of the breasts will be similar to their current appearance and not change drastically, but will be larger. Breast implants cannot predictably make precise shape changes in your breast.

❏ You may be able to feel the edges or shell of your implant after surgery, depending on the thickness of your tissues and how carefully you try to feel the implant.

❏ Your tissues are thin and stretchy. As a result, you may be at higher risk for visible rippling in areas of the breast, or at a higher risk of the lower breast stretching excessively following surgery, regardless of the implant you choose.

❏ Due to the width of your breasts and the stretch of your tissues, a significant amount of volume is required to just fill your breast to a level that will not leave you with an empty upper breast. Your tissues have already shown that they stretch, so they may not support the amount of volume required to get a good result, and you may have excessive stretching or thinning in the future, with the same risks as listed in the previous item above.

❏ Breast implants cannot predictably control the specific SHAPE of your breast or areas of your breast, so IF YOU CHOOSE TO HAVE BREAST AUGMENTATION, ALL YOU SHOULD PREDICTABLY EXPECT IS AN INCREASE IN THE SIZE OF YOUR BREASTS.

❏ Other: _____

❏ Other: _____

❏ Other: _____

Patient: Please initial below to document your understanding and acceptance of the above.

_____ Dr. [Surgeon's Name] has reviewed my patient images with me in detail. I have seen, understand, and accept each of the factors listed above that will not change or may be only partially improved following my augmentation. I totally understand and accept that my breasts or components of my breasts WILL NEVER MATCH ON THE TWO SIDES, and that perfection is not an option, and I only expect an INCREASE IN THE SIZE of my breasts.

No woman has two breasts that are the same, and no surgeon can make two breasts the same

"No woman has two breasts that are the same, and no surgeon can make two breasts the same." The surgeon asks the patient to choose and initial which breast is larger. The surgeon then explains: "No surgeon can make breasts match by placing a larger implant in the smaller breast to make it match the larger breast. The smaller breast, by definition, has less skin, and attempts to place excessive volume in that breast will result in a bulging upper pole and shape differences that are often more noticeable compared to the size difference that every woman has."

2. L/R breast is higher on chest–BREAST LEVELS ON THE CHEST WILL NEVER MATCH ON THE TWO SIDES.

   L/R nipple–areola higher on chest—NIPPLE LEVELS WILL NEVER MATCH ON THE TWO SIDES.

   Nipple position on the breast mounds is different on the two sides–NIPPLE POSITION AND DIRECTION WILL NEVER MATCH ON THE TWO SIDES.

   L/R fold beneath breast higher on chest–LEVEL OF MY BREASTS ON THE CHEST WILL NOT MATCH ON THE TWO SIDES.

Breasts are never located at the same level on the torso

   "Breasts are never located at the same level on the torso." One breast always appears higher on the torso compared to the other (this may result from the patient standing with one shoulder higher, a patient with scoliosis, and other causes, but augmentation does not correct any of these causes). One nipple is always higher than the other. The surgeon then asks the patient to choose and acknowledge that one breast is higher on the torso compared to the other, and one nipple is higher and positioned more medially or laterally on the breast compared to the other.

3. The position of the entire breast on the chest wall will not change, and nipple position will not change. If one fold beneath the breast is lower than the other, it will also be lower after your augmentation.

When we perform routine breast augmentation, we do not relocate the level of your breasts on your torso, and we do not reposition your nipples on your breast or torso. As a result, differences you see now will still be present following your augmentation

   "When we perform routine breast augmentation, we do not relocate the level of your breasts on your torso, and we do not reposition your nipples on your breast or torso. As a result, differences you see now will still be present following your augmentation, and may be more noticeable to you because you will be looking at your breasts much more following your augmentation."

4. The gap between the breasts will be similar to what it is now in order to avoid risks of visible implant edges and traction rippling in the cleavage area, both of which can be uncorrectable.

The gap between the breasts will be similar to what it is now in order to avoid risks of visible implant edges and traction rippling in the cleavage area, both of which can be uncorrectable

"In the gap between your breasts which many refer to as the cleavage area, your sternal bone is covered only by skin and a very thin layer of fat. If we move the inside edges of your implants inward under this thin skin in an attempt to narrow this gap, you will very likely be able to see edges of your implants. When the weight of your implants pulls on this thin overlying skin over time, you also will likely develop visible traction rippling in the cleavage area. Visible edges and traction rippling are unsightly, and are often uncorrectable. To avoid these uncorrectable deformities, you will have the same width gap following your augmentation that you have now. When you wish to narrow the gap between your breasts, you should use a push up bra, which is a much better alternative compared to visible, uncorrectable deformities."

5. Chest wall differences exist on the two sides that cannot be corrected and will affect breast shape.

"Every patient has subtle or not-so-subtle differences in the shape of the chest wall on the two sides, and many patients have some degree of spinal curvature or scoliosis. Breast augmentation does not change these underlying differences in shape or spinal curvature, and these conditions always affect breast shape to varying degrees."

6. The basic shape and configuration of the breasts will be similar to their current appearance and not change drastically, but will be larger. Breast implants cannot predictably make precise shape changes in your breast.

"A breast augmentation predictably does only one thing: it predictably makes your breasts larger. Other more subtle changes may occur, but they are not predictable, and no surgeon can predictably guarantee other subtle changes."

7. You may be able to feel the edges or shell of your implant after surgery, depending on the thickness of your tissues and how carefully you try to feel the implant.

"If you are planning to have breast augmentation, you should understand that you may be able to feel portions of your implant when you put your hands on your breasts. Many factors, including the thickness of your tissues, the type of implant you choose, and how carefully you feel may affect whether you can feel your implants. No surgeon can guarantee that you won't feel your implants, and there is no significant difference in how much you might feel your implants. If you feel them, you feel them, and that's a certain possibility if you choose to have breast augmentation."

A breast augmentation predictably does only one thing: it predictably makes your breasts larger

No surgeon can guarantee that you won't feel your implants, and there is no significant difference in how much you might feel your implants

For patients who have thin or "stretchy" skin, the following additional considerations may apply:

8. *For patients with thin and stretchy tissues*: Your tissues are thin and stretchy. As a result, you may be at higher risk for visible rippling in areas of the breast, or at a higher risk of the lower breast stretching excessively following surgery, regardless of the implant you choose.

   "Neither you nor your surgeon can change the characteristics of your tissues. Even if we make the best possible decisions and you choose to have breast augmentation, the effects of the implant on surrounding tissues may place you at a higher risk of deformities relating to excessive stretch or thinning of your tissues, some of which may not be correctable surgically."

9. *For patients with wide breasts (>13 cm), stretchy skin (anterior pull skin stretch >3 cm), and a long nipple to inframammary fold distance (>9.0 cm)*: Due to the width of your breasts and the stretch of your tissues, a significant amount of volume is required to just fill your breast to a level that will not leave you with an empty upper breast. Your tissues have already shown that they stretch, so they may not support the amount of volume required to get a good result, and you may have excessive stretching or thinning in the future, with the same risks as listed in the previous item above.

   "Again, neither you nor your surgeon can change the characteristics of your tissues. If your tissues have already shown that they stretch excessively, and a large volume is required to adequately fill your breast for an optimal aesthetic result and full upper breast, you may experience excessive stretching after augmentation."

10. Breast implants cannot predictably control the specific SHAPE of your breast or areas of your breast, so IF YOU CHOOSE TO HAVE BREAST AUGMENTATION, ALL YOU SHOULD PREDICTABLY EXPECT IS AN INCREASE IN THE SIZE OF YOUR BREASTS.

At the conclusion of this discussion with the surgeon and patient viewing an anteroposterior image of the patient's breasts, the surgeon asks the patient to initial the sheet to confirm that she understands and accepts each item on the sheet. This record is invaluable postoperatively when patients frequently question residual asymmetries, and enables surgeon personnel to re-read the document with the patient to resolve any issues without requiring surgeon time commitment.

Breast implants cannot predictably control the specific shape of your breast or areas of your breast, so if you choose to have breast augmentation, all you should predictably expect is an increase in the size of your breasts

▥ DEFINING WHAT SURGEONS CANNOT CONTROL AND POTENTIAL EVENTUALITIES

Clearly defining factors that surgeons cannot control and documenting patient accountability for understanding and accepting these realities are critical to minimize postoperative misunderstandings and potential medicolegal actions. If a misunderstanding occurs postoperatively, the patient educator can schedule a meeting with the patient in the office and ask the patient to review the documents and discussions that occurred preoperatively regarding these topics. During this discussion, the patient educator can tactfully present and review each of the documents signed by the patient preoperatively, asking the patient to read and review what she signed preoperatively, and asking if the patient has additional questions. This discussion can often avoid the necessity of a confrontational situation between the surgeon and the patient, and is invaluable to document the patient's awareness of these facts and her willingness to assume responsibility for them by her signatures on preoperative documents.

Table 3-3 is an excerpt from the "My Preferences and Information I Fully Understand and Accept" document. One of the final portions of the document, these paragraphs clearly specify factors that surgeons can and cannot control, potential eventualities, who will make decisions, and who will be responsible for costs associated with possible future surgical procedures.

> Clearly defining factors that surgeons cannot control and documenting patient accountability for understanding and accepting these realities are critical to minimize postoperative misunderstandings and potential medicolegal actions

▥ DEFINING THE ROLE AND INVOLVEMENT OF OTHER INDIVIDUALS

One of the most difficult areas of patient management is defining and managing the roles of other individuals in making decisions preoperatively or in judging and responding to outcomes or problems postoperatively. Every experienced surgeon has encountered situations in which a patient makes preoperative requests that may not be her own wishes, but instead represent the wishes of other individuals. If the surgeon and staff are not aware of the involvement of another individual in preoperative requests and decisions, significant misunderstandings can occur postoperatively when the patient's results do not match the expectations or desires of a husband, boyfriend, or significant other.

> One of the most difficult areas of patient management is defining and managing the roles of other individuals in making decisions preoperatively or in judging and responding to outcomes or problems postoperatively

To minimize and manage these potential problems, surgeons must constantly assure that the patient and any other person involved in decisions have an opportunity to participate

Table 3-3. Factors surgeons cannot control and potential eventualities

Factors Following My Augmentation that Dr. Tebbetts Cannot Control

I (please print and sign)_____ have read Dr. Tebbetts' informational materials and his entire book entitled *The Best Breast* and have had an opportunity to visit with Dr. Tebbetts' patient educator_____. The following is essential information that I must understand and accept before having Dr. Tebbetts perform my breast augmentation. I have discussed each of these items with my patient educator and fully understand and accept the tradeoffs, risks, costs, and outcomes associated with each item.

_____ From my reading of Dr. Tebbetts' book *The Best Breast*, and after my patient educator consultation, I understand and accept that there are several factors related to my individual tissue characteristics, how I heal, and how my tissues respond to my breast implants that Dr. Tebbetts cannot predict by tests before surgery, and cannot control after surgery.

INFECTION

_____ I fully understand and accept that if I develop an infection following my augmentation, Dr. Tebbetts will remove both of my breast implants, and will never replace either implant to minimize further reoperations, risks, and costs to me. I further understand and accept that, if implant removal is ever required for any reason, that deformities may result that may not be totally correctable.

_____ I understand and accept that Dr. Tebbetts must work with what I bring him to work with, and that he cannot change the qualities of the tissues of my breasts that affect stretch following surgery or how I will heal. I also understand and accept that Dr. Tebbetts cannot perform tests before surgery, or in any other way predict (1) how my skin will stretch following my augmentation, and (2) how my body will heal or not heal following my augmentation.

TISSUE STRETCH

My tissue characteristics and stretch of tissues following my augmentation: How they can affect my results, need for additional surgery, and costs

_____ If my tissues stretch excessively in any area following my augmentation, deformities can result over which Dr. Tebbetts has no control. These deformities include the following:

1. Excessive sagging or "bottoming out" of the breast with the implant too low and the nipple pointing excessively upwards
2. Shift of the implants to the sides with widening of the gap between the breasts
3. Thinning of tissues over the implant allowing the implant to become visible or palpable (able to be felt) in any area, and
4. Visible rippling in any area that can result when the implant pulls on the overlying tissues.

_____ I understand and accept that any or all of these deformities can occur in one or both breasts, and do not occur equally on the two sides. I also understand and accept that the larger breast implant I choose or my breasts require for optimal aesthetic results, the greater the risk of these deformities occurring. Although breasts never match exactly on the two sides, if any of these deformities occur, differences in the two breasts may be more noticeable and may not be correctable.

_____ I understand and accept that if any or all of the deformities caused by tissue stretch listed above should occur, even though the deformity may be visible, that Dr. Tebbetts alone will determine whether additional surgery is needed. Dr. Tebbetts will base this decision on whether he feels the potential benefits outweigh the potential risks of additional surgery and whether he feels I will get predictable improvement from additional surgery. I agree to abide by Dr. Tebbetts' decisions in all matters pertaining to whether or not additional surgery is performed.

Table 3-3. **Factors surgeons cannot control and potential eventualities—cont'd**

_____ I understand and accept that if my tissues stretch excessively for any reason following my augmentation, that additional surgery will not change the qualities of my tissues that allowed them to stretch in the first place. As a result, additional surgery to correct stretch deformities is unpredictable at best due to the limitations my tissues impose, and that surgery for any of the stretch deformities listed above may not successfully correct the deformity, and that any or all of these deformities can occur again if my tissues stretch again.

HEALING CHARACTERISTICS

My healing characteristics following my augmentation: How they can affect my results, need for additional surgery, and costs

_____ I understand and accept that Dr. Tebbetts has absolutely no control over how my body heals following my breast augmentation, and that he cannot predict (by tests prior to surgery) or control my individual healing characteristics.

_____ I understand and accept that my body will form a lining (capsule) around my breast implant following my augmentation, and that the capsule around the implant may contract (tighten) excessively, causing a variety of deformities that may require additional surgery and despite additional surgery, may be uncorrectable and require implant removal. The capsules that form and the amount that they tighten are never equal on both sides, so the effects of the capsule on each breast are usually different.

_____ I understand and accept that there are no tests or medical information that can accurately predict whether my capsules will tighten excessively, and that following my augmentation, Dr. Tebbetts has no control over how my body forms the capsule or how much the capsule will tighten or cause deformity.

_____ I understand and accept that any or all of the following deformities can result from how the capsule forms and tightens, and that Dr. Tebbetts cannot predict, prevent, or control the occurrence of any of these deformities:

5. Closing of a portion of the lower implant pocket (can be mild or severe), causing slight or significant upward displacement of the implant, and raising the fold under the breast leaving the incision scar below the fold (if the incision was made under the breast).
6. Closing of a portion of the outside of the implant pocket, causing flattening of areas of the outside contour of the breast and inward displacement of the implant.
7. Excessive firmness of the implant or breast.
8. Visible edges or bulging deformities in any area of the breast.
9. The quality of the scar that I will form wherever my incision is located.
10. The effects of my body healing and scarring in the area of the incision, adjacent areas to the incision or breast, or any area of the breast.
11. Discomfort or pain in areas of the breast.
12. Change in sensation or loss of sensation in any area of the breast or adjacent areas.
13. Occurrence of lymph node enlargement or small bands near the incision caused by incision or obstruction of small lymph vessels (both of which usually subside without treatment in 3–6 weeks).

_____ I understand and accept that any or all of these deformities can occur in one or both breasts, and do not occur equally on the two sides. Although breasts never match exactly on the two sides, if any of these deformities occur, differences in the two breasts may be more noticeable and may not be correctable.

Table 3-3. **Factors surgeons cannot control and potential eventualities—cont'd**

_____ I understand and accept that if any or all of the deformities caused by my healing characteristics or the characteristics of the capsule (lining) around my implants occur, even though the deformity may be visible, that Dr. Tebbetts alone will determine whether additional surgery is needed. Dr. Tebbetts will base this decision on whether he feels the potential benefits outweigh the potential risks of additional surgery and whether he feels I will get predictable improvement from additional surgery. I agree to abide by Dr. Tebbetts' decisions in all matters pertaining to whether or not additional surgery is performed.

_____ I understand and accept that if any of the deformities listed above occur following my augmentation, that additional surgery will not change the qualities of my tissues and healing characteristics that caused the deformity in the first place. As a result, additional surgery to correct these deformities (a) is unpredictable at best due to the limitations of my tissues and healing characteristics, (b) that surgery for any of the deformities listed above may not successfully correct the deformity, and (c) that any or all of these deformities can occur again after additional surgery because of my healing characteristics.

RESPONSIBILITY FOR COSTS ASSOCIATED WITH ADDITIONAL SURGERIES

_____ Since Dr. Tebbetts cannot predict or control my tissue characteristics or healing characteristics and how they will affect my chances of developing any of the deformities listed above related to tissue stretch and thinning or capsule or scar tissue formation following my augmentation, I understand and accept that should any of the deformities listed above (1–13) occur, if surgery is necessary to try to improve any of the following conditions, that _I will be personally responsible for all costs associated with any surgery that is performed (please initial beside each number indicating your complete understanding and acceptance of all costs associated with surgery for each deformity)_:

1. Excessive sagging or "bottoming out" of the breast with the implant too low and the nipple pointing excessively upwards
2. Shift of the implants to the sides with widening of the gap between the breasts
3. Thinning of tissues over the implant allowing the implant to become visible or palpable (able to be felt) in any area, and
4. Visible rippling in any area that can result when the implant pulls on the overlying tissues.
5. Closing of a portion of the lower implant pocket (can be mild or severe), causing slight or significant upward displacement of the implant, and raising the fold under the breast leaving the incision scar below the fold (if the incision was made under the breast).
6. Closing of a portion of the outside of the implant pocket, causing flattening of areas of the outside contour of the breast and inward displacement of the implant.
7. Excessive firmness of the implant or breast.
8. Visible edges or bulging deformities in any area of the breast.
9. Discomfort or pain in areas of the breast.
10. The effects of my body healing and scarring in the area of the incision, adjacent areas to the incision or breast, or any area of the breast.
11. Discomfort or pain in areas of the breast.
12. Change in sensation or loss of sensation in any area of the breast or adjacent areas.
13. Occurrence of lymph node enlargement or small bands near the incision caused by incision or obstruction of small lymph vessels (both of which usually subside without treatment in 3–6 weeks).

Table 3-3. Factors surgeons cannot control and potential eventualities—cont'd

_____ I understand and accept that Dr. Tebbetts does not accept insurance or any third party reimbursement for any type of additional surgery that may be necessary following my augmentation, and that I will be personally responsible for prepaying all costs of any additional surgery at least 2 weeks prior to the scheduled surgery. If I choose to pay by credit card, I understand and accept that I agree to sign additional documents authorizing full payment by my credit card company. Dr. Tebbetts will provide me with copies of my operative note from my surgery, but I assume all responsibility for any filing of insurance and understand that Dr. Tebbetts and his staff will not pursue payments from any third party.

_____ I understand and accept that costs of any additional surgery following my augmentation will likely exceed the costs of my original augmentation surgery, and that costs are determined by the complexity and length (time) of the surgery required. Fees for additional surgery will include laboratory fees, electrocardiogram fees if I am over 40 or have any heart condition, possible mammogram or magnetic resonance imaging fees, Dr. Tebbetts' surgeon fees, anesthesia fees, surgical facility fees, and costs of take home medications. I accept personal responsibility for all of these fees and, in addition, I understand and accept that I may have additional costs associated with time off work or normal activities.

_____ I understand and accept that Dr. Tebbetts alone sets his fees for all surgeries he performs, that these fees are not negotiable for any reason by any party, and must be prepaid at least 2 weeks prior to surgery.

_____ If following my breast augmentation, any additional surgery for the reasons listed above becomes necessary, and I later choose to dispute any of the items above for which I have indicated my full understanding and acceptance, I agree to pay any and all of Dr. Tebbetts' costs, including any attorney's fees, court costs, or any other costs associated with resolving the dispute.

_____ I have read all of Dr. [Surgeon's Name]' informational materials and have had an opportunity to visit with Dr. [Surgeon's Name]' patient educator_____. I have had an opportunity to ask questions and have had all of my questions answered to my satisfaction. I will have an additional opportunity to ask Dr. [Surgeon's Name] questions during our consultation.

I feel fully informed, and have had an opportunity to have all of my questions answered to my satisfaction.

Signed this _____day of the month of _____, 200_____ in the presence of the witness listed below.

_____   _____
Patient: (Please print)   Witness: (Please print)

_____   _____
Patient: (Please sign)   Witness: (Please sign)

in all preoperative education, and signs informed consent documents that specify each person's role in patient decision making and evaluation of postoperative results.

Two documents are critical to this process: (1) Will Anyone Else Be Involved in Your Choices or Decision Making—Part 1, and (2) Will Anyone Else Be Involved in Your Choices or Decision Making—Part 2. Table 3-4 contains the Part 1 document and Table 3-5 contains the Part 2 document. By incorporating these documents into their

Table 3-4. **Documenting the role of parties making decisions, Part 1**

Will Anyone Else Be Involved in Your Choices or Decision Making?
Part 1

If any other person will be involved in the choices or decisions you will make regarding your augmentation, or will be involved in any discussions with Dr. [Surgeon's Name] or his staff following surgery regarding your choices or your result, they will need to be as informed as you are to prevent their misinterpreting your choices, your decisions, or your result. They will need to understand all of the choices, tissue limitations, tradeoffs, and risks that we discuss with you. We will provide you with the necessary information and copies of your documents to review and discuss with them, but you are responsible for encouraging them to become familiar with your information and choices.

Will **_anyone else_** be involved in the choices or decisions you will make regarding your augmentation, or in any discussions with Dr. [Surgeon's Name] or his staff following surgery regarding your choices or your results?

Yes /No _____ (Please circle one and initial)

If yes, please specify: Name: _____Relationship: _____.

Please read and if you understand and accept the statements, initial each of the following items:

_____ Prior to my patient educator consultation, I was asked if anyone else would be involved in the choices or decision making process for my breast augmentation, and I was encouraged to bring them with me during each consultation visit or have them participate in patient educator telephone calls.

_____ If I do not specify in this document another person who will be involved in my choices or decision making, I specifically request Dr. [Surgeon's Name] and his staff to have no discussions following surgery about any aspect of my care or results with anyone other than me. I understand and accept that Dr. [Surgeon's Name] and his staff will not discuss any aspect of my choices, decisions, requests, or result following surgery with anyone who was not educated, informed, or who did not answer all of the items in the second section of this document.

_____ If I do not specify another person who will be involved, following surgery I accept total and complete responsibility for dealing with other people's opinions regarding my choices or my result. I will not involve anyone else in discussions with Dr. [Surgeon's Name] or his staff following surgery regarding any aspect of my result if I did not specify and involve that person to assure that they are educated and informed prior to my surgery.

_____ If I choose to involve anyone else in my choices, decision making, or in any evaluation or comment on my results, I will be personally responsible for providing that person with a copy of the book *The Best Breast*, a copy of Dr. [Surgeon's Name]' choices documents, informed consent documents, operative consent forms, and my breast implant manufacturer's information and operative consent forms. Further, I will encourage that person to read the documents in detail so that we reach a common understanding and acceptance of choices, risks, and tradeoffs prior to my surgery. Lastly, I will invite and encourage that person to participate in all of my consultations with my patient educator (in person or by phone) and in person for my consultation with Dr. [Surgeon's Name].

_____ I understand and accept that I alone am ultimately responsible for the decisions I make and the requests that I make of Dr. [Surgeon's Name]. If I involve anyone else in my decisions, it is my responsibility alone to reconcile their wishes and thoughts with what I choose for my own body. **Dr. [Surgeon's Name] will rely solely on my written requests that I will complete during my education and consultation process, and any other person's input must be included in my written requests prior to surgery.** Prior to surgery, I alone am responsible for making my choices and decisions. Following surgery, I alone will accept responsibility for my choices and decisions, and I alone will discuss any concerns I have with Dr. [Surgeon's Name] and his staff.

Table 3-4. **Documenting the role of parties making decisions, Part 1—cont'd**

Please ask the person you choose to involve in your choices or decision making prior to your breast augmentation procedure to please complete and sign the document entitled **Will Anyone Else Be Involved—Part 2**. You are then responsible for returning the form to our office at least 2 weeks prior to your surgery date. If you have specified a person to be involved, and this form is not returned to us at least 2 weeks prior to surgery, we will be unable to perform your surgery.

_____ I have been given a copy of **Will Anyone Else Be Involved—Part 2** and am aware that it must be returned to Dr. [Surgeon's Name]' office 2 weeks prior to my surgery date.

Signed this _____day of the month of _____, 200_____ in the presence of the witness listed below.

_____   _____
Patient: (Please print)   Witness: (Please print)

_____   _____
Patient: (Please sign)   Witness: (Please sign)

Table 3-5. **Documenting the role of parties making decisions, Part 2**

Will Anyone Else Be Involved in Your Choices or Decision Making?
Part 2

Please ask the person you choose to involve in your choices or decision making prior to your breast augmentation procedure to please complete and sign the following form. You are then responsible for returning the form to our office at least 2 weeks prior to your surgery date. If you have specified a person to be involved, and this form is not returned to us at least 2 weeks prior to surgery, we will be unable to perform your surgery.

Patient's name: _____

The person I choose to involve in my choices and decision making for breast augmentation is _____, my _____(relationship).

Patient's signature: _____Date: _____

Witness: _____Date: _____

Please ask the person listed above to initial each item and sign the following:

I _____, will be involved in the choices and decision making process prior to breast augmentation for _____, my _____ (relationship).

We appreciate your involvement and support in our patient's choices and decision making process for breast augmentation. In order for you to become familiar with essential information regarding the many choices and decisions that we must make, you will need to carefully read and consider all of the information that we have provided our patient and which she will provide you. We strongly encourage you to attend consultation visits so that we all understand and agree on the patient's choices and desires, and the inherent tradeoffs, limitations, and risks that are involved. Each patient has different tissues and tissue limitations and tradeoffs, and we individualize our decisions to try to achieve the best possible long-term results with the fewest risks and tradeoffs. Only by being involved can you thoroughly understand choices and decisions, and the reasons behind those decisions.

Table 3-5. Documenting the role of parties making decisions, Part 2—cont'd

Please circle the appropriate choice and initial each line.

_____ I have/have not completely read all information materials sent to the patient.

_____ I have/have not completely read Dr. [Surgeon's Name]' Patient Choices Document.

_____ I have/have not completely read Dr. [Surgeon's Name]' How Did We Do Informing You Document.

_____ I have/have not completely read Dr. [Surgeon's Name]' Operative Consent Forms.

_____ I have/have not completely read the breast implant manufacturer's information and consent forms.

_____ I have been given an opportunity to attend all consultation visits with Dr. [Surgeon's Name] and Dr. [Surgeon's Name]' patient educator, or to participate in patient education telephone calls. I chose to accept/decline these opportunities.

_____ I understand and accept that any input I have into choices or decisions must be reconciled with the patient having surgery, and that Dr. [Surgeon's Name] will only consider the specific written requests of the patient alone when making all surgical and implant choice decisions.

_____ I have absolutely no specific preferences or desires regarding any aspect of the patient's surgery or implant choices, including implant size or type or desired breast size or appearance that are not clearly expressed on the Patient Choices Document and the How Did We Do Informing You Document listed above. I understand that Dr. [Surgeon's Name] cannot read my mind or the patient's mind, and that in order for our desires to be met, we must be totally honest and forthright in our written requests of Dr. [Surgeon's Name] prior to surgery.

_____ I have been provided opportunities by Dr. [Surgeon's Name] and his staff to read all informational materials, patient choice forms, and informed consent documents, and I understand and accept all risks, limitations, and patient choices as listed on these forms. I am satisfied that I have been provided all information necessary for me to understand and I am satisfied that Dr. [Surgeon's Name] and his staff have satisfactorily answered all of my questions regarding breast augmentation. I am/am not totally comfortable with the choices made by the patient, _____, who is my _____ (relationship). I clearly understand that Dr. [Surgeon's Name] does not wish to proceed with any surgery if I have any unsatisfied concerns or questions until those concerns are addressed and I become totally comfortable.

_____ If I am not totally comfortable with any of the above items, I have made my concerns known to Dr. [Surgeon's Name] personally (or through notification of _____, a member of his staff, on _____ date).

_____ Following surgery, I understand and accept that any criticism or disagreement that I may have regarding the results of surgery will be discussed by Dr. [Surgeon's Name] or his staff only in terms of the **written choices made by the patient prior to surgery**. My input must be through the patient and must be expressed clearly on the documents listed above. I am totally comfortable that all of my concerns and input are expressed in the written choices made by the patient, and I will not express any concerns following surgery regarding breast size or appearance that are not clearly specified in the documents prior to surgery.

Signed this _____ day of the month of _____, 200_____ in the presence of the witness listed below.

_____   _____
Patient: (Please print)   Witness: (Please print)

_____   _____
Patient: (Please sign)   Witness: (Please sign)

preoperative patient education and informed consent process, surgeons can minimize chances of postoperative misunderstandings and optimally manage them should they occur.

ADDITIONAL DOCUMENTS IN THE EDUCATION AND INFORMED CONSENT SYSTEM

Several additional documents that address other specific issues and clinical situations are included in the Resources folder on the DVDs that accompany this book for surgeons to review and revise to accommodate individual practice needs and preferences. The author strongly encourages surgeons to read and review each document in detail, because each of these documents has evolved over a 30 year practice career in response to actual clinical situations that have occurred in the author's practice.

MINIMIZING POTENTIAL MEDICOLEGAL CHALLENGES

Thorough patient education and detailed, written documentation, signed paragraph by paragraph by the patient on multiple occasions, are the most predictable methods to minimize medicolegal challenges. When problems, misunderstandings, and challenges occur, the behavior and response of the surgeon and the surgeon's staff when the problem first occurs are critical. If the system detailed in this chapter has been used, the surgeon and staff can, with assurance, approach the situation positively with the patient. If the surgeon or staff attempt to explain or explain away postoperative occurrences that have not been defined and documented preoperatively, the patient often interprets the explanations as excuses. Patients who have been thoroughly educated preoperatively and who have documented their acceptance of responsibility for their decisions react more positively and predictably when untoward events or outcomes occur postoperatively. Legal review of patient records can be a positive or negative process from the surgeon's perspective, depending on the content, processes, and documentation that the patient encountered preoperatively.

Building a valid, comprehensive infrastructure of patient education and informed consent is invaluable to every surgeon's practice: no surgeon's technical skills can compensate for deficiencies in patient education and informed consent. That realization in the author's practice prompted the evolution of the system of patient education and informed consent presented in this chapter. As surgeons allocate their most precious resource . . . time . . . to specific objectives in their clinical practices, they should prioritize the importance of

---

Thorough patient education and detailed, written documentation, signed paragraph by paragraph by the patient on multiple occasions, are the most predictable methods to minimize medicolegal challenges

Building a valid, comprehensive infrastructure of patient education and informed consent is invaluable to every surgeon's practice: no surgeon's technical skills can compensate for deficiencies in patient education and informed consent

the patient education and informed consent infrastructure, and recognize that the system requires constant revision and updating for the entire duration of their clinical practices.

■ REFERENCES

1. Tebbetts JB: An approach that integrates patient education and informed consent in breast augmentation. *Plast Reconstr Surg* 110(3):971–978, 2002.

2. Food and Drug Administration. U.S. Food and Drug Administration. Product labeling data for Mentor and Allergan/Inamed core studies of saline implants. Online. Available: http://www.fda.gov/cdrh/breastimplants/labeling/mentor_patient_labeling_5900.html.

3. Food and Drug Administration. U.S. Food and Drug Administration. Product labeling data for Mentor and Allergan/Inamed core studies of conventional silicone gel implants. Online. Available: http://www.fda.gov/cdrh/breastimplants/labeling.html.

4. Health Canada. Transcript of expert advisory panel meeting on silicone filled breast implants. Online. Available: http://www.hc-sc.gc.ca/dhp-mps/md-im/activit/sci-consult/implant-breast-mammaire/eapbi_rop_gceim_crd_2005–09–29_e.html.

Anatomy for Augmentation: Cadaver and Surgical

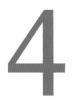

A detailed knowledge of the surgical anatomy pertaining to primary breast augmentation is essential for surgeons to deliver optimal, state-of-the-art results and long-term outcomes. Offering patients a range of incision and implant pocket alternatives to best suit individual tissue requirements and aesthetic preferences requires that surgeons thoroughly understand surgical relational anatomy of the breast, chest wall musculature, and axillary region.

A detailed knowledge of the surgical anatomy pertaining to primary breast augmentation is essential for surgeons to deliver optimal, state-of-the-art results and long-term outcomes

Essentials of surgical anatomy are included in Chapters 11, 12, and 13 that address inframammary, axillary, and periareolar incision approaches in detail. This chapter details principles of anatomy that apply to all incision approaches. Unembalmed (fresh) cadaver dissections are invaluable for surgeons to investigate details of surgical anatomy by performing surgical procedures and then dissecting the respective surgical fields with wide exposure to define specific tissue trauma that may occur with each approach. This approach to an in-depth understanding of what actually occurs as the result of specific surgical maneuvers is essential to help surgeons base their impressions on factual information instead of subjective opinions.

■ ANATOMIC TISSUE LAYERS OF THE BREAST AND CHEST

Figure 4-1 is the right breast in a fresh cadaver dissection. For wide exposure of the underlying tissue planes, an incision along the midline of the sternum connects with an incision that parallels the inframammary fold approximately 3 cm below the inframammary fold.

Figure 4-1. Right breast in fresh cadaver specimen. Incision along sternal midline connects to incision 3 cm below inframammary fold (IMF) and parallels the fold.

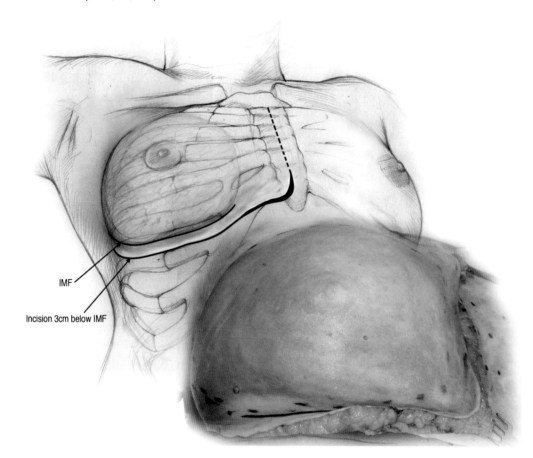

IMF

Incision 3cm below IMF

Dissection in the plane just deep to the deep subcutaneous fascia over the breast exposes the breast parenchymal mass (Figure 4-2) which consists of fatty infiltration of breast tissues with a whiter, fibroglandular tissue connection in the subareolar area. This tissue plane is largely irrelevant in primary breast augmentation unless the surgeon is combining a significant mastopexy procedure with the breast augmentation. When elevating skin flaps off underlying breast tissue, the plane of dissection is critical. Many surgeons,

Figure 4-2. Breast parenchymal mass with fatty infiltration of breast tissues (white arrow) and fibroglandular tissue in subareolar area (black arrow).

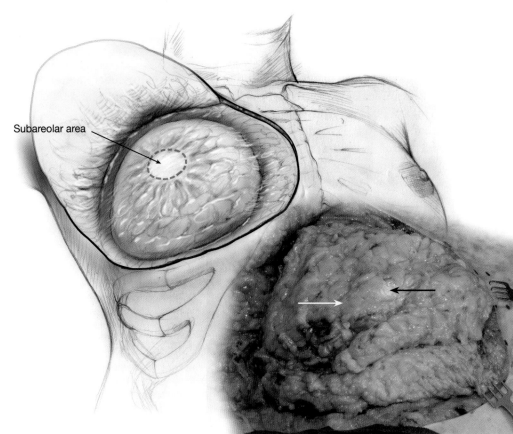

Subareolar area

concerned about preserving vascularity to the skin flaps, dissect too deeply, leaving breast parenchyma attached to the skin flaps, when the ideal plane of dissection is immediately deep to the deep subcutaneous fascia. In the correct plane, skin flap elevation preserves optimal suprafascial (to the deep subcutaneous fascia) arterial supply and venous drainage, while minimizing a parenchymal burden deep to the flap that "steals" blood supply from the flaps. Conversely, dissecting excessively superficially when elevating skin flaps compromises critical arterial supply and even more critical

In the correct plane, skin flap elevation preserves optimal suprafascial (to the deep subcutaneous fascia) arterial supply and venous drainage, while minimizing a parenchymal burden deep to the flap that "steals" blood supply from the flaps venous drainage from skin flaps. The optimal plane of dissection for skin flap elevation, immediately deep to the deep subcutaneous fascia, is well known to surgeons who have performed a large number of mastectomies and to plastic surgeons who must work with the results of these dissections when performing breast reconstruction.

Reflecting the entire skin, subcutaneous tissue, and breast parenchyma superolaterally exposes the anterior surface of the pectoralis major muscle and the serratus muscle inferolaterally (Figure 4-3). During this dissection, a major objective was to leave pectoralis fascia attached to the anterior surface of the pectoralis major muscle in order to examine the thickness of this fascia in various areas beneath the breast. As a result, remnants of breast parenchyma and fat remain on the anterior surface of the pectoralis major muscle.

If the surgeon leaves all pectoralis major origins intact along the inframammary fold, the muscle covers at most two-thirds of the breast implant intraoperatively, leaving the inferolateral one-third of the implant beneath skin and subcutaneous tissue

Medially, the pectoralis major muscle origins arise from the sternum and costal cartilages. While pectoral and clavicular heads of the muscle are defined in anatomy books, these segments are indistinguishable surgically. The relationship of the pectoralis muscle to a breast implant that a surgeon places deep to the muscle is particularly important. While the pectoralis major muscle in this typical cadaver dissection would appear to cover more than three-fourths of a subpectorally placed implant, in the clinical setting the implant tents the pectoralis major anteriorly and the muscle slides medially. If the surgeon leaves all pectoralis major origins intact along the inframammary fold, the muscle covers at most two-thirds of the breast implant intraoperatively, leaving the inferolateral one-third of the implant beneath skin and subcutaneous tissue.

Total muscle coverage, elevating serratus anterior and approximating it to the lateral border of the pectoralis, predictably blunts the inferior and lateral inframammary folds, and is unnecessary and undesirable in primary breast augmentation

The serratus anterior muscle is located inferolateral to the pectoralis major muscle (Figure 4-3). While some surgeons claim to place implants completely beneath muscle using blunt, blind dissection techniques, elevating the serratus anterior muscle and preserving robust vascularity is challenging under direct vision with wide exposure, and is impossible using blunt, blind dissection techniques. Total muscle coverage, elevating serratus anterior and approximating it to the lateral border of the pectoralis, predictably blunts the inferior and lateral inframammary folds, and is unnecessary and undesirable in primary breast augmentation. The serratus muscle, overlying a breast implant, often suffers vascular compromise and fibrous infiltration over time. The serratus muscle provides unpredictable soft tissue coverage laterally, and often atrophies and blunts delicate lateral and inferolateral breast contours.

Figure 4-3. Breast parenchyma reflected laterally exposes the pectoralis major (black arrow) and serratus anterior (white arrow) muscles.

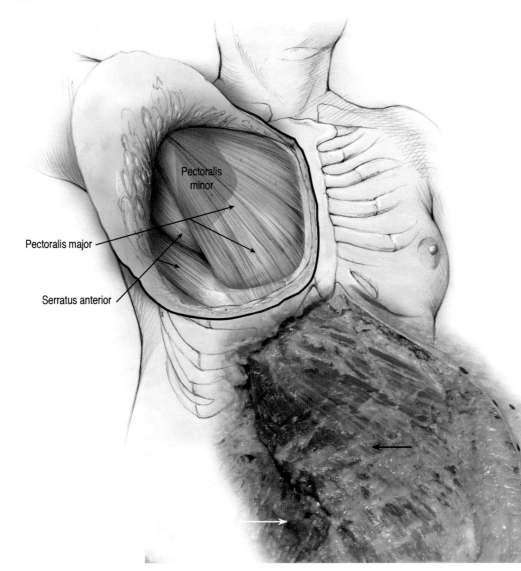

Figure 4-4. Pectoralis major muscle reflected superiorly to reveal pectoralis minor muscle beneath (long white arrow). The thoracoacromial artery (TAA) and pedicle are visible in the fat pad on the deep surface of the pectoralis major (black arrow). The pectoralis minor (long white arrow) and serratus anterior muscles (short white arrow) remain attached to the chest wall deep to the pectoralis major.

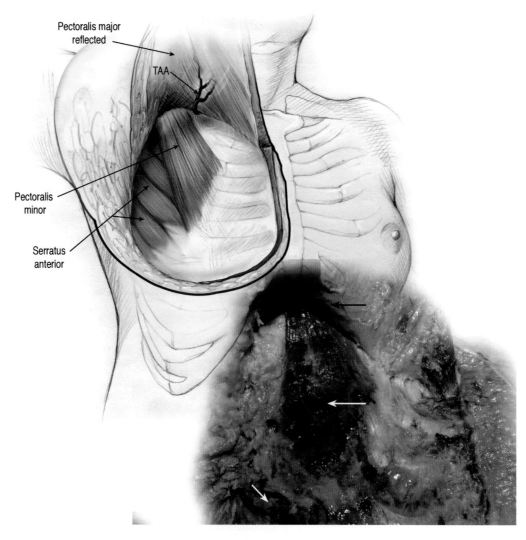

Reflecting the pectoralis major muscle superiorly (Figure 4-4) exposes the thoracoacromial pedicle on the deep surface of the pectoralis major muscle, and the pectoralis minor muscle and serratus anterior muscle attached to the chest wall deep to the pectoralis major muscle.

CRITICAL STRUCTURES IN THE SUBPECTORAL TISSUE PLANE

In another fresh cadaver specimen (Figure 4-5), viewing from medially over the sternum, the pectoralis major muscle is reflected laterally to expose structures deep to the pectoralis major. The lateral pectoral nerve courses with the thoracoacromial artery and vein through a fat pad deep to the pectoralis major and into the pectoralis major. The medial pectoral nerve in this specimen exits from deep to the pectoralis minor muscle at its superolateral border and courses anteriorly to innervate the lateral oblique portion of the pectoralis major muscle.

The location of the medial pectoral nerve can vary, with the nerve sometimes penetrating the pectoralis minor instead of exiting at the lateral border of the muscle. Clinically, the size of this nerve varies considerably. In most cases, surgeons can preserve this nerve when dissecting a subpectoral pocket, but occasionally the nerve exits through the

Figure 4-5. Subpectoral plane left breast, viewed from medially. The lateral pectoral nerve and thoracoacromial artery and vein exit the intercostal space and course anteriorly through the fat pad into the pectoralis major. The medial pectoral nerve exits from beneath the superolateral border of the pectoralis minor muscle to innervate the inferior oblique portion of the pectoralis major muscle. Anterior branches of lateral intercostal nerves (black arrows in cadaver photo) exit the intercostal spaces laterally for sensory innervation of the lateral chest and breast.

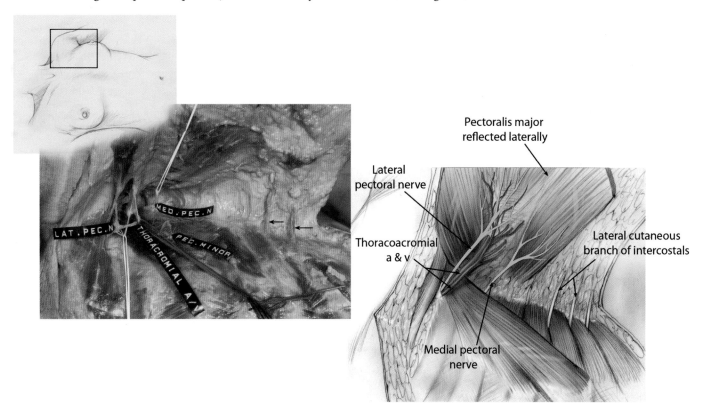

Figure 4-6. Structures deep to the pectoralis muscle, viewed from inferiorly in the left breast. The thoracoacromial artery and vein and lateral pectoral nerve exit the intercostal space and enter the pectoralis major muscle through the fat pad on its deep surface. The medial pectoral nerve exits lateral to the superior border of the pectoralis minor to innervate the inferior oblique portion of the pectoralis major muscle. A blunt dissector in an axillary tunnel demonstrates proximity of the medial pectoral nerve to axillary access.

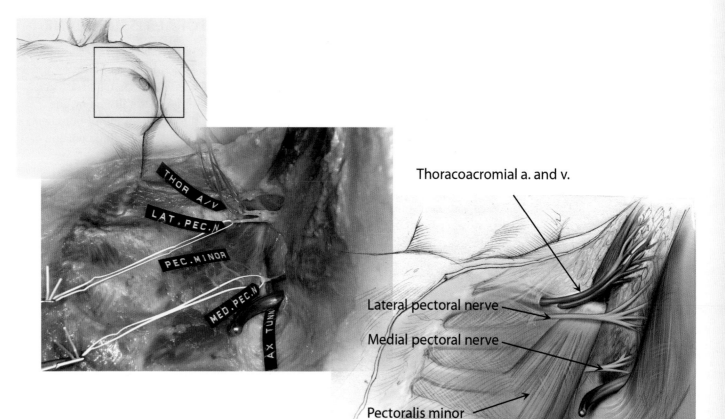

pectoralis minor more inferiorly and can restrict optimal soft tissue redraping over an implant. Division of the medial pectoral nerve, while not optimal, does not produce clinically significant weakness of the pectoralis that causes symptoms in most patients. Laterally, anterior intercostal nerve branches (black arrows) exit the intercostal spaces and course anteriorly to innervate the breast.

In the same fresh cadaver specimen, viewing the subpectoral plane from inferiorly provides a different perspective of critical structures (Figure 4-6). Superiorly, the thoracoacromial artery and vein and lateral pectoral nerve exit the intercostal space and enter the fat pad on the deep surface of the pectoralis major muscle. The medial pectoral nerve exits lateral to the superolateral border of the pectoralis minor muscle. A urethral

Division of the medial pectoral nerve, while not optimal, does not produce clinically significant weakness of the pectoralis that causes symptoms in most patients

sound blunt dissector placed into an axillary incision access tunnel illustrates the proximity of the medial pectoral nerve to the tunnel for axillary augmentation. The pectoralis minor muscle remains attached to the chest wall deep to the pectoralis major. The lateral border of the pectoralis minor muscle is an important landmark to limit initial lateral pocket dissection for partial retropectoral and dual plane pockets in order to avoid overdissection of the lateral pocket.

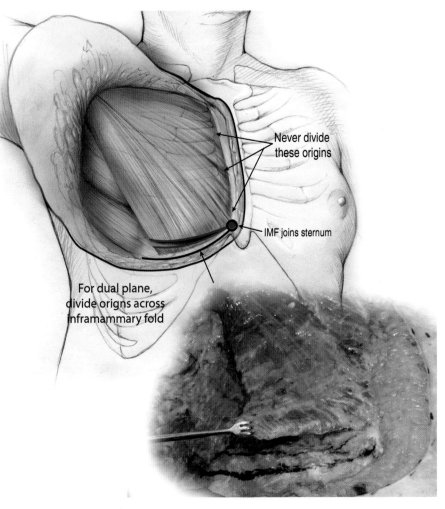

Figure 4-7. Right breast and pectoralis viewed from inferiorly. Inferior origins of pectoralis major muscle divided (blue line) 2 cm above inframammary fold (black line), beginning laterally and stopping where the inframammary fold (IMF) joins the sternum (black arrow), avoiding any muscle division whatever where medial pectoralis origins arise from the sternum medially.

Never divide these origins

IMF joins sternum

For dual plane, divide origins across inframammary fold

■ PECTORALIS MAJOR MUSCLE ANATOMY FOR DUAL PLANE AND PARTIAL RETROPECTORAL POCKETS

To create a dual plane pocket, the surgeon divides pectoralis muscle origins across the inframammary fold (Figure 4-7), from the lateral border of the pectoralis inferiorly across to the point where the inframammary fold joins the sternum, and *always stopping all division at that point.* Surgeons should never perform any division of pectoralis origins along the sternum, because even slight division of these origins can allow excessive upward migration of the pectoralis, sacrificing medial coverage, causing potential banding and window shading deformities superiorly, and risking longer-term implant edge visibility and traction rippling medially as the weight of the implant pulls on the capsule which is attached to thin overlying tissues.

Surgeons should always avoid division of medial pectoralis origins from the sternum. Division of these origins violates the number one priority in augmentation—to provide optimal thickness of soft tissue coverage over as many areas of the implant as possible

Surgeons should always avoid division of medial pectoralis origins from the sternum (Figure 4-8). Division of these origins violates the number one priority in augmentation—to provide optimal thickness of soft tissue coverage over as many areas of the implant as possible. The slightest division of these origins over only 1 or 2 cm superior to the junction of the inframammary fold with the sternum allows the inferior edge of the pectoralis major muscle to move excessively superiorly and when the muscle contracts,

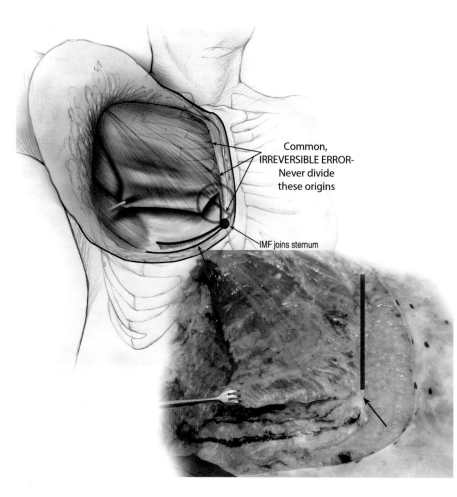

Common, IRREVERSIBLE ERROR- Never divide these origins

IMF joins sternum

Figure 4-8. Surgeons should not divide *any* origins of the pectoralis origins superior to the junction of the inframammary fold (IMF) with the sternum (no division in any area indicated by the red line in the photograph). Even slight divisions medially in this area sacrifice critical soft tissue coverage and massively increase risks of visible traction rippling long-term as the weight of the implant pulls on the capsule attached to thin overlying soft tissues.

risks severe and uncorrectable banding and window shading deformities. More importantly, division of origins along the sternum sacrifices critical soft tissue coverage in the intermammary space medially (Figure 4-9), increasing risks of implant edge visibility and visible traction rippling that are largely uncorrectable.

Figure 4-9. Dividing medial pectoralis origins along the sternum obliterates muscle cover of medial implant edges in the intermammary space, risking uncorrectable implant edge visibility and visible traction rippling (black arrows).

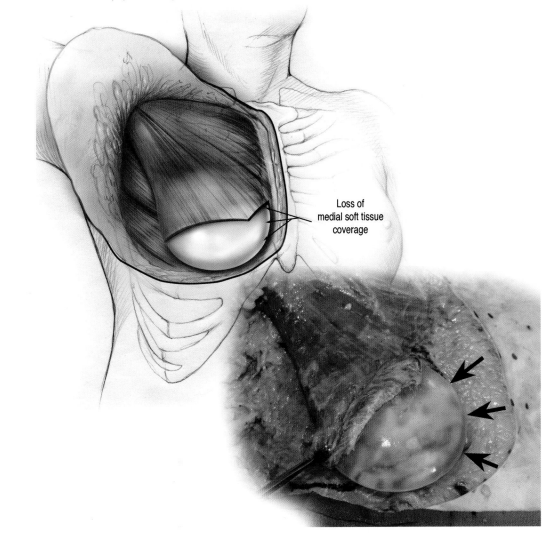

Loss of medial soft tissue coverage

To prioritize optimal soft tissue coverage medially, but also narrow the intermammary distance as much as possible, surgeons can identify and divide individual, pinnate origins of the pectoralis major that are located lateral to the main body of pectoralis origins along the sternum

To prioritize optimal soft tissue coverage medially, but also narrow the intermammary distance as much as possible, surgeons can identify and divide individual, pinnate origins of the pectoralis major that are located lateral to the main body of pectoralis origins along the sternum (Figure 4-10). These origins often have white, tendinous attachments to the ribs. Dividing these origins opens and smooths the borders of the medial pocket without sacrificing the coverage of the main body of pectoralis origins attached to the sternum. Before dividing these pinnate origins, surgeons should assure that the main body of pectoralis origins is visible and intact medial to the pinnate origins.

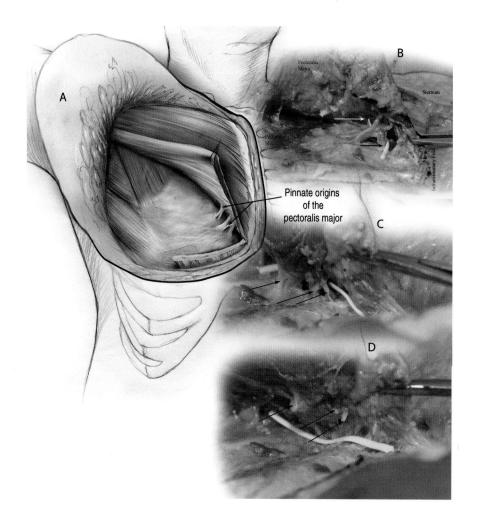

Figure 4-10. Medial subpectoral pocket viewed from laterally. The pectoralis major is reflected medially to expose pinnate origins of the pectoralis (white arrow in 4–10, *B*; pinnate origins lie lateral to yellow band in 4–10, *B*, *C*, and *D*). The surgeon can divide these pinnate origins (*D*) to open and smooth the medial pocket provided the surgeon guarantees that the main body of the pectoralis origins along the sternum remain intact.

■ MINIMIZING BLEEDING IN THE SUBMAMMARY AND SUBPECTORAL PLANES

Prospective hemostasis is a term that describes preventing bleeding instead of creating bleeding and then achieving hemostasis. Prospective hemostasis prevents blood staining of tissues that increases inflammation and pain postoperatively. Prospective hemostasis requires that surgeons anticipate the location of all significant blood vessels in the plane of pocket dissection, and control the vessels before cutting them. The location of perforating vessels in the mid pocket of submammary and subpectoral augmentations is described in detail in Chapter 11 where the vessels are more clearly visible in the clinical setting compared to a fresh cadaver dissection.

Understanding the location and course of medial perforating arteries and veins along the sternum (Figure 4-11) allows surgeons to totally avoid risks of interrupting these large vessels during dissection of submammary and subpectoral pockets. Medial perforators exit the

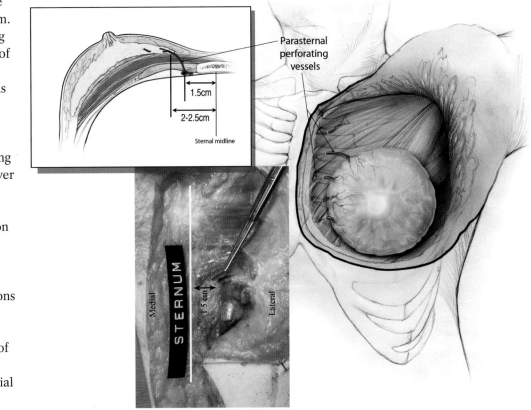

Figure 4-11. Medial anterior surface of pectoralis viewed from laterally. Large perforating arteries and veins (at tip of forceps) exit the intercostal space approximately 1.5 cm lateral to the midline of the sternum (inset cross sectional view). As the perforators course anteriorly, they enter the subpectoral space and submammary space 1–1.5 cm lateral to the midline. If the surgeon marks an intermammary distance of 3 cm, 1.5 cm lateral to the midline of the sternum on each side and limits medial pocket dissection to this point, the surgeon will rarely encounter a medial perforator. Dissection in the subpectoral plane that stops 1.5 cm lateral to the midline (tip of dissector visible in subpectoral space) prevents interruption of these perforators.

Defining an intermammary distance that is never narrower than 3 cm and avoiding any dissection medial to the medial pocket borders 1.5 cm lateral to the midline prevents inadvertent division of medial perforators

intercostal spaces approximately 1–1.5 cm lateral to the midline in the subpectoral space and then course anterolaterally to enter the submammary plane approximately 0.5 cm more lateral compared to their position in the subpectoral plane. Surgeons can totally avoid disrupting medial perforators by drawing a midline series of dots preoperatively on the skin, and defining the medial pocket borders by marking 1.5 cm lateral to the midline on the skin. Defining an intermammary distance that is never narrower than 3 cm and avoiding any dissection medial to the medial pocket borders 1.5 cm lateral to the midline prevents inadvertent division of medial perforators. A very large vein is usually present 1.5–2.5 cm lateral to the midline at the second intercostal space that surgeons can avoid by limiting superomedial pocket dissection in this area.

In the lateral pocket, anterior branches of lateral intercostal nerves (Figure 4-12) exit the intercostal spaces and course laterally for sensory innervation of the lateral chest wall and

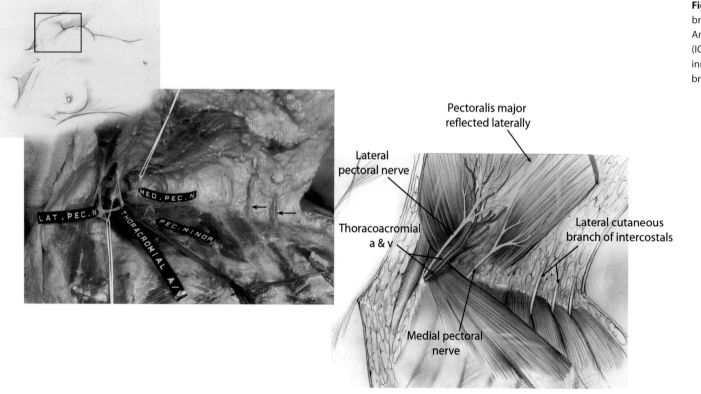

Figure 4-12. Lateral pocket left breast, viewed from inferiorly. Anterior intercostal nerve branches (ICN) exit the intercostal spaces to innervate the lateral chest wall and breast.

LAT. PEC. N

MED. PEC. N

PEC. MINOR

THORACROMIAL A/V

Pectoralis major reflected laterally

Lateral pectoral nerve

Thoracoacromial a & v

Lateral cutaneous branch of intercostals

Medial pectoral nerve

breast. These nerves can be interrupted by a blunt dissector or by sharp or electrocautery dissection. The larger or greater base width of a breast implant, the greater the risks of traction on lateral intercostal nerve branches or division of the branches when creating wider pockets for larger implants. The clinical consequences of dividing these nerves are unpredictable. While surgeons should attempt to preserve anterior intercostal nerve branches laterally, division of one or more of these nerve branches does not necessarily produce clinical symptoms that patients notice. While the role of these branches seems apparent in dissections and anatomy books, the size and role of these branches to sensory innervation is much less defined and predictable in the clinical setting.

▪ RELATIONSHIPS OF THE PECTORALIS MAJOR AND RECTUS ABDOMINIS AT THE INFRAMAMMARY FOLD

Figure 4-13 is a view of the medial inframammary fold junction with the sternum in the left breast of a fresh cadaver specimen. When surgeons blunt dissect a partial retropectoral pocket inferiorly along the inframammary fold, leaving all pectoralis major origins intact along the fold, the dissector passes deep to the pectoralis major muscle. Depending on the level of pectoralis origins and whether the surgeon intends to lower the inframammary fold, as dissection proceeds inferiorly the dissector avulses pectoralis origins off ribs in the lower pocket, and then continues inferiorly in two different planes. Medially, the dissector usually avulses pectoralis origins and may pass deep to the rectus sheath as illustrated in Figure 4-13. At the lateral border of the rectus sheath, the deep subcutaneous fascia fuses with the rectus sheath. As the dissector proceeds laterally and inferiorly across the inframammary fold, it usually avulses the deep subcutaneous fascia from its fusion with the lateral rectus sheath and then continues laterally deep to the deep subcutaneous fascia.

Dual plane pocket dissections under direct vision divide pectoralis origins above the inframammary fold and when lowering the fold, allow direct vision dissection deep to the pectoralis fascia and deep subcutaneous fascia under direct vision.

Figure 4-13. Medial inframammary fold area, left breast, viewed from laterally. The inferior pectoralis major fascia fuses with the anterior rectus sheath medially. The lateral anterior rectus sheath fuses with the deep subcutaneous fascia. A blunt dissector deep to the pectoralis major muscle, visible in the dissection photograph (black arrow), if used for blunt dissection via the axillary approach, usually avulses the pectoralis fascia from its fusion with the anterior rectus sheath medially, and avulses the deep subcutaneous fascia from its fusion with the lateral border of the anterior rectus sheath.

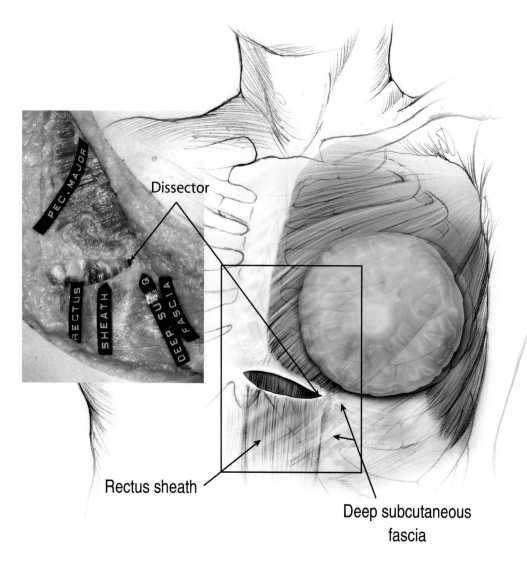

CRITICAL STRUCTURES IN THE AXILLARY REGION

Figures 4-14 and 4-15 demonstrate critical structures in the right axillary region in a fresh cadaver dissection. An Army–Navy retractor exposes the lateral border of the pectoralis major muscle overlying an axillary access tunnel for axillary subpectoral augmentation. The axillary artery and vein and brachial plexus are located in proximity to the access tunnel, superior and deep to the plane of dissection for axillary access. Branches of the intercostobrachial and medial brachial cutaneous sensory nerves to the arm course superficially in the axillary fat pad just posterior to the tunnel for axillary augmentation access. The locations of the intercostobrachial and medial brachial cutaneous nerves emphasize the importance of surgeons avoiding any dissection whatever in the axillary fat pad, constantly staying anterior to the fat pad for access to both submammary

The locations of the intercostobrachial and medial brachial cutaneous nerves emphasize the importance of surgeons avoiding any dissection whatever in the axillary fat pad, constantly staying anterior to the fat pad for access to both submammary and subpectoral pockets via the axillary approach

Figure 4-14. Right axillary region. An Army–Navy retractor exposes the lateral border of the pectoralis major muscle in the cadaver dissection, overlying an axillary access tunnel. The axillary artery (red Vesseloop) and vein (blue Vesseloop) and the brachial plexus (white Vesseloop) are in proximity to the axillary tunnel, coursing superolateral and deep in the axillary fat. Branches of the medial brachial cutaneous (MBCN) and intercostobrachial nerves (ICBN) course inferior to the axillary tunnel in the axillary fat pad.

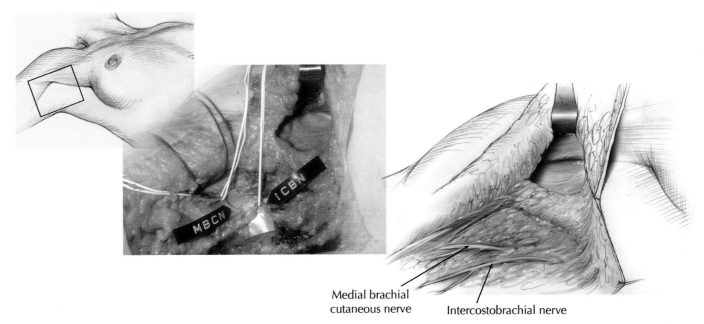

Medial brachial cutaneous nerve

Intercostobrachial nerve

Figure 4-15. Right axillary region. Branches of the intercostobrachial nerve (ICBN) and medial brachial cutaneous nerve (MBCN) course superficially in the axillary fat pad immediately posterior to the tunnel for axillary access.

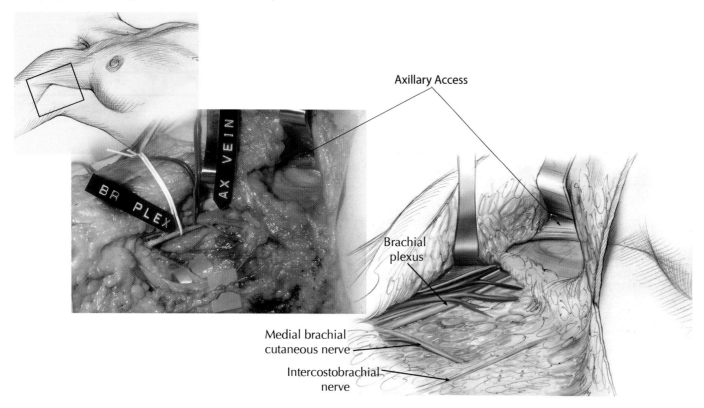

and subpectoral pockets via the axillary approach. The location of the axillary vessels and brachial plexus emphasizes the need to avoid traction on these structures by hyperabduction of the arm, and to avoid any retractor pressure on these structures during dissection.

Chapter 12 details specific methods that enable surgeons to gain excellent axillary access for submammary and subpectoral augmentation while protecting the critical structures in the axillary region.

■ IS THE PECTORALIS FASCIA A MEANINGFUL TISSUE LAYER FOR SOFT TISSUE COVERAGE?

A key question for surgeons is whether placing an implant beneath the pectoralis fascia adds meaningful soft tissue coverage compared to placing the implant in the submammary plane. Other key questions are: (a) how much of the implant can the pectoral fascia cover; and (b) what are the chances of any surgeon elevating this layer intact using any surgical technique?

Figures 4-16 and 4-17 illustrate the thickness of the pectoralis fascia over the lower and upper pectoralis major muscle respectively. Over the upper and lower pectoralis, the maximal thickness of the pectoral fascia is less than 0.2 mm, and probably less than 0.1 mm. Simple clinical observation during primary breast augmentation and reconstruction procedures confirms these thickness findings and illustrates the difficulty or impossibility of predictably elevating this tissue layer through any surgical approach. The

Adding less than 0.2 mm of additional coverage with filmy, flimsy pectoralis certainly does not address tissue coverage priorities and certainly does not provide additional, meaningful coverage or support for any breast implant

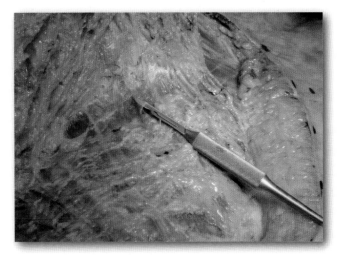

Figure 4-16. Wide view of entire right pectoralis major muscle with pectoral fascia overlying the muscle. The #15 scalpel blade has incised the pectoralis fascia and lies beneath the fascia over the middle upper portion of the muscle where the fascia is reported to be thickest.

Figure 4-17. Left: Closeup of the scalpel blade in Figure 4-16, illustrating the exceedingly thin, flimsy characteristics of the pectoralis fascia, even when substantial fragments of breast tissue have been left adherent to prevent damaging the pectoralis fascia during dissection. The caliper tips (middle and right) are set at 1 mm, demonstrating that in the mid portion of the pectoralis, the fascia is less than 0.2 mm thick.

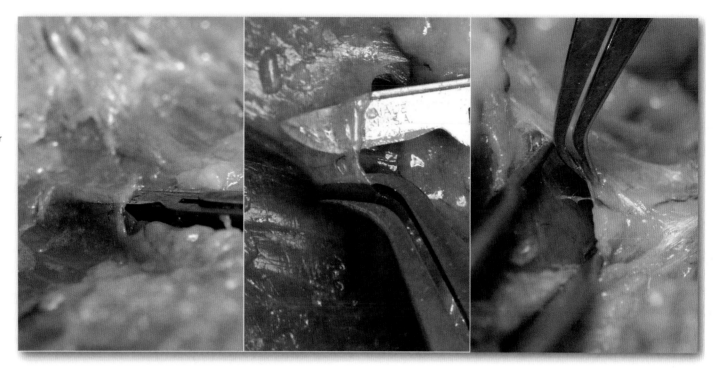

first priority in breast augmentation is to optimize long-term soft tissue coverage of the implants to reduce long-term reoperation rates and uncorrectable deformities. Adding less than 0.2 mm of additional coverage with filmy, flimsy pectoralis certainly does not address tissue coverage priorities and certainly does not provide additional, meaningful coverage or support for any breast implant.

Photographic Imaging of the Breast

■ WHAT PICTURES CAN AND CANNOT DO

Photographs, digital images, and pictures from other sources serve several functions for patients and surgeons. Patients frequently bring pictures to their surgical consultations to demonstrate to surgeons a result they desire from breast augmentation. Many surgeons actually encourage patients to bring pictures for this purpose, and most surgeons allow patients to browse before and after photographs from "brag books" to select the type of result they desire. Some surgeons use imaging software to morph patients' preoperative pictures into a representation of a possible postoperative result.

Surgeons have varying perspectives for these practices:

- "Seeing pictures selected by a patient gives me an idea of what the patient is thinking or what the patient wants."

- "From looking at a picture selected by a patient, I can tell what size the patient would like to be."

- "Provided a written disclaimer is included on morphed pictures saying that the images do not represent a guarantee of a result, morphed pictures help demonstrate possible results to a patient."

While each of these statements may be partially true, each is also partially untrue and inaccurate.

Using Pictures to Estimate Desired Breast Size

It is categorically impossible for any patient or surgeon to accurately determine the size of any breast from any picture, unless the picture contains rulers or other measurements of breast dimensions and skin stretch

It is categorically impossible for any patient or surgeon to accurately determine the size of any breast from any picture, unless the picture contains rulers or other measurements of breast dimensions and skin stretch. The two most important quantitative, non-subjective breast measurements to accurately estimate optimal breast volume are the base width of the breast and the degree of skin stretch. Neither of these critically important, objective parameters can be accurately defined from any photograph.

When surgeons and patients view pictures and relate breast size to apparent chest, torso, or body proportions, inherent inaccuracies make these relationships invalid and virtually useless in most cases. The critical parameters of the type of lens used to capture the image and the camera lens to subject distance are usually unknown to patient and surgeon, and are often inconsistent from image to image in a series of breast views. These critical parameters drastically affect visual proportions of breast size and proportional relationship of the breasts to the torso and body.

Assuming that a surgeon or patient "knows" (has an opinion that has no basis in measurement or science) what cup size a breast is in a photograph, the assumption by definition is flawed, because no surgeon or patient can accurately define any cup size by photographic or any other method

Assuming that a surgeon or patient "knows" (has an opinion that has no basis in measurement or science) what cup size a breast is in a photograph, the assumption by definition is flawed, because no surgeon or patient can accurately define any cup size by photographic or any other method. If the surgeon allows a patient to believe that the patient can accurately define breast size from a picture, the surgeon is misleading the patient. Whether viewing an image from a magazine or any other source, if a surgeon allows any patient to believe that the surgeon can even approximate a similar result in the patient, the surgeon is selling something that the surgeon may not be able to deliver. Even if the surgeon delivers what the surgeon thinks is a similar result, what if the patient sees the result differently? What if the patient thinks that the result is a bit too large or a bit too small compared to the picture? Once a patient is allowed to fix any image in her mind, nothing a surgeon or staff member can say will ever predictably dissuade her from that image. Nothing is likely to ever convince such a patient that what the surgeon is saying is correct and what she is saying is incorrect.

Photographs allow patients and surgeons to distort or avoid reality

Photographs allow patients and surgeons to distort or avoid reality. "Oh, her body looks like mine, and if I can just get breasts that look like hers, I'll be happy." From the surgeon's perspective: "She knows what she wants, and I need to deliver it . . ." (but without assuring that the patient realizes the consequences of her requests over her lifetime). Reality is that the patient's breasts can only be a larger version of her preoperative breasts. Inadequately informed and educated, the patient will deal with potentially negative consequences of her requests and choices while the surgeon consistently rationalizes, "That's what the patient wanted." Allowing the patient to believe otherwise, without optimal information, education, and informed consent process is misleading, and the surgeon is responsible for not educating or misleading the patient.

Using photographs preoperatively encourages patients to ignore their own tissue restrictions, limitations imposed by their individual breast dimensions and tissue characteristics, and focus on a result image that may be unrealistic to assure an optimally safe long-term result with minimal tradeoffs. Patients' breast dimensions and tissue characteristics never match the tissue characteristics of any other woman in a picture. Instead of focusing on the realities of the individual patient's personal breast dimensions and tissue characteristics, pictures often distract the patient and surgeon from realities and encourage patient and surgeon to prioritize photographic wishes over tissue realities. The result is often predictable. Instead of acknowledging each patient's individual tissue characteristics and breast dimensions and selecting an implant to *fit and fill* the patient's breast envelope for an optimal long-term result, wishes based on faulty photographic assumptions often encourage surgeons to "force" tissues to a desired result. When surgeons force tissues to a desired result instead of prioritizing soft tissue coverage and filling existing breast dimensions to an optimally safe result, the patient is much more likely to experience long-term tissue compromises such as parenchymal atrophy, chest wall distortions, skin thinning, visible implant edges, and visible traction rippling.

> Patients' breast dimensions and tissue characteristics never match the tissue characteristics of any other woman in a picture. Instead of focusing on the realities of the individual patient's personal breast dimensions and tissue characteristics, pictures often distract the patient and surgeon from realities and encourage patient and surgeon to prioritize photographic wishes over tissue realities

Despite any disclaimers, patients use photographs to shop for their desired result. Using images to discuss possible results is easy, but the practice is inaccurate and misleading. Patients should have an opportunity to view surgeon before and after results, but only to assure themselves that the surgeon can produce a result that is different compared to the preoperative photograph. Any other conclusion or inference the patient draws is largely inaccurate for all the reasons stated previously, and because all surgeon photographs are selected by the surgeon or staff and do not represent a random sample of the surgeon's results or experience.

> Using images to discuss possible results is easy, but the practice is inaccurate and misleading

Pictures are a poor, inaccurate, and invalid method of defining desired breast size preoperatively. A more realistic method of defining breast size alternatives for any patient is to measure the patient's breast base width and skin stretch using methods described in

> Pictures are a poor, inaccurate, and invalid method of defining desired breast size preoperatively

detail in Chapter 6, and to demonstrate to the patient the safe limits of her own tissue stretch during the surgeon consultation examination.

Using Photographs to Discuss Possible Changes in Breast Shape

Photographs are categorically inaccurate and misrepresenting as a method of discussing breast size or shape with patients. Photographs are even more inaccurate to discuss and predict postoperative breast shape. While certain implant types and sizes in certain clinical settings may effect shape changes in a breast, shape changes are usually subtle, rarely predictable, and have unpredictable longevity. Every patient should understand that the only guarantee from a breast augmentation is a larger breast and that any other changes that might occur are not predictable and should not be part of patient expectations.

In specific clinical situations such as a patient with constricted lower pole breasts, surgeons can realistically advise the patient what is required surgically to give the tissues a chance to stretch in the lower pole, aided by the pressure of a properly chosen implant. The surgeon certainly cannot predict or guarantee the extent to which any improvements might occur. Instead of showing a patient pictures of an optimally corrected constricted lower pole breast, or even a range of corrections, the surgeon can avoid the patient's predictably fixing the best image in her mind by assuring in signed documents that the patient acknowledges that the surgeon will attempt to expand the lower pole of the breast, but the degree to which expansion will occur is unpredictable, and that tradeoffs are inevitable. Similar principles apply to a wide range of other breast types and deformities.

Using Photographs as a Decision Aid in Operative Planning

For many years, the author believed that photographs were one of the most valuable tools during operative planning. Developing comprehensive, predictable measuring (TEPID[TM,1]) and decision support systems (High Five[TM,2]) helped the author realize that objective parameters and systems are always more helpful, accurate, and valid compared to subjective systems.

Photographs are largely subjective with respect to surgical planning and decisions; measurements are objective. The more any surgeon uses objective measurements and decision support systems, the more the surgeon will recognize that countless aspects of photographic images can be extremely misleading to even the most experienced surgeon.

Photographs are categorically inaccurate and misrepresenting as a method of discussing breast size or shape with patients

Photographs are largely subjective with respect to surgical planning and decisions; measurements are objective

Even the highest quality, most standardized breast photographs are currently two dimensional. No current three dimensional imaging system has been shown to produce greater reliability, reproducibility, or decision support in any valid scientific study. The breast is three dimensional. Photographic images are static, and do not reflect dynamic parameters of the breast tissues that directly impact critically important decisions in breast augmentation. The most important of these dynamic characteristics is skin stretch. Two different patients' breasts may appear virtually identical in a picture, but the degree of measurable skin stretch may differ dramatically between the patients. A correct decision based on photographs in one patient, therefore, is a suboptimal or incorrect decision in the other patient.

For optimal accuracy in surgical planning, surgeons should rely first on measurements, and use photographs as a secondary reference, avoiding conclusions from photographs that are not confirmed by objective measurements.

For optimal accuracy in surgical planning, surgeons should rely first on measurements, and use photographs as a secondary reference, avoiding conclusions from photographs that are not confirmed by objective measurements

Using Photographs as a Decision Aid in the Operating Room

Photographs can be helpful in the operating room, provided they are used in conjunction with objective preoperative measurements that are simultaneously available in the operating room. Other portions of this book will address specific decision processes in the operating room in more detail. To the extent that photographs may clarify very basic information for the surgeon in the operating room, they are useful. But surgeons must recognize that regardless of how carefully a patient is positioned on the operating table in any position, variables between what the surgeon's eye sees on the operating table and what the surgeon's eye sees in photographs are massive. As a result, surgeons must exercise extreme care in interpreting what they see during surgery and relating that impression to their impression from viewing preoperative photographs.

Surgeons must recognize that regardless of how carefully a patient is positioned on the operating table in any position, variables between what the surgeon's eye sees on the operating table and what the surgeon's eye sees in photographs are massive

■ VALID AND PRODUCTIVE USES OF PHOTOGRAPHIC IMAGES

Valid and productive uses of photographic images are described in Chapter 3: (a) using the patient's preoperative photographs to point out to the patient various differences and aspects of her breasts that *will not be predictably corrected or improved by breast augmentation*; and (b) documenting the appearance of the patient's breasts preoperatively and at intervals postoperatively to clarify issues and misunderstandings and to meet medicolegal requirements and challenges.

Valid and productive uses of photographic images are described in Chapter 3: (a) using the patient's preoperative photographs to point out to the patient various differences and aspects of her breasts that will not be predictably corrected or improved by breast augmentation; and (b) documenting the appearance of the patient's breasts preoperatively and at intervals postoperatively to clarify issues and misunderstandings and to meet medicolegal requirements and challenges

Patients rarely appreciate the many differences between their breasts when they view themselves in a mirror. Following a breast augmentation, patients "wear out" the mirror, and frequently discover differences that they incorrectly assume resulted from their augmentation procedure. If one nipple is higher than the other, or one breast is larger than the other, patients who were not thoroughly counseled using methods described in Chapter 3 blame differences on a suboptimal surgical procedure. Having preoperative photographs and the Images Analysis Sheet initialed item by item by the patient is invaluable when questions arise postoperatively. Instead of requiring valuable surgeon time to address the questions, the patient educator can view the images with the patient and simultaneously review each item that the surgeon discussed preoperatively with the patient. In most cases, this discussion ends with the patient saying: "Oh yes, now I remember those differences. I just wanted to be sure that nothing was wrong." In rare cases, further discussion with the surgeon may be necessary, but in either case, the combination of quality preoperative images and thoroughly documented discussions is invaluable.

Photographic images are a critically important part of the medical record in breast augmentation. From the most basic perspective, the quality of photographs reflects the quality of the surgeon's habits in other areas of the practice. Absent preoperative photographs and measurements, a patient could claim postoperatively that "there is no difference in my breasts", and short of declaring the presence of a breast implant in the breast, the surgeon could face challenges that photographic documentation could have prevented. While most surgeons recognize the importance of preoperative photographs, some surgeons neglect two other categories of photographs that are equally important: interval photographs postoperatively, and photographs of problems or complications.

Interval postoperative photographs are important for several reasons. Patients often develop their own perspective and conclusions for when and why various things occurred. If a patient develops a late grade 4 capsular contracture more than 6 months postoperatively, the patient might challenge the surgeon with: "It's been like this ever since surgery." If the surgeon had 3 month postoperative photographs that showed no breast distortion, the surgeon's explanation of late capsular contracture would more likely resonate with the patient. Absent interval photographs in this and many other situations, the surgeon's explanations may seem more like excuses and no more valid than the patient's preconceptions.

Interval photographs are also invaluable for documenting the effects of time, pregnancies, and nursing on patients' tissues and the resultant visual changes in the appearance of the breasts. Combined with signed informed consent documents which clearly state that the appearance of all breasts, augmented or not, usually declines over time or following pregnancy and nursing, interval photographs vividly document the predictable negative effects of aging, pregnancy, and nursing on breast appearance.

No surgeon enjoys photographing problems or complications, but documenting challenges is equally important compared to documenting successful results. If a complication occurs that is within the standard of practice and the surgeon successfully treats the problem, the patient may nevertheless experience some compromise in the result compared to an optimal result. When challenges arise, if the surgeon can show by interval photographs that the appearance of the problem improved markedly as the result of appropriate treatment, any visual compromise in the result often seems less drastic when observers compare the final compromise to the magnitude of the problem before successful treatment. Photographs of problems or complications are also invaluable education aids to the surgeon, both personally and in professional education forums.

Table 5-1 summarizes the potential strengths and limitations of breast imaging, listing what photographs can do best and what pictures cannot predictably deliver.

Photographic Documentation for Breast Augmentation

Imaging for breast augmentation requires basic hardware and software that is readily available to all plastic surgeons. Specific methodologies for photographic imaging vary widely among surgeons. This chapter focuses on current equipment and methodologies in

Table 5-1. Strengths and limitations of breast photographic images

Photographs can:	Photographs cannot:
1. Preoperatively document differences in the patient's breasts that will not be corrected by basic breast augmentation	1. Accurately and objectively define or predict breast size
2. Document the preoperative appearance of the patient's breasts	2. Accurately and objectively define or predict breast shape
3. Document the interval appearance of the patient's breasts postoperatively	3. Provide optimal information for decisions in preoperative planning without concomitant objective measurements
4. Document complications and problems	4. Provide optimal information for decisions during surgery without concomitant objective measurements

the author's practice that have evolved over a 30 year clinical practice. One of the challenges in photographic imaging is evolving and maintaining state-of-the-art equipment and image output while maintaining the ability to closely match images that were captured years earlier.

Hardware and software for breast photographic imaging

Digital photography has largely replaced conventional film photography for virtually all plastic surgery applications, so this chapter focuses entirely on digital solutions and workflow

Essential components of a photographic imaging system for breast augmentation include a camera or cameras to capture images, one or more light sources, a uniform background, equipment and methods for storage and retrieval of patient images, and dedicated or multiuse office space for patient imaging. Digital photography has largely replaced conventional film photography for virtually all plastic surgery applications, so this chapter focuses entirely on digital solutions and workflow.

Image resolution considerations

The quality and resolution capabilities of the camera system depend on the intended use of the output images. The human eye cannot detect the individual square pixel blocks of color in a color print if the print has a resolution of 300 dots per inch (dpi). For this reason, any images that a surgeon might want to print in a professional journal or magazine must have a resolution of 300 dpi. The larger the image a surgeon needs to print at 300 dpi, the higher quality, higher resolution camera the surgeon must purchase. Surgeons rarely need to print output larger than 5 inches by 7 inches at 300 dpi. Multiplying 5 inches and 7 inches respectively by 300 dpi yields a total pixel resolution of 1500×2100 pixels for a total pixel count of $3\,150\,000$ or 3.1 megapixels (1 megapixel equals 1 million pixels). Hence a 3.1 megapixel camera is capable of producing a 1500×1200 pixel print (5×7 inches) at 300 dpi resolution. Cropping to optimize an image discards pixels, so for most plastic surgery applications, a camera capable of delivering at least 4 megapixels is desirable. Cost per pixel is rapidly decreasing, hence surgeons should consider purchasing a 5 or 6 megapixel camera that enables 300 dpi output at larger print sizes if desired.

Cropping to optimize an image discards pixels, so for most plastic surgery applications, at least a camera capable of delivering 4 megapixels is desirable

Cameras

In addition to the resolution considerations discussed in the previous paragraph, other camera features facilitate surgeon and personnel workflow and optimize use of valuable time resources. Ideally, digital image capture, labeling with patient data, and transfer to a digital database should be a seamless process that occurs each time the surgeon captures an image. If a camera requires that surgeon or personnel remove a memory card, transfer the card to a card reader or computer, and then open and label each patient image individually, surgeon or personnel time waste is massive.

Before purchasing a camera, surgeons should define image capture and storage workflow, identifying and purchasing software that includes drivers for specific cameras that enable the camera to transfer sequential images via Firewire or wirelessly to a computer database that contains patient demographic and clinical data that automatically "attach" to captured images. Before purchasing camera or software, surgeons should always insist on a demonstration of the camera and software actually functioning in a realistic clinical setting to allow the surgeon to actually use the equipment and assess realistic capabilities.

A visible grid on the computer display or in the camera viewfinder allows the photographer to align specific points on the grid with specific anatomic landmarks to assure consistency of the patient image within the frame. Although image modification software such as Adobe Photoshop can adjust image size, color balance, and other parameters, a higher quality image captured by the camera assures the highest quality in the final printed image.

The camera lens should always be level with the patient's breasts in every view. Mounting the camera on a high quality tripod with adjustable elevation assures optimal leveling and camera stability. A variety of adjustable tripod heads allow surgeons to choose adjustment mechanisms that are most comfortable for the surgeon or photographer.

Imaging room setups and equipment

Although surgeons can use an on camera flash for lighting and a wall of an exam room for a background, state-of-the-art practices have a dedicated photo or image capture room with high quality studio lighting and seamless paper backgrounds. Surgeons whose practices span the technology change from film to digital photography must duplicate lighting systems to obtain reproducible, long-term followup pictures from patients from the film based era. The critical importance of accurate and reproducible photo documentation is neglected by many surgeons. Even surgeons who never plan to publish a single paper on breast augmentation should realize the importance of accurate, reproducible imaging for patient education, dealing with postoperative issues, and addressing medicolegal issues. The lesson is better learned earlier than later.

Before purchasing camera or software, surgeons should always insist on a demonstration of the camera and software actually functioning in a realistic clinical setting to allow the surgeon to actually use the equipment and assess realistic capabilities

The camera lens should always be level with the patient's breasts in every view

Figure 5-1. Dedicated imaging room with dual lighting systems for digital and legacy film based imaging.

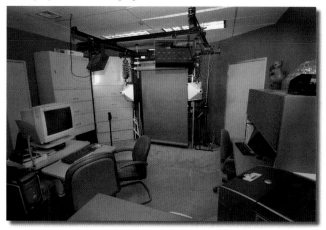

Figure 5-2. Two television studio lights (white arrows) and a similar overhead light directly over the patient position are used for digital imaging. Legacy strobe soft boxes (black arrows) and an overhead boom hairlight are used for film photography to closely match long-term followup pictures on patients who were originally imaged on film. The entire lighting system is mounted on a rail system (red arrows) that enables rapid reconfiguration of lighting if needed. Various color background papers accommodate the color tastes of associates who also use the room.

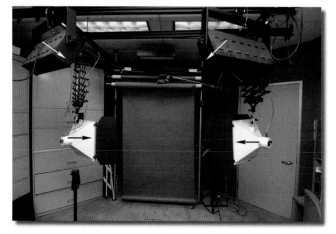

Figures 5-1 and 5-2 show the author's dedicated imaging room lighting and background configuration that uses three television studio lights (two at 45 degree angles in front of the patient and an overhead for highlighting and elimination of background shadows). Legacy lighting is suspended from a rail system to assure consistency with film images from the predigital era. The room is multipurpose for file storage. Television studio lights are mounted on an overhead rail system that also supports legacy strobe soft boxes and strobe boom hairlight to allow the author to match lighting for long-term followup photographs of patients from the film era. Seamless rolls of background paper are mounted on a spring loaded pole support system that spans from floor to ceiling. All of these components are available online from professional photography suppliers or distributors. Figure 5-3 is a wide field view of the entire image capture room from the area of the computer display terminal where surgeon and patient view the captured images and complete the Patient Images Analysis Sheet.

Views of the breast

A minimum of five views of the breast (Figure 5-4, A–E) are essential for imaging documentation in breast augmentation: anteroposterior, right and left oblique views, and right and left lateral views. Additional views that some surgeons use include squeeze views (Figure 5-4, F, G) and supine views (Figure 5-4, H). Squeeze views are extremely inconsistent and virtually useless from the standpoint of scientific objectivity, but at least indicate whether a breast has a grade 3 or 4 contracture. Supine views can provide important information. Most breast augmentation patients do not want their implants to shift laterally into the armpit, leaving a totally flat, preaugmented appearance. A supine view documents the position of the implant when the patient is supine. This

A minimum of five views of the breast are essential for imaging documentation in breast augmentation: anteroposterior, right and left oblique views, and right and left lateral views

view also dispels misconceptions such as the misconception that a form stable implant in a tailored pocket must have an undesirable, fixed appearance when the patient is supine. The patient in Figure 5-4 was augmented with an Allergan Style 410FM 270 gram form stable implant.

Although professional journals have elevated the requirements for the resolution of published images (to 300 dpi resolution with a minimum horizontal dimension of 3–3.5 inches), no indexed journals currently require all five standard views of patients in breast augmentation publications, allowing surgeons to publish selected views in lieu of full disclosure provided by all five standard views (Figure 5-4, A–E). Hopefully the more respected journals in plastic surgery will require that all augmentation

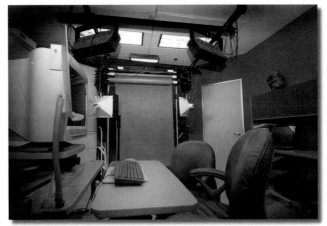

Figure 5-3. Imaging room viewed from computer display desk where surgeon and patient review the patient's images and complete and sign the Patient Images Analysis Sheet described in Chapter 3 and included in the Resources folder on the DVDs that accompany this book.

Figure 5-4. Views *A–E*, top row, left to right, are the five essential standardized views for primary breast augmentation. The squeeze and supine views (*F–H*, bottom row, left to right) are additional, optional views.

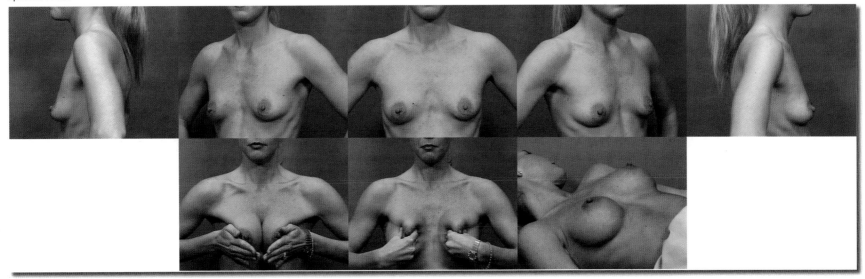

publications that include patient before and after images also include at least the five standard views described previously.

Image capture methods

The process of capturing patient images should be efficient and assure high quality images. The surgeon or an assistant can bring the patient to the photo room and ask her to stand facing for a left lateral photograph. A location marked on the floor for the patient's feet and for the tripod mounted camera assures a more constant lens-to-subject distance. The surgeon or assistant enters essential patient data in the photographic database or searches the database for existing data, and opens the patient's file in the database.

Patient positioning varies according to surgeon preference. The author prefers images captured with the patient's hands on her hips to clearly expose lateral thoracic and axillary areas. The surgeon encourages the patient to stand comfortably, never instructing her to level her shoulders or assume any position other than her natural standing position, because postoperatively at home, the patient will always view her breasts from her normal standing position.

As the surgeon or assistant captures each image, the camera transfers the image to the computer and the database tags and files the image. The surgeon then sequentially asks the patient to turn to the left oblique, anteroposterior, right oblique, and right lateral positions and captures an image in each position. When image capture is complete, the surgeon asks the patient to move to the chair adjacent to the surgeon in front of the computer display.

Archiving patient images and assuring data backup

All patient images are stored on the computer terminal's hard disk in the photo room, and copied to an archive file on the office servers. Nightly backup of all files to tape backup and weekly off site backup to tape and to hosted servers assure integrity of data. The regrettably common failure to establish rigid standards for data backup can be disastrous for a surgeon's practice. Regardless of established standards, constant, meticulous monitoring of data transfer by an independent third party consultant is usually more predictable and effective compared to systems that rely on surgeon or surgeon staff to assure data backup.

Printing patient images

For routine documentation in the patient's chart, color laser printers deliver rapid print output at a reasonable cost; color dot matrix printers produce higher quality prints on

All patient images are stored on the computer terminal's hard disk in the photo room, and copied to an archive file on the office servers. Nightly backup of all files to tape backup and weekly off site backup to tape and to hosted servers assure integrity of data

For routine documentation in the patient's chart, color laser printers deliver rapid print output at a reasonable cost; color dot matrix printers produce higher quality prints on glossy paper stock at slightly increased costs

glossy paper stock at slightly increased costs. Color printer technologies have increased quality while decreasing costs for high quality print output. Most surgeons will utilize both color laser and dot matrix printers. Providing patients high quality before and after images reinforces a positive image in the patient's mind, and reminds her of the level of change the augmentation produced.

▓ REFERENCES

1. Tebbetts JB: A system for breast implant selection based on patient tissue characteristics and implant–soft tissue dynamics. *Plast Reconstr Surg* 109(4):1396–1409, 2002.

2. Tebbetts JB, Adams WP: Five critical decisions in breast augmentation using 5 measurements in 5 minutes: the high five system. *Plast Reconstr Surg* 116(7):2005–2016, 2005.

Implants and Implant–Soft Tissue Dynamics

Implant–soft tissue dynamics impact short- and long-term results in breast augmentation. The more a surgeon understands the complex interactions between the implant device and the surrounding and supporting soft tissues, the more predictable the surgeon's results, and the more optimal the patient's experience and long-term outcome.

Understanding breast implant design and choosing optimal implant size, type, and dimensions requires that surgeons understand (1) the relationship of fill volume to each patient's individual breast dimensions and tissue characteristics, (2) how specific implant designs and characteristics affect distribution of fill in the breast, and (3) the complex interactions of the implant with the tissues of the breast (implant–soft tissue dynamics) short- and long-term. When surgeons objectively assess individual patient tissue characteristics, prioritize long-term soft tissue coverage of the implant, and base implant size and type selection on objective, quantified, proved processes, optimal long-term outcomes result.

Two categories of breast augmentation exist: breast enlargement (breast stuffing), and breast enlargement (filling and shaping the breast) with optimal control of distribution of fill and long-term aesthetics, while minimizing tissue compromises and reoperations. Stated another way, augmentation can either *optimally fill a breast acknowledging breast dimensions and tissue characteristics ("fit and fill")*, or the operation can *force tissues to a desired result*. Optimal long-term aesthetics with minimal tissue compromises and reoperations result when patients and surgeons adopt the "fit and fill" approach, understanding that the dimensions and tissue characteristics of the breast determine optimal implant volume and type. When patients and surgeons do not prioritize *tissues*

Two categories of breast augmentation exist: breast enlargement (breast stuffing), and breast enlargement (filling and shaping the breast) with optimal control of distribution of fill and long-term aesthetics, while minimizing tissue compromises and reoperations. Stated another way, augmentation can either optimally fill a breast acknowledging breast dimensions and tissue characteristics ("fit and fill"), or the operation can force tissues to a desired result

above arbitrary *wishes*, the surgeon may create a desired size and aesthetic appearance, but long-term, the patient may experience compromised aesthetics, additional reoperations, irreversible tissue consequences, and uncorrectable deformities.

OPTIMAL BREAST FILL—WHAT IS IT?

Optimal long-term breast aesthetics require appropriate fill of the breast soft tissue envelope, based on the dimensions and tissue characteristics of the breast. Appropriate fill of the breast soft tissue envelope varies according to the desired aesthetic result. If a patient desires a result that mimics the aesthetic characteristics of a normal breast with fewest compromises, total fill cannot exceed an amount that fills the upper pole to no more than slight convexity and keeps the borders of the breast within areas of optimal soft tissue coverage. If a patient desires a much larger breast that exceeds the capability of the skin envelope to accommodate, the surgeon must add excessive fill, create pocket boundaries outside of the areas of optimal soft tissue coverage, and fill to produce an excessively bulging and unnatural appearing upper breast.

Optimal fill is an amount of fill that recognizes and respects each individual patient's tissue characteristics

Optimal fill is different in every breast. The wider a breast and the greater the skin stretch, the greater fill is required for an optimal aesthetic result (Figure 6-1). Optimal fill, however, is more than simply the aesthetic result, regardless of whether the aesthetic result appears "natural" or not. The word optimal implies an amount of fill that addresses issues that are equally important compared to any aesthetic considerations. Optimal fill is an amount of fill that recognizes and respects each individual patient's tissue characteristics, balancing aesthetic considerations with the more important priorities of protecting and preserving the patient's tissue over her lifetime, and prioritizing optimal soft tissue coverage for the implants long-term. *Optimal breast fill is the least amount of fill that will produce the desired aesthetic appearance with the least long-term tissue compromises and the lowest long-term reoperation rates.*

Optimal breast fill is the least amount of fill that will produce the desired aesthetic appearance with the least long-term tissue compromises and the lowest long-term reoperation rates

DEFINING DESIRED BREAST SIZE PREOPERATIVELY

Neither surgeons nor patients can define any cup size, and surgeons certainly cannot predictably deliver what they cannot define

Patients frequently attempt to describe their desired breast size by specifying a cup size. Neither surgeons nor patients can define any cup size, and surgeons certainly cannot predictably deliver what they cannot define. Many surgeons also are aware that following augmentation, patients rapidly adjust to their new breast size and then wish they had requested a larger breast. This "if a little is good, more is better" tendency is perhaps a reflection of human nature, but it certainly has been a reality in breast augmentation for

Figure 6-1 A, B. The greater the base width of a breast, and the greater the degree of anterior pull skin stretch, the greater the volume required to fill the breast for an optimal aesthetic result.

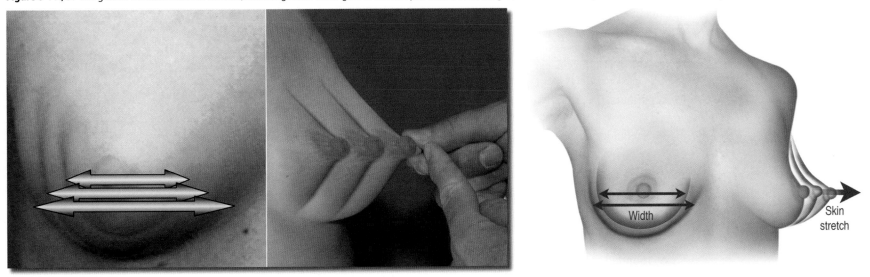

decades and has prompted many surgeons to "push" breast size at the primary operation to discourage patients from requesting larger implants postoperatively. This entire line of reasoning by patients and surgeons is severely flawed for several reasons:

1. Human nature is unlikely to change as the result of a breast augmentation; hence no defined end point limits repeated requests for larger breasts.

2. These methodologies seek to deliver a result based on indefinable parameters such as cup size or subjective appearance.

3. The methodologies prioritize forcing tissues to a subjectively desired result while ignoring the potential tissue compromises and uncorrectable deformities that can result from attempting to force tissues into a place they were never intended or genetically equipped to go.

Acknowledging these reasoning and decision process flaws, patients nevertheless need to have some understanding of what their result might be before having a breast augmentation. Surgeons are challenged to provide a realistic perspective while attempting to reconcile patients' wishes with their tissues. While many methods try to achieve these goals, no current methods are optimal based on current reoperation rates for size exchange following breast augmentation. How can surgeons provide a realistic perspective regarding the realities of breast fill and breast size that provides patients an opportunity to elect optimal fill, respecting their tissues, or request and assume full responsibility for a breast size that exceeds the capabilities of their tissues and risks severe tissue compromises?

Most patients, if optimally educated, understand the following concepts:

> The wider a breast and the greater amount the skin stretches forward when pulled away from the chest, the greater the volume required to fill the breast envelope

1. The wider a breast and the greater amount the skin stretches forward when pulled away from the chest, the greater the volume required to fill the breast envelope.
2. For any given width and skin stretch, if the surgeon could pour fluid into the breast through a funnel in the upper breast, the lower breast would fill first, then the middle, then the upper, and at some point the breast would appear ideally filled. If the surgeon continued to pour more fluid into the breast, the upper breast would begin to bulge excessively, and eventually would assume an exaggerated, bulging, rounded shape in the upper breast.
3. Based on concepts 1 and 2 above, once the breast is full, it is full. Attempting to put excess volume in the breast envelope distorts the breast, precluding a natural appearance, and poses irreversible risks to the tissues, including thinning of the skin, atrophy of breast parenchyma, and even chest wall depressions or deformities.

Key to the patient understanding and accepting these concepts are two questions that each patient must answer in a written document:

1. Do you want a breast that is attractive and that is not empty in the upper breast?
2. Do you want a breast that looks like an attractive but *normal* breast with a full upper breast, or do you want a breast with an excessively bulging and unnatural appearing upper breast? (This question must be an either/or question, nothing in between.)

These questions are absolutely key to the decision making process, because if the patient requests a breast that looks like a normal, natural breast with a full upper pole, then the patient must accept that when the breast envelope is full, it is full, and adding more volume will produce excessive upper bulging that is unnatural and not what she requested. At the same time, if the patient requests a breast that is not empty in the upper pole, the surgeon must place adequate volume in the envelope to fill it, otherwise, the upper breast will be empty.

The amount of fill required to adequately fill the breast to prevent an empty upper breast is essentially the same volume required to deliver a full but natural upper breast that looks like a normal breast rather than a round, globular, bulging, "Baywatch" appearing upper breast. By asking these two simple questions and documenting the patient's answers, the surgeon can assure the patient that the surgeon has placed the maximal amount of fill in the breast that the envelope can accommodate and continue to look like a normal but full breast. Simultaneously, the surgeon can assure the patient that the amount placed is the minimal amount to adequately fill the breast and produce optimal upper fill. This black and white approach with the patient eliminates the grays of in between wishes and sizes that no surgeon can deliver, and provided the surgeon has documented the patient's answers in writing, serves as an excellent reminder to the patient postoperatively of what she requested preoperatively if any discussion of size issues occurs postoperatively.

> The amount of fill required to adequately fill the breast to prevent an empty upper breast is essentially the same volume required to deliver a full but natural upper breast that looks like a normal breast rather than a round, globular, bulging, "Baywatch" appearing upper breast

◼ HELPING PATIENTS UNDERSTAND BREAST SIZE AND FILL—THE FUNNEL ANALOGY

We previously discussed the basic concepts of using the funnel analogy to help patients understand principles of breast fill. This concept and discussion technique are so effective and helpful that they deserve a more detailed discussion.

The most effective way to demonstrate these concepts to a patient is to ask the patient to look down while seated in an examination chair. The surgeon grasps the areolar skin and after advising the patient that she may experience some discomfort, pulls the areolar skin maximally anteriorly until the patient experiences discomfort, then marks this point of maximal stretch with the index fingernail of the opposite hand. Releasing the skin, the surgeon then cups the hand around the lower breast at a distance equal to the point of maximal stretch. The dialog with the patient is: "Can you feel that I am pulling your skin as far forward as it is possible to go?" When the patient, wincing, acknowledges positively, the surgeon says: "If I now cup my hand at that maximum stretch distance from your breast, do you understand that your tissues will not stretch much more than what I am showing you?" When the patient acknowledges, the surgeon continues: "As you look down at this approximate amount of enlargement of your breast, do you understand that the amount of expansion of your skin that I am demonstrating is about

The surgeon emphatically reminds the patient that although it may be possible to force implant size to further stretch the skin over time, this approach virtually guarantees atrophy or loss of the patient's breast parenchyma, sacrificing critical coverage over the implant that maximizes risks of visible implant edges and traction rippling, and potentially eliminating the ability of the patient to nurse

the maximum stretch your skin can safely tolerate?" The patient, at this point, is acutely aware of the meaning of maximal stretch, based on what she just felt when the surgeon stretched her skin maximally. The surgeon emphatically reminds the patient that although it may be possible to force implant size to further stretch the skin over time, this approach virtually guarantees atrophy or loss of the patient's breast parenchyma, sacrificing critical coverage over the implant that maximizes risks of visible implant edges and traction rippling, and potentially eliminating the ability of the patient to nurse.

Mentally recording the patient's reply, the surgeon continues: "If we had a funnel and could simply pour fluid into your breast from above, the lower breast would fill first, then the middle, and finally the top (Figure 6-2). If we stop before we put adequate fill in the breast, the upper breast will not be filled optimally. Once the breast is full and looks perfect, if we continue to add filler, you will have an increasingly bulging and unnaturally appearing upper breast. So, based on the width of your breast and the stretch of your

Figure 6-2 A, B. Using a funnel analogy with increments of fill into the breast helps patients understand that a specific amount of fill is required to fill the breast envelope. That same amount of fill is the maximum, safest amount of fill the breast can tolerate without creating an excessively full upper breast.

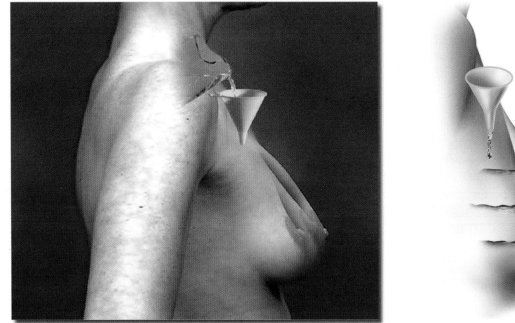 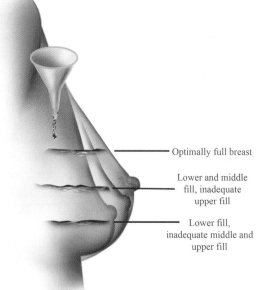

Optimally full breast

Lower and middle fill, inadequate upper fill

Lower fill, inadequate middle and upper fill

tissue, there is a limit to what we can safely put in your breast and end up with a breast that looks more like a breast compared to a basketball. If you like the rounded, bulging, basketball look, then we must overfill your breast using an excessively large implant, and you must assume full responsibility for tissue changes that might occur over time. These tissue changes can include shrinkage of your breast tissue, thinning of your skin and soft tissue over the implant that allows you to see edges of the implant, tissue thinning that may allow you to see visible traction rippling, and even deformities of your chest wall due to excessive pressure by the implant."

"If you want a breast that looks like a breast, the width of your breast and the amount of skin stretch that you have defines a maximum amount of fill that we can safely put in your breast. You should look at what I show you when I cup my hand at the maximal stretch distance. If that size looks too large to you, we have to put less fill in your breast, but remember that if we stop short while pouring fluid into the breast, you may have an empty upper breast. If that size I am showing you looks too small, then we must force more fill into your breast, and remember that once the breast is full, pouring more fill produces a more bulging upper breast that looks less like a normal breast."

> If you want a breast that looks like a breast, the width of your breast and the amount of skin stretch that you have defines a maximum amount of fill that we can safely put in your breast

Obviously, the surgeon must use professional judgment and communicate effectively with the patient during this process, but these simple concepts and the simple funnel analogy are very effective to help patients understand realities and define "black and white" choices instead of indefinable "shades of gray" choices. The surgeon concludes this part of the discussion by saying: "By now, I'm sure you understand that we want to fill your breast maximally to a degree that your tissues will tolerate, nothing less and nothing more, if you want a breast that looks like a breast. When we agree to fill your breast maximally to this level, you should also be aware that unless medical reasons arise later, we are not willing to change and increase the size of your implants because we have already maximally filled your breast to a safe level, and going beyond that point is obviously not in the best interests of you and your tissues."

■ CONTROLLING DISTRIBUTION OF FILL AND BREAST SHAPE

All surgeons address the basic objective of enlarging the breast when they perform breast augmentation. In addition to enlarging the breast, some surgeons also wish to try to improve specific areas of breast shape. Two factors largely determine breast shape: the dimensions and stretch characteristics of the envelope, and the distribution of fill (parenchyma) within the breast envelope. Surgeons cannot change the genetic characteristics of breast skin and the effects of pregnancy on a patient's breast skin envelope. Surgeons can, however, impact the distribution of fill within the breast and therefore affect breast shape provided they understand three absolute requirements to control breast shape:

1. *The surgeon must control distribution of fill within the breast.*

2. *In order to control distribution of fill within the breast, the surgeon must first control the position of the implant in the soft tissue pocket, and*

3. *implant design and fill must enable the surgeon to control distribution of fill within the implant.*

A practical example clarifies these principles. Using any currently manufactured round, smooth, gel or saline breast implant, if the surgeon or manufacturer fills the implant to current manufacturer recommended volumes and the surgeon then performs a tilt test[1] on the implant (Figure 6-3, A), the upper pole of the implant collapses because the recommended or actual fill volume of the implant is less than the displacement volume of the mandrel used to manufacture the implant. Manufacturers have traditionally designated round implant recommended fill volumes less than mandrel volume to allow the upper implant to collapse and avoid an excessively round or bulging appearance in the upper breast. While these design and fill parameters may accomplish that goal, surgeons cannot control the distribution of fill within that type of implant. Depending on the degree of "back pressure" on the implant from overlying tissues, the filler within the implant shell can displace in any direction, and in doing so, uncontrollably affect breast shape. With all current round implants, the surgeon cannot control the distribution of the filler within the *implant*, and because the implant has a *smooth outer shell*, the surgeon cannot control the *position of the implant within the breast pocket*. Hence all current round, smooth breast implants fail to satisfy either of the essential criteria that may allow surgeons to control breast shape because surgeons cannot control distribution of fill within the device and they cannot control the position of the device within the breast. In contrast, by increasing the fill to mandrel ratio and refining implant shape, an anatomically shaped, saline filled implant, the Allergan Style 468, does not experience upper shell collapse when tilt tested (Figure 6-3, B). By not experiencing upper shell collapse, the anatomic implant allows the surgeon better control of upper pole fill, and decreases risks of shell folding or collapse that shorten shell life.

To attempt to control breast shape more effectively, surgeons must first control distribution of fill within the implant device. One method of accomplishing this goal is to add more filler to approximate the mandrel volume of the implant. The problem with this method, especially with round implant designs, is that increasing fill produces a shape in

To predictably control breast shape, surgeons must control distribution of fill within the breast, and control position of the implant; to control distribution of fill within the breast, the surgeon must control distribution of fill within the breast implant

With all current round implants, the surgeon cannot control the distribution of the filler within the implant, and because the implant has a smooth outer shell, the surgeon cannot control the position of the implant within the breast pocket

Figure 6-3 A. This 300 cc round implant, filled to maximum manufacturer's recommended fill, demonstrates severe upper shell collapse when subjected to the tilt test by tilting the implant upright.

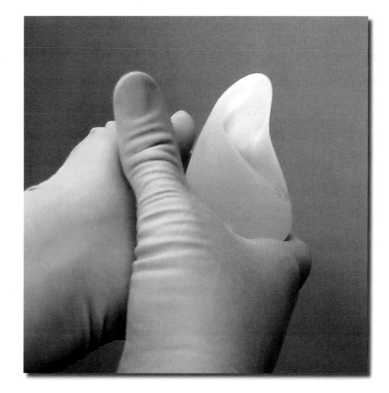

Figure 6-3 B. Comparison of a round saline implant filled to manufacturer's recommended fill (left) to an anatomic saline implant also filled to manufacturer's recommended fill (right), demonstrates that the anatomic implant, with a higher fill to mandrel ratio, does not experience upper shell collapse and does not lose vertical height when subjected to the tilt test.

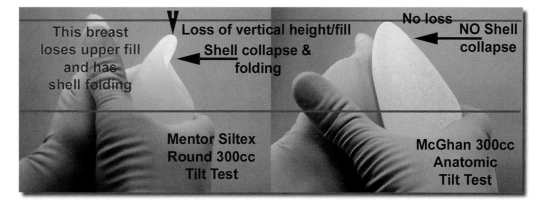

the device that is excessively round and causes excessive bulging in the upper breast, compromising surgeons' ability to produce a natural appearing augmentation result. A second problem, more minor, is an increase in firmness of the device as fill volume increases relative to mandrel volume. Although a concern for some surgeons, peer reviewed and published studies indicate that patients understand and tolerate slight increased firmness if the firmness provides more opportunity to control breast shape and position, and more importantly, to minimize shell collapse and folding that shorten implant shell life.[2]

> The most effective method of controlling distribution of fill within the implant device is to increase the cohesiveness of the filler material

The most effective method of controlling distribution of fill within the implant device is to increase the cohesiveness of the filler material. Various materials have been added to saline to attempt to increase its cohesiveness, and all have failed or have caused undesirable side effects that resulted in withdrawal of the products from the market. In contrast, manufacturers can formulate silicone gel to produce a wide range of cohesiveness. A key question is whether increasing cohesiveness of silicone gel filler materials increases control over the distribution of fill within the implant device. The answer is no, unless the degree of cohesiveness increases to a point where the implant becomes *form stable* when it is subjected to the tilt test. A *form stable implant* is an implant that experiences no shell folding and minimal, if any, shell collapse, and less than 0.5 cm vertical dimension shortening when a surgeon places the implant in the hand, supports the lower pole without pressing on it, and tilts the implant to an upright position (the tilt test, Figure 6-3, *B*, right).

> A form stable implant is an implant that experiences no shell folding and minimal, if any, shell collapse, and less than 0.5 cm vertical dimension shortening when a surgeon places the implant in the hand, supports the lower pole without pressing on it, and tilts the implant to an upright position (the tilt test)

The word "cohesive" has become an implant manufacturer marketing buzzword that means little, if anything at all, to the two objectives most important to surgeons and patients: (1) prolonging the life of the implant shell by reducing shell collapse and folding (thereby reducing unnecessary reoperations to replace failed implants), and (2) providing surgeons a device that allows control of distribution of fill within the device that in turn offers more opportunity to control distribution of fill and shape of the breast. One manufacturer, in advertisements, claims that all of their silicone gel implant designs are "all cohesive, all the time". What the manufacturer does not specify is the actual differences in cohesiveness between their various silicone gel implant products, and how those differences may affect the life of the devices, reoperation rates, and the efficacy of the devices with respect to providing surgeons a better opportunity to control shape in the breast. Even the term "form stable" is becoming polluted by marketing jargon, but implants that meet the criteria for form stability defined previously at least demonstrate

Figure 6-4. All currently manufactured smooth, round implants, regardless of filler material or shell profile, demonstrate some degree of upper shell sagging, collapse, or folding when upright in a tilt test. All smooth shell implants displace to the most dependent portion of the pocket, depending on the position of the patient. Surgeons cannot control the position of smooth shell implants and therefore cannot control distribution of fill in the breast with smooth shell implants.

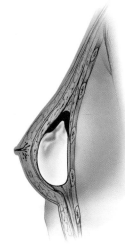

control of distribution of fill within the implant shell, and therefore provide surgeons a better opportunity to more accurately control breast shape.

Implant shell characteristics can dramatically affect surgeons' ability to control the position of the implant in the periprosthetic pocket, and therefore control the distribution of fill in the breast that defines breast shape. Smooth shell implants, regardless of the characteristics of the implant filler material, fall to the most dependent portion of the implant pocket, and provide surgeons virtually no control over distribution of fill within the breast (Figure 6-4), especially the upper breast. Surgeons can increase breast fill by selecting a larger size, smooth shell implant, but surgeons cannot control the distribution of fill within the pocket or within the breast using smooth shell implants.

Many surgeons believe the misconception that controlling implant position requires tissue adherence to a large portion of the implant shell surface, especially with anatomic or shaped implants. Absent this adherence, most surgeons believe that shaped implants experience a high rate of implant malposition. Neither of these beliefs is accurate, and neither has been proved by valid scientific data. To understand the factors that determine the degree to which surgeons can control the position of the implant device in the periprosthetic pocket, surgeons must understand the shell–tissue interactions of textured shell implants, and must also understand biological factors independent of shell surface characteristics that impact the position of the device in the pocket.

■ BREAST IMPLANT SHAPES

Two basic categories of implant shapes are currently available— round and anatomic or shaped (Figure 6-5). Terms describing implant shape are somewhat confusing. The term

Implant shell characteristics can dramatically affect surgeons' ability to control the position of the implant in the periprosthetic pocket, and therefore control the distribution of fill in the breast that defines breast shape. Smooth shell implants, regardless of the characteristics of the implant filler material, fall to the most dependent portion of the implant pocket, and provide surgeons virtually no control over distribution of fill within the breast, especially the upper breast

Many surgeons believe the misconception that controlling implant position requires tissue adherence to a large portion of the implant shell surface, especially with anatomic or shaped implants

Figure 6-5. Basic profile shapes of anatomic or shaped implants and round implants.

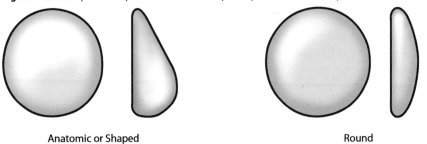

Anatomic or Shaped   Round

Figure 6-6. The term "profile" refers to the anterior–posterior dimension or projection of both round and shaped or anatomic implants. The higher the profile or projection of any implant, the more pressure it exerts anteriorly on parenchyma and posteriorly on the chest wall, increasing risks of parenchymal atrophy and chest wall deformities with high and extremely high profile implants.

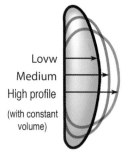

Lovw
Medium
High profile

(with constant volume)

"round" describes the shape of current round implants when viewed in anteroposterior view with the implant lying on a table, while the terms "shaped" and "anatomic" refer to the shape of the implant viewed laterally. Some current shaped implants are designed on a round base, while others are shaped or tapered in both anteroposterior and lateral views.

Profile is a term that describes the anteroposterior dimension of both round and shaped implants. Currently, low, medium, and high profile designs exist for both round and shaped implants (Figure 6-6). Round implants, by definition, have a vertical dimension or height that equals the base width of the implant. Shaped implants have varying heights relative to the width of the devices, hence the terms "low", "medium", and "full height" apply to shaped implants only (Figure 6-7). References to the height of the implant are meaningless if the implant is not form stable in the upright position, because if the upper pole of any implant collapses, it is impossible for the surgeon to predict the vertical height of the device in the breast. At the present time in the United States, the only form stable implant with stable height when tilted vertically is the Allergan Style 410 cohesive, form stable implant.

Round implants may or may not appear round in the breast, depending on the volume of implant fill relative to the mandrel volume of the implant. All current round implants, whether prefilled or adjustable saline devices, have manufacturer recommended (or actual) fill volumes that allow the upper implant shell to collapse in order for the round implant to produce a tapered, natural appearing upper breast. Surgeons can create a rounder appearing breast and rounder, more bulging upper breast by increasing the fill volume of adjustable saline implants or by selecting progressively larger size round implants (saline or silicone filled) that exceed a fill volume of the patient's breast envelope that produces a natural appearing upper breast.

Shaped implants may or may not confer their shape to the visual shape of the breast depending on several variables. The less breast parenchyma in the breast, and the less compliant the breast envelope, the more the postoperative appearance of the breast reflects the shape of the implant. Low and mid-height shaped implants create essentially the same shape as a collapsed upper pole round implant (includes virtually all current round implants filled to manufacturer recommended or actual fill volumes). A significant

Figure 6-7. Shaped implants are available in varying heights, but these heights are meaningless unless the device is adequately form stable to retain its full height when tilted to the upright position.

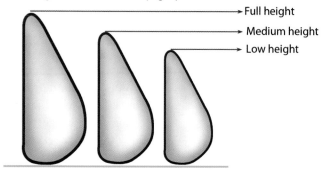

→ Full height
→ Medium height
→ Low height

References to the height of the implant are meaningless if the implant is not form stable in the upright position, because if the upper pole of any implant collapses, it is impossible for the surgeon to predict the vertical height of the device in the breast

The less breast parenchyma in the breast, and the less compliant the breast envelope, the more the postoperative appearance of the breast reflects the shape of the implant

difference is that although the breasts might appear similar with a conventional collapsed round implant and a reduced height shaped implant, if the shaped implant is form stable, the shell of the shaped implant may experience less collapse and shell folding and may have a longer shell life compared to the collapsed shell of the round implant (Figure 6-8). Full height, shaped implants can better control initial distribution and maintenance of fill in the upper breast, *provided the full height, shaped implant is truly form stable and does not experience upper shell collapse with the implant in the upright position* (Figure 6-9). Currently, the most form stable, full height anatomic or shaped implant is the Inamed/Allergan Style 410 device.

To provide a wider range of implants to surgeons, manufacturers have created "matrices" of implant designs that include low, medium, and high profile designs in round implants and the same range of profiles in varying heights in anatomic or shaped implants. The almost unending array of implant shapes, sizes, and dimensions are more important to address marketing concerns than to address real patient needs in breast augmentation, because only four basic implant shapes are necessary to deliver optimal results. Many surgeons select a certain shape and height implant to create a desired breast shape, when in reality, experienced surgeons can provide an optimal aesthetic result in virtually every type of primary breast augmentation using only four basic implant shapes and projections: (1) conventional round (if surgeon and patient are minimally concerned with implant shell collapse), (2) medium height, medium profile, form stable shaped implants that mimic collapsed round devices and are easier for surgeons to use compared to full height implants, (3) full height, low profile, form stable implants for optimal control of breast shape and upper breast fill in patients with less compliant envelopes (anterior pull skin stretch of 2 cm or less), and (4) full height, medium profile, form stable implants that optimize control of breast filler distribution and control of upper breast fill in a majority of breast types. While a large number of available implant designs increases surgeons' and patients' choices and is appealing from a marketing standpoint, a greater number of implant designs does not assure a greater number of optimal aesthetic results. Optimal aesthetic results and minimal negative long-term tissue consequences result more from surgeon evaluation, decision processes, the dimensions of the periprosthetic pocket, and an understanding of implant–soft tissue dynamics compared to the design of the implant device.

◼ IMPLANT EFFECTS ON BREAST TISSUES

Every breast implant, regardless of type, size, or shape, causes changes in the tissues of the breast. The extent to which those changes are positive or negative relates directly to the surgeon and patient decision making process. The positive experience of breast

Full height, shaped implants can better control initial distribution and maintenance of fill in the upper breast, provided the full height, shaped implant is truly form stable and does not experience upper shell collapse with the implant in the upright position

The almost unending array of implant shapes, sizes, and dimensions are more important to address marketing concerns than to address real patient needs in breast augmentation, because only four basic implant shapes are necessary to deliver optimal results

Every breast implant, regardless of type, size, or shape, causes changes in the tissues of the breast. The extent to which those changes are positive or negative relates directly to the surgeon and patient decision making process

Figure 6-8. Moderate height, shaped, form stable implants (left) produce a similar degree of fill as a round, low or moderate profile implant of similar size (right) that experiences upper shell collapse. Hence moderate height, shaped implants are often used by surgeons who are gaining initial experience with shaped devices before progressing to full height, form stable shaped implants that demand more accuracy in selecting implant size and in precisely locating the inframammary fold and positioning the implant.

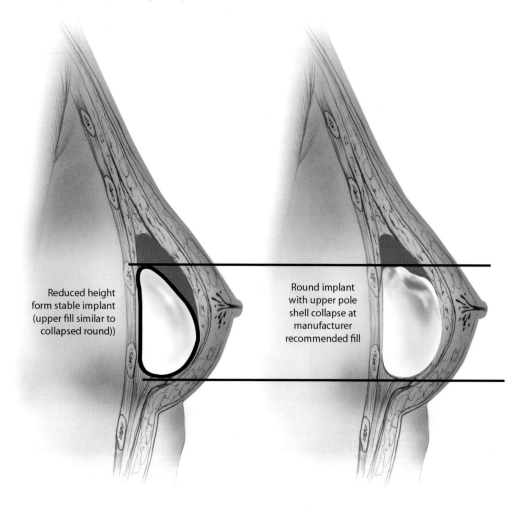

Reduced height form stable implant (upper fill similar to collapsed round))

Round implant with upper pole shell collapse at manufacturer recommended fill

Figure 6-9. Left: Full height, form stable implants offer surgeons the greatest degree of initial control of fill of the upper breast in all types of breast augmentation. Right: Shorter height implants that experience more upper shell collapse, even if claimed to be "form stable", do not offer surgeons as predictable control of upper breast fill. Many tissue factors can affect upper breast fill and its longevity.

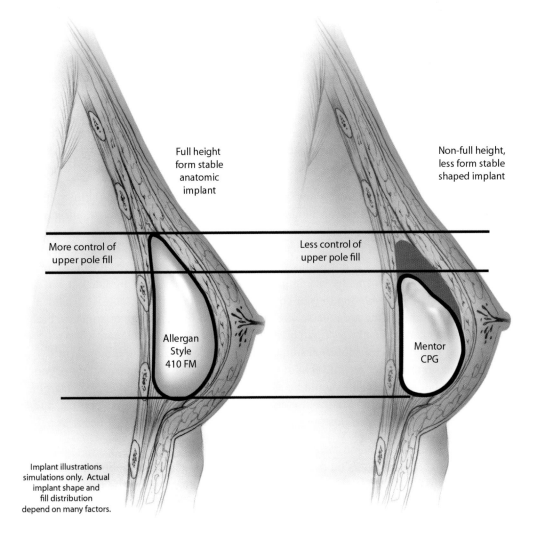

Full height
form stable
anatomic
implant

Non-full height,
less form stable
shaped implant

More control of
upper pole fill

Less control of
upper pole fill

Allergan
Style
410 FM

Mentor
CPG

Implant illustrations
simulations only. Actual
implant shape and
fill distribution
depend on many factors.

enlargement and enhancement short-term is predictable for most patients. Choices and decisions that the patient and surgeon make preoperatively, especially the size and projection of the implants, impact longer-term effects of the implant on the skin envelope and breast parenchyma that may cause negative tissue effects. Wound healing factors including capsular formation and contraction, and tissue stretch factors including skin stretch and thinning, are not totally predictable or controllable by the patient or the surgeon.

When discussing potential implant effects on tissues, and the decision processes to minimize potentially negative tissue effects, surgeons should distinguish breast augmentation considerations from breast reconstruction considerations. In breast augmentation, patients and surgeons have more flexibility and options compared to breast reconstruction in which the mastectomy defect and contralateral breast size and shape dictate options.

During the first 6 months postoperatively, short-term tissue effects include skin stretch to accommodate the implant and capsule formation around the implant. Genetic tissue characteristics vary among patients, and render each patient's tissue responses to breast implants different and not totally predictable. Skin stretch is predictable, but the degree to which the skin stretches is not totally predictable. Excessive skin stretch can occur in some patients, even with smaller size implants. Capsule formation is predictable, but the degree to which the capsule tightens or contracts is not totally predictable. Capsular tightening and skin stretch are inversely related, and invariably different from one breast to the other. One capsule always tightens slightly more than the other, and when a capsule tightens, it increases internal support of the implant, reducing the implant's stretch effects on the inferior pole skin of the breast. These effects can be subtle or more pronounced, but every patient should be aware preoperatively of genetic tissue factors related to wound healing and tissue stretch that no surgeon or patient can control, and anticipate the inevitability of postoperative differences in the breasts that occur as a result of those factors.

> One capsule always tightens slightly more than the other, and when a capsule tightens, it increases internal support of the implant, reducing the implant's stretch effects on the inferior pole skin of the breast

Long-term effects of implants on breast tissues are critically important, because those effects can cause irreversible changes, compromises, or deformities in the tissues of the breast and the chest wall. Patient requests and choices, and patient and surgeon preoperative decisions and implant choices largely determine the likelihood of negative tissue consequences long-term, including excessive skin stretch, thinning of subcutaneous tissues, atrophy of breast parenchyma, and pressure deformities of the chest wall. Most of these potentially negative tissue effects are not apparent in the first 1 or 2 years

> Long-term effects of implants on breast tissues are critically important, because those effects can cause irreversible changes, compromises, or deformities in the tissues of the breast and the chest wall

postoperatively, but become increasingly noticeable over many years. Preoperative patient education is critical to optimal decisions that reduce negative tissue consequences. Patients should be aware and accountable for the potential long-term effects of their preoperative requests and choices, and surgeons should provide information about potential long-term tissue effects to patients and provide optimal decision support preoperatively.

Implant Size Effects on Tissues

The larger a breast implant, the more potential negative long-term effects on the patient's breast tissues. While many factors may affect tissue response, implant size is clearly one of the most important factors that surgeons and patients can control. Implants predictably add weight to the breast, and the more weight in a breast, the more negative tissue effects are likely to occur over time. Surgeons and patients who prefer large implants attempt to justify large implants using various rationales including a patient's right to choose whatever size she wishes. When patient or surgeon chooses an implant larger than 350 cc, the important question is whether the patient not only knows preoperatively what she *wants*, but also what she is likely to *get* long-term as a consequence of large implants.

The term "large implants" in this book refers to implants larger than 350 cc volume or 350 grams in weight. Patients with wider breasts and greater skin stretch preoperatively may require more volume to adequately fill the breast envelope for optimal aesthetic results. When breast width and skin stretch require volumes greater than 350 cc or weights greater than 350 grams for adequate fill, patients should be aware preoperatively that the amount of volume/weight required for optimal aesthetics may cause potentially negative tissue effects over time. These tissue effects may include excessive skin stretch and thinning, visible traction rippling from the weight of the implant pulling on thin overlying soft tissues, visible implant edges, thinning of the subcutaneous tissue, thinning or atrophy of the breast parenchyma, and possible depression or concavity of the chest wall in extreme cases. Given this information preoperatively, patients and surgeons can make better decisions regarding benefit/risk considerations.

Negative tissue effects due to implant size also relate to the preoperative characteristics of the overlying soft tissues. Placing larger volumes in a previously stretched or large dimension breast envelope is completely different compared to placing large volume implants in a smaller or tighter skin envelope to force the breast tissues to a desired result. While negative tissue effects may occur as a result of larger volumes required to "fit and

The larger a breast implant, the more potential negative long-term effects on the patient's breast tissues

When patient or surgeon chooses an implant larger than 350 cc, the important question is whether the patient not only knows preoperatively what she *wants*, but also what she is likely to *get* long-term as a consequence of large implants

Placing larger volumes in a previously stretched or large dimension breast envelope is completely different compared to placing large volume implants in a smaller or tighter skin envelope to force the breast tissues to a desired result

fill" an already large envelope, placing large implants to force tighter, smaller dimension breast envelopes to an arbitrary result virtually guarantees more negative long-term tissue effects and possible irreversible tissue changes or deformities.

Implant Shape Effects on Tissues

The single most important factor of implant shape or dimensions that determines long-term tissue effects is implant projection—the anterior–posterior dimension of the implant. *High projection or high profile breast implants have two predictably negative effects on breast tissues: excessive pressure and excessive weight. High profile implants apply more anterior pressure to breast parenchyma and posterior pressure to the chest wall (causing potential parenchymal atrophy and chest wall depressions), and for any specific implant width, adding projection adds weight and all of the potential negative effects of implant weight listed previously, focused primarily on the lower pole tissues of the breast.*

Tissue effects of implant shape, similar to tissue effects of implant size, also relate to the dimensions and characteristics of the breast envelope and parenchyma. One of the most potentially damaging decisions that patients and surgeons can make preoperatively is choosing high projection or high profile implants to force tissues to a more projecting breast result in a patient with a less compliant (anterior pull skin stretch less than 3 cm) breast envelope. While many patients may request a more projecting breast, and a high profile or projection implant may produce the desired result short-term, long-term parenchymal atrophy and chest wall depressions can easily reduce projection over time, negating the more projecting result and leaving the patient with a result that could have been achieved with a less projecting implant and without irreversible negative tissue consequences (Figure 6-10). The pressure effects of highly projecting implants on overlying and underlying tissues over time are impressive, but many surgeons do not recognize the gravity of these effects until they have been in practice for many years, and only if they have seen significant numbers of patients with high profile implants in long-term followup.

In primary breast augmentation, high profile implants are rarely an optimal choice when balancing potential aesthetic benefits with potential negative long-term tissue consequences. Without optimal preoperative patient education, patients' *wishes* may result in negative long-term effects on patients' *tissues*. While patients and some surgeons think that high profile implants invariably produce increased projection in the postoperative breast, this assumption is not necessarily true. The longer-term loss of parenchymal thickness, subcutaneous tissue thickness, and potential chest wall depression often exceeds the increased anterior–posterior dimension of the implant, resulting in a net

> High projection or high profile breast implants have two predictably negative effects on breast tissues: excessive pressure and excessive weight

> One of the most potentially damaging decisions that patients and surgeons can make preoperatively is choosing high projection or high profile implants to force tissues to a more projecting breast result in a patient with a less compliant (anterior pull skin stretch less than 3 cm) breast envelope

Figure 6-10. Left: Normal thickness of breast parenchyma is (center) compressed by every breast implant, but (right) is markedly compressed and subsequently frequently shrinks or atrophies in response to high profile and extremely high profile implants which can also cause chest wall depressions or deformities.

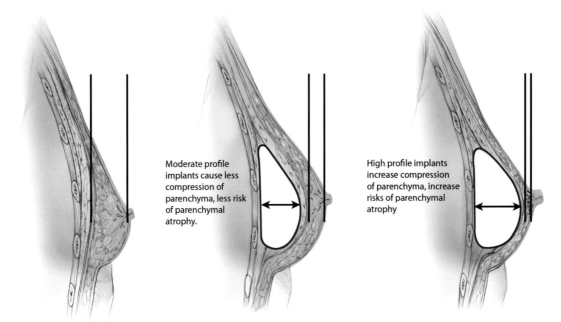

Moderate profile implants cause less compression of parenchyma, less risk of parenchymal atrophy.

High profile implants increase compression of parenchyma, increase risks of parenchymal atrophy

loss of breast projection long-term, with tissue thinning that often results in visible traction rippling and implant edge visibility (Figure 6-10).

■ HIGH PROFILE IMPLANTS FOR PRIMARY AUGMENTATION—QUESTIONABLE LOGIC

High profile implants have limited, logical applications in primary breast augmentation. When anterior pull skin stretch exceeds 3 cm and nipple-to-inframammary fold distance measured under maximal stretch is between 9 and 10 cm, a high projection or high profile device may provide more anterior "push" on the envelope to expand the stretched envelope anteriorly. Breasts with these tissue dimensions are sometimes termed "glandular ptotic" breasts, and surgeons sometimes advise patients that a more projecting implant produces more breast and nipple–areolar "lift" compared to less projecting implants. Breast implants, regardless of their projection, categorically do not lift the

> High profile implants have limited, logical applications in primary breast augmentation

breast, and any change in nipple–areola position is more apparent than real. Often the result is a "pseudo-lifted", larger breast that remains relatively low on the torso. When breast width is 12 cm or greater combined with the dimensions described previously for skin stretch and nipple-to-fold distance, selecting a high profile implant to provide "lift" adds substantially more volume and weight to the implant for each base dimension. The added weight, over time, usually negates any "lift" effect of the high profile implant, and simultaneously causes additional stretch and thinning of the lower breast envelope that may increase ptosis, traction rippling, and implant edge visibility.

Grades 3 and 4 capsular contracture around any breast implant cause a predictable change in implant shape to a more spherical configuration. As the capsule tightens and distorts implant shape to a rounder configuration, implant projection increases relative to implant base width. As a result, grades 3 and 4 capsular contracture make any implant a more highly projecting implant, and long-term untreated capsular contracture may result in increased risks of parenchymal atrophy and chest wall deformities. More form stable implants with highly cohesive silicone gel may resist spherical distortion from capsular contracture more effectively compared to non-form stable implants, but the difficulty of controlling for a large number of variables precludes valid scientific studies to verify this assumption.

■ IMPLANT SHELL LONGEVITY AND IMPLANT FILL VOLUME TO MANDREL VOLUME RATIOS

Implant fill volume relative to mandrel volume (the water displacement volume of the mandrel used to manufacture the implant shell) is an important determinant of implant shell longevity. Silicone implant shells are manufactured by dipping a mandrel (a solid molded model of the desired size of the implant shell) into formulated fluid silicone solutions multiple times to achieve the desired shell thickness. The water displacement volume of the mandrel is the actual volume inside the shell that was manufactured on the mandrel.

The actual volume of filler material that the manufacturer places into the shell of prefilled implants varies substantially compared to the water displacement volume of the mandrel, depending on the desired characteristics and dimensions of the final product. With conventional (non-cohesive, non-form stable) silicone gel filled implants, manufacturers used lower fill volume to mandrel volume ratios to make the final implant softer, more compliant, and more "natural" to palpation. This practice continues with somewhat more cohesive, but non-form stable implants today. With current round, smooth and textured

Implant fill volume relative to mandrel volume is an important determinant of implant shell longevity

saline filled implants, manufacturers specify recommended fill volumes that are less than the mandrel volume of the implant for similar reasons. Lower fill volume to mandrel volume ratios in round implants also allow the upper shell of the implant to collapse in order to achieve a more natural appearance in the breast.

Decreasing the fill volume of any implant relative to its mandrel volume makes the implant feel softer, but inevitably allows the upper and mid portions of the implant shell to collapse and/or fold. Implant shell collapse and folding creates stress on the implant shell that can cause shell "fold flaw" fatigue and shell failure. Historically, implants with relatively lower fill volume to mandrel volume ratios have had substantially higher shell failure rates and shorter implant life spans.

> Implant shell collapse and folding creates stress on the implant shell that can cause shell "fold flaw" fatigue and shell failure

For more than three decades, a majority of the surgeon market has focused on surgeons' perceived "naturalness" of implants pre- and post implantation. Surgeon feedback to implant manufacturers has consistently prompted manufacturers to prioritize marketing concerns and palpability characteristics of implants over other considerations such as implant shell longevity during the implant design process. To the author's knowledge, no objective, scientific studies have ever been done by any manufacturer to objectively and prospectively assess fill volume to mandrel volume effects on implant shell life during the implant design process. The vast majority of all breast implants have been designed to address specific marketing considerations, and implant shell life has defined itself over time after the devices have been implanted.

■ POLYURETHANE COVERED IMPLANTS AND THE PRICE OF A LOW FILL TO MANDREL VOLUME RATIO

In the 1980s, surgeons implanted significant numbers of Replicon, polyurethane covered, silicone gel implants. These shaped, silicone gel filled implants (Figure 6-11, top) had an extremely low fill volume to mandrel volume ratio, and relatively thin silicone shells with an overlying layer of polyurethane foam. Tissue ingrowth into the polyurethane foam occurred over several months, and the polyurethane separated from the implant shell and became incorporated into the surrounding capsule. While the implant had an exceedingly low rate of capsular contracture, the low fill volume to mandrel volume ratio allowed marked collapse and shell folding following breakdown of the polyurethane (Figure 6-11, bottom left), and the implant design had an extremely high shell failure rate (Figure 6-11, bottom right) and reoperation rate. Other round, silicone gel and alternative filler designs with low fill to mandrel volume ratios have had similarly high shell failure rates. Experience using and subsequently replacing these devices prompted the author to

Figure 6-11. Polyurethane covered implants and the price of a low fill to mandrel volume ratio. Top: The Meme (top left) and Replicon (top right) polyurethane covered implants appeared to be quite form stable preoperatively. In the body, the polyurethane shell degraded within approximately 2 years (2 year explant, bottom left), leaving a thin, markedly underfilled silicone gel shell that experienced marked collapse, folding, and a high shell failure rate (bottom right).

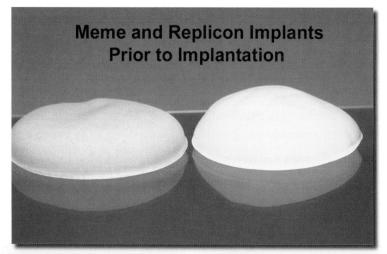

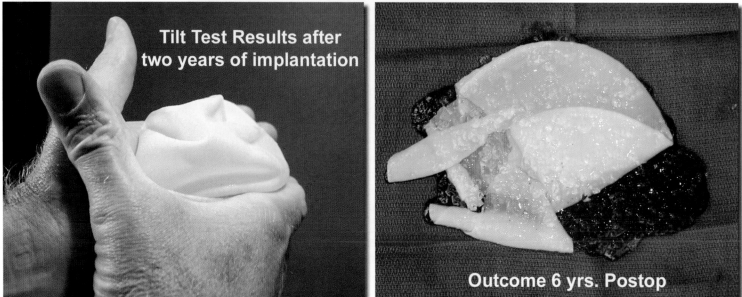

question low fill to mandrel volume ratios with respect to shell longevity and question whether other filler formulations might decrease the likelihood of gel migration when shell failure occurred.

Increasing implant shell longevity and decreasing gel migration in the event of shell failure were the author's two highest priorities when designing the first highly cohesive, form stable, anatomically shaped, silicone gel filled implant, the McGhan/Inamed Style 410. Increasing the fill volume to mandrel volume ratio required designing an implant with a tapered upper pole, because increasing fill volumes adequately to prevent shell collapse in a round implant design produced a consistently unnatural and excessively bulging upper breast in many patients. The Style 410 was the first implant design that did not experience upper shell collapse and/or folding with the implant upright. It was also the first implant to utilize a highly cohesive, form stable gel filler formulation that allowed control of distribution of fill within the implant shell. These design characteristics, implemented more than a decade ago, have been validated by substantially lower implant shell failure rates in the United States Food and Drug Administration (FDA) premarket approval (PMA) study of the 410 device and over a decade of use internationally since its introduction in 1993. The track record of the 410 and 468 implants and their design characteristics have prompted manufacturers to increase fill to mandrel volume ratios in a wide range of implant products to promote longer implant shell life.

Increasing implant shell longevity and decreasing gel migration in the event of shell failure were the author's two highest priorities when designing the first highly cohesive, form stable, anatomically shaped, silicone gel filled implant, the McGhan/Inamed Style 410

■ THE TILT TEST, ADEQUACY OF IMPLANT FILL, AND CAUSES OF VISIBLE RIPPLING

In 1996, the author wrote an editorial in the journal *Plastic and Reconstructive Surgery* entitled "What is adequate fill? Implications in breast implant surgery".[1] In addition to discussing the filler volume considerations relative to implant shell life, this editorial introduced a simple tilt test that allows surgeons to rapidly and easily assess adequacy of implant fill volume in a clinical setting. With either prefilled silicone or saline filled implants, the surgeon places the implant in the palm of the hand (Figure 6-12). If necessary, the surgeon can support the lower pole without pressing on it with the opposite hand, and then the surgeon tilts the implant upright to assess the degree of upper shell collapse or folding. A form stable implant, regardless of the filler material, does not experience upper shell collapse or folding as the implant is tilted upright, as indicated by the Allergan Style 468 anatomic saline implant on the left of Figure 6-12 and Allergan Style 410 form stable anatomic silicone gel implant on the right. If the upper shell collapses significantly or if any folding occurs, the fill volume of the device, in the author's opinion, is not optimal to maximally prevent shell stress that could decrease the

A form stable implant, regardless of the filler material, does not experience upper shell collapse or folding as the implant is tilted upright, as indicated by the Allergan Style 468 anatomic saline implant and Allergan Style 410 form stable anatomic silicone gel implant

Figure 6-12. A form stable implant, regardless of the filler material, does not experience upper shell collapse or folding as the implant is tilted upright, as indicated by the Allergan Style 468 anatomic saline implant on the left and Allergan Style 410 form stable anatomic silicone gel implant on the right.

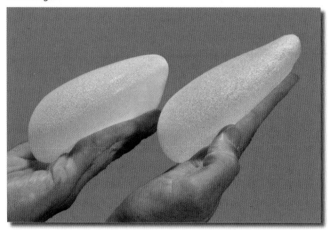

shell life of the device. These are currently the only two implant devices that exhibit this level of form stability.

This editorial also introduced the terms "underfill rippling" and "traction rippling" to distinguish two different etiologies of visible rippling post augmentation: *underfill rippling* is rippling caused by a low implant fill volume relative to the mandrel volume of the implant, whether in a prefilled or saline filled device; *traction rippling* is rippling that can be caused by the weight of any implant (regardless of filler volume to mandrel volume ratio) pulling on the implant capsule that is attached to thin overlying soft tissues. Traction rippling can be caused by any implant in the presence of suboptimal overlying soft tissue coverage, and can be largely prevented by decisions and techniques that prioritize and optimize long-term soft tissue coverage over the implant. Preventing underfill rippling requires that surgeons and manufacturers prioritize higher fill volume to mandrel volume for all implant designs.

> Underfill rippling is rippling caused by a low implant fill volume relative to the mandrel volume of the implant, whether in a prefilled or saline filled device; traction rippling is rippling that can be caused by the weight of any implant (regardless of filler volume to mandrel volume ratio) pulling on the implant capsule that is attached to thin overlying soft tissues

▪ PATIENT ACCEPTANCE OF ADEQUATELY FILLED IMPLANTS

For decades, surgeons have assumed that patients' number one priority when choosing a breast implant was the "naturalness" of the device. As a result, surgeons encouraged manufacturers to design maximally "natural" devices that utilized a combination of thin implant shells with a very liquid, non-cohesive form of silicone gel or saline, and a low fill volume to mandrel volume ratio. These design characteristics, while "natural", were distinctly suboptimal with respect to maximizing implant shell life.

Increasing fill volume to mandrel volume ratio causes any implant to feel firmer. A large percentage of surgeons assumed that patients would not want anything other than maximal softness in a breast implant, but unfortunately, for more than two decades, no surgeon actually studied patients' choices and priorities with respect to breast implant fill ratios. In 2000, the author published a study entitled "Patient acceptance of adequately filled breast implants using the tilt test" in the journal *Plastic and Reconstructive Surgery*.[2] In a series of 667 breast augmentations, when educated about implant fill issues and given a choice of implant preoperatively, 609 of 667 patients chose an adequately filled implant, the McGhan/Inamed Style 468 textured, anatomic saline implant over softer implants with lower fill to mandrel volume ratios. These 609 patients accepted the potential tradeoff of a slightly firmer implant to help minimize risks of earlier shell failure due to shell collapse and folding. Of the 609 patients followed up to 5.5 years, no patient requested exchange to a softer implant. Using an adequately filled implant to prevent shell collapse and folding according to the tilt test, no patient in the series experienced underfill wrinkling or rippling that required reoperation. The reoperation rate for deflation for the Style 468 implant over the 6 year period of the study was 9 of 1218 implants or 0.739%, lower than reported for any other saline filled device. The results of this study demonstrate conclusively that patients who are thoroughly educated preoperatively about all implant options and potential tradeoffs of underfilled implants certainly accept slight increased implant firmness as a tradeoff for possible increased implant shell life.

> Patients who are thoroughly educated preoperatively about all implant options and potential tradeoffs of underfilled implants certainly accept slight increased implant firmness as a tradeoff for possible increased implant shell life

■ TEXTURED IMPLANT SURFACES AND SHELL–TISSUE INTERACTIONS

Currently in the United States, two implant textured shell surfaces share a majority of the textured silicone shell implant market—the Siltex™ textured surface manufactured by Mentor Corporation, and the Biocell™ textured surface manufactured by Inamed/Allergan Corporation. These two surfaces differ significantly in manufacturing methodologies, characteristics of the surface, and tissue interactions with the surface.

During the 1980s, surgeons noticed that polyurethane covered implants had a markedly lower incidence of capsular contracture compared to smooth silicone gel filled implants, but a high shell failure rate. When polyurethane covered implants were removed from the market, manufacturers developed textured silicone surfaces to attempt to duplicate the dramatic reduction in capsular contracture that occurred with polyurethane covered implants. Tissue interaction with a polyurethane covering is drastically different compared to tissue interaction with any textured silicone surface ever developed.

The author has 30 years' clinical experience with textured and smooth implant surfaces, including both textured surfaces mentioned previously, as well as other textured surfaces including polyurethane covered surfaces and Dow Corning Silastic MSI (limited experience). This discussion will focus on the two most common surfaces currently in the United States, Biocell™ and Siltex™.

Tissue actively "grows into" *polyurethane* sheeting that is fixed with silicone adhesive to the outer surface of implants. The active tissue ingrowth occurs in the first few weeks following implantation, and during this period, polyurethane implants feel "fixed" to surrounding tissue. After ingrowth is complete and the capsule matures, breakdown of the polyurethane occurs over an extended period of months to years. As the polyurethane begins to break down, it separates from the silicone outer shell of the implant, and the implant, for practical purposes, behaves like a smooth shell implant with increasing mobility and decreasing ability to control distribution of fill within the breast. Early generations of polyurethane covered devices had extremely thin shells, and the silicone gel fill volumes were relatively low compared to mandrel volumes. As a result, dramatic shell folding occurred with these devices and caused an extremely high rate of shell failure (see Figure 6-11).

The Allergan Biocell™ textured surface manufacturing process uses salt crystals washed away near the end of the manufacturing process to create an open pore network that is deeper compared to the Mentor Siltex™ surface that utilizes a stamping process to produce the texturing on the outer shell. Detailed specifications of each of these surfaces are available from the respective implant manufacturers. The observations and comments that follow are based on more than 15 years' experience with both of these surfaces in both primary augmentation and reoperation procedures.

When discussing tissue interactions with current textured silicone surfaces, surgeons should clearly define terms and distinguish non-adherence from adherence, and distinguish adherence from tissue ingrowth. Despite many surgeons' belief that tissues "grow into" textured silicone surfaces, especially the deeper Biocell™ textured surface, the author is not aware of any valid scientific studies that demonstrate *active tissue ingrowth into any silicone surface. Tissue does not actively "grow into" any silicone surface on any currently manufactured implant. Adherence to the Biocell™ surface is primarily a mechanical process, not an active tissue ingrowth process.* Surgeons routinely notice the marked degree of tissue adherence that occurs with Biocell™ textured tissue expanders, and often translate that observation into a belief that similar adherence and tissue ingrowth occur with Biocell™ textured implants in primary breast augmentation.

■ ADHERENCE AND TISSUE INGROWTH IN PRIMARY BREAST AUGMENTATION

In primary breast augmentation, any adherence to the Biocell™ surface is a mechanical phenomenon, not the result of active tissue ingrowth. Many factors affect the degree of adherence that occurs in any individual case, including implant size and projection, the relative "tightness" of the breast skin envelope, tissue pressures of the pectoralis muscle

Tissue does not actively "grow into" any silicone surface on any currently manufactured implant. Adherence to the Biocell™ surface is primarily a mechanical process, not an active tissue ingrowth process

In primary breast augmentation, any adherence to the Biocell™ surface is a mechanical phenomenon, not the result of active tissue ingrowth

in subpectoral augmentation, the amount of fluid present in the pocket postoperatively, and many other factors. The larger the implant, and the tighter the overlying soft tissues, the more adherence occurs with the Biocell™ surface. In the vast majority of primary breast augmentation cases, tissue adherence to the Biocell™ surface occurs over 20–50% of implant surface, but certainly not over 100% of the surface except in rare cases of patients with exceedingly tight overlying tissues and pockets dissected to very tightly fit the implant. Tissue adherence is more predictable with Biocell™ implants when surgeons minimize bleeding and tissue trauma that promote more postoperative inflammation and transudation in the periprosthetic pocket. Predictable adherence occurs without the use of drains in a majority of cases where the surgeon selects the implant to fit the patient's individual tissue characteristics[3,4] and uses optimal surgical techniques to minimize trauma and bleeding.[5] These techniques are detailed in subsequent chapters of this book.

Periprosthetic tissues virtually never adhere to or "grow into" the Mentor Siltex™ surface. If a surgeon places a *very* large Siltex™ implant into a patient with an exceedingly tight breast skin envelope, the Siltex™ surface may appear to adhere, but true adherence does not occur with this surface. Even with the dramatic pressures created by a textured tissue expander with the Siltex™ surface, true adherence does not occur. In primary breast augmentation, adherence to the Siltex™ surface virtually never occurs.

Is tissue adherence to textured implant surfaces important and, if so, why is adherence important? Some surgeons believe that reducing capsular contracture with textured surface implants requires tissue adherence to the implant surface. That misconception has been conclusively disproved by similar capsular contracture rates in FDA PMA study data for saline filled implants.[6–8] A more important role for tissue adherence to a textured silicone implant shell is to better predict and control the position of anatomic or shaped implants within the implant pocket.

■ SURFACE TEXTURING TO CONTROL POSITION OF ANATOMIC OR SHAPED IMPLANTS

Control of breast shape requires control of distribution of fill within the breast and control of distribution of fill within the implant. Anatomic or shaped, form stable implant devices offer surgeons an opportunity to approach primary breast augmentation in a more sophisticated manner compared to implanting underfilled (relative to mandrel volume) round smooth implants into a breast with virtually no control over distribution of fill. Many current implants being marketed as "cohesive and form stable" may possess some cohesive characteristics, but many are certainly not form stable. Truly form stable, shaped implants provide surgeons an opportunity to more accurately put filler into specific areas of the breast at the time of surgery. Postoperatively, tissue adherence to the implant surface helps maintain the desired implant position and thereby provide a better opportunity to control distribution of fill within the breast.

Tissue adherence to the implant shell of shaped implants, while desirable, is not essential to maintain position of the implant. The author has reoperated on patients with Inamed/ Allergan Style 468 full height, anatomic, saline filled implants with Biocell™ textured shells and found no adherence whatever to the Biocell™ surface, yet perfectly normal position of the implants. How could that occur? *The mechanisms by which the Biocell™ surface most predictably maintains the position of shaped implants are a combination of friction and partial adherence.* The deeper texturing of the Biocell™ surface creates more friction against tissues adjacent to the implant in the immediate postoperative period compared to the shallow texturing of Siltex™ implants. Friction at the shell–tissue interface, combined with accurate, dry, atraumatic pocket dissection, creates an environment in which the periprosthetic capsule forms around the implant while the friction of the implant holds the implant in place. Friction at the shell–tissue interface maintains implant position as the capsule forms. Logically, deeper or more aggressive shell texturing produces more friction at the shell–tissue interface, and is more likely to maintain implant position as the capsule forms compared to textured surfaces that produce less friction. Friction during capsule formation is a completely different mechanism compared to actual tissue adherence to a textured implant surface, and tissue adherence to current silicone textured surfaces is not an active tissue ingrowth process. Capsular formation occurs in every case, with or without adherence to the implant shell. The capsule may form on the inner surface of the implant pocket, on the surface of the implant, or both. Adherence may or may not occur at varying degrees, but in any case, adherence occurs later, and adherence does not require active tissue ingrowth.

■ TISSUE INTERACTIONS AND ADHERENCE WITH THE BIOCELL™ SURFACE

How can adherence occur without "active" tissue ingrowth? Fluid transudate accumulates around every breast implant in the early postoperative period, regardless of whether surgeons place drains into the pocket. This transudate contains cells that are in constant contact with tissue surfaces, the implant surface, and with other cells. With the Biocell™ surface, cells migrate into the interstices of the open pore network where the cells *do not*

> Tissue adherence to the implant shell of shaped implants, while desirable, is not essential to maintain position of the implant

> The mechanisms by which the Biocell™ surface most predictably maintains the position of shaped implants are a combination of friction and partial adherence

"actively" attach to the silicone surfaces (no study has shown an active process of cells actively adhering to a silicone surface). Instead, cells "attach" to each other within the interstices. Cells attaching to each other create a matrix within the interstices of the open pore network that produce adherence without actual "active" tissue ingrowth into a silicone surface, but only in areas where *adjacent capsular or soft tissue intimately contacts the implant shell surface. In other words, adherence with Biocell™ requires two processes: (1) cells attaching to each other within the open pore network, and (2) soft tissue immediately adjacent to the matrix of cells forming in the textured surface so that the cells can also attach to the adjacent soft tissue.* If soft tissue is not in contact with the Biocell™ surface as the capsule forms, one "capsule" forms on the Biocell™ surface of the implant as described previously, and a second capsule forms on exposed tissue surfaces within the pocket that are not in contact with the Biocell™ surface. A "double capsule" is of no clinical significance, and simply indicates that, during capsular formation, portions of the pocket soft tissues were not in direct contact with the Biocell™ surface. In fact, a double capsule is desirable because it virtually always includes attachments from the capsule on the tissue side of the pocket to the "capsule" on the implant, further stabilizing implant position.

> In fact, a double capsule is desirable because it virtually always includes attachments from the capsule on the tissue side of the pocket to the "capsule" on the implant, further stabilizing implant position

■ COMMON MISCONCEPTIONS REGARDING TEXTURED SURFACE IMPLANTS

All textured surface implants are not the same. When surgeons opine about implant failure rates or malposition rates of shaped implants, they frequently lump all textured implants into a single category and comment globally on textured surface implants as if all of those implants were the same. Frequently, those global opinions are globally inaccurate and do not reflect peer reviewed and published data on different textured devices.

The following are common misconceptions about textured, anatomic implants compared to round implants that surgeons often hear or promote:

1. Anatomic implants have higher malposition rates compared to round implants
2. Textured, anatomic implants have a higher failure rate compared to round implants
3. Textured, anatomic implants cause more seromas
4. Textured and textured, anatomic implants cause more visible rippling compared to round, smooth implants.

Table 6-1. Reoperation and complication rates for round versus anatomic implants

	*Averaged inamed/ mentor saline PMAs 2002[2-4]	**Tebbetts studies PRS 2000–2002 combined data[5-7]	% difference
Number of patients	2165	1662	
Length of followup	3 years	Up to 7 yrs	
Capsular contractures Grade 3–4 (patients)	9.0%	0.7%	1260%
Hematomas #/%	2.0%	0.2%	1008%
Seromas #/%	3.0%	0.1%	2393%
Infections #/%	2.5%	0.3%	731%
Deflations #/%	4.0%	0.8%	411%
Malposition reoperations #/%	2.0%	0.1%	1562%
Size exchange reoperations #/%	8.7%	0.2%	4568%
Size adjustment reoperations #/%	—	0.0%	—
Visible rippling or wrinkling upright #/%	15.5%	0.0%	15500%
Reoperations all causes #/%	17.0%	3.0%	465%

*PMA study patients included predominately smooth and textured round implants.

**Patients in these combined studies had Inamed Style 468, full height, textured, anatomic, saline filled implants.

PMA and peer reviewed and published data do not support these common misconceptions.

Table 6-1 compares summary averaged data from FDA saline implant PMA studies of Mentor and McGhan[6-8] to data from three large series[2,5,9] of patients who received textured, anatomic implants with respect to complications and reoperation rates. The patients in the PMA study had only 3 year followup, while the patients in the other combined series had up to 7 year followup. These data strongly dispute the generalized misconceptions listed previously with peer reviewed and published data which suggest that textured, anatomic implants, used in conjunction with optimal planning and surgical techniques, have as low or lower rates of complications or reoperations compared to any type of round implants.

■ THE ROLE OF BREAST IMPLANTS IN BREAST AUGMENTATION OUTCOMES

Breast implants affect patient outcomes in breast augmentation, but each of the following affects patient outcomes more than the implant device itself: patient education, patient choices and the patient decision process; the surgeon's skill set; surgeon decision processes; surgical planning based on objective rather than subjective parameters, and surgical techniques that are capable of delivering rapid recovery.

No breast implant design can compensate for suboptimal patient education, decision processes, decision support, and surgical execution. Absent optimal information and knowledge, patients cannot make optimal decisions and assume responsibility for their choices and decisions. No implant device can compensate for suboptimal, subjective preoperative planning that forces tissues to a result instead of matching the implant to patient tissue characteristics and accepting a degree of improvement that the tissues will allow without causing irreversible negative tissue consequences. No implant device can create an optimal tissue environment or compensate for compromised tissue characteristics, and no type of implant can improve the patient's surgical experience and recovery.

> No breast implant design can compensate for suboptimal patient education, decision processes, decision support, and surgical execution

> No implant device can create an optimal tissue environment or compensate for compromised tissue characteristics, and no type of implant can improve the patient's surgical experience and recovery

Implant longevity is critically important to all patients, and should be a high priority for all surgeons. Surgeons should insist that implant manufacturers provide device failure and device problem data for each specific implant style, model, or product code, not grouped data that make objective evaluation of individual implant types impossible. Surgeons should provide these data to patients preoperatively, and allow patients to participate in implant selection decisions, instead of the surgeon having a "preferred" type of implant and encouraging patients to select that particular device based on partial or suboptimal information. All patients should be aware preoperatively that every breast implant device can and will experience shell failure at some point, and that placing any implant device in the body virtually assures that the patient will have additional surgical procedures with attendant costs and risks in the future.

> Implant longevity is critically important to all patients, and should be a high priority for all surgeons

Serving patients' best interests requires that surgeons continually update their knowledge and understanding of breast implant design and implant soft tissue dynamics. This knowledge and the continual updating of implant performance data are essential to help patients make optimal preoperative decisions to minimize the potential negative impact of breast implant devices on patients' tissues long-term.

■ REFERENCES

1. Tebbetts JB: What is adequate fill? Implications in breast implant surgery. *Plast Reconstr Surg* 97(7):1451–1454, 1996.

2. Tebbetts JB: Patient acceptance of adequately filled breast implants using the tilt test. *Plast Reconstr Surg* 106(1):139–147, 2000.

3. Tebbetts JB: A system for breast implant selection based on patient tissue characteristics and implant–soft tissue dynamics. *Plast Reconstr Surg* 109(4):1396–1409, 2002.

4. Tebbetts JB, Adams WP: Five critical decisions in breast augmentation using 5 measurements in 5 minutes: the high five system. *Plast Reconstr Surg* 116(7):2005–2016, 2005.

5. Tebbetts JB: Achieving a predictable 24 hour return to normal activities after breast augmentation Part II: Patient preparation, refined surgical techniques and instrumentation. *Plast Reconstr Surg* 109:293–305, 2002.

6. Food and Drug Administration. U.S. Food and Drug Administration. General and Plastic Surgery Devices Panel Meeting Transcript. Washington, D.C. October 14–15, 2003. Online. Available: http://www.fda.gov/ohrms/dockets/ac/03/transcripts/3989T1.htm.

7. Food and Drug Administration. U.S. Food and Drug Administration. General and Plastic Surgery Devices Panel Meeting Transcript. Washington, D.C. February 18, 1999.

8. Food and Drug Administration. U.S. Food and Drug Administration. General and Plastic Surgery Devices Panel Meeting Transcript. Washington, D.C. March 1–3, 2000. Online. Available: http://www.fda.gov/cdrh/gpsdp.html#030100.

9. Tebbetts JB: Dual plane (DP) breast augmentation: optimizing implant–soft tissue relationships in a wide range of breast types. *Plast Reconstr Surg* 107:1255, 2001.

Tissue Assessment, Decision Processes, and Operative Planning

■ BACKGROUND AND IMPORTANCE OF TISSUE BASED, QUANTITATIVE SYSTEMS AND DECISION PROCESSES

Breast augmentation outcomes are largely determined by preoperative decisions. The quality of preoperative decisions is directly related to the information on which the decisions are based and the prioritized decision making processes that surgeon and patient use preoperatively. This chapter focuses on the logic and published data that validate tissue based, quantitative preoperative patient assessment and decision processes, and the clinical application of those processes.

Preoperative Parameters and the Scientific Validity of Breast Augmentation Studies

Scientific validity of any prospective or retrospective study in breast augmentation requires that a study address variables that affect outcomes, defining those variables preoperatively, collecting objective, quantified data, and analyzing that data to test a hypothesis. A consistent weakness of most published studies in breast augmentation is a failure to define critical variables preoperatively and collect objective data pre- and postoperatively that relate to those variables. More than 53 variables affect the outcome of every breast augmentation. Table 7-1 lists surgeon and implant variables that exist in every breast augmentation.[1]

The extent to which surgeons address these 53 variables by recording objective, quantifiable pre- and intraoperative data for subsequent analysis largely determines the scientific validity of any clinical breast augmentation study. If a study fails to address these variables preoperatively, no amount of sophisticated statistical postoperative analysis can create scientific validity. Any statistical analysis is only as scientifically valid as the data which the process analyzes. A majority of published studies on breast augmentation are scientifically weak because of failure to address critical preoperative variables.

Breast augmentation outcomes are largely determined by preoperative decisions. The quality of preoperative decisions is directly related to the information on which the decisions are based and the prioritized decision making processes that surgeon and patient use preoperatively

More than 53 variables affect the outcome of every breast augmentation

Table 7-1. **Variables that impact outcomes in breast augmentation**	
Clinical and tissue variables	**Surgeon variables**
Genetic factors	Incision approach
Hormonal factors	Parenchymal dissection
Pregnancy history	Location Extent
Nursing history	Pocket dissection method
Age	Pocket dissection technique
Medications (especially birth control pills and hormones)	Degree of tissue trauma
Skin and subcutaneous tissue thickness	Bleeding intraoperatively
Skin compliance	Blood remaining in tissues Blood remaining in pocket
Breast parenchyma	Pocket dimensions
Amount	Pocket dissection plane—submammary or subpectoral
Base width	Division of pectoralis origins
Height	Location
Consistency and distribution	Extent
Attachments to pectoralis	Method of implant leak testing
Attachments to serratus	Method of implant fill
Attachments to deep subcutaneous fascia	Implant fill accuracy
Capsule	Implant insertion method
Thickness	Implant positioning method
Compliance	Tissue closure method
Degree of contracture	Postoperative bandaging methods
Age of capsule	Postoperative implant motion exercises
Attachments to pectoralis	Postoperative activity regimen
Attachments to serratus	
Pectoralis major muscle	Postoperative drug regimen
Thickness	
Compliance	
Degree of contraction	
Degree of passive tension	
Size of periprosthetic pocket	
Shape of periprosthetic pocket	
Patient arm position	
Patient degree of pectoralis contraction (passive or active)	
Implant fill volume	
Air in implant	
TOTAL TISSUE VARIABLES: 31	TOTAL SURGICAL VARIABLES: 22
TOTAL VARIABLES, TISSUES AND SURGICAL: 53	

To be scientifically valid, any study that compares methodologies, surgical techniques, or implants must prospectively create comparative cohorts of patients that acknowledge and control for the 53 variables listed in Table 7-1

To be scientifically valid, any study that compares methodologies, surgical techniques, or implants must prospectively create comparative cohorts of patients that acknowledge and control for the 53 variables listed in Table 7-1. Regardless of the methods, techniques or implants the study attempts to compare, conclusions are scientifically invalid if the investigator does not preoperatively define two groups of patients, with each of the two groups having similar variables to those listed in Table 7-1. Addressing a small percentage of these variables is not adequate to validate conclusions—the two groups must have similar age, pregnancy, and tissue characteristics, quantified objectively, to achieve scientific validity.

Subjective Versus Objective Assessment of Variables

Objectivity is essential to scientific validity

Objectivity is essential to scientific validity. Analysis of quantifiable, objective data yields scientifically valid conclusions. Analysis of subjective parameters, regardless of the sophistication of statistical analysis, generates opinions, but does not generate scientifically valid conclusions. Terms such as "thin", "thick", "stretchy", "tight", "minimal" and "moderate" frequently appear in scientific discussions and presentations. These terms are totally subjective and vary over a wide range of interpretations by individual surgeons. None of these terms is quantifiable, and none can be tested scientifically. The methods described in this chapter enable surgeons to address similar variables objectively instead of subjectively, recording specific measurements that are objective and quantifiable. Surgeons can use these objective data to make decisions of pocket location, implant selection, and surgical techniques. Scientific evaluation of outcomes data can then draw scientifically valid conclusions of the efficacy of the decision processes, implant devices, and surgical techniques. When surgeons use subjective impressions instead of objective, quantifiable measurements and data to make decisions and select implants and techniques, scientifically valid evaluation and conclusions are impossible.

When surgeons use subjective impressions instead of objective, quantifiable measurements and data to make decisions and select implants and techniques, scientifically valid evaluation and conclusions are impossible

Impact of Surgeon Education on Patients' Experience and Outcomes

Surgeon education in breast augmentation and many other surgical disciplines is based on a preceptor model. Resident plastic surgeons learn breast augmentation principles and techniques from their professors and attending physicians. In many academic plastic surgery programs, resident experience in breast augmentation is limited, and attending academic surgeons may perform very few breast augmentations compared to plastic surgeons in private practice. When academic and private practice surgeons who teach residents refer to breast augmentation as a "simple" operation, it is not surprising that for more than three decades, reoperation rates of 15–20% in just 3 years[2–4] following breast augmentation have changed minimally, and for many patients, the patient experience (recovery and outcomes) remains largely unchanged.

Improvement in patient outcomes in breast augmentation relates directly to the development and dissemination of improved methodologies and scientifically proved processes. The extent to which surgeon residency education programs and professional society education programs effectively disseminate new information about proved processes and the extent to which surgeons implement proved processes determine future improvements in patient outcomes. Improving patient outcomes requires that those who define content for educational programs or venues prioritize dissemination of proved processes that have objectively documented superior outcomes in peer reviewed and published studies. When surgeons use attendee evaluation form data and prioritize maximizing numbers of surgeons on a program with short presentations in lieu of thorough delivery of proved process content, the result is often more entertaining than educational. Ultimately, the degree to which surgeons choose to learn, improve, and implement proved processes, allocating time and financial resources, determines the experience and outcomes of their patients.

The extent to which surgeon residency education programs and professional society education programs effectively disseminate new information about proved processes and the extent to which surgeons implement proved processes determine future improvements in patient outcomes

Redefining the Patient Experience in Breast Augmentation

The current decade has produced quantum improvements in surgeons' approach to breast augmentation and has redefined the potential patient experience, outcome, and reoperation rates. Advances in tissue assessment, preoperative decision processes, surgical techniques, implant devices, and postoperative management now allow surgeons to routinely enable patients to return to full normal activities within 24 hours following breast augmentation with an overall reoperation rate of 3% over 7 years postoperatively.[5–7] For the first time in the history of Food and Drug Administration (FDA) premarket approval (PMA) studies of breast implants, refined decision processes, methodologies, and techniques produced a zero percent reoperation rate in 50 consecutive patients in an FDA study of Inamed/Allergan Style 410 form stable, cohesive gel anatomic breast implants.[8] These methods, which have redefined the surgeon and patient experience in breast augmentation, are peer reviewed and published in the journal *Plastic and Reconstructive Surgery*, and are available to surgeons worldwide. The specific tissue assessment, preoperative decision processes, and operative planning methodologies are the subject of this chapter.

For the first time in the history of Food and Drug Administration (FDA) premarket approval (PMA) studies of breast implants, refined decision processes, methodologies, and techniques produced a zero percent reoperation rate in 50 consecutive patients in an FDA study of Inamed/Allergan Style 410 form stable, cohesive gel anatomic breast implants

Evolution of Preoperative Planning and Implant Selection Methods

In plastic surgery, artistry is an invaluable adjunct to science. Artistry is a complement to science, not a substitute for quantifiable objectivity and the scientific method. Even Michelangelo and Leonardo—consummate artists—were consummate believers in the value and necessity of extensive measurements and planning before embarking on any artistic endeavor.

For decades, surgeons and patients have based choices and decisions about breast implant size and type on subjective parameters—patients' wishes for a particular bra cup size, requests to look like a particular photograph from a magazine or another patient's photographic outcome, or a volume to mimic a test implant placed into a bra. While each of these methods may appeal to some patients and surgeons, none is quantifiable, none is objective, and none is scientific.

Optimizing outcomes for patients requires developing processes of decision making that can be refined, optimized, and transferred to other surgeons—systems that use quantifiable parameters to make objective decisions, providing data that can be used to scientifically test hypotheses. A measurement system for breasts is similar to other measurement systems in common use in plastic surgery—systems that define optimal dimensions for cleft lip or palate repair, craniofacial surgery, and virtually every reconstructive procedure where quantifying a dimension helps a surgeon deliver a more accurate product.

While plastic surgeons routinely use and insist on quantifiable parameters in a wide range of reconstructive and cosmetic procedures, a relatively small percentage of surgeons currently base decisions in breast augmentation on quantifiable tissue dimensions and parameters. Quantitatively based systems do not dictate to surgeons or patients what they can choose, nor do they dictate a standard of practice. Systems for implants based on quantifiable parameters to define individual patient tissue characteristics offer surgeons additional tools to help make decisions more objective than subjective, make outcomes more predictable, and reduce reoperation rates.

Table 7-2 summarizes the evolution of quantitative, tissue based systems and decision process support for patient assessment and critical decisions in breast augmentation since their inception in 1992.

Artistry is a complement to science, not a substitute for quantifiable objectivity and the scientific method

Optimizing outcomes for patients requires developing processes of decision making that can be refined, optimized, and transferred to other surgeons—systems that use quantifiable parameters to make objective decisions, providing data that can be used to scientifically test hypotheses

Quantitatively based systems do not dictate to surgeons or patients what they can choose, nor do they dictate a standard of practice

Table 7-2. Evolution of quantitative, tissue based systems and decision process support for patient assessment and critical decisions in breast augmentation.

Date	System	Functions	Limitations	Published and Peer Reviewed References
1992	Dimensional System (licensed by McGhan/Inamed as the BioDimensional™ System)	■ Allowed patients to define desired intermammary distance (IMD) and cup size ■ Based selection of implant on desired breast base dimensions to create desired IMD ■ Selected implant to force patient tissues to a desired result with desired intermammary distance ■ DEFINED DESIRED RESULT AND FORCED TISSUES TO THAT RESULT BY SELECTING APPROPRIATE IMPLANT	■ Prioritized a desired result instead of prioritizing long-term optimal coverage and minimal patient tissue compromises ■ Two dimensional, did not consider tissue stretch, a critical third dimension ■ System did not define implant volume limits or projection limits ■ DID NOT QUANTITATE AND PRIORITIZE SOFT TISSUE COVERAGE LONG-TERM	Tebbetts JB: *Dimensional augmentation mammaplasty using the BioDimensional™ System*. Santa Barbara: McGhan Medical Corporation, 1994, pp 1–90.
2001	TEPID™ System	■ Quantified thickness of soft tissue coverage on which to base preoperative decisions of pocket location ■ Added and quantified the third critical dimension of tissue stretch to previous two dimensional system ■ Based implant selection on quantified, individual patient tissue characteristics ■ DEFINED AND LIMITED IMPLANT SIZE ACCORDING TO INDIVIDUAL PATIENT TISSUE CHARACTERISTICS	■ Did not define critical decisions in augmentation ■ Did not prioritize and order critical decisions ■ Did not define OPTIMAL PROCESSES by scientifically validated, peer reviewed and published data ■ Did not provide definitive patient and surgeon decision support processes based on proved processes validated by peer reviewed and published outcomes data	Tebbetts JB: A system for breast implant selection based on patient tissue characteristics and implant–soft tissue dynamics. *Plast Reconstr Surg* 109(4):1396–1409, 2002.
2005	High Five™ Decision Process and System	■ Integrates all aspects of the TEPID™ System, adds decision process priorities and support ■ Selects implant volume to meet quantified needs for optimal fill and breast envelope dimensions ■ Limits implant size and base dimensions to minimize negative long-term tissue compromises and uncorrectable deformities ■ DEFINES AND PRIORITIZES THE FIVE CRITICAL DECISIONS IN AUGMENTATION ■ PRIORITIZES OPTIMAL LONG-TERM SOFT TISSUE COVERAGE AND MINIMAL PATIENT TISSUE COMPROMISES ■ BASES CRITICAL DECISIONS FOR OPTIMAL LONG-TERM OUTCOMES ON QUANTIFIED, INDIVIDUAL PATIENT TISSUE CHARACTERISTICS (Allows individual surgeon and patient to deviate from system recommendations—provides a template for individual decisions)	■ Impact on widespread patient outcomes limited by voluntary surgeon implementation of proved processes ■ Although peer reviewed and published, proved, prioritized processes not currently prioritized in educational venues of surgeon professional organizations ■ A majority of patients are not aware of the existence and impact on outcomes of the proved processes in the system	Tebbetts JB, Adams WP: Five critical decisions in breast augmentation using 5 measurements in 5 minutes: the high five system. *Plast Reconstr Surg* 116(7):2005–2016, 2005.

Objectives and Limitations of the First Generation Dimensional System

To attempt to increase the reliability and predictability of results to patients, in 1990 the author developed a dimensional system that enabled a more quantitative method of assessing a patient's breasts and selecting appropriate implants to deliver the patient's desired result. This first dimensional system was published in a monograph in 1994,[9] and was licensed by McGhan Medical Corporation as the BioDimensional™ System and subsequently distributed worldwide. During the past decade, the BioDimensional™ System has become the most widely accepted and used dimensional system worldwide by providing surgeons with a more objective, quantitative, and scientific approach to breast evaluation and decision making in breast augmentation.

When first introduced in 1994, the BioDimensional™ System[9] allowed patients to define their desired intermammary distance by displacing the breasts medially, then using measurements of the existing breast width and the desired breast width to determine the base width of the implant required to deliver the patient's desired result. The original dimensional system functioned in two dimensions (base width and height), and focused on forcing tissues to a desired result (delivering the desired base width to achieve the patient's goals for desired intermammary distance). This system is still in use as the Allergan BioDimensional™ System. This first generation dimensional system produced a paradigm shift in surgeons' approach to patient assessment and decision making in breast augmentation. For the first time, surgeons could design a desired result using a quantitative assessment and decision making methodology instead of relying on bra stuffing, photographs, or subjective cup size methods to define objectives.

> The original dimensional system functioned in two dimensions (base width and height), and focused on forcing tissues to a desired result

While this first generation system reoriented many surgeons' thinking toward a more quantitative, reproducible, scientific approach to patient assessment and implant selection, the system has evolved two more generations with more than a decade of experience in a wide range of breast types. The strengths of the first generation system were (1) attempting to quantify dimensions and patient tissue characteristics, (2) basing decisions on quantifiable parameters, (3) enabling more scientific evaluation of quantified parameters, and (4) encouraging more consistent and predictable results.

An additional decade of clinical experience and longer-term followup of larger numbers of patients have pointed out limitations of this first generation system: (1) the system prioritized achieving a specific result instead of prioritizing optimal soft tissue coverage long-term (did not include specific, quantifiable parameters that mandate optimal tissue coverage, (2) the system and current revisions by other surgeons have no guidelines or restrictions on volume limits, (3) the system is two dimensional, omitting a critical third dimension—tissue stretch—that affects decisions about optimal volume for a specific patient's envelope and provides information about risks of excessive stretch with bottoming or traction rippling, and (4) the system was originally designed to be specific to one manufacturer's family of anatomic implant products.

In summary, the first generation BioDimensional™ System allows patients and surgeons to design a desired result by width and height dimensions, and then select an implant of appropriate dimensions to *force the tissues to the desired result*. In contrast to the first generation system, next generation systems do not force tissues to a desired result; instead, they recognize and quantify what the tissues will allow or what the tissues require to achieve an optimal long-term result with minimal negative tissue consequences.

Priorities for the Next Generation Measurement and Decision Process System

Priority 1 is preserving the patient's tissues over time by making *optimal decisions of volume and coverage* based on quantifiable parameters, not prioritizing an arbitrary implant size that may compromise the patient's tissues over time. An optimal system for tissue analysis and implant selection should prioritize the quality and integrity of patients' tissues long-term above all other considerations by defining quantifiable guidelines for total weight (volume) of the breast implant based on tissue coverage considerations. Patients often arrive at their consultation "knowing" what they want, and one of the responsibilities of the surgeon is to meet a patient's expectations. An equally important question, however, is whether the patient is adequately educated to understand *how what she wants is likely to affect what she is realistically likely to get* long-term—the potential long-term tissue consequences of her current wishes. Absent guidelines built into a system that integrates patient education and informed consent systems with quantifiable tissue assessment, patients and surgeons will likely continue to select implant size and type based on subjective and arbitrary considerations of breast size without acknowledging responsibility for the potential longer-term tissue consequences of their choices. The ultimate goal for the welfare of the patient is *prioritizing her tissues over her wishes* if she desires an optimal long-term result with minimal tissue compromises, reoperations, and uncorrectable tissue deformities.

The ultimate goal for the welfare of the patient is prioritizing her tissues over her wishes if she desires an optimal long-term result with minimal tissue compromises, reoperations, and uncorrectable tissue deformities

To avoid implant palpability, visibility, visible traction rippling, and extrusion risks long-term, the surgeon must prioritize *optimal, long-term soft tissue coverage* of the implant and *preservation of the patient's existing breast parenchyma* long-term, above all other considerations. Some of the most preventable complications of breast augmentation occur when surgeons and patients fail to prioritize optimal soft tissue coverage of the implant or decide to select implants with excessive size or projection that stretch, thin, and compromise tissues, and increase risks of parenchymal atrophy long-term.

Priority 2 is to provide *quantitative* data regarding patient tissue characteristics—data that enable surgeons to make objective decisions and allow scientific evaluation of outcomes.

Priority 3 is that all measurements concerning implant weight (size, volume) and coverage be made *on the breast*, not from landmarks on the breast to other landmarks on the chest, torso, or abdomen. *The ultimate consequences and aesthetics of any breast implant to the tissues of the breast are within the boundaries of the breast.* When performing primary augmentation, surgeons do not relocate the breast on the torso. While some surgeons may be tempted to base implant dimensions (especially implant height) on measurements such as sternal notch-to-nipple distance, these measurements and the subsequent decisions may be overly simplistic and inaccurate, depending on the filler distribution dynamics and implant–soft tissue dynamics of the implant selected.

> The ultimate consequences and aesthetics of any breast implant to the tissues of the breast are within the boundaries of the breast

Principles of Breast Aesthetics and Implant–Soft Tissue Relationships

Specific characteristics and relationships define an aesthetic breast. Every breast has a specific amount of skin that defines the dimensions—base width, stretch, and height—of the skin envelope. The skin envelope has specific tissue characteristics—base width, thickness, and stretch—that determine how much the envelope will stretch in response to adding fill (an implant). A funnel analogy is helpful when discussing these issues with patients. If the surgeon could pour filler into a funnel in the top of the breast, the lower breast would fill first until it reached its limit of anterior stretch, then the middle portion of the breast would fill, and finally the upper pole of the breast would fill to create an optimal breast contour and optimal transition of the breast from the chest. If the surgeon adds inadequate fill to any breast, the lower breast will be fuller compared to the middle or upper breast. When the breast is full with an optimal contour, adding additional volume creates excessive fullness in the upper breast, desired by some patients and surgeons, but also adding weight that ultimately causes more stretching of the lower envelope and loss of upper fill.

The wider the base width (BW) of the existing parenchyma, and the greater the skin stretch measured by anterior pull skin stretch (APSS), the greater volume required to fill the envelope for optimal aesthetics. Two components define optimal fill postoperatively: the patient's existing parenchyma and the implant. To predict optimal implant volume, the surgeon must estimate the parenchyma's contribution to stretched envelope fill (PCSEF). If the envelope is adequately filled preoperatively with the patient's existing parenchyma (>80%) and the skin stretches minimally, less volume is required in the implant. Conversely, if the skin stretches significantly, and minimal parenchyma (<20%) is present, more implant volume is required for optimal fill of the envelope.

*Optimal fill is defined as the **minimal** amount of fill required to produce an optimal aesthetic result while minimizing potential negative tissue consequences.* In a parous breast, more volume is often required due to the width or increased stretch characteristics of the envelope. Conversely, in a nulliparous breast with APSS < 2 cm (a tight envelope) and PCSEF > 80% (an envelope already full with parenchyma), much less volume is required for optimal fill.

When selecting an implant device, surgeons must consider not only the effects of volume/weight, but also the effects of focusing that volume in a specific area to achieve projection. For any given base width breast implant, increasing projection means adding weight and adding pressure directly behind the existing parenchyma (usually to satisfy a patient or surgeon's desire for a more projecting breast). Pressure focused on lower pole parenchyma can produce parenchymal atrophy over time. Currently there are no scientifically valid studies that define amounts of parenchymal atrophy that occur with varying projection implants, but experienced surgeons who have long-term followup of more than 10 years with highly projecting or high profile devices are aware that highly projecting implant devices can have negative tissue consequences to the parenchyma and lower pole skin envelope over time that include irreversible skin stretch and parenchymal atrophy. A high profile implant may temporarily create a more projecting breast, but lose the projection over time due to parenchymal atrophy, resulting in a permanent, uncorrectable compromise to the patient's tissues with loss of parenchyma.

The wider the base width of a patient's parenchyma, the longer the nipple-to-inframammary fold measurement for optimal aesthetics. Stated another way, the optimal

---

Optimal fill is defined as the *minimal* amount of fill required to produce an optimal aesthetic result while minimizing potential negative tissue consequences

---

The wider the base width of a patient's parenchyma, the longer the nipple-to-inframammary fold measurement for optimal aesthetics

position of the inframammary fold depends on the width of the breast. If the breast is excessively wide compared to the nipple-to-fold measurement, the breast appears boxy. If nipple-to-fold distance is too great compared to the width of the breast, the breast appears narrow, tubular, or ptotic. When increasing the width of the breast during augmentation, the optimal level to set the inframammary fold intraoperatively depends on the planned base width of the postoperative breast.

Two Basic Approaches to Breast Augmentation

Surgeons currently use two basic approaches to breast augmentation: (1) defining a desired result (using dimensions or subjective parameters) and selecting implants to force the tissues toward the desired result, and (2) allowing the tissues to define optimal fill by the dimensions and stretch characteristics of the envelope.

The first approach—forcing the tissues to a desired result—often produces larger breasts, especially in younger, nulliparous patients, compared to the latter, by forcing tighter tissues to stretch more than they stretch under manual measurement (APSS), and by widening the breast using an implant with a base width that exceeds the base width of the existing parenchyma. When patients and surgeons choose this approach to achieve a desired result, patients should be aware and acknowledge in informed consent documents that forcing their tissues to the desired result may produce negative tissue consequences long-term, including tissue stretch and thinning, parenchymal atrophy, visible or palpable implant edges, visible traction rippling, and ptosis. Some of those tissue consequences may be irreversible.

The second approach—allowing the tissues to define optimal fill by the dimensions and stretch characteristics of the envelope—attempts to minimize negative tissue consequences long-term in a wide variety of breasts. The simplest of approaches—selecting an implant with a base width less than the base width of the existing parenchyma and a projection less than or equal to the limit of manual stretch of the breast skin (APSS)—can avoid a very large number of uncorrectable tissue consequences and complications of breast augmentation.

No system is without tradeoffs. Even with a system that allows tissue dimensions and stretch to define volume requirements, some wide, parous breasts with minimal to moderate parenchyma require very large implants in order to adequately fill the envelope for an optimal aesthetic result. In these cases, patients must be aware that the amount of

The simplest of approaches—selecting an implant with a base width less than the base width of the existing parenchyma and a projection less than or equal to the limit of manual stretch of the breast skin (APSS)—can avoid a very large number of uncorrectable tissue consequences and complications of breast augmentation

volume required for an optimal result may add enough weight to cause negative consequences to their tissues over time such as tissue stretch and thinning, parenchymal atrophy, visible or palpable implant edges, visible traction rippling, and ptosis. Some of those tissue consequences may be irreversible.

Requirements of a Clinically Practical Measurement and Decision Assist System

A system for implant selection should address each of these critical decision areas and present the surgeon with specific, quantifiable data on which to base each decision. For efficiency, the system should not include any parameters that are not essential to one of these decisions and the system should enable the surgeon to perform all measurements and make all of these decisions in 5 minutes or less. The system that has evolved from the original dimensional system meets all of these criteria, has been adopted and used by a large number of surgeons, and with minor modifications, is used routinely by patients in the author's practice.

Tissue Coverage Priorities and Measurements

Assuring optimal soft tissue coverage requires surgeons to quantify soft tissue coverage in critical areas over the implant and use quantified criteria for pocket selection and additional soft tissue cover.

Traditional methods of subjective tissue assessment (e.g. thick, thin, tight, loose) are impossible to quantify, and therefore cannot be used to make objective decisions based on criteria determined by data. Without quantified criteria, surgeons cannot scientifically evaluate outcomes and derive outcomes based treatment algorithms.

> Traditional methods of subjective tissue assessment (e.g. thick, thin, tight, loose) are impossible to quantify, and therefore cannot be used to make objective decisions based on criteria determined by data

Specific measurements of tissue coverage parameters should include measurements of pinch thickness of skin and subcutaneous tissue superior to the breast parenchyma (STPTUP, soft tissue pinch thickness of the upper pole) and at the inframammary fold (STPTIMF). Patients whose tissues are thin (less than 2 cm pinch thickness above the existing parenchyma) are at risk short- and long-term for visible edges of the implant superiorly and superior traction rippling caused by traction of the implant on the capsule attached to the thin overlying soft tissues.

The system should set a quantified criterion to suggest additional muscle coverage (e.g. STPTUP < 2 cm) by placing the implant in either a traditional partial retropectoral or a dual plane (dividing origins of pectoralis along the inframammary fold) position. The system should also set a quantified criterion that suggests preserving muscle origins of the pectoralis intact along the inframammary fold when patient tissues along the fold are exceedingly thin (e.g. STPTIMF < 0.5 cm), choosing a traditional subpectoral pocket instead of a dual plane pocket that divides pectoralis origins along the inframammary fold.

To assure optimal pectoralis coverage medially when additional coverage is indicated, the system should remind surgeons to avoid any division of pectoralis origins medially along the sternum, from the xiphoid inferiorly to the junction with the medial inframammary fold.

Most importantly, the system should always specify an implant base width that is less than or equal to the base width of the patient's existing parenchyma in order to assure parenchymal coverage of implant edges. If surgeons applied only a single dimensional criterion when selecting an implant, this criterion alone could avoid many complications that occur as the result of inadequate tissue coverage. The only exception to this specification is in very narrow base width breasts with base widths less than 11 cm, including constricted lower pole breasts and tubular breasts. In these cases, widening the base width of the breast may be required for optimal correction of the deformity, but the patient should understand and accept the potential coverage compromises that might occur in the future and acknowledge these possible consequences in informed consent documents preoperatively.

Implant Volume Parameters

The system should suggest an optimal volume for the patient's envelope dimensions and tissue characteristics. Optimal volume is defined as the volume of implant required to adequately fill the existing envelope and produce the desired result with minimal long-term tissue consequences.

Minimal objective measurements to predict volume include base width of the breast and skin stretch. Additional measurements that refine optimal volume requirements include measurements of lower pole skin quantity and the quantity of existing parenchyma. Additional measurements add little to a system that has proved itself over a decade in over 4500 augmentations with up to 15 year followup. These optimal, essential measurements include *base width* (BW) of the existing breast parenchyma, quantitative

> Optimal volume is defined as the volume of implant required to adequately fill the existing envelope and produce the desired result with minimal long-term tissue consequences

measurement of *anterior pull skin stretch* (*APSS*), quantitative measurement of *nipple-to-fold distance under maximal stretch* (*N:IMF$_{max\ stretch}$*), and an *estimate of parenchymal contribution to stretched envelope fill* (*PCSEF*).

Surgeons can optionally add implant height and projection measurements to planning considerations, but making these measurements on the patient is challenging, because landmarks are indistinct and the measurements are difficult to reproduce.

Useless and potentially misleading measurements and measurement concepts

Sternal notch to nipple (SN:N) measurements are largely useless in primary breast augmentation for the following reasons: (1) the inframammary fold is the only fixed landmark of the breast and defines the position of the breast on the torso, (2) optimal breast aesthetics require a specific nipple-to-inframammary fold (N:IMF) distance that is proportionate and quantitatively related to the base width (BW) of the breast, (3) in primary breast augmentation, surgeons do not routinely reposition the inframammary fold cephalad, and (4) SN:N is a byproduct of (1) and (2) above that if considered individually can lead to surgeons creating disproportionate N:IMF distances.

When nipple levels are markedly different bilaterally, surgeons may consider SN:N, but should remember that primary augmentation does not reposition the breast on the torso. Altering SN:N without assuring that the resulting N:IMF is appropriate for breast width can create aesthetic disasters that are difficult or impossible to correct. Virtually every patient has one breast that is located slightly higher on the torso compared to the opposite breast. This means that the levels of the inframammary folds on the two sides are different. If a surgeon attempts to lower one fold to match the other without considering effects on nipple position, the result is often an excessively upward displaced nipple-areola on the side where the surgeon lowers the inframammary fold and often an excessively long N:IMF. Similarly, if the surgeon moves one nipple-areola complex (NAC) to a level to match the other when the locations of the inframammary folds are different on the two sides, one side will have an excessively long N:IMF compared to the other with a "bottomed out" appearance of the breast on that side, even though SN:N matches on the two sides. The author's indications for nipple-areola repositioning are (1) SN:N measurement > 1.5 cm different on the two sides, (2) the patient is concerned about the nipple level differences and accepts all risks, costs, and tradeoffs of nipple-areola repositioning, and (3) NAC levels can be adjusted to maintain similar BW to N:IMF distances bilaterally. *A key concept for surgeons to remember is that the most important relationship to optimize aesthetics is an N:IMF distance that is proportionate to BW; this requires making N:IMF distance symmetric bilaterally, regardless of any other considerations.* Surgeons must thoroughly educate patients preoperatively that (1) breast augmentation does not reposition the breast on the torso, (2) NAC positions and the levels of the inframammary folds never match before or after a breast augmentation, and (3) the best compromise for optimal aesthetics is to try to create similar N:IMFs bilaterally that are proportionate to the width of the breast.

> A key concept for surgeons to remember is that the most important relationship to optimize aesthetics is an N:IMF distance that is proportionate to BW; this requires making N:IMF distance symmetric bilaterally, regardless of any other considerations

■ OPTIMIZING OUTCOMES USING QUANTITATIVE TISSUE ASSESSMENT AND DECISION PROCESS SYSTEMS

Essentials to Achieve Optimal Outcomes

Preoperative decisions and intraoperative execution determine results and outcomes. The quality of surgeon and patient decisions relates directly to the quality and quantity of information (data) used to make decisions. Optimal outcomes with minimal complications and reoperations occur when patients and surgeons use *optimal decision processes* (decision algorithms) and *objective, quantifiable, tissue based data* to make the critical decisions that determine outcomes. The best opportunity to optimize outcomes is preoperatively, by insisting on objective quantifiable data to use in the decision making process, and by implementing proved decision processes to make decisions of implant pocket location, implant volume and type, optimal location of the inframammary fold, and incision location.

Optimal decisions require an orderly, prioritized approach to decision making that is algorithmic, not random—a defined decision making approach that prioritizes and orders the decisions that most impact outcomes. *Making decisions does not optimize outcomes unless surgeons and patients base decisions on objective, quantifiable data and unless they used proved, optimal decision processes that prioritize and order decisions in a manner that has been scientifically tested, peer reviewed and published, and implemented by other surgeons.* An optimal decision making process is a process that has been thoroughly tested by surgeons in valid scientific studies that are peer reviewed and published in the most respected journal in plastic surgery. Most surgeons have an individual "system" for making decisions relating to breast augmentation, but optimal outcomes for large numbers of patients require that surgeons identify and implement

> Optimal decisions require an orderly, prioritized approach to decision making that is algorithmic, not random—a defined decision making approach that prioritizes and orders the decisions that most impact outcomes

"best practices" or proved processes that have been clearly shown to deliver superior outcomes.

Adopting Successful Business Principles and "Best Practices" to Improve Outcomes

The world's most successful businesses use highly paid consultants to identify proved processes or "best practices" that other businesses have successfully implemented to deliver high performance and a track record of success. A company develops a "best practice" by using process engineering principles to perform detailed examinations and analyses of the processes that the company uses to manufacture a product, improve efficiency, or address customer needs. Every process can be improved, and the most successful companies commit substantial resources to constant reexamination and improvement of critical processes.

When a refined process delivers consistent, predictable, and long-term desired outcomes (greater efficiency, productivity, and profits), the process or processes become a "best practice" that consultants and other businesses recognize. To successfully compete, other companies want to learn and implement these "best practices" to improve their own bottom lines. Adopting proved processes or best practices is a win–win situation for businesses and their customers—the business delivers a superior product with greater efficiency, lower cost, and a higher profit margin, and the customer receives all of the benefits of a better product with fewer malfunctions, problems, and a longer product life span.

A similar win–win situation occurs when plastic surgeons adopt and implement "best practices" and proved processes in breast augmentation. The surgeon becomes more efficient by focusing on key processes that have been proved to affect outcomes, while minimizing time waste addressing variables that have not been shown to affect outcomes. More importantly, by following a proved template of prioritized decisions, the surgeon is less likely to overlook key decisions or base key decisions on less than optimal data. Suboptimal decisions produce suboptimal outcomes that in turn require large commitments of surgeon time to treat complications or deal with untoward results and unhappy patients. The same decisions and processes that increase surgeon efficiency shorten operative times, reduce the amount of anesthetic drugs that a patient receives, improve key surgical techniques, dramatically reduce postoperative morbidity, and allow patients to be out to dinner the evening of their breast augmentation and return to full normal activities within 24 hours with long-term reoperation rates at up to 9 years of 3% or less.[5–8,10] Refinement and implementation of proved processes in breast augmentation has, in peer reviewed and published studies, redefined the surgeon and patient experience in breast augmentation. Tissue based, quantitative preoperative assessment and decision making requires less than 5 minutes of surgeon time while applying the most state-of-the-art processes that produce the most rapid recovery in published literature. Operative times are shorter, surgery center costs and costs to patients decrease, surgeons can perform more procedures in less time, patients' recovery is dramatically faster, morbidity is less, and long-term reoperation rates dramatically decrease.

Integrating Quantifiable Tissue Based Assessment with Proved Decision Support Processes

Optimal outcomes and minimal reoperation rates require (1) a tissue based, quantitative preoperative assessment system to provide objective data, and (2) a decision process that prioritizes and orders decisions that most impact outcomes. By integrating a quantitative tissue assessment system with a proved decision process system, surgeons and patients have optimal data to make optimal decisions for optimal outcomes. In order to effectively address these requirements, the author recognized the need for two integrated systems, and the result was the development of the TEPID™ System[1] for implant selection based on quantitative tissue characteristics, and the High Five™ System,[11] a prioritized decision assist system that integrates the TEPID™ System.

By integrating a quantitative tissue assessment system with a proved decision process system, surgeons and patients have optimal data to make optimal decisions for optimal outcomes

In the April 2002 issue of *Plastic and Reconstructive Surgery*, the author published a system for breast implant selection based on patient tissue characteristics and implant–soft tissue dynamics, the TEPID™ System.[1] TEPID is an acronym for tissue characteristics of the breast (T), the envelope (E), parenchyma (P), implant (I), and the dimensions (D) and dynamics of the implant relative to the soft tissues. This study of 627 consecutive breast augmentations using the system conclusively demonstrated the efficacy of the system. The system eliminated the need for intraoperative sizer implants, and dramatically reduced the number of implants that were ordered for each case, with only six cases requiring more than one size implant ordered for the procedure. Only two reoperations for size change were performed in the study, a rate dramatically lower compared to previous FDA PMA studies,[2–4] and in only eight cases did the surgeon deviate at all from the implant volume recommended by the system.

The TEPID™ System provided the first objective, quantitatively based tissue assessment system that based implant size selection on patient tissue characteristics

The TEPID™ System provided the first objective, quantitatively based tissue assessment system that based implant size selection on patient tissue characteristics. Experience using the system in the author's practice now includes more than 3500 consecutive breast augmentations, with no reoperations for size exchange in the last 1700 cases, and an overall reoperation rate up to 9 year followup of less than 3%. Other surgeons, including the author's associates, have adopted the system with similar results.[11] In the author's practice, patients are performing self measurements and using the system during the patient education process to help them understand reasonable ranges of implant size based on their individual tissue characteristics and breast dimensions. The system is simple, effective, and individualizes implant and pocket selection criteria to maximize soft tissue coverage and minimize long-term uncorrectable tissue changes and deformities.

The High Five™ System,[11] published in the December 2005 issue of *Plastic and Reconstructive Surgery*, prioritizes the five most critical decisions in preoperative planning for augmentation mammaplasty. Integrating the quantitative tissue assessment data from the TEPID™ System, the High Five™ System uses the objective, quantified data to make decisions in order of priority of impacting outcomes. This proved process template has enabled the author and colleagues in the United States and Europe to deliver a predictable, consistent return to normal activities in 24 hours or less with a long-term reoperation rate in large series of less than 3%. This level of transferable, reproducible recovery and long-term outcomes is unmatched by any series in the published medical literature over the past four decades. Most recently, implementation of these proved processes enabled the author to report zero percent reoperation rate in 50 consecutive patients in an FDA study of Inamed/Allergan Style 410 form stable, cohesive gel anatomic breast implants,[8] a first in the history of FDA PMA studies for breast implants.

The High Five™ Tissue Assessment and Decision Support System

The High Five™ tissue assessment and decision support process for breast augmentation is a third generation decision support process that prioritizes five critical decisions, identifies five key measurements, and completes all preoperative assessment and operative planning decisions in breast augmentation in 5 minutes or less.

When planning and performing primary breast augmentation, surgeons must make decisions that consider variables and choose alternatives that ultimately determine outcomes. If critical preoperative decisions and choices are suboptimal, suboptimal long-term outcomes are almost certain, and uncorrectable tissue compromises and deformities can occur. Preoperative choice of implant pocket location determines the adequacy of

The High Five™ tissue assessment and decision support process for breast augmentation is a third generation decision support process that prioritizes five critical decisions, identifies five key measurements, and completes all preoperative assessment and operative planning decisions in breast augmentation in 5 minutes or less

soft tissue coverage over all areas of the implant for the patient's lifetime. Choice of implant volume and size defines the amount of weight and pressure the implant exerts on adjacent and overlying tissues over time, and determines the extent of potentially negative tissue consequences that the implant can produce.

While more than 50 tissue and surgeon variables listed in Table 7-1 occur in every breast augmentation, a clinically practical and adoptable preoperative decision process must prioritize the most critical decisions that determine long-term outcomes. Surgeons can improve outcomes, reduce reoperation rates, and improve practice efficiency by integrating quantitative preoperative tissue assessment with a systematic approach to five critical decisions in breast augmentation. The High Five™ decision support process adds a defined decision support component to the established TEPID™ System of implant selection based on individual patient tissue characteristics.

Five Critical Decisions in Breast Augmentation Planning

Surgeons must make decisions in five critical areas when planning a breast augmentation (Table 7-3). Each of these decisions should be based on quantifiable measurements or data. In order of priority, these decisions define:

1. Optimal soft tissue *coverage/pocket location for the implant*

2. Implant *volume* (weight)

3. *Implant* type, shape, dimensions

4. Optimal *location for the inframammary fold* based on the width of the implant selected for augmentation

5. *Incision* location.

Surgeons must make decisions in five critical areas when planning a breast augmentation

Table 7-3. **Five prioritized decisions of the High Five™ System.**

1. Soft tissue coverage: Pocket location

2. Implant size (weight)

3. Implant type, shape, dimensions

4. Imframammary fold position (N:IMF)

5. Incision location

Each of these decisions directly impacts outcomes in breast augmentation and determines potential consequences to the patient's tissues over time:

- Optimal soft tissue *coverage/pocket location for the implant* determines future risks of visible traction rippling, visible or palpable implant edges, and possible risks of excessive stretch or extrusion. Providing and maintaining optimal long-term soft tissue coverage is the number one priority in breast augmentation if avoiding reoperations and uncorrectable deformities and tissue compromises is a priority.

- Implant *volume* (weight) determines implant effects on tissues over time, and risks of excessive stretch, excessive thinning, visible or palpable implant edges, visible traction rippling, ptosis, and parenchymal atrophy. Implant volume and weight directly impact the degree of potential negative effects of a breast implant on patient tissues over time.

- *Implant type, size, dimensions* determine control over distribution of fill within the breast, adequacy of envelope fill, and risks of excessive stretch, excessive thinning, visible or palpable implant edges, visible traction rippling, ptosis, and parenchymal atrophy. Implant dimensions or projection that force tissues to a desired result that exceeds tissue tolerances risk uncorrectable tissue compromises including excessive skin stretch and thinning, parenchymal atrophy, and chest wall deformities.

- Optimal *location for the inframammary fold* based on the width of the implant selected for augmentation determines the position of the breast on the chest wall, the critical aesthetic relationship between breast width and nipple-to-fold distance, and distribution of fill (especially upper pole fill). For optimal aesthetics and to avoid "boxy" or "bottomed out" appearing breasts, nipple-to-inframammary fold distance must be proportionate to the base width of the augmented breast.

- *Incision* location determines degree of trauma to adjacent soft tissues, exposure of implant to endogenous bacteria in the breast tissue, surgeon visibility and control, potential injury to adjacent neurovasculature, and potential postoperative morbidity or tradeoffs.

Clinical Experience with the High Five™ Tissue Assessment and Decision Support Process

The clinical experience in the published report of the High Five™ process in 2005[11] was over 2300 consecutive breast augmentations with up to 7 year followup, with an overall

The clinical experience in the published report of the High Five™ process in 2005[11] was over 2300 consecutive breast augmentations with up to 7 year followup, with an overall reoperation rate of 2.9% and a reoperation rate for implant size exchange of 0.3%.

reoperation rate of 2.9% and a reoperation rate for implant size exchange of 0.3%. These results strongly suggest a benefit of using quantitative assessment and proved decision processes when compared with averaged data from McGhan and Mentor FDA PMA studies for saline implants which reported overall reoperation rates of 17% and reoperation rates for size exchange or adjustment of 8.7% at just 3 years postoperatively.

Since publication of the High Five™ process, clinical experience with the system has increased exponentially as associates and colleagues in the United States and internationally have implemented the system. The simplicity, efficiency, reproducibility, and transferability of the system have been consistently noted by colleagues, and colleagues have reported dramatic improvements in patient recovery, outcomes, and practice efficiency as they have implemented the system.

Clinical Evaluation and Patient Record Forms

Table 7-4 is a High Five™ Clinical Evaluation and Operative Planning Form, and Table 7-5 is a comprehensive Clinical Evaluation Form that integrates the High Five™ form with additional patient medical history information and documentation of patient choices following the patient education and informed consent process. Both of these forms are provided in the Resources folder on the accompanying DVDs in Microsoft Word™ and Adobe Acrobat™ pdf formats for surgeon use and modification to address individual preferences and needs.

Clinical Measurements and Methods for High Five™

The High Five™ process requires only five clinical measurements that a surgeon can perform and record in less than 5 minutes (Table 7-6). Each measurement relates directly to a critical decision that impacts outcomes and determines tissue consequences of breast augmentation over time.

Measurements are always better than subjective assessment, because measurements provide quantifiable data that are required for valid scientific analysis. Measurements that do not directly impact a decision are inefficient and can be misleading, leading to compromised decisions. The utmost "surgeon artistry" and "artistic eye" cannot substitute for objective measurements. Artistry complements but cannot substitute for objectivity if optimal, scientifically valid, long-term outcomes are a priority.

Surgeons can perform these measurements with the patient sitting upright or standing. Each measurement need not be accurate to the millimeter, and measurements may vary

The High Five™ process requires only five clinical measurements that a surgeon can perform and record in less than 5 minutes

Measurements are always better than subjective assessment, because measurements provide quantifiable data that are required for valid scientific analysis

Table 7-4. **High Five™ Clinical evaluation and operative planning form**

High Five™ Tissue Analysis and Operative Planning

Patient Name:		Date:	

1. COVERAGE- Selecting Pocket Location to Optimize Soft Tissue Coverage Short- and Long-Term

STPTUP		If <2.0 cm., consider dual plane (DP) or partial retropectoral (PRP, pectoralis origins intact across IMF)	DP
STPTIMF		If STPTIMF <0.5 cm, consider subpectoral pocket and leave pectoralis origins intact along IMF	PRP RM

POCKET LOCATION SELECTED BASED ON THICKNESS OF TISSUE COVERAGE

2. IMPLANT VOLUME- Selecting an Estimated Implant Volume for Optimal Envelope Fill

Estimating Desired Breast Implant Volume Based on Breast Measurements and Tissue Characteristics

Base Width		B.W. Parenchyma (cm)	10.5	11.0	11.5	12.0	12.5	13.0	13.5	14.0	14.5	15.0	cc
		Initial Volume (cc)	200	250	275	300	300	325	350	375	375	400	
APSS$_{MaxStr}$		[2]If APSS <2.0, −30 cc; If APSS >3.0, +30 cc; If APSS >4.0, +60 cc Place appropriate number in blank at right											cc
N:IMF$_{MaxSt}$		If N:IMF >9.5, +30 cc Place appropriate number in blank at right											cc
PCSEF %		If PCSEF <20%, +30 cc; If PCSEF >80%, −30 cc Place appropriate number in blank at right											cc
Pt. request													cc

[7]**NET ESTIMATED VOLUME** TO FILL ENVELOPE BASED ON PATIENT TISSUE CHARACTERISTICS ... cc

3. IMPLANT DIMENSIONS, TYPE, MANUFACTURER- Selecting specific implant characteristics

Implant Manufacturer	Implant Style/Shape/Shell/Filler Material	Implant Vol (cc)	*Implant Base Width	Breast Base Width[1]	Implant Projection
		cc	cm.	cm.	cm.

*For optimal long-term coverage, implant base width should not exceed base width of patient's existing parenchyma, even if wider IMD results.

4. INFRAMAMMARY FOLD LOCATION- Estimating desired postoperative inframammary fold position

(Circle Volume closest *to net estimated implant volume* calculated above, and *circle suggested N:IMF* in the cell beneath that volume)

		Volume closest to calculated "total estimated implant volume" above	200	250	275	300	325	350	375	400
		Recommended new N:IMF distance (cm.) under maximal stretch▶	7.0	7.0	7.5	8	8	8.5	9.0	9.5
*Planning Level of New Inframammary Fold**	Transfer the patient's N:IMF$_{MaxSt}$ measurement from above to corresponding cell at right. Then transfer the TEPID™ recommended new N:IMF to the corresponding cell at right. If the patient's preop N:IMF is shorter than the TEPID™ recommended new N:IMF, consider lowering the fold. If the patient's preop N:IMF is equal to or greater than the TEPID™ recommended new N:IMF, no change in IMF position is indicated.		Patient's Preoperative N:IMF$_{MaxSt}$		TEPID™ Recommended N:IMF$_{MaxSt}$	Change In Fold Position	Lower Fold		
				cm.		cm.	Yes/No	cm.		

*Other factors may affect optimal IMF level and require surgeons to modifiy the TEPID™ System recommendations for N:IMF

5. INCISION LOCATION- Selecting desired incision location

Inframammary	Axillary	Periareolar	Umbilical

Table 7-5. Augmentation Mammaplasty Clinical Evaluation for _____ Patient Preferences, Objectives, Preparation, History, Limitations, Exam, Surgical Choices

Size: Pt. Desires: ❏ Natural appearing breast ❏ Unnatural, bulging upper breast ❏ Proportionate to protect tissues ❏ Very large *Approximate* Desired Cup _____ Requests specific cc's:

_____

❏ Pt. Chooses Size ❏ Pt. Leaves Size Choice to Dr. Tebbetts
Implant: ❏ Round ❏ Anatomic ❏ Smooth ❏ Textured
❏ Saline ❏ Silicone ❏ Pt. Leaves Type Choice to Dr. Tebbetts
Pocket Location: ❏ PRP ❏ RM ❏ Dr. Tebbetts to decide
Incision Location: ❏ IM ❏ PA ❏ AX ❏ UMB
❏ Pt. Leaves Incision Choice to Dr. Tebbetts Pts. Initials _____

Capsular Contracture and Tissue Stretch Factors:
❏ Implant choice may affect risk
❏ Pt. accepts full responsibility for all costs for any surgery necessary to treat any capsule or tissue stretch deformities and costs exceed costs of original surgery
Pts. Initials _____

Patient Has Completed, Read and Signed:
❏ Pt. Educator Consult ❏ Choice Documents
❏ The Best Breast Book Pt. Ed. Initials: _____
Discussed/Patient Accepts That:
❏ Implants will be removed/not replaced if one infection or 2 capsular contractures occur
❏ The larger the implant, the more risks of sensory loss, tissue damage, and need for reoperations
Pts. Initials _____

Age _____
Height _____ Wt. _____ lbs
Frame: ❏ Sm ❏ Med ❏ Lrg
Torso: ❏ Nl ❏ Wide ❏ Nr
Gravida _____
Para _____
Bra **Band** Size: 32, 34, 36
Breast **Cup** Size (Approx.)
Prior to pregnancy _____
Largest with preg _____
Current Cup Size _____
Desired Cup Size _____
Previous Breast Disease:
❏ None
Biopsies: ❏ No ❏ Yes
_____
Family Hx. Breast Cancer
❏ No ❏ Yes
Mother Grandmother Aunt
❏ Maternal ❏ Paternal

Previous Mammograms:
❏ No ❏ Yes
Date: _____
Interpretation: ❏ Normal
❏ Other: _____
Pertinent Medical History:
❏ None
_____
_____
Smoker: ❏ No ❏ Yes _____
Allergies: ❏ NKA
_____
Current Meds, Herbs, Vits:
_____
Companion: _____
Relation: _____

Specific Limitations Discussed with Patient:
❏ Your breasts will never match
❏ You may lose some or all sensation
❏ You may see or feel edges of your implant due to thin tissues
❏ You may require reoperations and additional costs in the future due to implant size requested, your tissue stretch characteristics or capsule you form
❏ We give no guarantee of cup size
❏ Any reoperation may require an inframammary incision
❏ Other:
_____
❏ Patient vocalizes understanding and acceptance of all items checked above. Pt. Initials _____

Breast Masses
❏ None
❏ Size and Location:
_____

Larger Breast:
❏ Left ❏ Right
Est. Vol. Diff. _____ cc
TBD
Nipple Level
Discrepancy _____ cm
N/A
IMF Level
Discrepancy _____ cm
N/A
Envelope Compliance
❏ Nl ❏ Inc ❏ Dec
❏ Constricted Lower Env.
❏ Short, fixed IMF
❏ Other:
_____

The High Five™ measurements and decisions data chart from Table 7-4 can be combined on a single page with the clinical evaluation data in Table 7-5 for optimal surgeon efficiency during the surgeon consultation. This combined document is available in MS Word™ and Adobe Acrobat™ pdf formats on the DVDs that accompany this book.

Table 7-6. Five simple measurements of the High Five™ System.

| 1. Soft tissue pinch thickness upper pole **(STPTUP)** |

| 2. Soft tissue pinch thickness at IMF **(STPTIMF)** |

| 3. Base width (BW) |

| 4. Anterior pull skin stretch (APSS) |

| 5. Nipple-to-inframammary fold distance (N:IMF) |

slightly among surgeons or from one measuring session to another. The system is designed to accommodate these variances while providing essential information for decision making. Every surgeon becomes more consistent with the measurements with increasing experience and repetition. When measurements approach limits that suggest a decision change, the surgeon should consider all additional variables that are present in the case before making definitive decisions.

The High Five™ process includes five clinical measurements:

1. Base width (BW) of the existing breast parenchyma
2. Anterior pull skin stretch (APSS)
3. Soft tissue pinch thickness of the upper pole (STPTUP)
4. Soft tissue pinch thickness at the inframammary fold (STPTIMF)
5. Nipple-to-inframammary fold distance under maximal stretch ($N:IMF_{max\ stretch}$).

For additional accuracy, surgeons should estimate the existing parenchyma's contribution to stretched envelope fill (PCSEF) as a percentage of final desired volume. Optimal accuracy requires that surgeons use a flexible tape measure and calipers to perform the measurements. If calipers are not available, surgeons and patients can perform the measurements with only a flexible tape measure, but the measurements may be slightly less accurate.

Each of the five clinical measurements is critical to the five prioritized decisions in the High Five™ process. Table 7-7 is an illustrated flowchart that details each measurement

Text continued on p. 163

Table 7-7. High Five™ tissue assessment and decision processes flowchart.

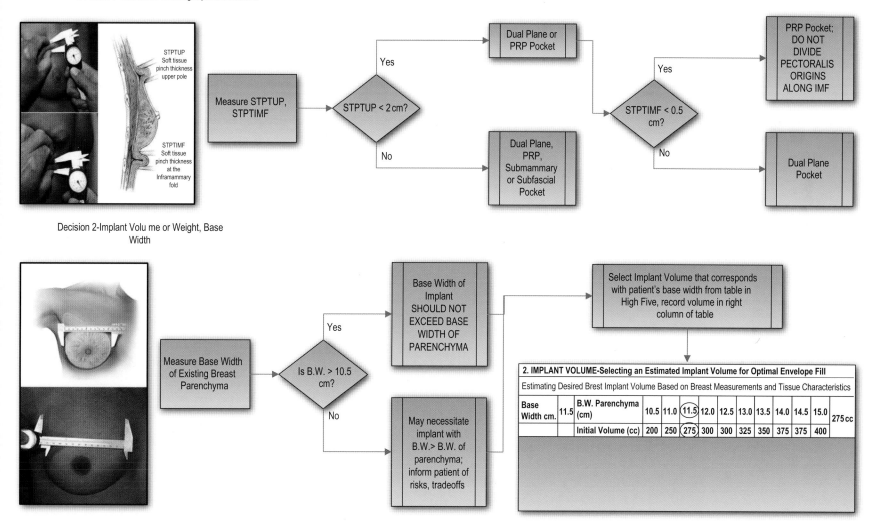

Decision 1-Soft tissue coverage; pocket location

- STPTUP Soft tissue pinch thickness upper pole
- STPTIMF Soft tissue pinch thickness at the Inframammary fold

Measure STPTUP, STPTIMF

STPTUP < 2 cm?

Yes → Dual Plane or PRP Pocket

No → Dual Plane, PRP, Submammary or Subfascial Pocket

STPTIMF < 0.5 cm?

Yes → PRP Pocket; DO NOT DIVIDE PECTORALIS ORIGINS ALONG IMF

No → Dual Plane Pocket

Decision 2-Implant Volu me or Weight, Base Width

Measure Base Width of Existing Breast Parenchyma

Is B.W. > 10.5 cm?

Yes → Base Width of Implant SHOULD NOT EXCEED BASE WIDTH OF PARENCHYMA

No → May necessitate implant with B.W.> B.W. of parenchyma; inform patient of risks, tradeoffs

Select Implant Volume that corresponds with patient's base width from table in High Five, record volume in right column of table

2. IMPLANT VOLUME-Selecting an Estimated Implant Volume for Optimal Envelope Fill

Estimating Desired Brest Implant Volume Based on Breast Measurements and Tissue Characteristics

Base Width cm.	11.5	B.W. Parenchyma (cm)	10.5	11.0	11.5	12.0	12.5	13.0	13.5	14.0	14.5	15.0	275 cc
		Initial Volume (cc)	200	250	275	300	300	325	350	375	375	400	

Table 7-7. High Five™ tissue assessment and decision processes flowchart, Page 2—cont'd

Decision 2-Implant Volume or Weight, APSS

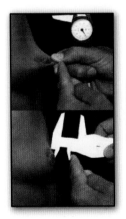

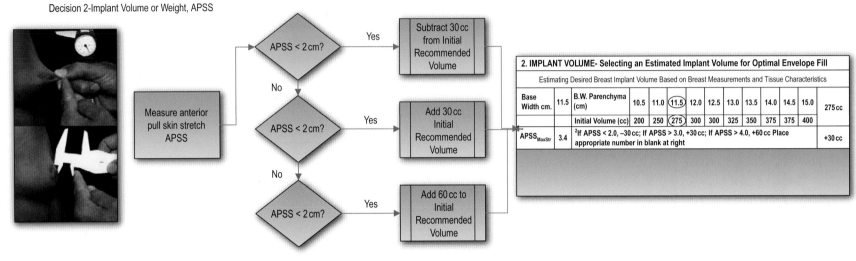

```
Measure anterior
pull skin stretch
APSS
```

```
APSS < 2 cm?  ──Yes──▶  Subtract 30 cc
                          from Initial
                          Recommended
                          Volume
   │
   No
   │
APSS < 2 cm?  ──Yes──▶  Add 30 cc
                          Initial
                          Recommended
                          Volume
   │
   No
   │
APSS < 2 cm?  ──Yes──▶  Add 60 cc to
                          Initial
                          Recommended
                          Volume
```

2. IMPLANT VOLUME- Selecting an Estimated Implant Volume for Optimal Envelope Fill

Estimating Desired Breast Implant Volume Based on Breast Measurements and Tissue Characteristics

Base Width cm.	11.5	B.W. Parenchyma (cm)	10.5	11.0	(11.5)	12.0	12.5	13.0	13.5	14.0	14.5	15.0	275 cc
		Initial Volume (cc)	200	250	(275)	300	300	325	350	375	375	400	
APSS$_{MaxStr}$	3.4	[2]If APSS < 2.0, −30 cc; If APSS > 3.0, +30 cc; If APSS > 4.0, +60 cc Place appropriate number in blank at right											+30 cc

Decision 2-Implant Volume or Weight, N:IMF

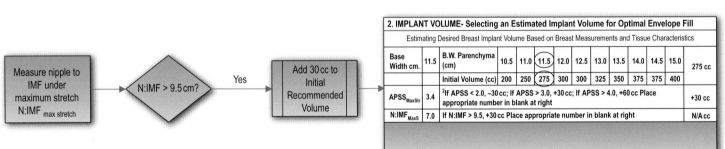

```
Measure nipple to
IMF under
maximum stretch
N:IMF max stretch
```

```
N:IMF > 9.5 cm?  ──Yes──▶  Add 30 cc to
                             Initial
                             Recommended
                             Volume
```

2. IMPLANT VOLUME- Selecting an Estimated Implant Volume for Optimal Envelope Fill

Estimating Desired Breast Implant Volume Based on Breast Measurements and Tissue Characteristics

Base Width cm.	11.5	B.W. Parenchyma (cm)	10.5	11.0	(11.5)	12.0	12.5	13.0	13.5	14.0	14.5	15.0	275 cc
		Initial Volume (cc)	200	250	(275)	300	300	325	350	375	375	400	
APSS$_{MaxStr}$	3.4	[2]If APSS < 2.0, −30 cc; If APSS > 3.0, +30 cc; If APSS > 4.0, +60 cc Place appropriate number in blank at right											+30 cc
N:IMF$_{MaxS}$	7.0	If N:IMF > 9.5, +30 cc Place appropriate number in blank at right											N/A cc

Table 7-7. High Five™ tissue assessment and decision processes flowchart, Page 3—cont'd

Decision 2-Implant Volume or Weight, PCSEF

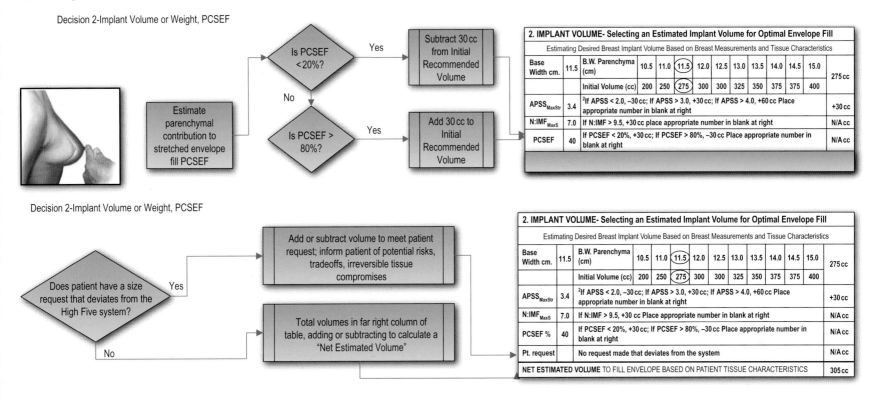

Is PCSEF <20%? — Yes → Subtract 30 cc from Initial Recommended Volume

No

Estimate parenchymal contribution to stretched envelope fill PCSEF

Is PCSEF > 80%? — Yes → Add 30 cc to Initial Recommended Volume

2. IMPLANT VOLUME- Selecting an Estimated Implant Volume for Optimal Envelope Fill

Estimating Desired Breast Implant Volume Based on Breast Measurements and Tissue Characteristics

Base Width cm.	11.5	B.W. Parenchyma (cm)	10.5	11.0	(11.5)	12.0	12.5	13.0	13.5	14.0	14.5	15.0	275 cc
		Initial Volume (cc)	200	250	(275)	300	300	325	350	375	375	400	
$APSS_{MaxStr}$	3.4	[2]If APSS < 2.0, –30 cc; If APSS > 3.0, +30 cc; If APSS > 4.0, +60 cc Place appropriate number in blank at right											+30 cc
$N{:}IMF_{MaxS}$	7.0	If N:IMF > 9.5, +30 cc place appropriate number in blank at right											N/A cc
PCSEF	40	If PCSEF < 20%, +30 cc; If PCSEF > 80%, –30 cc Place appropriate number in blank at right											N/A cc

Decision 2-Implant Volume or Weight, PCSEF

Does patient have a size request that deviates from the High Five system? — Yes → Add or subtract volume to meet patient request; inform patient of potential risks, tradeoffs, irreversible tissue compromises

No

Total volumes in far right column of table, adding or subtracting to calculate a "Net Estimated Volume"

2. IMPLANT VOLUME- Selecting an Estimated Implant Volume for Optimal Envelope Fill

Estimating Desired Breast Implant Volume Based on Breast Measurements and Tissue Characteristics

Base Width cm.	11.5	B.W. Parenchyma (cm)	10.5	11.0	(11.5)	12.0	12.5	13.0	13.5	14.0	14.5	15.0	275 cc
		Initial Volume (cc)	200	250	(275)	300	300	325	350	375	375	400	
$APSS_{MaxStr}$	3.4	[2]If APSS < 2.0, –30 cc; If APSS > 3.0, +30 cc; If APSS > 4.0, +60 cc Place appropriate number in blank at right											+30 cc
$N{:}IMF_{MaxS}$	7.0	If N:IMF > 9.5, +30 cc Place appropriate number in blank at right											N/A cc
PCSEF %	40	If PCSEF < 20%, +30 cc; If PCSEF > 80%, –30 cc Place appropriate number in blank at right											N/A cc
Pt. request		No request made that deviates from the system											N/A cc
NET ESTIMATED VOLUME TO FILL ENVELOPE BASED ON PATIENT TISSUE CHARACTERISTICS													305 cc

Decision 3-Implant Type, Dimensions, Shape, Filler Material

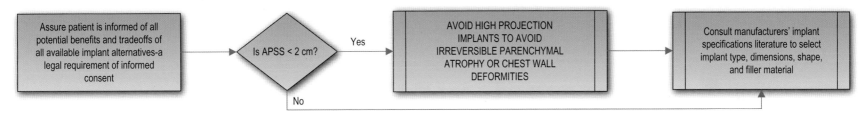

Assure patient is informed of all potential benefits and tradeoffs of all available implant alternatives-a legal requirement of informed consent

Is APSS < 2 cm? — Yes → AVOID HIGH PROJECTION IMPLANTS TO AVOID IRREVERSIBLE PARENCHYMAL ATROPHY OR CHEST WALL DEFORMITIES → Consult manufacturers' implant specifications literature to select implant type, dimensions, shape, and filler material

No

Table 7-7. High Five™ tissue assessment and decision processes flowchart, Page 4—cont'd

Decision 4-Determining optimal position for the inframammary fold

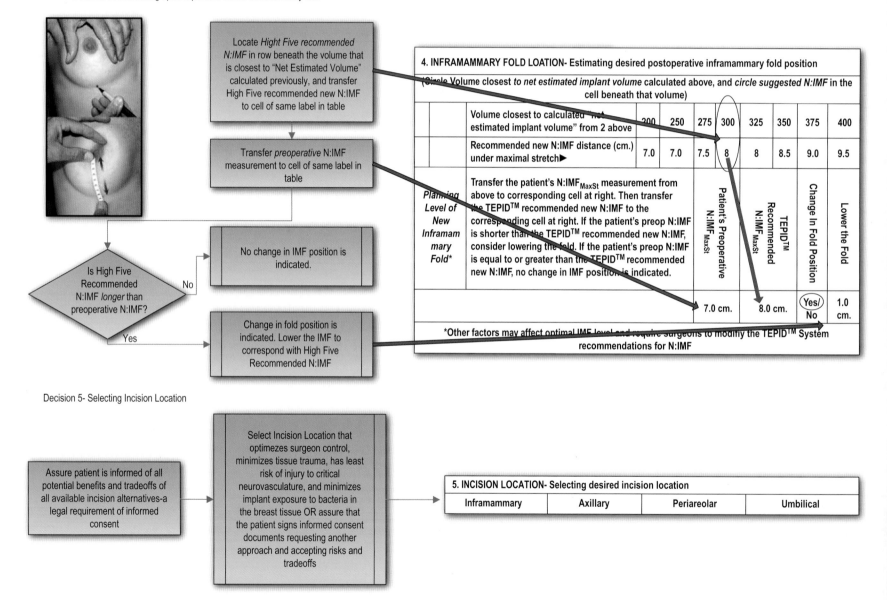

Locate *Hight Five recommended N:IMF* in row beneath the volume that is closest to "Net Estimated Volume" calculated previously, and transfer High Five recommended new N:IMF to cell of same label in table

Transfer *preoperative* N:IMF measurement to cell of same label in table

Is High Five Recommended N:IMF *longer* than preoperative N:IMF?

No → No change in IMF position is indicated.

Yes → Change in fold position is indicated. Lower the IMF to correspond with High Five Recommended N:IMF

4. INFRAMAMMARY FOLD LOATION- Estimating desired postoperative inframammary fold position

(Circle Volume closest *to net estimated implant volume* calculated above, and *circle suggested N:IMF* in the cell beneath that volume)

	Volume closest to calculated "net estimated implant volume" from 2 above	200	250	275	300	325	350	375	400
	Recommended new N:IMF distance (cm.) under maximal stretch▶	7.0	7.0	7.5	8	8	8.5	9.0	9.5

Planning Level of New Inframam mary Fold*	Transfer the patient's N:IMF_MaxSt measurement from above to corresponding cell at right. Then transfer the TEPID™ recommended new N:IMF to the corresponding cell at right. If the patient's preop N:IMF is shorter than the TEPID™ recommended new N:IMF, consider lowering the fold. If the patient's preop N:IMF is equal to or greater than the TEPID™ recommended new N:IMF, no change in IMF position is indicated.	Patient's Preoperative N:IMF_MaxSt	TEPID™ Recommended N:IMF_MaxSt	Change In Fold Position	Lower the Fold
		7.0 cm.	8.0 cm.	Yes/ No	1.0 cm.

*Other factors may affect optimal IMF level and require surgeons to modify the TEPID™ System recommendations for N:IMF

Decision 5- Selecting Incision Location

Assure patient is informed of all potential benefits and tradeoffs of all available incision alternatives-a legal requirement of informed consent

Select Incision Location that optimezes surgeon control, minimizes tissue trauma, has least risk of injury to critical neurovasculature, and minimizes implant exposure to bacteria in the breast tissue OR assure that the patient signs informed consent documents requesting another approach and accepting risks and tradeoffs

5. INCISION LOCATION- Selecting desired incision location

Inframammary	Axillary	Periareolar	Umbilical

and associated decision in the High Five™ process by using example measurements to complete the High Five™ Clinical Evaluation Form in a stepwise progression.

Since the number one priority is providing and maintaining optimal soft tissue coverage over all areas of the implant long-term, the first measurement, *soft tissue pinch thickness of the upper pole* (STPTUP) quantifies soft tissue coverage in the upper breast where upper pole implant edge visibility is most likely long-term. To measure STPTUP (Figure 7-1, upper), the surgeon grasps the skin and subcutaneous tissue superior to the patient's

Figure 7-1. Upper: Soft tissue pinch tissue measurement of the thickness of the subcutaneous tissue that would be covering the implant with a submammary or subfascial pocket location. If less than 2 cm, surgeons should choose dual plane or partial retropectoral pocket location to optimize long-term soft tissue coverage. Lower: The surgeon measures STPTIMF by firmly pinching soft tissues at the inframammary fold and measuring with calipers.

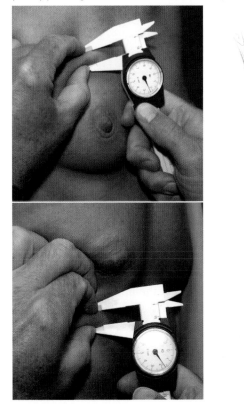

STPTUP
Soft tissue
pinch thickness
upper pole

STPTIMF
Soft tissue
pinch thickness
at the
inframammary
fold

When STPTUP is less than 2 cm, in order to provide optimal long-term soft tissue coverage surgeons should prioritize a traditional subpectoral or dual plane pocket location instead of a submammary or subfascial pocket location

breast parenchyma in the upper pole of the breast, pinches it firmly, and measures the pinched thickness of skin and subcutaneous tissue with calipers. When measuring patients with very little subcutaneous tissue, the surgeon must avoid inadvertently pinching and lifting the pectoralis major muscle when performing this measurement. *When STPTUP is less than 2 cm, in order to provide optimal long-term soft tissue coverage surgeons should prioritize a traditional subpectoral or dual plane pocket location instead of a submammary or subfascial pocket location.* Surgeons can avoid inadvertently including the pectoralis muscle either by asking the patient to tense the pectoralis by pushing the hands together at the umbilicus, or by grasping pectoralis with soft tissue and then releasing gently and regrasping only subcutaneous tissue.

The second measurement, soft tissue pinch thickness at the inframammary fold (STPTIMF), quantifies thickness of skin and soft tissue at the fold to assist in deciding whether dividing pectoralis major muscle origins along the inframammary fold in dual plane techniques to minimize tradeoffs of traditional partial subpectoral pocket locations will leave the patient with adequate soft tissue coverage at the inframammary fold. To measure STPTIMF (Figure 7-1, lower), the surgeon grasps the skin and subcutaneous tissue at or immediately adjacent to the inframammary fold, pinches it firmly, and measures the pinched thickness of skin and subcutaneous tissue with calipers. *When STPTIMF is less than 0.5 cm (and the surgeon is already considering a subpectoral or dual plane pocket with STPTUP less than 2.0 cm), the surgeon should leave inferior origins of the pectoralis major along the inframammary fold intact* and select the traditional subpectoral pocket instead of a dual plane pocket in which the surgeon divides the pectoralis origins along the inframammary fold.

When STPTIMF is less than 0.5 cm (and the surgeon is already considering a subpectoral or dual plane pocket with STPTUP less than 2.0 cm), the surgeon should leave inferior origins of the pectoralis major along the inframammary fold intact

The third measurement, base width (BW), quantifies the base width of the patient's existing parenchyma. This measurement is the single most important measurement, because it provides information for two critical decisions. The wider the breast, the more volume is required for optimal fill or the more volume the breast can accommodate without excessive skin stretch or parenchymal atrophy, hence this measurement is critical to estimate optimal implant volume. If the base width of the implant exceeds the base width of the patient's existing parenchyma (and as a rule it should not in over 95% of primary augmentations), edges of the implant are covered only by skin and subcutaneous tissue that stretches and often thins with aging. When implant base width exceeds the base width of the existing parenchyma, risks of implant edge visibility, palpability, and visible traction rippling increase exponentially. When BW is less than 11 cm in rare cases of constricted or "tubular" breasts, optimal aesthetic results may require selecting an implant with a base width greater than the 10 cm base width of the patient's existing parenchyma. In each case, surgeons should thoroughly inform the patient of potential tradeoffs, long-term tissue compromises or uncorrectable tissue changes that might result from prioritizing aesthetics to achieve a desired aesthetic result. To measure BW (Figure 7-2), the surgeon uses the calipers to measure the width of the patient's existing breast parenchyma in anteroposterior view. This is a linear measurement, not a curved measurement over the surface of the breast. The surgeon places the medial caliper tip at the point where the visible upslope of the breast begins, and laterally at the lateral profile line of the breast. The base width is the first measurement that will be used later in the High Five™ decision process.

The fourth measurement, anterior pull skin stretch (APSS), quantifies the degree of maximal anterior stretch of the areolar skin with manual traction anteriorly. Combined with base width, skin stretch is a major determinant of optimal volume required to fill an envelope. APSS also provides a quantitative measurement of limits of stretch when skin compliance is limited. To measure APSS, the surgeon advises the patient that strong skin stretching is necessary. Holding the caliper in the palm of the hand, the surgeon uses the thumb and index finger of the same hand to grasp the skin of the areola adjacent to the

Figure 7-2 A, B. Base width is the base width of the patient's existing breast parenchyma, a linear measurement from the initial upslope of the breast mound medially to the lateral visual border of the breast. Surgeons should assure that this measurement is conservative and actually measures the base width of existing parenchyma. To completely avoid an excessively wide measurement of base width, surgeons can simply measure base width and subtract 0.5 cm to assure that the implant is not wider than existing parenchyma.

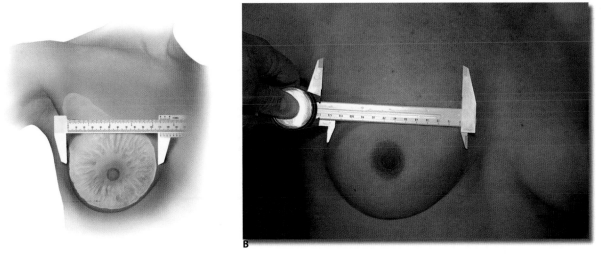

A   B

nipple and pull it maximally anteriorly until the skin will stretch no further anteriorly (Figure 7-3). The surgeon marks the point of maximal anterior pull skin stretch with the index fingernail of the other hand (Figure 7-3, *A*), then releases the skin and uses the caliper to measure from the marked maximal point of stretch at the fingernail back to the resting surface of the areola (Figure 7-3, *B*). APSS is a very useful parameter, because it is an excellent indicator of a point past which the skin simply will not stretch short-term. The mild discomfirt of maximally stretching the skin to its limit powerfully demonstrates to the patient a point which her skin simply will not stretch without potentially damaging the tissues.

The fifth and final measurement is nipple-to-inframammary fold distance measured under maximal stretch or N:IMF$_{max\ stretch}$. This measurement quantifies the amount of skin from the nipple to the existing inframammary fold. As the amount of inferior pole skin increases in the breast, the volume required to optimally fill the envelope also increases. N:IMF serves three important purposes: (1) to remind surgeons to add additional volume to the volume recommend by High Five™ when N:IMF is 9.5 cm or greater, (2) to remind surgeons that when N:IMF approaches 9 cm, larger volumes usually exceeding 350 cc may be required to optimally fill the breast but also require advising the patient of potential long-term tradeoffs of larger implants, and (3) to remind surgeons that N:IMF distances at or above 10 cm mandate careful consideration of mastopexy. To measure

> N:IMF distances at or above 10 cm mandate careful consideration of mastopexy

Figure 7-3 A, B. To measure anterior pull skin stretch (APSS), the surgeon grasps the periareolar skin and pulls maximally anteriorly (upper and middle), and then marks that point with the index fingernail of the opposite hand. Releasing the skin, the surgeon then (bottom) caliper measures the distance from the point marked by the index fingernail back to the skin of the areola.

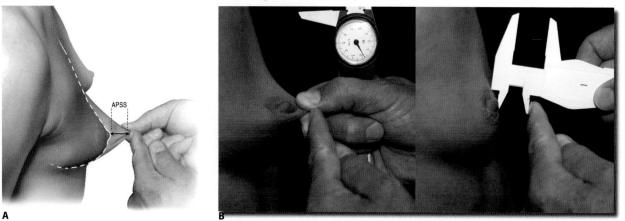

A

B

N:IMF (Figure 7-4), the surgeon lifts the breast and marks a dot at the 6 o'clock position of the inframammary fold. Placing the tip of a flexible tape measure exactly opposite the midpoint of the nipple, the surgeon then grasps the tip of the tape measure with the areola, maximally lifts and stretches the skin of the lower pole of the breast cephalad and measures from the nipple to the marked point at the inframammary fold.

To further refine the estimate of optimal volume for a patient's breast envelope, the surgeon should consider how much of the maximally stretched envelope the patient's existing parenchyma will fill. The difference between the total volume of the stretched envelope and the volume of the patient's existing parenchyma is the implant volume required for optimal aesthetics and tissue safety:

Final volume of optimally filled envelope = existing parenchyma + implant volume

Defining parenchymal contribution to stretched envelope fill or PCSEF requires that the surgeon envision the maximally stretched envelope after augmentation. The surgeon can

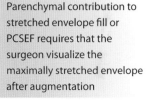

Parenchymal contribution to stretched envelope fill or PCSEF requires that the surgeon visualize the maximally stretched envelope after augmentation

Figure 7-4. Left: After placing a dot at the 6 o'clock position of the inframammary fold, the surgeon places the tip of a flexible tape measure exactly beside the center of the nipple (right), and lifting to maximally stretch the lower pole skin, the surgeon measures from the nipple to the dot at the inframammary fold.

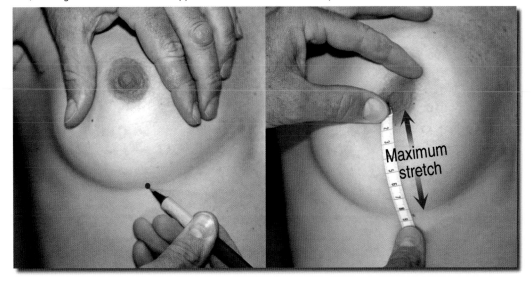

make this estimate while measuring APSS by cupping the hand equidistant from the lower pole of the breast at a distance equal to APSS and envisioning a straight line from the point of APSS up to the chest wall to define the upper pole. While envisioning the outline of the maximally stretched envelope (Figure 7-5), the surgeon estimates the percentage of fill of the stretched envelope that the patient's existing parenchyma will contribute. This estimate is only pertinent to the decision process if PCSEF is less than 20% or greater than 80%. A PCSEF of less than 20% indicates minimal existing parenchyma and/or an extremely large or stretchy envelope, in which case the surgeon should add an additional 30 cc of volume to the initial volume High Five™ recommends. When PCSEF is greater than 80%, indicated by a breast envelope that is already filled with good aesthetics, the patient's existing parenchyma is already near optimally filling the envelope, and the surgeon should subtract at least 30 cc or more from the initial volume the system recommends based on breast base width. Referring back to the funnel analogy described previously, if a funnel were present in the upper breast through which the surgeon introduces fill, and the breast is already full, evidenced by excellent preoperative aesthetics, and optimal upper pole fill adding additional volume is likely to produce excessive upper pole fullness with bulging and rounding of the upper pole and more likelihood of upper implant edge visibility.

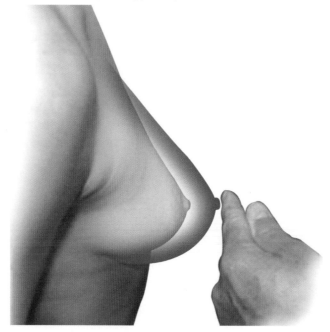

Figure 7-5. After determining the maximal anterior stretch of the patient's envelope when measuring anterior pull skin stretch (APSS), the surgeon envisions the capacity of the maximally stretched envelope by cupping the hand equidistant from the lower pole at the APSS distance (left photo), and defining a visual line from the APSS point to the chest wall in the upper pole (right photo). The surgeon then estimates the existing parenchyma's contribution to stretched envelope fill by asking what percentage of the maximally stretched envelope (pink in illustration) is filled by existing parenchyma.

Applying the High Five™ Decision Process Clinically

Table 7-4 is a clinical form that contains all of the necessary information to apply the High Five™ decision process. A clinical example is an excellent method to rapidly learn to apply the system. This example includes measurements from a 32 year old, gravida 2, para 2 patient who had a 34C cup breast prior to pregnancy, enlarged to a maximal 34D cup with pregnancy, and presented with a 34B cup breast requesting a full but natural appearing breast with adequate volume for optimal aesthetic fill, but avoiding excessive volume that might compromise her tissues long-term. Excerpts from Table 7-4 accompany a step-by-step description of applying the system during the surgeon's clinical examination.

1. Soft tissue coverage and pocket selection

Table 7-4. **A- Soft tissue coverage measurements and implant pocket selection**			
1. COVERAGE- Selecting Pocket Location to Optimize Soft Tissue Coverage Short- and Long-Term			
STPTUP	**1.4 cm.**	**If < 2.0 cm., consider dual plane (DP) or partial retropectoral (PRP, pectoralis origins intact across IMF)**	(DP) (1),2,3 PRP RM
STPTIMF	**0.8 cm.**	**If STPTIMF < 0.5 cm, consider subpectoral pocket and leave pectoralis origins intact along IMF**	
POCKET LOCATION SELECTED BASED ON THICKNESS OF TISSUE COVERAGE			

The surgeon performs the first two measurements and records the measurements on the evaluation sheet.

1. STPTUP—soft tissue pinch thickness of the upper pole (skin and subcutaneous tissue superior to the breast parenchyma)—1.4 cm.
2. STPTIMF—soft tissue pinch thickness at the inframammary fold—0.8 cm.

Implant pocket selection is based on quantified soft tissue coverage to assure optimal long-term coverage over the implant. If soft tissue pinch thickness of the upper pole (STPTUP) is less than 2.0 cm, providing optimal long-term coverage requires that the surgeon choose either a dual plane (dividing pectoralis origins only along the inframammary fold) or partial retropectoral (pectoralis origins along the inframammary fold left intact) pocket location to assure optimal soft tissue coverage. If STPTIMF is less than 0.5 cm, the surgeon should forego the potential advantages of a dual plane pocket

When selecting a dual plane or partial retropectoral pocket location to optimize coverage, the surgeon never divides origins of the pectoralis major from the sternal notch to the sternal junction with the inframammary fold in order to assure optimal coverage in this critical area, regardless of a patient's desired intermammary distance

and preserve the origins of the pectoralis major along the inframammary fold for additional coverage, selecting a traditional partial subpectoral pocket. Adding fascial coverage of less than 1 mm thickness with a retromammary or subfascial pocket is inconsequential coverage long-term when pectoralis muscle coverage is available and when dual plane techniques enable surgeons to minimize tradeoffs of traditional retropectoral placement. When selecting a dual plane or partial retropectoral pocket location to optimize coverage, the surgeon *never divides origins of the pectoralis major from the sternal notch to the sternal junction with the inframammary fold in order to assure optimal coverage in this critical area, regardless of a patient's desired intermammary distance.*

Considering the quantified measurements of soft tissue thickness, the surgeon chooses either dual plane 1, 2, 3, partial retropectoral, or retromammary pocket location, and circles the choice on the form. This patient's STPTUP is 1.4 cm, and her STPTIMF is 0.8 cm, therefore a submammary or subfascial pocket location would not provide her the maximal, optimal soft tissue coverage long-term. Since STPTIMF is greater than 0.5 cm, the patient can have a dual plane 1 pocket with division of pectoralis origins along the inframammary fold, enabling her to avoid the tradeoffs of a traditional subpectoral pocket that include increased distortion with contraction, lateral displacement over time with widening of the intermammary distance, cephalad implant displacement, and a less predictable shape and position of the inframammary fold.

2. Implant volume

Table 7-4. **B- Selecting an estimated implant volume for optimal envelope fill**

2. IMPLANT VOLUME- Selecting an Estimated Implant Volume for Optimal Envelope Fill												
Estimating Desired Breast Implant Volume Based on Breast Measurements and Tissue Characteristics												
Base Width cm.	11.5	B.W. Parenchyma (cm)	10.5	11.0	11.5	12.0	12.5	13.0	13.5	14.0	14.5	15.0	275 cc
		Initial Volume (cc)	200	250	275	300	300	325	350	375	375	400	
APSS$_{MaxStr}$	3.4	[2]If APSS <2.0, −30 cc; If APSS >3.0, +30 cc; If APSS >4.0, +60 cc Place appropriate number in blank at righ											+30 cc
N:IMF$_{MaxS}$	7.0	If N:IMF >9.5, +30 cc Place appropriate number in blank at right											N/A cc
PCSEF %	40	If PCSEF <20%, +30 cc; If PCSEF >80%, −30 cc Place appropriate number in blank at right											N/A cc
Pt. request		No request made that deviates from the system											N/A cc
NET ESTIMATED VOLUME TO FILL ENVELOPE BASED ON PATIENT TISSUE CHARACTERISTICS													305 cc

Next, the surgeon measures and records the following parameters:

3. BW—base width of the existing breast parenchyma, a linear measurement—11.5 cm.

4. APSS (skin stretch)—anterior pull skin stretch, a measurement of maximal anterior skin stretch by manual traction comfortably tolerated by an awake patient—3.4 cm.

5. N:IMF$_{max\ stretch}$—nipple-to-inframammary fold distance, measured under maximal stretch—7.0 cm.

6. PCSEF (parenchyma fill)—an estimate of the contribution of the patient's existing breast parenchyma to stretched envelope fill—40%. To estimate PCSEF, the surgeon pulls the periareolar skin maximally anteriorly (APSS), then cups the hand or envisions the envelope stretched this same amount over the entire breast and estimates the amount of fill as a percentage that the patient's existing parenchyma will provide to the maximally stretched envelope.

The surgeon then locates the base width that corresponds with the patient's base width in the row to the right. In the cell immediately beneath, the surgeon circles the initial estimated desired implant volume for that base width breast, and transfers this number to the blank space at the far right of the row.

This volume represents an *estimated initial desired implant volume* based on the breast base width. These volumes were derived from data described in the initial TEPID™ report.[1] These initial recommended volumes were derived from average base widths of a large number of different moderate profile implants to assure that the base width of the implant did not substantially exceed the base width of the patient's existing parenchyma in order to assure optimal implant edge coverage. Individual surgeons can adjust these starting volumes for each base width as desired and are adjustable by the surgeon depending on other parameters including patient wishes. Next, the surgeon adjusts the estimated starting volume depending on skin stretch.

If anterior pull skin stretch (APSS) is less than 2 cm (very tight envelope), the surgeon subtracts 30 cc (or another increment of the surgeon's preference) from the estimated starting volume. If APSS is >3 cm (in this patient example APSS is 3.4 cm), the surgeon adds 30 cc, and if APSS is >4 cm the surgeon adds 60 cc to the starting volume, recording the appropriate addition or subtraction in the cell at the far right of the "APSS" row.

If the nipple-to-inframammary fold distance (N:IMF$_{max\ stretch}$) is greater than 9.5 cm when measured under maximal stretch (in this case N:IMF$_{max\ stretch}$ is 7.0 cm), the surgeon adds

30 cc (or another increment of the surgeon's preference) to the starting volume to provide adequate additional fill volume for a larger lower envelope. If applicable, the surgeon records this additional volume in the far right cell of the "N:IMF$_{max\ stretch}$" row. In this example case, N:IMF$_{max\ stretch}$ is not applicable to increasing the initial recommended volume.

The PCSEF (parenchymal contribution to stretched envelope fill) estimate is necessary to adjust volume for patients whose skin envelopes are tighter (APSS < 2 cm) and already filled with parenchyma (PCSEF > 80%), or for patients with very lax skin envelopes (APSS > 3 cm) who have very little breast parenchyma (PCSEF < 20%). If PCSEF is >80% (already full envelope), the surgeon subtracts 30 cc from the initial estimated volume, and if PCSEF is <20% (empty envelope), the surgeon adds 30 cc and records applicable additions or subtractions in the cell to the far right of the "PCSEF" row. In this case, the patient's existing parenchyma contributes approximately 40% to stretched envelope fill, so no volume adjustment is required.

When patient or surgeon desires a larger or smaller implant volume compared to what the system recommends, the surgeon can use the "Patient request" line in the system to add or subtract desired volume

If the patient or surgeon desires a greater or lesser volume than the system recommends, the surgeon can add or subtract an additional volume increment and record it in the space provided in the far right cell of the "Patient request" row. *The High Five^{TM} system does not replace patient or surgeon preferences or choices.* The system provides guidelines based on quantified tissue characteristics of each individual patient. When patient or surgeon desires a larger or smaller implant volume compared to what the system recommends, the surgeon can use the "Patient request" line in the system to add or subtract desired volume.

The surgeon calculates net estimated volume by adding or subtracting increments described above from the initial estimated volume and records the appropriate number in the cell at the far right of the "Net Estimated Volume" row.

3. Implant type and dimensions

Table 7-4. **C- Selecting specific implant characteristis**

3. IMPLANT DIMENSIONS, TYPE, MANUFACTURER- Selecting specific implant characteristics					
Implant Manufacturer	**Implant Style/Shape/Shell/Filler Material**	**Implant Vol (cc)**	***Implant Base Width**	**Breast Base Width**[1]	**Implant Projection**
		cc	cm.	cm.	cm.

*For optimal long-term coverage, implant base width should not exceed base width of patient's existing parenchyma, even if wider IMD results.

The High Five™ system applies to a wide range of implant types, sizes, and dimensions. Having derived a net estimated implant volume based on quantified tissue parameters, the surgeon can then consult size and dimension charts for any type of implant, and select implant dimensions (width, height, projection) that the surgeon feels are most appropriate. Surgeons should always prioritize long-term, optimal soft tissue coverage by assuring that implant base width does not exceed the base width of the patient's existing parenchyma, even at the expense of a wider intermammary distance. In rare cases of breasts with less than a 10 cm base width (narrow base width breasts, tubular or severely constricted lower pole breasts), surgeons may need to select an implant base width that exceeds the base width of the existing parenchyma.

The surgeon records the implant volume, the base width of the implant selected, the base width of the patient's existing parenchyma (BW measured previously), and implant projection. *For optimal long-term coverage, the base width of the implant selected should not exceed the base width of the patient's existing parenchyma, except in cases of tubular breasts, severely constricted lower pole breasts, or breasts with a base width less than 11 cm.* In these rare cases and any other elective situation in which implant base width exceeds base width of the existing parenchyma, surgeons should thoroughly inform patients of potential long-term tissue consequences, including implant edge visibility and visible traction rippling, and informed consent documents should clearly reflect surgeon and patient acceptance of responsibility for these decisions that can produce uncorrectable problems in the future. Implant projection is an important dimension that may affect distribution of fill and tissue consequences postoperatively, and is included only for postoperative reference. Surgeons should consider potential irreversible parenchymal atrophy effects when selecting highly projecting implants.

Surgeons may consider additional, more detailed tissue considerations and implant–soft tissue interactions when selecting implants, but should always prioritize selecting implant devices that provide significant aesthetic improvements while minimizing negative soft tissue consequences, minimizing risks of inadequate coverage long-term, and minimize uncorrectable deformities. When patient requests conflict with optimal safety for patient tissues long-term, surgeons should strongly emphasize these potential risks to patients and decline to perform procedures that may compromise patient tissues long-term.

> For optimal long-term coverage, the base width of the implant selected should not exceed the base width of the patient's existing parenchyma, except in cases of tubular breasts, severely constricted lower pole breasts, or breasts with a base width less than 10.5 cm

4. Inframammary fold location

Table 7-4. **D- Estimating desired postoperative inframammary fold position**											
4. INFRAMAMMARY FOLD LOCATION- Estimating desired postoperative inframammary fold position											
(Circle Volume closest *to net estimated implant volume* calculated above, and *circle suggested N:IMF* in the cell beneath that volume)											
		Volume closest to calculated "net estimated implant volume" from 2 above	200	250	275	(300)	325	350	375	400
		Recommended new N:IMF distance (cm.) under maximal stretch▶	7.0	7.0	7.5	(8)	8	8.5	9.0	9.5
Planning Level of New Inframammary Fold*	Transfer the patient's N:IMF$_{MaxSt}$ measurement from above to corresponding cell at right. Then transfer the TEPID™ recommended new N:IMF to the corresponding cell at right. If the patient's preop N:IMF is shorter than the TEPID™ recommended new N:IMF, consider lowering the fold. If the patient's preop N:IMF is equal to or greater than the TEPID™ recommended new N:IMF, no change in IMF position is indicated.			Patient's Preoperative N:IMF$_{MaxSt}$		TEPID™ Recommended N:IMF$_{MaxSt}$		Change In Fold Position	Lower the Fold
					7.0 cm.		8.0 cm.		(Yes)/No	1.0 cm.

*Other factors may affect optimal IMF level and require surgeons to modifiy the TEPIDTM System recommendations for N:IMF

The ideal nipple-to-inframammary fold distance to mark preoperatively and set intraoperatively depends on the projected width of the postoperative breast. For optimal aesthetics, the wider the breast, the longer the nipple-to-inframammary fold distance

The ideal nipple-to-inframammary fold distance to mark preoperatively and set intraoperatively depends on the projected width of the postoperative breast. For optimal aesthetics, the wider the breast, the longer the nipple-to-inframammary fold distance. If N:IMF is excessively short compared to BW, the breast will have a "boxy" or transversely rectangular appearance, with inadequate fill and rounding of the lower pole. Conversely, if N:IMF is excessively long compared to BW, the breast will have a "bottomed out" appearance of the lower pole, with excessive fill in the lower pole often accompanied by nipple-areola malposition. Surgeons who "always" or "never" lower or reposition the inframammary fold when widening the breast with a breast augmentation create suboptimal aesthetic results that could be prevented by using proved, quantitative methods to determine optimal position of the inframammary fold.[1,11] Whether repositioning of the inframammary fold is indicated or not depends entirely on (a) the preoperative N:IMF measurement, and (b) the volume/width of the proposed implant for augmentation.

To estimate the optimal level of the inframammary fold, the surgeon first locates the volume closest to the previously calculated "net estimated implant volume" (Table 7-4D). In the cell immediately beneath, the system lists a "High Five™ recommended new N:IMF distance measured under maximal stretch". The surgeon circles the recommended number, and then transfers that number to the cell in the row below labeled "High Five™ recommended N:IMF$_{max\ stretch}$". Next, the surgeon transfers the preoperative N:IMF$_{max\ stretch}$ measurement to the cell labeled "Patient's Preoperative N:IMF$_{max\ stretch}$" in the same row.

If the recommended N:IMF$_{intraop}$ for the planned volume implant is greater than the patient's preoperative N:IMF$_{max\ stretch}$, the surgeon should lower the fold to the recommended level by drawing a new inframammary fold at the appropriate distance from the nipple during preoperative marking. If the recommended N:IMF$_{max\ stretch}$ is the same or longer than the patient's preoperative N:IMF$_{max\ stretch}$, no lowering of the fold is indicated. After comparing the preoperative N:IMF with the recommended N:IMF, the surgeon decides whether to lower the fold, and circles either "Yes" or "No". If the choice is to lower the fold, the surgeon then records the appropriate number of centimeters to lower the fold in the cell below "Lower Fold".

When repositioning the inframammary fold is indicated, during preoperative marking the surgeon first marks the existing inframammary fold. Next, placing the lower pole skin under maximal stretch, the surgeon measures downward from the nipple the prescribed, new N:IMF distance, and places a dot at the 6 o'clock position of the inframammary fold (Figure 7-6, left). This dot represents the level of the desired, new inframammary fold.

Figure 7-6. Left: The surgeon first marks the existing inframammary fold (violet dots). The violet arrow represents the level of the preoperative inframammary fold. Right: Next, the surgeon places the lower pole skin under maximal tension and measures from the nipple a distance prescribed by the High Five™ System directly down to or below the 6 o'clock position of the inframammary fold and places a dot (large red dot). This dot represents the desired, new inframammary fold level. The surgeon then outlines the new inframammary fold (red dots), changing curvature as necessary to optimize aesthetics. The red arrow indicates the level of the new inframammary fold. The surgeon places an inframammary incision exactly at the desired, new fold level (red dots).

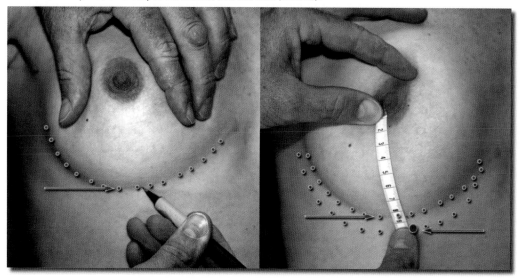

The surgeon then draws the desired, new inframammary fold, correcting or improving any existing fold contour irregularities (Figure 7-6, right). Regardless of the incision approach the surgeon selects, this new inframammary fold topographic marking defines the desired inferior extent of implant pocket dissection. If the surgeon chooses an inframammary incision, the surgeon marks the incision exactly at the level of the desired, new inframammary fold, not above the desired new fold.

Shortening N:IMF or raising the inframammary fold is virtually never indicated in primary breast augmentation, because adding volume to the breast widens the breast, necessitating a long N:IMF for optimal aesthetics. Even in cases that have a relatively long N:IMF preoperatively, the tradeoffs and uncontrollable variables of surgically attempting to raise the fold make this maneuver undesirable in primary breast augmentation.

5. Incision location

Table 7-4. E- Selecting desired incision location

5. INCISION LOCATION- Selecting desired incision location			
Inframammary	Axillary	Periareolar	Umbilical

Incision location is based on patient preference, patient considerations of degree of surgical control, tissue trauma, and tradeoffs, and surgeon preferences and skill set. The surgeon records the planned incision location in the appropriate space in Table 7-4E.

The entire High Five™ clinical assessment and operative planning sequence described in this chapter requires less than 5 minutes once a surgeon is familiar with the system. Most surgeons gain this level of familiarity after using the system in five clinical cases. The system is highly reproducible and transferable, and many surgeons including the author have learned that these five measurements are much more helpful in making optimal clinical decisions compared to clinical photographs. In e-mail communications regarding clinical cases, these measurements enable surgeons to communicate with quantifiable data and criteria instead of relying on subjective opinions derived from photographs.

The High Five™ clinical assessment and operative planning system is incorporated into a comprehensive, one page clinical evaluation form that the surgeon uses during the surgeon consultation, a combination of Tables 7-4 and 7-5. This form is available in

Microsoft Word™ and Adobe Acrobat™ pdf formats in the Resources folder on the DVDs accompanying this book for individual surgeon modification and use.

Using High Five™ to Establish Realistic Patient Expectations

The surgeon clinical assessment using the High Five™ process provides an excellent opportunity for surgeons to help patients understand what their individual tissues will realistically allow them to have without causing irreversible negative tissue changes and deformities that are surgically uncorrectable. Chapter 6 details basic concepts of implant–soft tissue interactions, and defines methods for surgeons to demonstrate these concepts to patients during the clinical examination. Specific methods to emphasize key concepts during the High Five™ clinical assessment deserve additional comment.

When performing measurements, surgeons should ask the patient to look down at her breasts while the surgeon performs each measurement. As the surgeon performs the soft tissue thickness measurements, the surgeon should explain the critical long-term importance of providing the best possible soft tissue coverage—not selecting a breast implant pocket that *may* provide adequate coverage for a while, but selecting an implant pocket location that puts the most possible soft tissue over the implant for the longest possible time. Surgeons should explain to patients that the idea that a dual plane or partial retropectoral pocket location causes more postoperative pain has been conclusively disproved by developing optimal surgical techniques,[7] and that dual plane techniques[6] virtually eliminate the tradeoffs of traditional retropectoral placement, including postoperative pain, distortion on contraction, lateral displacement over time, upward implant displacement, and breast contour limitations. If STPTIMF is less than 0.5 cm, the surgeon should point out to the patient that to assure optimal long-term coverage, the patient should consider accepting any tradeoffs of traditional subpectoral placement and leave the inferior origins of the pectoralis major intact along the inframammary fold.

When measuring base width, surgeons should explain to the patient that this measurement defines the width of her existing breast tissue. Grasping and lifting the skin medial to the parenchyma in the gap between the breasts, the surgeon can point out that if an implant edge is located beneath this thin skin, edge visibility and visible traction rippling can occur and are largely uncorrectable. To avoid these uncorrectable consequences, it is necessary to limit width and size of a breast implant to a width no greater than the width of the existing breast tissue, and accept a wider gap between the breasts in lieu of uncorrectable problems in the future. Surgeons must realistically

The surgeon clinical assessment using the High Five™ process provides an excellent opportunity for surgeons to help patients understand what their individual tissues will realistically allow them to have without causing irreversible negative tissue changes and deformities that are surgically uncorrectable

Surgeons should explain to patients that the idea that a dual plane or partial retropectoral pocket location causes more postoperative pain has been conclusively disproved by developing optimal surgical techniques

question the level of understanding and motivations of patients who continue to insist on implant sizes and narrowing of the intermammary distance that are likely to produce uncorrectable tissue consequences.

When performing the measurement of anterior pull skin stretch (APSS), surgeons can emphasize the limitations of tissue stretch. At the point of maximal stretch while pulling anteriorly on the areolar skin, the surgeon can add additional pull to the point of discomfort and point out to the patient that the skin simply will not stretch further than a certain point. The surgeon can further emphasize that attempting to force excessive stretch with an excessively large or excessively projecting implant can cause irreversible skin thinning, visible implant edges, traction rippling, atrophy of breast tissue, and possible chest wall deformities that are largely uncorrectable.

These three simple demonstrations during clinical assessment help patients understand that if they wish to avoid uncorrectable tissue compromises and deformities, *they must reconcile what they want with what their tissues will realistically allow them to have,* and that what any surgeon can safely deliver is limited by the tissue thickness, base width, and skin stretch of their existing tissues. A vast majority of patients clearly understand and appreciate this in-depth information that defines choices to prevent negative consequences long-term, and delivering this critical information requires no additional time commitment by the surgeon if the surgeon integrates these conversations into the clinical assessment process.

OPERATIVE PLANNING AND METHODS TO OPTIMIZE THE SURGICAL EXPERIENCE

Surgeons should make every possible decision in breast augmentation before entering the operating room. Optimizing the operative experience for a patient requires that the surgeon use anesthetic and operative time efficiently, eliminating unnecessary and undesirable steps that unnecessarily prolong anesthesia time, increase doses of anesthetic drugs, and introduce variables that prolong recovery and add unnecessary morbidity to the postoperative experience. Eliminating unnecessary intraoperative maneuvers and postoperative adjuncts requires that surgeons discard preconceptions and practice and adopt more efficient, proved processes. Change is uncomfortable to many surgeons, but improving patient outcomes and the patient experience require change.

Peer reviewed and published studies conclusively demonstrate that current quantitative tissue assessment and implant selection methods including TEPID™ and High Five™

Peer reviewed and published studies conclusively demonstrate that current quantitative tissue assessment and implant selection methods including TEPID™ and High Five™ totally eliminate the need to use intraoperative sizers in primary breast augmentation

totally eliminate the need to use intraoperative sizers in primary breast augmentation.[1,11] Sizer use increases costs by increasing operating times, increases drug doses and costs, increases risks of pocket contamination, increases tissue trauma and bleeding, and introduces variables that can compromise decisions. Sizers and subjective visual observations are not as accurate as quantified measurements and defined, objective decision processes, proved by extensive peer reviewed and published data.[1,6-8,11] Using defined decision processes and quantitative tissue assessment also obviates a need for ordering and stocking multiple sizes of implants for each case, drastically reducing costs of shipping implants and manufacturer inventory costs.

Chapter 15 contains detailed descriptions of methods that enable surgeons to allow patients to be out to dinner the evening of their breast augmentation and return to full normal activities within 24 hours. Critical to this process, and often omitted from operative planning, is the necessity to define and deliver specific protocols for anesthetic and post anesthetic recovery care. The author's protocols are included in Chapter 15 and in electronic files in the Resources folder on the DVDs that accompany this book. Surgeons can deliver optimal efficiency and outcomes only if they can control every aspect of the patient's operative experience, including the types and amounts of drugs that patients receive intraoperatively and during the recovery process. Defining protocols for anesthesia and recovery care and working with anesthesia and recovery colleagues and personnel to assure consistent delivery of these protocols is essential to deliver optimal recovery and outcomes.

■ ADOPTING AND IMPLEMENTING QUANTITATIVE TISSUE ASSESSMENT TO IMPROVE OUTCOMES

The number of patients who will benefit from improved methodologies depends on the number of surgeons who implement quantitative tissue assessment and defined decision processes. The methodologies described in this chapter represent a quantum change in preoperative planning and assessment that have significantly redefined the patient experience and outcomes in breast augmentation.

■ REFERENCES

1. Tebbetts JB: A system for breast implant selection based on patient tissue characteristics and implant–soft tissue dynamics. *Plast Reconstr Surg* 109(4):1396–1409, 2002.

2. Food and Drug Administration. U.S. Food and Drug Administration. General and Plastic Surgery Devices Panel Meeting Transcript. Washington, D.C. October 14–15, 2003. Online. Available: http://www.fda.gov/ohrms/dockets/ac/03/transcripts/3989T1.htm.

3. Food and Drug Administration. U.S. Food and Drug Administration. General and Plastic Surgery Devices Panel Meeting Transcript. Washington, D.C. February 18, 1992.

4. Food and Drug Administration. U.S. Food and Drug Administration. General and Plastic Surgery Devices Panel Meeting Transcript. Washington, D.C. March 1–3, 2000. Online. Available: http://www.fda.gov/cdrh/gpsdp.html#030100.

5. Tebbetts JB: Patient acceptance of adequately filled breast implants using the tilt test. *Plast Reconstr Surg* 106(1):139–147, 2000.

6. Tebbetts JB: Dual plane (DP) breast augmentation: optimizing implant–soft tissue relationships in a wide range of breast types. *Plast Reconstr Surg* 107:1255, 2001.

7. Tebbetts JB: Achieving a predictable 24 hour return to normal activities after breast augmentation Part II: Patient preparation, refined surgical techniques and instrumentation. *Plast Reconstr Surg* 109:293–305, 2002.

8. Tebbetts JB: Achieving a zero percent reoperation rate at 3 years in a 50 consecutive case augmentation mammaplasty PMA study. *Plast Reconstr Surg* 118(6):1453–1457, 2006.

9. Tebbetts JB: *Dimensional augmentation mammaplasty using the BioDimensional™ System.* Santa Barbara: McGhan Medical Corporation, 1994, pp 1–90.

10. Tebbetts JB: Achieving a predictable 24 hour return to normal activities after breast augmentation Part I: Refining practices using motion and time study principles. *Plast Reconstr Surg* 109:273–290, 2002.

11. Tebbetts JB, Adams WP: Five critical decisions in breast augmentation using 5 measurements in 5 minutes: the high five system. *Plast Reconstr Surg* 116(7):2005–2016, 2005.

Implant Pocket Locations

Implant pocket location determines the quality and quantity of long-term soft tissue coverage of breast implants, the number one priority in breast augmentation. Assuring optimal soft tissue coverage of implants for the patient's lifetime is the number one priority in breast augmentation in order to avoid irreversible tissue compromises and uncorrectable deformities such as visible implant edges and visible traction rippling. No decision in breast augmentation is more important than selection of implant pocket location.

Breast augmentation is a medically unnecessary operation designed to improve breast aesthetics. Every elective, non-essential, aesthetic procedure should deliver substantial improvements with minimal risks and negative tissue consequences long-term. While breast augmentation patients almost uniformly experience substantial short-term benefits and a high rate of patient satisfaction, a small but significant percentage of patients experience deformities and tissue compromises that are often uncorrectable, including implant edge visibility superiorly and medially and visible traction rippling medially in the cleavage area. These difficult or uncorrectable deformities often result from choosing a pocket location that does not maximize soft tissue coverage over the implant, and could be almost totally avoided by more appropriate preoperative selection of pocket location based on quantified tissue parameters and proved decision processes. The first priority in every primary breast augmentation is to assure *optimal*, not marginal, soft tissue coverage in every area of the implant for the patient's lifetime, by selecting pocket location based on objective criteria for each patient's individual tissue thickness in areas overlying their breast implants.

Assuring optimal soft tissue coverage of implants for the patient's lifetime is the number one priority in breast augmentation in order to avoid irreversible tissue compromises and uncorrectable deformities such as visible implant edges and visible traction rippling. No decision in breast augmentation is more important than selection of implant pocket location

The first priority in every primary breast augmentation is to assure optimal, not marginal, soft tissue coverage in every area of the implant for the patient's lifetime

Choice of pocket location and surgical techniques determines the thickness of soft tissue overlying the superior, medial, and inferior areas of every patient's breast implants for the patient's lifetime. Inferolaterally and laterally, surgeons have fewer options to increase soft tissue coverage. In areas where additional soft tissue coverage options are available, surgeons should prioritize providing maximal soft tissue coverage above all other considerations or perceived tradeoffs of one pocket location over another.

■ SUBJECTIVE VERSUS OBJECTIVE SELECTION OF POCKET LOCATION

Surgeons have traditionally based opinions regarding implant pocket location largely on subjective parameters that relate to the relative benefits and tradeoffs of one pocket location compared to another. While these subjective comparisons are valid, they do not prioritize optimal, long-term soft tissue coverage and are not based on analysis of quantifiable data to derive scientifically valid conclusions. For example, whether or not a patient experiences some degree of breast distortion with contraction of the pectoralis major muscle and the degree of perceived distortion that results are inconsequential compared to the potential uncorrectable deformities and tissue compromises that can result from failure to provide optimal long-term coverage. Similarly, creating a very narrow intermammary distance or cleavage is not as high a priority as assuring optimal soft tissue coverage medially to prevent the often uncorrectable deformities of visible implant edges and visible traction rippling medially.

Objective selection of implant pocket location requires that surgeons do the following:

1. Prioritize optimal, long-term soft tissue coverage over all other considerations in primary breast augmentation.

2. Educate patients regarding the critical importance of optimal, long-term soft tissue coverage to avoid irreversible tissue compromises and uncorrectable deformities that can occur many years after their breast augmentation.

3. Select pocket location to assure optimal, long-term soft tissue coverage rather than satisfying perceived, short-term goals such as larger size/width implants or narrower intermammary distance, using peer reviewed and published, proved decision processes.[1-3]

> Creating a very narrow intermammary distance or cleavage is not as high a priority as assuring optimal soft tissue coverage medially to prevent the often uncorrectable deformities of visible implant edges and visible traction rippling medially

4. Objectively measure and quantify soft tissue thicknesses in lieu of subjective impressions of "thick" or "thin" tissue coverage.

5. Set specific, objective, quantifiable criteria on which to base decisions of pocket location.

6. Base decisions of pocket location on the defined, peer reviewed and published criteria of soft tissue thickness and coverage, not on subjective, perceived tradeoffs in pocket locations.

▓ IMPLANT POCKET LOCATION OPTIONS

Implant pocket location options currently include submammary, subfascial, partial retropectoral, dual plane, and totally submuscular pockets. Each of these pocket locations can provide specific amounts of soft tissue coverage in specific areas of the breast, and each location has a unique set of potential benefits and tradeoffs.

Many preconceptions and misconceptions exist regarding implant pocket locations, evidenced by the frequency of inaccurate statements in professional publications and presentations by plastic surgeons. Defining truth about implant pocket locations requires an objective analysis of each pocket location based on quantified, peer reviewed and published outcomes data that scientifically define benefits and tradeoffs. Critical outcomes data that define which pocket locations are really best for patients must include: (a) objective data that define and quantify the thickness of patient tissues preoperatively, (b) incidence of visible implant edges or visible traction rippling with at least 10 year followup, and (c) reoperation rates for these deformities long-term. Absent objective, quantified data regarding preoperative tissue thickness preoperatively and the specific, objective criteria the surgeon used to select pocket location, any discussion of implant pocket selection becomes a subjective expression of non-scientific opinions that is not scientifically valid and that cannot credibly derive recommendations that optimize outcomes.

Retromammary Pocket Location

A submammary or retromammary pocket locates the breast implant posterior to the patient's breast parenchyma and anterior to the pectoralis major muscle and fascia (Figure 8-1). An often quoted advantage of the subpectoral pocket is that it locates the implant in the same tissue plane as the patient's existing breast parenchyma where the implant is not subject to tissue pressures and tissue dynamics of an overlying muscle tissue layer. Absent additional tissue thickness layers on the implant, the implant can exert more direct and predictable fill and pressure to more predictably control breast shape, especially fill in the upper and medial breast areas. The decades long problem with this argument in favor of the submammary pocket location is that it ignores the most important single priority in breast augmentation—maximizing soft tissue cover over the implant for the patient's lifetime to avoid uncorrectable tissue compromises and tissue deformities that occur with aging, including tissue thinning, skin stretch, implant edge visibility, and visible traction rippling.

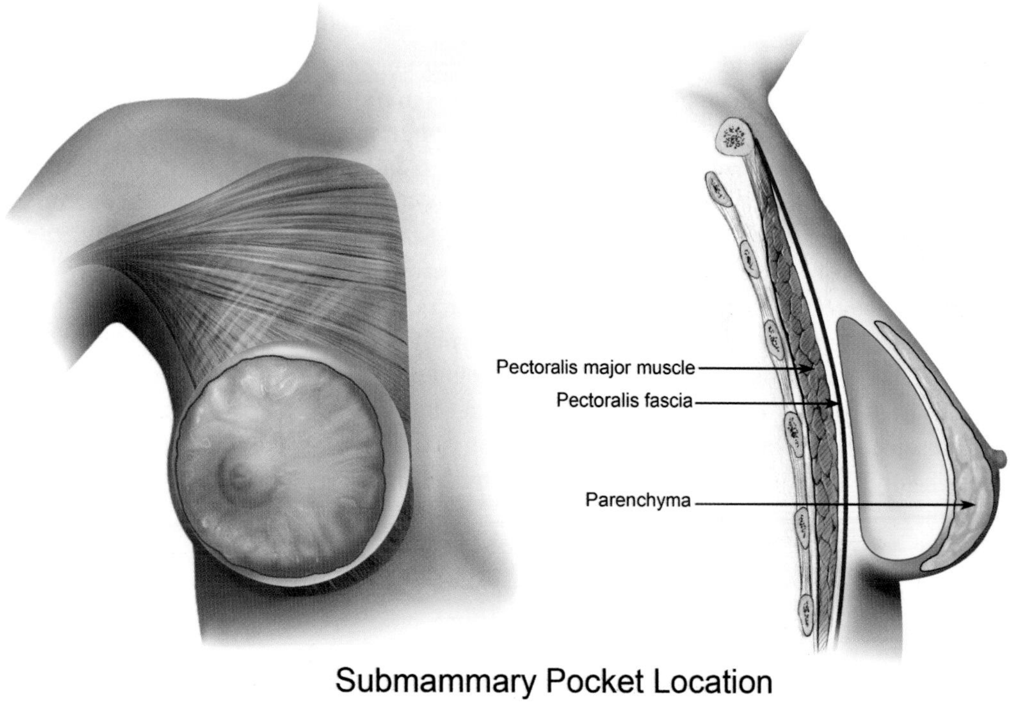

Figure 8-1. The submammary or retromammary pocket location locates the breast implant posterior to breast parenchyma and anterior to the pectoralis major muscle and fascia.

Pectoralis major muscle
Pectoralis fascia
Parenchyma

Submammary Pocket Location

Dual plane placement releases the origins of the pectoralis along the inframammary fold and almost totally obviates these tradeoffs of traditional partial retropectoral placement when compared to submammary placement while providing maximal additional soft tissue coverage medially and superiorly

Retromammary placement also theoretically avoids other tradeoffs of muscle pressure on the implant in the subpectoral plane. With traditional partial retropectoral placement, intact pectoralis origins along the inframammary fold allow the pectoralis muscle to transmit more pressure to the implant, and can contribute to upward implant displacement (or failure of the implant to rest at exactly the lower border of the pocket), less control of upper and medial fill, and lateral displacement of the implant over time. Dual plane placement,[1] discussed in more detail later in this chapter, releases the origins of the pectoralis along the inframammary fold and almost totally obviates these tradeoffs of traditional partial retropectoral placement when compared to submammary placement while providing maximal additional soft tissue coverage medially and superiorly.

Surgeons have traditionally advised patients that pocket dissection in a submammary plane, because it does not involve dissection beneath the pectoralis muscle, causes less postoperative pain; however, with the development of the dual plane pocket[1] and documented 24 hour recovery[4,5] using a dual plane pocket, this potential advantage of submammary augmentation is no longer true. Development of the dual plane pocket[1] and surgical techniques that minimize trauma to the pectoralis and bleeding,[5] combined with tissue based implant selection,[2,3] now allow patients with subpectoral and dual plane augmentations to be out to dinner the evening of surgery and return to full normal activities in 24 hours,[4,5] a recovery that is indistinguishable from retromammary augmentations. More importantly, for the first time in history a peer reviewed and published study has shown that surgeons can achieve a zero percent reoperation rate in a consecutive series of primary augmentations in an Food and Drug Administration (FDA) premarket approval (PMA) study,[6] emphasizing the importance of combining optimal soft tissue coverage, decision processes, and surgical techniques.

Development of the dual plane pocket[1] and surgical techniques that minimize trauma to the pectoralis and bleeding,[5] combined with tissue based implant selection,[2,3] now allow patients with subpectoral and dual plane augmentations to be out to dinner the evening of surgery and return to full normal activities in 24 hours,[4,5] a recovery that is indistinguishable from retromammary augmentations

In the submammary plane, surgeons can more effectively control the intermammary distance or cleavage gap by dissecting the pockets medially to a desired location that defines a desired intermammary distance. In order to accomplish the same objective in a submuscular plane, surgeons must divide the origins of the pectoralis major muscle medially. In both cases, this apparent benefit can also be a curse longer term. When the medial or inferomedial edge of the implant is covered only by skin and subcutaneous tissue, the thickness of this coverage largely determines whether a patient will experience visible implant edges in the future, and whether visible traction rippling will occur when the weight of the implant pulls on the capsule attached to thin overlying tissues medially. These deformities can sometimes be corrected by changing a submammary implant to a retropectoral pocket location, but at the expense of dealing with additional risks and variables. If a surgeon disrupts or divides the medial origins of the pectoralis muscle along

If a surgeon disrupts or divides the medial origins of the pectoralis muscle along the sternum at any location from sternal notch to xiphoid, visible implant edges and traction rippling are common deformities that are largely uncorrectable

the sternum at any location from sternal notch to xiphoid, visible implant edges and traction rippling are common deformities that are largely uncorrectable. When surgeons markedly narrow the intermammary distance, synmastia risks increase, and synmastia deformities can be extremely difficult or impossible to optimally correct. Patients should be informed and aware that absent extremely thick tissues in the intermammary gap or cleavage gap between the breasts (a very rare occurrence), it is much safer to live with a slightly wider intermammary distance, keeping the medial edge of the implant under existing parenchyma or the pectoralis muscle, rather than living with uncorrectable deformities in the cleavage area.

Three specific issues are associated with the submammary pocket location: (1) this location exposes the implant to a maximal surface area contact with breast parenchyma that contains endogenous bacteria, (2) soft tissue thickness behind and peripheral to the patient's existing parenchyma is often inadequate to assure maximal, optimal, long-term soft tissue coverage over all areas of the implant, and (3) an implant in the submammary plane may interfere more with breast imaging compared to subpectoral placement.

Over the past 25 years, most surgeons with extensive experience in submammary and subpectoral augmentation have experienced higher rates of capsular contracture with both smooth and textured surface implants placed in the submammary compared to the subpectoral plane. While conflicting data exist in the literature, a large body of evidence over many years suggests that a greater exposure of the implant to endogenous bacteria in the breast occurs with the implant in a submammary plane, and this exposure likely contributes to a somewhat higher rate of capsular contracture with submammary augmentation. In recent years, the differences in rates of capsular contracture between the submammary location and the subpectoral have decreased, and with implementation of improved surgical techniques and antibacterial irrigation regimens, differences may be negligible.

When capsular contracture rates were extremely high in the 1970s and 1980s with smooth shell implants placed in a submammary location, surgeons began seeking alternatives that included a submuscular pocket location and textured surface implant devices. Over the next three decades, as surgeons used more submuscular pocket locations, an incredibly beneficial byproduct of the first objective to reduce capsular contracture was a dramatic decrease in the incidence of uncorrectable visible implant edges and traction rippling laterally. Uncorrectable deformities that result when surgeons place implants under inadequate or suboptimal soft tissue coverage have occurred since the beginning of breast augmentation, but the direct link between the surgeon prioritizing soft tissue coverage to prevent these problems during the preoperative decision process did not occur until much more recently.[1-4]

High profile implants placed in the submammary plane place more direct pressure on the breast parenchyma, and are likely to cause more parenchymal atrophy over time when placed submammary compared to subpectoral. The larger the implant and the tighter the overlying skin, the greater the potential extent of parenchymal atrophy. Even moderate profile implants in the submammary plane can cause parenchymal atrophy if implant size is excessive for the dimensions and stretch characteristics of the overlying envelope. These potentially negative effects of implant pressure on parenchyma are actually beneficial when surgeons attempt to correct constriction deformities of the breast, including constricted lower pole breasts and tubular breasts. More direct pressure of the breast implant on constricted parenchyma and the overlying soft tissue envelope promotes stretching and correction of the constricted lower pole tissues, regardless of the type of tissue release the surgeon performs. The dual plane approach discussed later in this chapter facilitates correction of these types of deformity while adding significant additional pectoralis major muscle coverage for the implant superiorly and medially.

The tissue plane for submammary pocket dissection contains more perforating vessels compared to partial retropectoral and dual plane pockets, but these vessels pose no significant differences in ease of pocket dissection for surgeons using electrocautery dissection. Some surgeons believe that dissection in the submammary plane poses more risks to nipple-areola innervation compared to submuscular pockets, but this belief is illogical anatomically, assuming precise surgical techniques and a knowledge of the innervation of the breast.

Table 8-1 summarizes the potential benefits and inherent tradeoffs of the submammary pocket location.

Even moderate profile implants in the submammary plane can cause parenchymal atrophy if implant size is excessive for the dimensions and stretch characteristics of the overlying envelope

Table 8-1. Potential advantages and tradeoffs of the submammary pocket location

Potential advantages*	Potential tradeoffs
More direct implant pressure to shape the breast	Inadequate soft tissue coverage superiorly and medially
More precise control of upper and medial breast fill	Higher rate of capsular contracture with resultant higher reoperation rates
Less risk of lateral displacement of implants due to pectoralis pressure	Greater interference with mammography
Less risk of upward displacement of implants due to pectoralis pressure	Increased risk of synmastia with marked narrowing of the intermammary distance
Less risk of breast distortion with pectoralis contraction	

*All of these potential advantages are also achievable using a dual plane pocket location, and the dual plane location maximizes tissue coverage.

Subfascial Pocket Location

A subfascial pocket locates the breast implant posterior to the patient's breast parenchyma and posterior to the pectoralis major fascia but anterior to the pectoralis major muscle (Figure 8-2). The subfascial pocket concept was introduced by Graf and associates in 2002.[7] In their publication the authors state that potential advantages of a subfascial pocket include: (1) avoiding implant deformation or distortion (as seen in the retromuscular position), (2) leaving additional soft tissue between the implant and the skin, and (3) minimizing implant edge prominence that is, according to the authors, inherent to subglandular placement.

Fresh cadaver anatomy of the pectoralis fascia

The characteristics of the pectoralis fascia are best illustrated in fresh cadaver dissections where the anatomy can be exposed widely under direct vision, facilitating exposure and

Figure 8-2 A, B. The subfascial pocket location locates the breast implant posterior to the pectoralis major muscle fascia and anterior to the pectoralis major muscle.

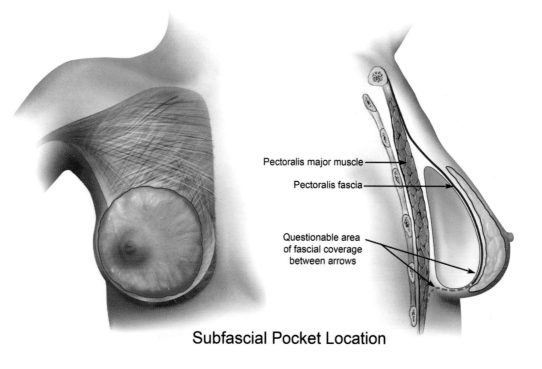

Pectoralis major muscle

Pectoralis fascia

Questionable area of fascial coverage between arrows

Subfascial Pocket Location

elevation of the pectoralis fascia unhindered by blood in an operating field which can make the layer almost imperceptible. Embalmed cadaver analysis of the pectoralis fascia is virtually useless as it pertains to clinical reality, because the embalming process totally changes the characteristics of the pectoralis fascia. Analysis of the thickness of the pectoralis fascia, especially in embalmed cadavers, has little pertinence to the key clinical question of whether any surgeon can predictably elevate the pectoralis fascia intact, and even if the surgeon can do that, whether the pectoralis fascia provides scientifically verifiable soft tissue coverage that is really any different compared to a submammary pocket. To date, despite numerous anecdotal reports of clinical series using a subfascial pocket location, no published study has compared scientifically valid cohorts of patients with various pocket locations because no comparative study has controlled for the 53 tissue and surgical variables that exist in every breast augmentation patient.[2]

Figure 8-3 is a lateral view of the right breast in a fresh cadaver dissection. The pectoralis fascia 3 cm above the inframammary fold has been incised and draped over the tips of Adson forceps. Figure 8-4 is a closeup view of the pectoralis fascia draped over the Adson forceps with the fascia resting between the tips of calipers set at 1 mm thickness. At this level, 3 cm above the inframammary fold, the pectoralis fascia is not more than 0.2 mm thick, and is difficult to maintain intact for draping between the caliper tips.

Figure 8-3. Lateral view of right breast, fresh cadaver dissection. Parenchyma and pectoralis fascia are incised 3 cm superior to the inframammary fold.

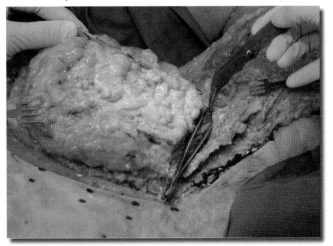

In the right breast of this cadaver, the author and an assistant attempted to elevate the breast tissue off the underlying pectoralis fascia under direct vision with wide exposure. Figure 8-5 shows the breast parenchyma reflected laterally, exposing the pectoralis major muscle and overlying pectoralis fascia. Small portions of breast and adipose tissue were left attached to the pectoralis fascia in an attempt to preserve the layer intact,

Figure 8-4. Closeup view of incised pectoralis fascia 3 cm superior to inframammary fold. Caliper tips are set 1 mm apart for comparison to thickness of pectoralis fascia which is less than 0.2 mm thick.

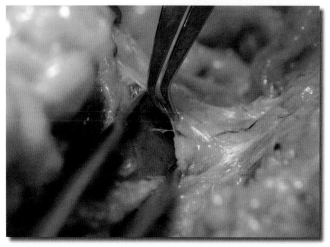

Figure 8-5. Breast parenchyma is reflected laterally and superiorly, attempting to leave intact pectoralis fascia overlying the pectoralis major muscle.

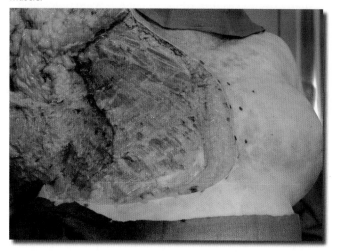

Figure 8-6. Small scalpel incision in pectoralis fascia overlying the upper one-third of the pectoralis where the fascia is supposedly thickest.

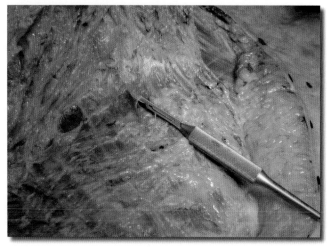

but even with this wide exposure under direct vision, it was exceedingly difficult to maintain the pectoralis fascia intact. Small disruptions of the fascia are apparent in several areas of the dissection.

The pectoralis fascia is supposedly thickest over the middle and upper portions of the pectoralis major muscle. In Figure 8-6, the scalpel has made a small incision in what appears to be the thickest portion of the fascia over the upper portion of the muscle. This area would be the thickest portion of pectoralis fascia overlying a subfascial breast implant. Figure 8-7 is a closeup photograph of the fascia draped over the tip of the scalpel blade. The fascia is so thin that it is transparent, allowing the cutting edge of the scalpel blade to show through the fascia. In Figure 8-8 the fascia on one side of the incision has been placed between caliper tips with the caliper set at 1 mm. The thickness of the pectoralis fascia over this upper portion of the pectoralis muscle is clearly in the range of 0.1–0.2 mm at most, and the filmy, flimsy tissue characteristics of the fascia are apparent.

Figure 8-7. Closeup of pectoralis fascia over scalpel blade over upper third of pectoralis major muscle, demonstrating the less than 2 mm thickness of the pectoralis fascia.

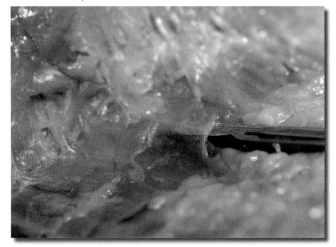

Figure 8-8. Pectoralis fascia over upper third of pectoralis draped between caliper tips set at 1 mm demonstrate thickness of pectoralis fascia at less than 0.2 mm.

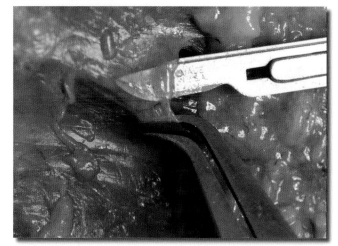

The photographs of fresh cadaver illustrations in this chapter, combined with basic clinical observation during breast augmentation and reconstruction, should convince any surgeon that the pectoralis fascia is not a tissue layer that provides any meaningful, additional soft tissue coverage over any breast implant compared to a submammary placement. In no area overlying a breast implant does the amount of coverage added by pectoralis fascia compare with pectoralis major muscle coverage. These observations can be confirmed in any clinical case of breast augmentation or reconstruction by simply examining the pectoralis fascia in various areas. The appeal of a subfascial pocket to some surgeons, regardless of the reasons, is anatomically illogical and scientifically unproved.

Advantages and tradeoffs of a subfascial pocket location

The potential positives of the subfascial pocket location are much more theoretical than real. The subfascial pocket is essentially a submammary pocket with at most 1 mm of additional fascial coverage. The pectoralis fascia is thickest superiorly (and less than 1 mm thick in that location), and thins significantly from the mid level of the muscle inferiorly to become almost non-existent near the inframammary fold. In most cases the pectoralis inferiorly is indistinguishable from the deep subcutaneous fascia at the level of the inframammary fold. Surgeons can readily observe the thickness and tissue

> The photographs of fresh cadaver illustrations in this chapter, combined with basic clinical observation during breast augmentation and reconstruction, should convince any surgeon that the pectoralis fascia is not a tissue layer that provides any meaningful, additional soft tissue coverage over any breast implant compared to a submammary placement

characteristics while performing breast augmentation or reconstruction procedures, and can easily appreciate the difficulty of raising this particularly thin and flimsy layer of fascia intact. In addition, the pressure and stretch forces exerted by even a moderate size breast implant render this tissue layer even thinner and of no significance whatever as additional soft tissue cover.

Currently, there is no proof in scientifically valid, peer reviewed and published studies that it is surgically possible to elevate the pectoralis fascia and have it remain intact over the entire anterior surface of a breast implant during any primary breast augmentation. Inferiorly and inferolaterally the fascia becomes so attenuated that predictable surgical elevation is improbable at best. An implant in the subfascial location has similar risks of interfering with mammography as a submammary implant. When surgeons attempt to substantially narrow the intermammary distance to less than 3 cm, risks of synmastia are similar for the subfascial and submammary pocket locations.

All currently published studies of clinical series that suggest benefits of the subfascial pocket locations are anecdotal and fail to establish comparative cohorts of patients that have similar quantified tissue characteristics preoperatively. Absent valid comparative cohorts, it is impossible to scientifically validate claims of advantages of the subfascial pocket location for breast augmentation.

Table 8-2 summarizes the potential benefits and inherent tradeoffs of the subfascial pocket location.

Currently, there is no proof in scientifically valid, peer reviewed and published studies that it is surgically possible to elevate the pectoralis fascia and have it remain intact over the entire anterior surface of a breast implant during any primary breast augmentation

All currently published studies of clinical series that suggest benefits of the subfascial pocket locations are anecdotal and fail to establish comparative cohorts of patients that have similar quantified tissue characteristics preoperatively

Table 8-2. Potential advantages and tradeoffs of the subfascial pocket location

Potential advantages	Potential tradeoffs
Less risk of lateral displacement of implants due to pectoralis pressure	Thin, flimsy tissue layer that provides no additional soft tissue coverage superiorly and medially—less than an additional 1 mm of fascia is not meaningful coverage
Less risk of upward displacement of implants due to pectoralis pressure	No proof that fascia can be dissected intact to provide complete implant coverage, especially inferiorly
Less risk of breast distortion with pectoralis contraction	Greater interference with mammography
1 mm or less additional coverage compared to submammary	Increased risk of synmastia with marked narrowing of the intermammary distance
Decreased risks of implant edge prominence compared to submammary	No published data with preop and postop tissue thicknesses documented to prove any advantage

In summary, the subfascial pocket location provides no proved advantages in valid scientific studies compared to the submammary pocket location, and the thin, flimsy layer of fascia provides no significant additional soft tissue coverage compared to the submammary pocket location.

Partial Retropectoral Pocket Location

A partial retropectoral pocket (traditional "subpectoral" pocket) locates the breast implant posterior to the patient's breast parenchyma and posterior to the pectoralis major muscle and fascia, and preserves all pectoralis major muscle origins across the inframammary fold area (Figure 8-9). Dempsey and Latham proposed a partial

Figure 8-9 A, B. The traditional retropectoral or subpectoral pocket preserves all origins of the pectoralis muscle intact along the inframammary fold, and provides muscle coverage over at least the upper two-thirds of the implant, but does not provide muscle coverage of the implant inferolaterally.

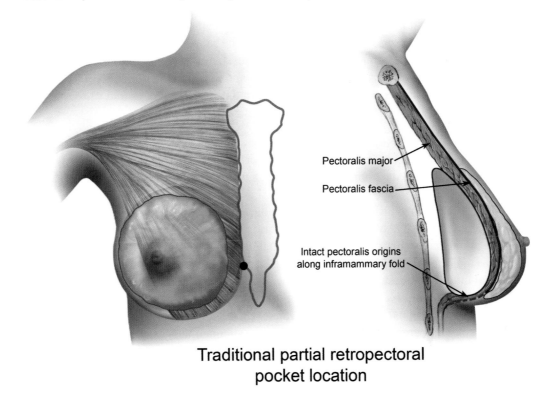

Pectoralis major

Pectoralis fascia

Intact pectoralis origins along inframammary fold

Traditional partial retropectoral pocket location

retropectoral or subpectoral pocket location in 1968[8] and during the next decade many surgeons noted a significant reduction in capsular contracture rates with smooth shell, silicone gel filled implants in the subpectoral location. When developing a traditional subpectoral or partial retropectoral pocket, the surgeon does not divide the inferior origins of the pectoralis major across the inframammary fold.

The author prefers the term "partial retropectoral" to describe the traditional subpectoral pocket location because the pectoralis major muscle never completely covers a breast implant placed in this pocket location. The pectoralis major muscle does not cover the inferolateral one-fourth to one-third of the breast implant. Even with a subpectoral pocket placement, the implant remains only "partial retropectoral" because it is not totally covered by muscle. Many patients and some surgeons continue to believe that the pectoralis major muscle provides complete muscle coverage of an implant, but it does not, hence the term "partial retropectoral" more accurately describes this pocket location compared to "subpectoral".

Surgeons have gained access for partial retropectoral placement through all available incision approaches. Most surgeons gained access to the subpectoral tissue plane by: (a) gaining access from the lateral border of the pectoralis major (via the inframammary and periareolar approaches), (b) splitting the pectoralis muscle along the direction of its fibers (via the periareolar approach), or (c) accessing from the superolateral border of the pectoralis (via the axillary approach).

The partial retropectoral (PRP) pocket location provides the greatest area and thickness of soft tissue coverage of breast implants of any pocket location, and therefore this pocket location best addresses the number one priority in primary augmentation—assuring optimal, maximal soft tissue cover for the longest possible time. By providing this additional coverage, the PRP pocket location reduces or eliminates risks of visible implant edges and visible traction rippling superiorly and medially, provided surgeons preserve all medial origins of the muscle intact along the sternum. Intact origins of the pectoralis major across the inframammary fold, according to some surgeons, provide additional inferior support for implants, reducing risks of inferior implant malposition and excessive inferior pole stretch. By interposing the muscle tissue plane between the implant and overlying parenchyma, the PRP pocket location interferes less with mammography and breast imaging compared to the submammary pocket location.

The advantages of a traditional partial retropectoral or subpectoral approach are compromised by the static and dynamic tissue forces that the pectoralis applies to the

> The partial retropectoral pocket location provides the greatest area and thickness of soft tissue coverage of breast implants of any pocket location, and therefore this pocket location best addresses the number one priority in primary augmentation—assuring optimal, maximal soft tissue cover for the longest possible time

> The advantages of a traditional partial retropectoral or subpectoral approach are compromised by the static and dynamic tissue forces that the pectoralis applies to the breast implant short- and long-term

breast implant short- and long-term. Intact inferior origins of the pectoralis across the inframammary fold apply pressure to the inferior portion of breast implants that produce two compromises: (1) intact muscle pressure prevents the implant resting at the inferior-most point of the pocket, leaving a triangular dead space that fills with fluid and undergoes fibrous tissue replacement until the space is obliterated, and (2) muscle pressure with intact inferior pectoralis origins may cause upward implant displacement in a relatively small percentage of patients. These muscle force effects detract from the accuracy of the position of the inframammary fold immediately post surgically, compromising the accuracy, shape, and time required for formation of the definitive inframammary fold compared to submammary augmentation. The constant pressure on the lower implant with closure of the triangular dead space by fibrous replacement can also produce varying degrees of inferior pocket closure that displace implant fill superiorly and result in bilateral asymmetries of upper pole fill that are noticeable to patients.

Constant muscle pressure in the PRP pocket transmits to the implant that is resting on the curved surface of the thoracic wall. The dynamics of muscle pressure on the implant resting on the curved thoracic wall can cause stretch of the lateral breast soft tissue envelope and gradual shift or displacement of the implant laterally, producing a widening of the intermammary distance that is objectionable to patients and surgeons. When inferior origins of the pectoralis are intact, dynamic pressure of pectoralis muscle contraction produces a range of distortion of breast shape and position, depending on the amount and location of pectoralis attachments to the periprosthetic capsule and soft tissue attachments to the overlying parenchyma. While these tradeoffs are acceptable to most patients who are thoroughly informed of tradeoffs preoperatively, the dynamic effects of the pectoralis are problematic for some patients and surgeons. Regardless of the potential tradeoffs, however, optimizing soft tissue coverage remains the number one priority in augmentation.

When the inferior origins of the pectoralis are intact across the inframammary fold, the larger the implant, the greater the stretch the implant places on the overlying pectoralis. Pectoralis stretch causes discomfort, and combined with many surgeons' preference for blunt dissection techniques that avulse muscle origins off the ribs in the central and lower pocket, PRP patients can experience more postoperative pain and require a longer postoperative recovery period compared to submammary augmentation patients. More refined surgical techniques[5] and the development of the dual plane approach and pocket[1] have eliminated all differences in pain and recovery, with subpectoral and dual plane patients routinely going out to dinner the evening of surgery and returning to full, normal activities within 24 hours.[4,5]

Fresh cadaver anatomy of the subpectoral pocket location

Figure 8-10 shows the right chest of a fresh cadaver with the skin and breast parenchyma reflected superolaterally to expose the pectoralis major muscle and overlying pectoralis fascia with fragments of attached fat and parenchyma. Elevation of the lateral edge of the pectoralis via inframammary or periareolar incision approaches (Figure 8-11) provides access to the subpectoral space. When a breast implant is located in a subpectoral pocket (Figure 8-12), the inferolateral one-third is not covered by pectoralis major muscle. In this cadaver demonstration, the lateral soft tissues have been reflected, allowing more exposure of the superolateral portion of the implant compared to the clinical situation in which only the inferolateral portion of the implant is uncovered by pectoralis. Pressure of the overlying muscle with intact inferior origins across the inframammary fold is causing an "overfill" effect with shell scalloping on a 250 cc smooth shell, saline implant filled to manufacturer's recommendations.

In Figure 8-13, the breast parenchyma has been replaced over the pectoralis to demonstrate the relationships between the tissue layers and the implant. This specimen

Figure 8-10. Right chest, fresh cadaver specimen, with skin and breast parenchyma reflected superolaterally to expose the pectoralis major muscle with overlying pectoralis fascia.

Figure 8-11. Elevation of the lateral border of the pectoralis major muscle for access to the subpectoral space.

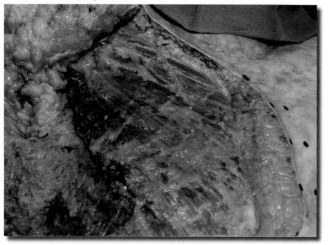

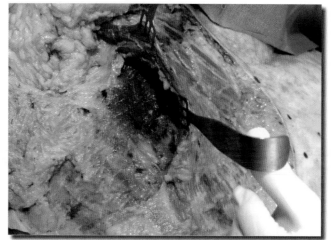

Figure 8-12. Degree of muscle coverage of an implant in a partial retropectoral pocket location. The implant "scalloping" is not due to overfill of the implant, but is instead a consequence of muscle pressure in the cadaver setting.

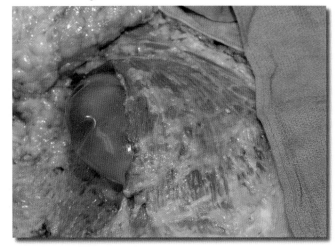

Figure 8-13. Viewed from lateral (left is superior, right is inferior), breast parenchyma has been replaced over partial retropectoral implant to demonstrate tissue layer relationships. Inframammary fold is on the right of the photograph.

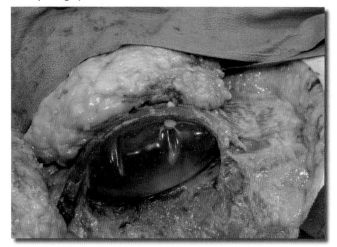

Figure 8-14. Lateral view of partial retropectoral implant. Note dead spaces in the pocket superiorly (white arrow, left) and inferiorly (white arrow, right) created by intact muscle origins across the inframammary fold.

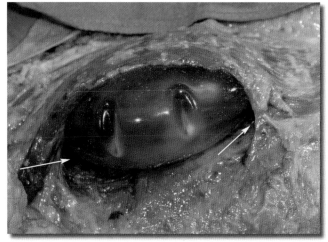

has considerable thickness of breast parenchyma and subcutaneous tissue, and would have had adequate soft tissue coverage for a submammary or subfascial pocket according to the 2 cm pinch thickness criterion of the TEPID[TM,2] and High Five[TM,3] systems. In the closeup lateral view of the subpectoral implant in Figure 8-14, the superior and inferior attachments of the muscle with accompanying muscle tension create a triangular dead space superior and inferior to the implant. Pressure of the inferior muscle origins across the inframammary fold at the right of the image prevents the implant resting at the inferior-most aspect of the pocket. The process of wound healing obliterating this dead space can result in unpredictable upward implant displacement or inframammary fold level or shape aberrations.

Figure 8-15 is a closeup lateral view of the breast implant with overlying pectoralis muscle. The pectoralis muscle is average thickness in this cadaver specimen. The scalpel blade is beneath the pectoralis fascia, gently lifting the fascia to demonstrate the drastic differences in thickness of the pectoralis fascia compared to pectoralis muscle overlying the implant. Compared to the soft tissue thickness of the pectoralis major muscle, the pectoralis fascia is inconsequential. The thin, flimsy pectoralis fascia provides no additional meaningful coverage compared to the thickness and consistency of the pectoralis major muscle.

Table 8-3 summarizes the potential benefits and inherent tradeoffs of the partial retropectoral pocket location.

The thin, flimsy pectoralis fascia provides no additional meaningful coverage compared to the thickness and consistency of the pectoralis major muscle

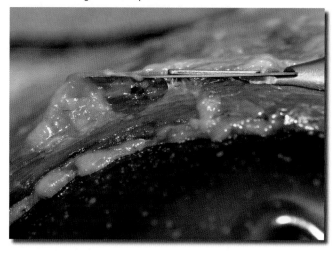

Figure 8-15. Closeup lateral view of partial retropectoral implant with overlying pectoralis major muscle and pectoralis fascia. The scalpel is lifting the thin layer of pectoralis fascia to demonstrate the drastic differences in thickness and soft tissue cover of the muscle compared to the fascia, which is inconsequential in terms of meaningful, long-term soft tissue coverage for the implant.

Table 8-3. Potential advantages and tradeoffs of the partial retropectoral* pocket location

Potential advantages	Potential tradeoffs
Provides the most additional long-term soft tissue cover of any available tissue layer, therefore best addresses the highest priority in primary breast augmentation	Tissue pressure of intact inferior muscle origins tends to displace implant upward
Less interference with mammograms compared to submammary	Tissue pressure of muscle with intact origins may displace implants laterally with time, widening the intermammary distance
Reduces reoperation risks for inadequate coverage deformities, especially superiorly and medially	With intact origins along the IMF, causes distortion of breast shape with pectoralis contraction
Reduces risks of uncorrectable implant edge visibility or visible traction rippling superiorly and medially if all medial origins are preserved	Tissue pressure of intact inferior origins makes precise shape and location of IMF less predictable compared to submammary, prolongs formation of definitive IMF
Intact inferior pectoralis origins reduce risks of inferior implant displacement	Tissue pressure on implant reduces surgeon control of fill in specific areas of the breast
With intact medial origins, eliminates risks of synmastia	
	Causes more postoperative discomfort compared to submammary, subfascial, and dual plane, especially when blunt dissection is used to create the pocket

*Pectoralis origins intact across the inframammary fold. IMF, inframammary fold.

Dual Plane Pocket Location

A dual plane pocket locates the breast implant posterior to the patient's breast parenchyma and posterior to the pectoralis major muscle and fascia in the upper breast and posterior to only breast parenchyma in the lower breast

A dual plane pocket locates the breast implant posterior to the patient's breast parenchyma and posterior to the pectoralis major muscle and fascia in the upper breast and posterior to only breast parenchyma in the lower breast. By dividing pectoralis major origins across the inframammary fold to allow the lower pectoralis muscle border to rotate superiorly, a dual plane pocket allows the implant to rest in a submammary location (posterior to breast parenchyma) in the lower breast (Figure 8-16). The dual plane pocket is designed to maximize long-term soft tissue coverage while minimizing the tradeoffs of the traditional partial retropectoral or subpectoral pocket location. By releasing the origins of the pectoralis across the inframammary fold and preserving all

The dual plane pocket is designed to maximize long-term soft tissue coverage while minimizing the tradeoffs of the traditional partial retropectoral or subpectoral pocket location

Figure 8-16. A dual plane pocket location provides maximal medial and superior soft tissue coverage while minimizing the muscle dynamics tradeoffs of the traditional subpectoral pocket. To create a dual plane pocket, the surgeon divides origins of the pectoralis major across the inframammary fold, but stops all muscle division where the fold meets the sternum at the red dot. Surgeons should never divide any origins of the main body of the pectoralis medially along the sternum.

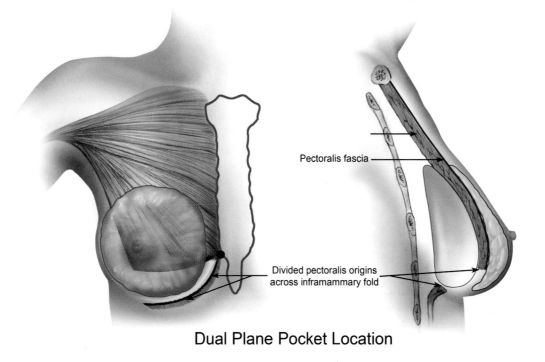

Pectoralis fascia

Divided pectoralis origins across inframammary fold

Dual Plane Pocket Location

muscle origins along the sternum, a dual plane pocket virtually eliminates all of the negative tradeoffs of a traditional partial retropectoral pocket and incorporates all of the advantages of a submammary or subfascial pocket.

Surgeons can precisely adjust the desired position of the lower border of the pectoralis major muscle by adjusting the degree to which they separate attachments of the pectoralis from the overlying parenchyma. The ability to precisely modulate the position of the pectoralis to optimize coverage while minimizing the static and dynamic tradeoffs of an intact pectoralis allow surgeons to (1) eliminate or dramatically reduce the negative tradeoffs associated with traditional partial retropectoral placement, and (2) correct deformities such as tubular breasts, glandular ptosis, and constricted lower pole breasts that previously required a submammary approach with compromised soft tissue coverage in order to optimally address the deformities.

> Surgeons can precisely adjust the desired position of the lower border of the pectoralis major muscle by adjusting the degree to which they separate attachments of the pectoralis from the overlying parenchyma

A dual plane pocket consists of a submammary pocket inferiorly and a partial retropectoral pocket superiorly (Figure 8-16). The surgeon divides the origins of the pectoralis muscle across the inframammary fold, 1 cm superior to the desired postoperative inframammary fold level, stopping precisely where the inframammary fold joins the sternum. *The surgeon never divides any portion of the main pectoralis origins along the sternum, not even 1 cm superior to the junction of the inframammary fold with the sternum.* Preserving all medial origins of the pectoralis along the sternum all the way to the junction of the inframammary fold (IMF) assures two objectives: (1) maximal, optimal, long-term medial coverage of the breast implant edges, and (2) a fixed rotation point for the muscle at the IMF–sternal junction that allows the inferior muscle edge to rotate superomedially while preventing superior retraction of the entire muscle to prevent muscle banding deformities that can result when the surgeon releases pectoralis origins along the sternum.

> The surgeon never divides any portion of the main pectoralis origins along the sternum, not even 1 cm superior to the junction of the inframammary fold with the sternum

The dual plane pocket provides the same degree of maximal long-term soft tissue coverage superiorly and medially as a partial retropectoral pocket. By releasing pectoralis origins along the inframammary fold, the surgeon dramatically decreases the muscle pressure on the lower implant that can cause upward implant displacement, and the unpredictable dead space at the inframammary fold area that occurs when muscle origins are intact. Dividing inferior origins across the inframammary fold also dramatically decreases stretch on the pectoralis, reducing patient discomfort to levels comparable to a submammary pocket. Without the constant pressure of intact pectoralis origins across the inframammary fold transmitted to the implant, lateral displacement of the implant with widening of the intermammary distance rarely occurs. When surgeons place excessively large implants in tight skin envelope breasts, lateral displacement is likely, even if the implant is in a submammary or subfascial plane, because pressure of the tight overlying tissues produces similar effects as pressure from an intact pectoralis major muscle over the implant.

In large series of patients with long-term followup of more than 3000 consecutive primary augmentations with up to current 10 year followup,[1-6,9] peer reviewed and published in the journal *Plastic and Reconstructive Surgery*, the dual plane pocket totally eliminated reoperations for implant edge visibility or visible traction rippling in any area of the breast. No equivalent data have ever been published for any other pocket location that delivers similar results. In addition, no patient in these series was ever reoperated for breast distortion created by muscle contraction. Implant malposition in these series was 0.2%, a rate equal to or better than any other pocket location.

Table 8-4 summarizes the potential benefits and potential tradeoffs of the dual plane pocket location.

> In large series of patients with long-term followup of more than 3000 consecutive primary augmentations with up to current 10 year followup,[1-6,9] peer reviewed and published in the journal *Plastic and Reconstructive Surgery*, the dual plane pocket totally eliminated reoperations for implant edge visibility or visible traction rippling in any area of the breast

Table 8-4. Potential advantages and tradeoffs of the dual plane* pocket location

Potential advantages	Potential tradeoffs
Provides the most additional long-term soft tissue cover of any available tissue layer in the upper and medial areas of the breast, therefore best addresses the highest priority in primary breast augmentation	Decreases coverage slightly at the IMF compared to leaving intact pectoralis origins with partial subpectoral placement (peer reviewed and published data[1-6,11] show no reoperations for inferior implant edge visibility, and 0.2% overall implant malposition at up to 10 year followup, equal to or better than data for any previous pocket location)
Optimizes soft tissue coverage while dramatically reducing or eliminating the potential tradeoffs of partial retropectoral (subpectoral) placement	
Minimal to no lateral implant displacement over time compared to partial retropectoral	
Minimal to no significant breast distortion with pectoralis contraction compared to partial retropectoral	
Reduces postoperative discomfort to levels that are no different compared to submammary, allows patients to be out to dinner the evening of surgery and return to full normal activities in 24 hours[5]	
Reduces reoperation risks for inadequate coverage deformities, especially superiorly and medially	
Reduces risks of uncorrectable implant edge visibility or visible traction rippling superiorly and medially if all medial origins are preserved	
Makes the location and shape of the inframammary fold more predictable compared to partial retropectoral	
Control of breast fill equal to submammary or subfascial location with aesthetically indistinguishable results	

*Pectoralis origins divided across the inframammary fold (IMF).

Dual plane 1, 2, and 3—varying the position of the pectoralis

Surgeons can adjust the position of the inferior border of the pectoralis major muscle using the dual plane approach. By dividing the inferior origins of the muscle from laterally across the inframammary fold, stopping where the fold joins the sternum, the surgeon creates a dual plane 1 pocket (Figure 8-17). In addition, if the surgeon incrementally separates the pectoralis muscle from the overlying parenchyma, the lower edge of the pectoralis rotates superomedially to create a dual plane 2 or 3 pocket. Varying the position of the inferior border of the pectoralis allows surgeons to maximize soft tissue coverage of the implant while allowing the inferior edge of the pectoralis to rotate superomedially and allow more direct pressure of the implant to be transmitted directly to the parenchyma and overlying skin envelope. The versatility of dual plane techniques allows surgeons to provide additional, optimal superior and medial coverage when addressing breast deformities such as constricted lower pole breasts and glandular ptotic breasts that previously could not be optimally treated with a partial

Figure 8-17. In a dual plane 1 (DP1) procedure, the surgeon divides the pectoralis origins across the inframammary fold, but does not separate the inferior muscle edge from overlying breast parenchyma. Incremental separation of the superior pectoralis muscle from overlying parenchyma allows the muscle to rotate superomedially for dual plane 2 and 3 pockets to treat glandular ptotic and constricted lower pole breasts.

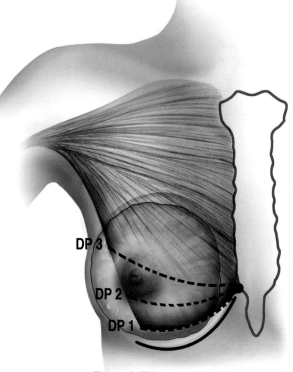

DP 3

DP 2

DP 1

Dual Plane 1, 2, and 3 Pocket Locations

The versatility of dual plane techniques allows surgeons to provide additional, optimal superior and medial coverage when addressing breast deformities such as constricted lower pole breasts and glandular ptotic breasts that previously could not be optimally treated with a partial retropectoral pocket

retropectoral pocket. A dual plane 1 pocket allows the inferior muscle edge to move cephalad 2–3 cm superior to the inframammary fold. A dual plane 2 pocket separates the cut muscle edge from overlying parenchyma in increments to allow the cut edge to move cephalad to approximately the lower border of the areola, and a dual plane 3 allows movement to the level of the nipple or top of the areola (Figure 8-17).

Surgeons can optimally treat over 90% of nulliparous and parous breasts with a dual plane 1 pocket, simply by dividing the inferior origins of the pectoralis across the inframammary fold, *without any additional separation of the cut edge of the pectoralis from the overlying parenchyma*. In most cases, when the surgeon divides the inferior origins of the pectoralis 1 cm above the desired postoperative inframammary fold for a dual plane 1 technique, the lower border of the muscle retracts cephalad approximately 2–3 cm (Figure 8-18). At this point, soft tissue attachments of the muscle to the overlying breast parenchyma tether and restrict further cephalad movement of the muscle edge.

Figure 8-18. Division of inferior pectoralis major muscle origins across the inframammary fold allows the inferior muscle border to rotate 2–3 cm superomedially without any separation of the pectoralis from overlying breast parenchyma.

In glandular ptotic breasts, breast parenchyma "slides off" the anterior surface of the pectoralis major muscle due to weak soft tissue attachments at the parenchyma–muscle interface (Figure 8-19, A). If surgeons create a traditional partial retropectoral pocket, preserving the inferior margins of the pectoralis intact and placing an implant beneath the muscle, the subpectoral implant creates one breast mound, and the existing parenchyma creates a

> Surgeons can optimally treat over 90% of nulliparous and parous breasts with a dual plane 1 pocket, simply by dividing the inferior origins of the pectoralis across the inframammary fold, without any additional separation of the cut edge of the pectoralis from the overlying parenchyma

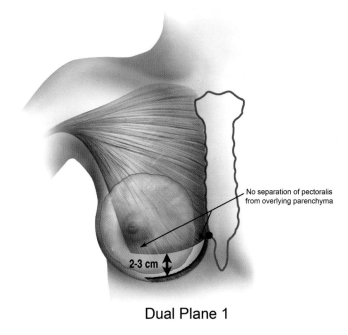

No separation of pectoralis from overlying parenchyma

2-3 cm

Dual Plane 1

Figure 8-19. A: Compliant attachments between breast parenchyma and underlying pectoralis major muscle allow glandular tissue to slide inferiorly off the surface of the pectoralis. B: When breast parenchyma slides inferiorly off the pectoralis, fixation at the inframammary fold level can produce a "double bubble" deformity in the lower breast. C: Dividing the pectoralis origins across the inframammary fold (dual plane 1) and then separating the muscle for an additional 1 cm from overlying breast parenchyma allows the inferior pectoralis edge to move superiorly, allowing implant pressure to further expand the lower pole of the breast and disrupting the overly mobile parenchyma–muscle interface that allowed the double bubble to form. D: Further separation of the superior pectoralis major from overlying parenchyma (dual plane 3) allows the inferior cut muscle edge to rotate superomedially to the nipple or superior areola to treat more severe lower pole constriction deformities by allowing additional implant pressure to expand the breast lower pole.

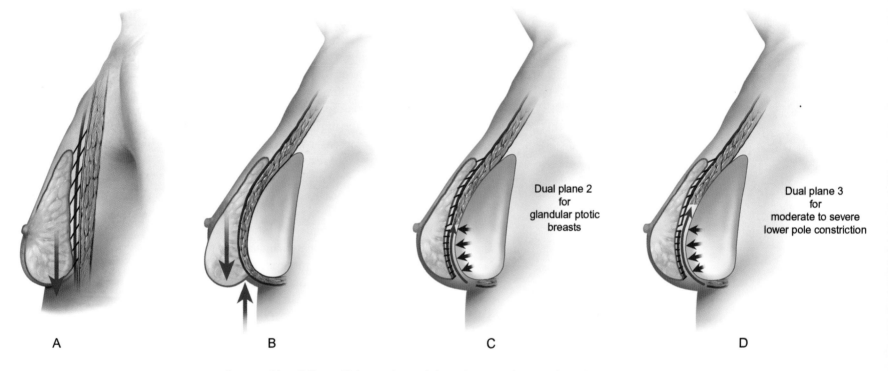

Dual plane 2
for
glandular ptotic
breasts

Dual plane 3
for
moderate to severe
lower pole constriction

A   B   C   D

second mound by sliding off the surface of the subpectoral mound. Traditional partial retropectoral implant placement preserves the parenchyma–muscle interface that allowed the breast tissue to slide off the pectoralis to create the glandular ptosis. If the surgeon does not disrupt the pectoralis–parenchyma interface, the parenchymal mass continues to slide off the surface of the pectoralis, creating a "double bubble" appearance with a secondary fold or indentation located cephalad to the inframammary fold (Figure 8-19, *B*).

When developing a dual plane 2 pocket, the surgeon not only divides pectoralis origins across the inframammary fold, but after dividing the origins, the surgeon then incrementally separates the inferior cut edge of the pectoralis from its attachments to the overlying parenchyma in 1 cm increments, allowing the muscle edge to move superiorly

To most accurately control the position of the pectoralis and preserve optimal coverage, surgeons should always develop the entire subpectoral pocket before performing any additional dissection for separation of pectoralis from overlying parenchyma to approximately the lower edge of the areola. *To most accurately control the position of the pectoralis and preserve optimal coverage, surgeons should always develop the entire subpectoral pocket before performing any additional dissection for separation of pectoralis from overlying parenchyma.*

When treating glandular ptotic breasts, allowing the muscle edge to move superiorly accomplishes two important functions: (1) it disrupts the preoperative parenchyma–muscle interface that allowed the parenchyma to slide off the pectoralis, and (2) it allows the implant, unrestricted by overlying pectoralis, to exert maximal anterior projecting force in direct contact with the parenchyma to optimally correct the glandular ptosis (Figure 8-19, C). When the periprosthetic capsule forms, the tightness of the parenchymal connections to the capsule determines whether the parenchyma can slide inferiorly, but the parenchymal–capsular adherence is usually a vast improvement compared to the preoperative parenchyma–muscle interface.

A dual plane 3 pocket is similar to a dual plane 2 pocket, but the surgeon continues to separate the cut inferior muscle edge from the overlying parenchyma in 1 cm increments until the lower border of the muscle moves superiorly to the level of the nipple or superior border of the areola (Figure 8-19, D). Moving the muscle border further cephalad (while preserving all medial pectoralis attachments to the sternum down to the level of the IMF–sternal junction) allows surgeons to remove pectoralis muscle restriction to implant projection in the lower pole to better stretch and correct tubular breast and constricted lower pole breast deformities.

When developing dual plane 2 or 3 pockets, surgeons should always begin by dividing only the pectoralis origins across the inframammary fold (dual plane 1) and checking the residual restricting effect of the pectoralis to full anterior expansion of the envelope by inserting the index and long fingers into the incision and lifting anteriorly. If the muscle edge is far enough cephalad to remove restriction to anterior expansion, and if the surgeon feels no banding restriction along the inferior cut edge of the pectoralis when pulling anteriorly, no further separation of the muscle from the overlying parenchyma is necessary. *A key principle is to perform the minimal amount of separation of the pectoralis from the overlying parenchyma to allow unrestricted anterior expansion and/ or parenchyma–muscle interface disruption to correct the deformity while preserving maximal soft tissue coverage.*

A key principle is to perform the minimal amount of separation of the pectoralis from the overlying parenchyma to allow unrestricted anterior expansion and/or parenchyma–muscle interface disruption to correct the deformity while preserving maximal soft tissue coverage

When surgically separating the cut edge of the muscle from the overlying parenchyma via the inframammary approach, the surgeon sweeps a needlepoint electrocautery instrument medially and laterally along the parenchyma–muscle interface to separate the attachments (Figure 8-20). It is extremely important to perform this separation to the furthest lateral extent of the cut edge of the pectoralis to prevent residual lateral attachments from restricting superomedial rotation.

Table 8-5 summarizes the surgical techniques and clinical indications for dual plane 1, 2, and 3 type pockets.

Summary of critical surgical principles for the dual plane pocket

The following important technical principles are essential to optimal outcomes using dual plane techniques:

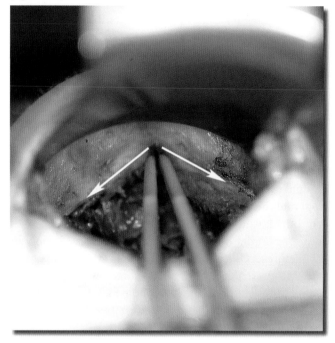

Figure 8-20. When surgically separating the cut edge of the muscle from the overlying parenchyma via the inframammary approach, the surgeon sweeps a needlepoint electrocautery instrument medially and laterally along the muscle–parenchyma interface to separate the attachments (Figure 8-22).

Pocket type	Inferior pectoralis origins divided across IMF	Pectoralis surgically separated from overlying parenchyma	Clinical indications
Dual plane type 1	Yes	No	90% of all breasts
Dual plane type 2	Yes	Yes	Glandular ptotic breasts
Dual plane type 3	Yes	Yes	Severe glandular ptosis Constricted lower pole Tubular deformities

Table 8-5. **Surgical techniques and clinical indications for dual plane 1, 2, and 3 pockets**

IMF, inframammary fold.

1. Optimizing soft tissue coverage long-term is the number one priority in breast augmentation. Subjective estimates of the thickness of soft tissue (terms such as "thick" or "thin") are unscientific, inaccurate, not transferable, and not subject to valid scientific analysis. Surgeons should quantify soft tissue coverage by objective measurements and base decisions of implant pocket location and surgical technique on objective data.[2,3] *When soft tissue pinch thickness at the inframammary fold is less than 0.5 cm, surgeons should not divide pectoralis origins along the inframammary fold*, because long-term benefits of the additional soft tissue coverage of the pectoralis in this area outweigh the tradeoffs of leaving the origins intact. These tradeoffs include more implant distortion with pectoralis contraction, more lateral displacement of the implant over time with widening of the intermammary distance, and slightly less accurate and predictable position and shape of the inframammary fold postoperatively.

2. Regardless of the incision approach, surgeons should *always try to dissect the entire subpectoral pocket before performing any dissection that separates attachments of pectoralis to the overlying parenchyma*. Leaving all pectoralis–parenchyma attachments intact greatly facilitates retraction and exposure for accurate dissection of the subpectoral pocket and avoids excessive release of pectoralis–parenchyma attachments that can allow the inferior edge of the pectoralis to move excessively superiorly.

3. Surgeons should *never divide any of the medial origins of the pectoralis from the sternum, from the sternal notch inferiorly to the junction of the inframammary fold with the sternum.* Any release of pectoralis origins from the sternum superior to the inframammary fold risks excessive superior retraction of the entire lower pectoralis and can cause banding or windowshading deformities when the pectoralis contracts. Risks of "partial" pectoralis division medially, or "attenuating" medial origins to additionally narrow the intermammary distance, far outweigh any possible benefits. "Partial" divisions and "attenuations" can easily become complete divisions, sacrificing critical medial coverage and risking often uncorrectable deformities such as implant edge visibility, visible traction rippling, or synmastia. Restoring soft tissue coverage medially that has been surgically destroyed by poor decisions or poor technique is often impossible, and can create uncorrectable deformities that are preventable by quantifying and preserving optimal soft tissue coverage.

When soft tissue pinch thickness at the inframammary fold is less than 0.5 cm, surgeons should not divide pectoralis origins along the inframammary fold, because long-term benefits of the additional soft tissue coverage of the pectoralis in this area outweigh the tradeoffs of leaving the origins intact

4. Intraoperatively, after dividing pectoralis origins along the inframammary fold, surgeons should be very conservative when separating the pectoralis from overlying breast parenchyma. *Very small increments of separation of pectoralis from overlying parenchyma allow significant upward movement of the inferior border of the pectoralis.* Surgeons should not decide preoperatively to perform a dual plane 2 or 3 procedure, except in cases with significant glandular ptosis or lower pole constriction. Instead, the surgeon should make the decision intraoperatively, after first dividing the inferior origins of the pectoralis and then inserting two or three fingers behind the muscle and breast and pulling anteriorly to assess the expansion of the lower pole and position of the inferior border of the pectoralis. Most cases of primary augmentation do not require additional separation of pectoralis from overlying parenchyma (dual plane 2 or 3). Careful, incremental decision making and release optimize coverage, reduce increased implant exposure to parenchyma, reduce surgical trauma and bleeding, and reduce risks of excessive release and cephalad migration of the pectoralis.

5. Surgeons can apply dual plane techniques via inframammary, periareolar, and axillary approaches, but the inframammary approach provides far superior surgical control compared to other incision approaches. Dual plane techniques are most accurate via the inframammary approach, because surgeons can develop the entire subpectoral pocket without first separating any of the attachments between the pectoralis and overlying breast parenchyma.

6. Via the periareolar approach, the surgeon must first dissect through breast parenchyma before dividing pectoralis origins along the inframammary fold. Regardless of whether surgeons aim directly for the pectoralis at the desired level of muscle division, dissection through breast parenchyma inevitably separates some of the attachments of the parenchyma to the pectoralis, making precise control of the position of the inferior border of the muscle technically more difficult. Suture reattachment of the pectoralis to the parenchyma may be helpful to more accurately position the inferior border of the pectoralis, but suturing muscle to parenchyma is not a highly accurate and reliable maneuver.

7. Via the axillary approach, whenever surgeons divide inferior origins of the pectoralis along the inframammary fold, they are performing a dual plane type 1 procedure, because the cut inferior edge of pectoralis moves superiorly and the implant contacts breast parenchyma in the lower pole of the breast. Although

> Dual plane techniques are most accurate via the inframammary approach, because surgeons can develop the entire subpectoral pocket without first separating any of the attachments between the pectoralis and overlying breast parenchyma

technically possible, surgeons should not attempt a dual plane 2 or 3 procedure via the axilla, because precise, incremental separation of pectoralis from overlying parenchyma requires a retrograde dissection that surgeons can more accurately perform via an inframammary or periareolar approach.

Fresh cadaver anatomy of the dual plane pocket

In Figure 8-21, *A*, a smooth shell saline implant is located in a partial retropectoral pocket with the inferior origins of the pectoralis major muscle intact along the inframammary fold (black line), and the level of proposed division of pectoralis origins across the inframammary fold for a dual plane 1 pocket marked by a purple line on the muscle. The surgeon divides the pectoralis origins across the inframammary fold, 1 cm superior to the fold, beginning at the lateral-most extent of the muscle and continuing medially to a point where the inframammary fold joins the sternum (Figure 8-21, *B*).

Surgeons should not attempt a dual plane 2 or 3 procedure via the axilla, because precise, incremental separation of pectoralis from overlying parenchyma requires a retrograde dissection that surgeons can more accurately perform via an inframammary or periareolar approach

Figure 8-21 A. To create a dual plane 1 pocket, surgeons should divide the inferior origins of the pectoralis muscle across the inframammary fold (purple line) 1 cm superior to the inframammary fold (black line).

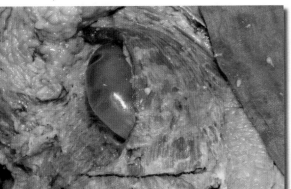

Figure 8-21 B. A retractor is lifting the inferior cut edge of the pectoralis major muscle which has been divided across the inframammary fold, always stopping where the fold meets the sternum.

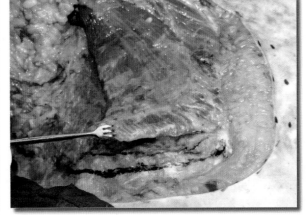

Figure 8-22 A. Position of the pectoralis for a dual plane 1 pocket with simulated implant.

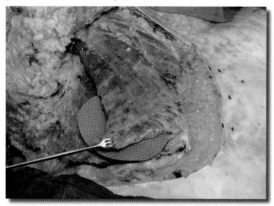

Figure 8-22 B. Position of the pectoralis for a dual plane 2 pocket with simulated implant.

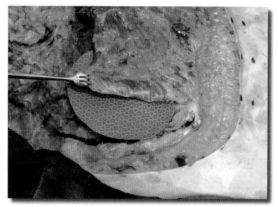

Figure 8-22 C. Position of the pectoralis for a dual plane 3 pocket with simulated implant.

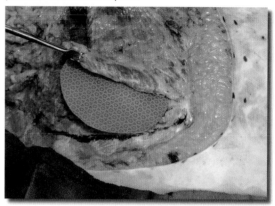

It is critically important for surgeons to preserve all medial origins of the pectoralis intact from the sternal notch to the junction of the sternum with the inframammary fold to assure optimal medial coverage, prevent muscle retraction and banding, and provide a fixed point inferiorly for muscle rotation

Figure 8-22, *A*, *B*, and *C* demonstrate the relative position of the pectoralis muscle overlying a simulated implant for dual plane 1, 2, and 3 pockets respectively. It is critically important for surgeons to preserve all medial origins of the pectoralis intact from the sternal notch to the junction of the sternum with the inframammary fold to assure optimal medial coverage, prevent muscle retraction and banding, and provide a fixed point inferiorly for muscle rotation. Division of pectoralis should never continue past the junction of the inframammary fold with the sternum into the area of pectoralis origins along the lower sternum indicated by the calipers in Figure 8-23.

Figure 8-23. Surgeons should never divide any of the main body of pectoralis origins along the sternum in the area between the tips of the caliper to avoid uncorrectable visible implant edges and traction rippling.

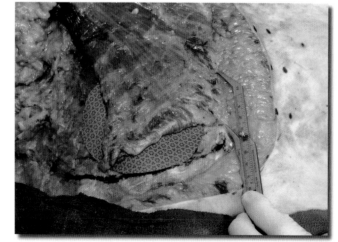

In Figure 8-24, *A*, the pectoralis is retracted superiorly to expose individual, pinnate origins of the pectoralis in the medial pocket. In most cases, a few of these pinnate origins are visible in the implant pocket, and some have white, tendinous attachments to underlying ribs (Figure 8-24, *B*). When these pinnate origins are clearly visible as separate origins apart from the body of the pectoralis origins that are attached medially to the sternum, the surgeon can safely divide these pinnate origins (Figure 8-24, *C*), provided the surgeon is absolutely certain division never risks the complete integrity of the main body of muscle origins along the sternum.

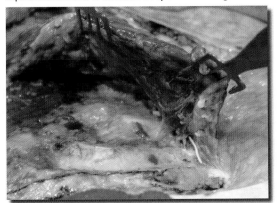

Figure 8-24 A. In the inferomedial portion of the dual plane pocket, a yellow band indicator is positioned between pinnate origins of the pectoralis and the main body of pectoralis origins along the sternum. The pinnate origins are separate and lateral to the main body of muscle origins.

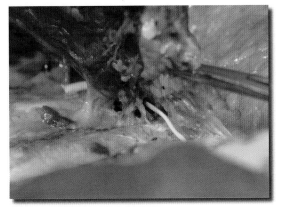

Figure 8-24 B. Pinnate origins of the pectoralis that are located lateral to the main body of pectoralis origins along the sternum often have a whitish or tendinous appearance that is visible in this closeup view.

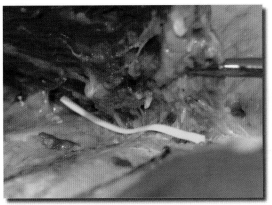

Figure 8-24 C. The pinnate origins in Figure 8-24, *B* have been divided, revealing the intact main body of pectoralis origins along the sternum, located to the right of the yellow indicator.

Dual plane compared to submammary or subfascial pocket locations

Peer reviewed and published data in the journal *Plastic and Reconstructive Surgery*[1,5,6,9] strongly support the following statements regarding the dual plane pocket location:

1. Optimal soft tissue coverage using dual plane principles dramatically reduces overall reoperation rates and reoperations for visible rippling and rippling.

2. Dividing pectoralis origins along the inframammary fold does not result in a higher incidence of inferior implant malposition when using optimal implant selection and surgical techniques.

3. Patients who are thoroughly educated preoperatively regarding tradeoffs of optimal muscle cover versus risks of reoperations or deformities that can result from inadequate cover overwhelmingly prefer maximal soft tissue cover and accept tradeoffs of dual plane placement compared to submammary or subfascial placement.

4. The dual plane approach that preserves all medial attachments of pectoralis to the sternum eliminated reoperations for visible implant edges, visible rippling, and synmastia at up to 12 years followup.

5. Applying optimal dual plane and 24 hour surgery techniques,[1,5,6] pain and recovery for subpectoral augmentation is no different compared to submammary or subfascial augmentation, enabling most patients to be out to dinner the evening of surgery and 96% of patients to return to full, normal activities within 24 hours.

6. The dual plane approach does not limit control of fill in any area of the breast, and consistently produces aesthetic results that are indistinguishable from optimal submammary or subfascial augmentation results while consistently providing maximal, long-term soft tissue coverage and reducing reoperation rates.

7. Patients who are optimally informed and educated preoperatively readily accept a wider intermammary distance (cleavage gap) in exchange for optimal, long-term soft tissue coverage and decreased risks of visible implant edges, visible traction rippling in the cleavage area, and possible synmastia.

8. The dual plane approach significantly reduces or eliminates the following tradeoffs associated with traditional subpectoral augmentation: increased postoperative pain, longer recovery interval, breast distortion during pectoralis contraction, and lateral displacement of the implant due to pectoralis pressure.

9. Using optimal dual plane[1] and 24 hour[5,6] techniques, surgeons can eliminate all of the following unnecessary adjuncts: all surgical bandages, special straps or bras for

> The dual plane approach that preserves all medial attachments of pectoralis to the sternum eliminated reoperations for visible implant edges, visible rippling, and synmastia at up to 12 years followup

> Optimal soft tissue coverage using dual plane principles dramatically reduces overall reoperation rates and reoperations for visible rippling and rippling

> Applying optimal dual plane and 24 hour surgery techniques,[1,5,6] pain and recovery for subpectoral augmentation is no different compared to submammary or subfascial augmentation, enabling most patients to be out to dinner the evening of surgery and 96% of patients to return to full, normal activities within 24 hours

implant positioning, implant motion exercises, drains, intercostal blocks, pain pumps, and narcotic strength pain medications.

No studies currently exist for submammary or subfascial breast augmentation that compare to the studies referenced in this chapter with respect to the size of the clinical series, length of followup, and long-term reoperation rates.

Total Submuscular Pocket Location

A total submuscular pocket locates the breast implant posterior to the patient's breast parenchyma and posterior to the pectoralis major muscle, pectoralis fascia, and posterior to the serratus anterior muscle laterally. This pocket location requires that the surgeon precisely elevate the serratus anterior muscle laterally and create continuity between the lateral edge of the pectoralis major and the medial edge of the serratus to assure complete muscle coverage of the implant.

It is virtually impossible to predictably create a totally submuscular pocket using blunt or blind (not under direct visualization) dissection. Elevating an intact serratus muscle laterally and assuring its continuity with the lateral border of the pectoralis requires precise, direct vision dissection. Many published reports that purport to create a "totally submuscular" pocket do not meet these criteria, and do not really deliver a totally submuscular pocket. Blunt or blind dissection to elevate the serratus muscle often fails to elevate an intact serratus, and often results in a partial retropectoral (pectoralis coverage only) pocket with a shredded serratus that does not provide meaningful coverage.

Assuming that a surgeon is able to precisely elevate an intact serratus muscle laterally, the muscle does not predictably survive to provide additional, significant tissue coverage laterally. When reoperating total submuscular cases for implant replacement years later, the author has noted marked atrophy or virtual absence of the serratus laterally, presumably the result of implant pressure and/or vascular compromise of the muscle. The pressure of the serratus muscle on the implant laterally also causes other significant tradeoffs including unpredictable and suboptimal contours of the lateral mammary fold, implant displacement medially with accompanying nipple-areola malposition, and suboptimal overall breast aesthetics.

> The total submuscular pocket location is not a logical option in primary breast augmentation

The total submuscular pocket location is not a logical option in primary breast augmentation.

◼ POCKET BORDERS AND CONTROL OF IMPLANT POSITION AND BREAST SHAPE

The size of the pocket and the location of pocket borders largely determine the position of smooth shell breast implants postoperatively. The periprosthetic capsule forms on the inner surface of the pocket with smooth shell implants. The position and potential displacement of all smooth shell implants are determined by (1) the size of the pocket the surgeon creates, (2) the areas and extent of pocket closure that occur during the wound healing process, (3) the size of the capsule that forms around the implant, and (4) the degree of contraction of the capsule that can decrease the size of the periprosthetic space.

From the earliest years of breast augmentation until the ban on silicone gel implants in 1994, most surgeons believed that one of the most effective ways to decrease the incidence of capsular contracture was to create a pocket that was much larger than the dimensions of smooth shell implants and instruct patients to perform various types of implant displacement maneuvers postoperatively. Theoretically, the displacement "exercises" would prevent adherence of pocket surfaces and decrease in pocket size, encouraging formation of a large capsular space that minimized risks of the capsule impinging on the implant. Additionally, many surgeons believed (and some continue to believe) that a large periprosthetic space is essential to allow implants to displace laterally and decrease projection with the patient supine for an optimally natural result. The author followed these principles until the mid 1980s, and published supine photographs of axillary augmentation patients to document the natural appearance of the breasts.[10]

While the practice of developing oversize pockets for smooth shell implants and using motion or displacement maneuvers may have some validity, these practices also have the following tradeoffs:

1. Creating a larger pocket creates much larger wound surface areas that are subject to all of the uncontrollable variables of wound healing.

2. Many patients complain about excessive implant displacement and many patients do not want their implants to displace laterally in the supine position (confirmed in a large patient survey in the author's practice).

3. If the pocket is large enough to allow significant loss of projection and lateral displacement with the patient supine, the pocket also allows lateral shift over the curvature of the thoracic wall with the patient upright, widening the intermammary distance (a significant negative to most patients).

4. Motion exercises have never been shown in valid comparative scientific studies to decrease the incidence of capsular contracture.

5. Patient compliance with motion or displacement exercises is variable and unpredictable.

6. Displacement exercises place additional requirements on patients postoperatively that are largely unnecessary.

7. Lastly, and most importantly, it is impossible to maximally control fill in specific areas of the breast to optimally control breast shape without controlling the position of the implant which, in turn, controls the distribution of fill in the breast and therefore controls breast shape.

Extensive clinical experience with a wide range of implant shell types (smooth, polyurethane covered, Biocell™ silicone textured, Siltex™ silicone textured, and others) in the author's practice over three decades, combined with dramatic improvements in surgical techniques, has substantially changed the author's perspective of implant–soft tissue relationships and interactions. The following concepts are derived from this experience:

1. Two levels of breast augmentation exist: breast enlargement and breast enlargement with shape control. Every breast augmentation enlarges the breast, but does not predictably control or improve shape. Controlling shape in a breast requires that the surgeon control the distribution of fill in the breast. To control distribution of fill in a breast, the surgeon must control the position of the breast implant and control distribution of fill within the breast implant. Shape control is impossible with smooth shell implants, especially smooth shell implants that experience upper shell collapse in the upright position when subjected to the tilt test.[11]

Two levels of breast augmentation exist: breast enlargement and breast enlargement with shape control

2. Surgeons cannot predictably control the position of a smooth shell implant because of the large number of uncontrollable variables associated with wound healing mechanisms and capsular formation and contraction. With smooth shell implants, surgeons can only control implant position by precisely creating implant pocket dimensions that only slightly exceed implant dimensions, with the tradeoff that smaller degrees of capsular contraction can impact implant shape, position, and feel.

Surgeons cannot predictably control the position of a smooth shell implant because of the large number of uncontrollable variables associated with wound healing mechanisms and capsular formation and contraction

3. Creating excessively large implant pockets significantly increases patient morbidity and decreases predictability of the result.

Creating excessively large implant pockets significantly increases patient morbidity and decreases predictability of the result

4. Large implant pockets are unnecessary for any type of implant to have adequate mobility to please 95% of patients, regardless of pocket location. In the absence of clinically significant capsular contracture (grades 3 and 4), movement at the capsule–soft tissue interface is completely adequate to achieve a degree of naturalness that satisfies most patients.

> Dissecting large pockets and recommending motion exercises are both totally unnecessary to achieve low rates of capsular contracture and a high degree of patient satisfaction

5. Dissecting large pockets and recommending motion exercises are both totally unnecessary to achieve low rates of capsular contracture and a high degree of patient satisfaction. Data in large series of patients with both saline[1-6] and form stable silicone gel[4] implants prove that optimal surgical techniques, with pockets dissected to precisely fit the base width of the implant, deliver 24 hour recovery, and have capsular contracture rates that are 0.7% up to 7 years with the Allergan/Inamed Style 468 textured, anatomic saline implant and zero percent in a consecutive series with 3 year followup with the Allergan/Inamed Style 410 textured, anatomic form stable silicone gel implant.

6. Based on the experience in the studies in item (5) above, for the past 5 years the author has limited pocket dissection with round, smooth saline implants and dissected pockets to fit the base width of the implant. The result has been a comparably low capsular contracture rate to the studies in item (5) with much better control of breast shape. Patients are more satisfied with better breast shape, naturalness, and avoiding motion exercises compared to the previous practice of dissecting large pockets and performing motion exercises with smooth shell implants.

▓ REFERENCES

1. Tebbetts JB: Dual plane (DP) breast augmentation: optimizing implant–soft tissue relationships in a wide range of breast types. *Plast Reconstr Surg* 107:1255, 2001.

2. Tebbetts JB: A system for breast implant selection based on patient tissue characteristics and implant–soft tissue dynamics. *Plast Reconstr Surg* 109(4):1396–1409, 2002.

3. Tebbetts JB, Adams WP: Five critical decisions in breast augmentation using 5 measurements in 5 minutes: the high five system. *Plast Reconstr Surg* 116(7):2005–2016, 2005.

4. Tebbetts JB: Achieving a predictable 24 hour return to normal activities after breast augmentation Part I: Refining practices using motion and time study principles. *Plast Reconstr Surg* 109:273–290, 2002.

5. Tebbetts JB: Achieving a predictable 24 hour return to normal activities after breast augmentation Part II: Patient preparation, refined surgical techniques and instrumentation. *Plast Reconstr Surg* 109:293–305, 2002.

6. Tebbetts JB: Achieving a zero percent reoperation rate at 3 years in a 50 consecutive case augmentation mammaplasty PMA study. *Plast Reconstr Surg* 118(6):1453–1457, 2006.

7. Graf RM, Bernardes A, Rippel R, Araujo LR, Damasio RC, Auersvald A: Subfascial breast implant: a new procedure. *Plast Reconstr Surg* 111(2):904–908, 2003.

8. Dempsey WC, Latham WD: Subpectoral implants in augmentation mammaplasty. Preliminary report. *Plast Reconstr Surg* 42(6):515–521, 1968.

9. Tebbetts JB: Patient acceptance of adequately filled breast implants using the tilt test. *Plast Reconstr Surg* 106(1):139–147, 2000.

10. Tebbetts JB: Transaxillary subpectoral augmentation mammaplasty: long-term follow-up and refinement. *Plast Reconstr Surg* 74:636–647, 1984.

11. Tebbetts JB: What is adequate fill? Implications in breast implant surgery. *Plast Reconstr Surg* 97(7):1451–1454, 1996.

Incision Approaches

Four incision approaches are currently used for primary breast augmentation: inframammary, axillary, periareolar, and umbilical (Figure 9-1). This chapter provides an overview and comparison of incision approaches, and Chapters 11, 12, and 13 address the inframammary, axillary, and periareolar approaches in detail.

Figure 9-1. Incision locations for primary breast augmentation.

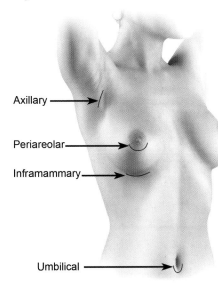

Axillary

Periareolar

Inframammary

Umbilical

■ ISSUES AND SELECTION CRITERIA FOR INCISION APPROACH

Patient selection of incision approach largely depends on the patient's knowledge of incision options and the relative advantages, tradeoffs and limitations of each approach. Most patients, prior to in-depth education from a surgeon, form opinions about incision locations based on the experience of friends who have had breast augmentation, from internet sources, or from surgeon marketing materials. Few patients have adequate information on which to make informed choices when they first contact a surgeon's office. Patients can form opinions based on information from internet sources or from other materials they have seen, but until they receive complete information about incision alternatives, they rarely have an in-depth perspective of the true positives or potential limitations of available incision alternatives.

Patients who have an optimal result from breast augmentation rarely express any concern whatever about the location of their scar, positively or negatively. Absent gross scar hypertrophy or scar malposition, educated patients understand that a scar is a necessary tradeoff of augmentation, that the location

Patients can form opinions based on information from internet sources or from other materials they have seen, but until they receive complete information about incision alternatives, they rarely have an in-depth perspective of the true positives or potential limitations of available incision alternatives

Patients who have an optimal result from breast augmentation rarely express any concern whatever about the location of their scar, positively or negatively

of the scar is not as important as the quality of the result, and that few normal observers of a beautiful breast pay much attention to any scar (just as few observers would pay much attention to a stretch mark). Incision location is much more a preoperative concern than a postoperative concern, provided the surgeon educates the patient and applies basic principles to optimize scar quality. The most important of principles to optimize scar quality in every case, regardless of skin type or other considerations, include: (1) adequate incision length to minimize trauma to skin edges for access and implant insertion, (2) avoiding trauma to skin edges during the procedure, (3) optimal incision location to minimize tension and stretch on the incision, and (4) optimal incision closure techniques that minimize tension on the skin while also minimizing the amount of suture left in the wound to stimulate inflammation.

Surgeons usually have a personal preference for incision location based on their individual training, personal experiences, or marketing beliefs. Few surgeons had extensive experience with multiple incision locations during their training, and understandably, surgeons tend to prefer the incision location that they learned during residency training or the incision with which they have the most clinical experience. Unfortunately, once surgeons gain a preference for a specific incision location, they sometimes tend to form and verbalize negative opinions about alternative incision locations that are not based on truth, scientific data, or logic.

> Surgeons usually have a personal preference for incision location based on their individual training, personal experiences, or marketing beliefs

Some surgeons base choice of incision on marketing concerns, promoting a specific incision location as superior because few competing surgeons in the same geographic area are using that incision location. Many surgeons market "short scar" in lieu of educating patients that an excessively short scar almost assures additional trauma to skin edges that compromises scar quality and makes the scar more apparent. Certain cultures or nationalities of surgeons and patients have strongly ingrained preferences for incision location that are based almost completely on perceptions instead of facts or logic.

> Many surgeons market "short scar" in lieu of educating patients that an excessively short scar almost assures additional trauma to skin edges that compromises scar quality and makes the scar more apparent

Logically, patients and surgeons should choose an incision alternative that is most likely to facilitate an optimal result for the patient, recognizing that an optimal breast augmentation outcome depends on many factors that are more important compared to the location of the scar. In order of priority, surgeons should include the following considerations when choosing incision location:

1. Surgeon skill set to perform the operation at an optimal level via the incision approach

2. Degree of overall control the incision location affords the surgeon to facilitate optimal control of surgical variables to achieve an optimal result in the patient's specific breast type

3. Ability to optimally insert the type of implant selected for the augmentation

4. Extent to which the location and required instrumentation facilitate the surgeon performing the operation with minimal tissue trauma and prospective hemostasis[1] (preventing bleeding before it occurs instead of creating bleeding and then achieving hemostasis to minimize inflammation and pain postoperatively)

5. Extent to which the incision approach traumatizes tissues for access to the surgical pocket for dissection and implant insertion

6. Patient preference after thorough patient education regarding all incision alternatives.

▓ INCISION LOCATION CHOICE IN THE DECISION PROCESS

Incision location is the fifth priority decision of the High Five™ decision process algorithm for primary breast augmentation.[2] Decisions to choose pocket location, implant volume (weight), implant type, and location of the inframammary fold decisions precede selection of incision location. Prioritizing incision location choice above any of the other considerations potentially compromises the outcome, especially the long-term outcome, because the incision location decision does not directly impact the quality of the patient's tissues long-term or the position of the breast on the chest.

Inappropriately prioritizing the choice of incision location can limit other options and compromise other decisions. For example, prioritizing a periareolar incision in a patient with a very small diameter areola limits implant options to inflatable or small non-inflatable implants, and prioritizing an umbilical incision location precludes the patient having options of prefilled, especially form stable, silicone gel implants and the accuracy and control of dissection under direct vision. Patients frequently prioritize incision location above more important decisions, and patient education is vitally important to help patients understand which decisions are most important to optimize results, minimize reoperations, and prevent uncorrectable deformities. A superb scar in the patient's desired location can never compensate for a suboptimal operation and outcome.

Patients frequently prioritize incision location above more important decisions, and patient education is vitally important to help patients understand which decisions are most important to optimize results, minimize reoperations and prevent uncorrectable deformities

In the United States, informed consent law requires that patients make choices regarding their medical care. Surgeons can provide information and assist in the decision process, but patients ultimately must choose the options for their care that they determine are best. Surgeons can easily influence a patient's choice of incision location through the content of information they provide the patient, but surgeons are legally responsible for providing the patient valid information about all options during the informed consent process and documenting that the patient understands the options. Informed consent law requires that the patient make the final decision of incision location.

■ POPULAR MYTHS REGARDING INCISION LOCATION

Many myths have evolved regarding incision location in breast augmentation. The following are *untrue statements* regarding incision locations:

1. *For patients with minimal breast tissue, the inframammary incision location is not a good choice because a shallow inframammary fold cannot conceal the scar.* This opinion is not necessarily true, and thousands of happy patients with this type of breast have had inframammary incisions. Surgeon placement of the incision is critical to minimize scar visibility in any incision location.

2. *Surgeons should place inframammary incisions slightly above the level of the projected postoperative inframammary fold.* One of the greatest determinants of scar quality is the degree of stretch that can cause scar widening. Breast implants exert maximal stretch on the skin of the breast lower pole. Minimal stretch forces occur when an inframammary incision is located precisely in the postoperative inframammary fold, not above the fold where stretch is likely to cause scar widening.

> Minimal stretch forces occur when an inframammary incision is located precisely in the postoperative inframammary fold, not above the fold where stretch is likely to cause scar widening

3. *A shorter scar is always preferable to a longer scar.* This assumption is inaccurate, because shorter scars limit visualization and accuracy, compromise results, and promote skin edge trauma that compromises scar quality.

4. *Incisions off the breast are always less noticeable compared to incisions on the breast.* The patient always notices a scar, regardless of where it is located. In the presence of a beautiful breast with an acceptable periareolar or inframammary scar, observers might equally notice a scar in the axillary or umbilical areas.

5. *One incision or another best preserves breast sensation.* The most common cause of sensory impairment following breast augmentation is an excessively large pocket or excessively large implant. Incision locations off the breast may cause less impairment of breast sensation immediately adjacent to the incision location on the

breast, but no valid scientific evidence documents superiority of any incision location with respect to long-term breast sensation.

■ OBJECTIVITY IN EVALUATING INCISION APPROACHES

Scientifically valid comparisons of incision locations are virtually impossible because the number of variables that affect scar width and quality preclude preoperatively establishing scientifically valid cohorts of patients with similar wound healing mechanisms. Any surgeon can select photographs to prove or disprove any opinion regarding scar quality outcomes in breast augmentation, but selected photographs do not provide objective, scientifically valid comparisons.

> Any surgeon can select photographs to prove or disprove any opinion regarding scar quality outcomes in breast augmentation

Other factors that complicate or obviate objective comparisons of incision locations are surgeons' willingness to verbalize opinions about incision location that are not based on significant clinical experience, or variations in surgeons' decision processes and technical skills that can affect scar location and quality.

The author's opinions and statements in this chapter derive from 30 years of clinical experience using inframammary, axillary, periareolar, and a limited number (six) of umbilical incision approaches. Comments regarding the umbilical incision approach are based on this limited experience and on logic derived from experience with the other incision approaches.

■ THE INFRAMAMMARY INCISION LOCATION—ADVANTAGES AND TRADEOFFS

1:7
1:12

The inframammary incision approach is the most widely used incision approach in breast augmentation. Based on published data and logic, the inframammary approach is the incision approach to which surgeons should objectively compare all other incision approaches. The inframammary incision approach provides a level of direct vision and surgical control that is unmatched by other incision locations, and enables surgeons to achieve greater control over a greater number of surgical variables that affect outcomes. The most important of these variables are the degree of tissue trauma and bleeding that occur during the operation, the degree of precision during pocket dissection, and the ease with which the surgeon can introduce the implant without damaging the device. No incision approach surpasses the inframammary approach with respect to these three important considerations.

> The inframammary incision approach provides a level of direct vision and surgical control that is unmatched by other incision locations, and enables surgeons to achieve greater control over a greater number of surgical variables that affect outcomes

Compared to all other
incision approaches, the
inframammary approach
causes the least trauma to
adjacent tissues for pocket
access and implant insertion

Compared to all other incision approaches, the inframammary approach causes the least trauma to adjacent tissues for pocket access and implant insertion. All areas of the implant pocket are directly visible and accessible through this approach, and surgeons can precisely complete pocket dissection in all pocket locations and place all types of breast implant via this approach. The inframammary approach requires no special instrumentation, and is the most efficient of all approaches with respect to minimizing operative times, thereby minimizing drug dosages and optimizing patient recovery.[1] In the author's published study detailing techniques that deliver predictable 24 hour recovery, comparable recovery was achieved via inframammary, periareolar, and axillary approaches, but operative times were longer for periareolar and axillary approaches compared to the inframammary approach.[1]

Adequate incision length, care
to avoid trauma to skin edges,
and precise closure techniques
produce equivalent quality
scars in all current incision
locations over a wide range of
patient skin types

The primary tradeoff of an inframammary incision is the presence of a visible scar on the aesthetic unit of the breast. Some surgeons believe that incisions in thinner skin of the areola or axilla result in uniformly superior scars compared to the inframammary scar, but this has not been the author's experience. Adequate incision length, care to avoid trauma to skin edges, and precise closure techniques produce equivalent quality scars in all current incision locations over a wide range of patient skin types. The location of the incision is less important than these other considerations. In over 3000 consecutive primary breast augmentations, the author has injected steroids into only two patients' scars, and has performed no surgical scar revisions for poor quality scars.

Another potential tradeoff of the inframammary scar is that in order to have the scar in an optimal location postoperatively, surgeons must plan the location of the postoperative inframammary fold (IMF) and locate the inframammary incision *precisely at the level of the planned postoperative inframammary fold.* If the surgeon routinely makes the incision in the *preoperative* IMF without considering and planning the level of the *postoperative* IMF, the resultant scar will usually be above the inframammary fold on the skin of the breast lower pole where it is subjected to greater stretch forces that cause scar widening. These two potential tradeoffs of the inframammary incision are minor and largely controllable compared to tradeoffs of the other incision approaches.

Virtually every type of breast can be optimally augmented via the inframammary approach, with few exceptions. Despite some surgeons' preference for a periareolar approach in constricted lower pole breasts and tubular breasts, if areolar asymmetry or areolar pseudoherniation is not present, and provided the surgeon knows how to plan the position of the postoperative inframammary fold,[2,3] the inframammary approach provides excellent access to address these deformities.

The inframammary incision is not an optimal choice in patients who have an extremely strong history of hypertrophic scarring, and is not ideal in any patient who has a phobia or great concerns about having a scar on the breast. If a patient strongly prefers a scar off the aesthetic unit of the breast, provided she is thoroughly educated and understands the tradeoffs, an axillary incision location is an excellent alternative.

> The inframammary incision is not an optimal choice in patients who have an extremely strong history of hypertrophic scarring, and is not ideal in any patient who has a phobia or great concerns about having a scar on the breast

■ THE AXILLARY INCISION LOCATION—ADVANTAGES AND TRADEOFFS

> The axillary incision approach is the most logical incision approach for patients who strongly desire an incision located off the visible aesthetic unit of the breast

The axillary incision approach is the most logical incision approach for patients who strongly desire an incision located off the visible aesthetic unit of the breast. The primary advantage of the axillary approach is that it locates the incision off the breast, and compared to the umbilical approach, it causes far less trauma to adjacent tissues for access to the surgical pocket. In addition, compared to the umbilical approach that currently utilizes blunt, blind dissection, the axillary approach enables surgeons to perform all pocket dissection under direct vision with electrocautery instruments and apply prospective hemostasis principles[1,4] that minimize tissue trauma and blood in the tissues. Technical refinements in endoscopically assisted axillary augmentation enable patients with submammary or subpectoral axillary augmentation to predictably experience 24 hour return to normal activities,[1] and allow surgeons to perform all dissection under direct vision.[4]

> Compared to the umbilical approach that currently utilizes blunt, blind dissection, the axillary approach enables surgeons to perform all pocket dissection under direct vision with electrocautery instruments and apply prospective hemostasis principles[1,4] that minimize tissue trauma and blood in the tissues

3:1

All current pocket locations are accessible via the axillary approach, and surgeons with optimal skill sets can place all types of currently available implants accurately and precisely via the axillary approach. A common misconception is that surgeons cannot precisely and accurately place anatomic or shaped implants via the axilla, especially shaped implants that contain form stable silicone gel. Peer reviewed and published reports confirm the ability to place shaped implants via the axilla,[1-4] and further confirm a rate of implant malposition at up to 7 year followup that is substantially lower compared to the malposition rate for round implants in Food and Drug Administration (FDA) premarket approval (PMA) studies.[1,3,5–8] Surgeons can insert form stable silicone gel implants via the axillary approach, but the inframammary approach provides better access and more control for placing form stable gel implants with less risk of damage to the devices.

Incision location is critical to minimize scar visibility in the axilla, orienting the scar transversely (anterior and posterior) in the apical, hair bearing hollow of the axilla, at least 2 cm posterior to the lateral edge of the pectoralis major muscle

Incision location is critical to minimize scar visibility in the axilla, orienting the scar transversely (anterior and posterior) in the apical, hair bearing hollow of the axilla, at least 2 cm posterior to the lateral edge of the pectoralis major muscle. Surgeons have direct vision access for dissection of the upper half of the implant pocket using electrocautery instruments, but the approach requires specialized endoscopic instrumentation described in Chapter 12 to eliminate blunt dissection that compromises recovery and outcomes. Critical neurovascular structures such as the axillary artery and vein and the brachial plexus are adjacent to the axillary incision site, and rare injuries to these structures have been reported in cases of axillary augmentation. The intercostobrachial and medial brachial cutaneous nerves course through the axillary fat, and injuries to these structures occur when surgeons dissect excessively posteriorly in the axillary fat pad.

Other potential tradeoffs of the axillary approach that are usually temporary but nevertheless cause postoperative morbidity include transient lymphadenopathy, axillary fluid collections, difficulty and delay in shaving the axilla, transient sensory loss in the axilla and upper arm, and lymphatic or fibrous bands in the axilla. The incidence of each of these potential tradeoffs is extremely low, but surgeons should inform patients of each of these tradeoffs when discussing incision alternatives. Although questions have been raised regarding this approach compromising sentinel node sampling or imaging, published studies indicate that accurate imaging sampling can be performed following axillary augmentation.

Although reports exist in the literature documenting some reoperations via the axilla, no reoperation via the axilla is as accurate, controlled, and provides as many intraoperative options compared to performing the reoperation via the inframammary or periareolar approach

An important and significant tradeoff that must be addressed with patients preoperatively is that most problems that necessitate a reoperation following axillary augmentation require an additional inframammary or periareolar incision to optimize control and accuracy during the reoperation. Although reports exist in the literature documenting some reoperations via the axilla, no reoperation via the axilla is as accurate, controlled, and provides as many intraoperative options compared to performing the reoperation via the inframammary or periareolar approach.

The axillary approach is not an optimal choice in patients with severe glandular ptosis, and does not provide optimal exposure and control for correction of tubular breasts and moderate to severe constricted lower pole breasts.

The axillary approach is not an optimal choice in patients with severe glandular ptosis, and does not provide optimal exposure and control for correction of tubular breasts and moderate to severe constricted lower pole breasts

■ THE PERIAREOLAR INCISION LOCATION—ADVANTAGES AND TRADEOFFS

The periareolar approach for breast augmentation provides excellent access for direct visualization and control of pocket dissection in all areas of the pocket. Proponents of this approach emphasize that all areas of the pocket are approximately equidistant from the incision, facilitating control and flexibility. Advocates of the periareolar approach often state that the periareolar location uniformly produces superior scar results compared to the inframammary approach, but no valid scientific studies confirm this opinion, and the author's clinical experience indicates equal scar results in all locations. The periareolar approach is particularly logical for patients who have areolar asymmetries, deformities, or nipple-areola malposition that require correction at the time of breast augmentation.

3:2

Surgeons can insert virtually all types of implant via the periareolar approach, provided the diameter of the patient's areola is adequate. Larger silicone gel implants, especially form stable gel implants, are more difficult to place via a periareolar incision, with greater risks of damaging the implant during insertion. No critical neurovascular structures are in close proximity to any area of dissection in this approach.

Regardless of whether surgeons attempt to tunnel over and around breast parenchyma or dissect directly through breast parenchyma, dissection through or around breast parenchyma causes significantly more tissue trauma compared to inframammary and axillary approaches. Although the author documented 24 hour return to normal activities following periareolar augmentation in both submammary and subpectoral pocket locations,[1] dissection through breast parenchyma undoubtedly results in more edema, occasional ecchymosis, and a longer time required for the breast tissues to return to normal compared to the inframammary approach which does not traumatize breast parenchyma.

Inserting any breast implant via a periareolar approach exposes the implant to more endogenous bacteria in the breast parenchyma compared to other approaches. Although scientific studies fail to confirm higher infection rates and capsular contracture rates for the periareolar approach, additional tissue trauma and exposure of the implant to bacteria are valid concerns that deserve surgeon consideration. Incising around or through the areola undoubtedly interrupts innervation in this area, but no scientifically valid studies document greater long-term sensory loss from the periareolar approach. Creation of a tunnel through breast parenchyma has resulted in a low incidence of cases

Advocates of the periareolar approach often state that the periareolar location uniformly produces superior scar results compared to the inframammary approach, but no valid scientific studies confirm this opinion

Regardless of whether surgeons attempt to tunnel over and around breast parenchyma or dissect directly through breast parenchyma, dissection through or around breast parenchyma causes significantly more tissue trauma compared to inframammary and axillary approaches

Inserting any breast implant via a periareolar approach exposes the implant to more endogenous bacteria in the breast parenchyma compared to other approaches

Creation of a tunnel through breast parenchyma has resulted in a low incidence of cases of herniation of the implant through the parenchymal defect, with or without surgical closure of the parenchyma at the time of augmentation

of herniation of the implant through the parenchymal defect, with or without surgical closure of the parenchyma at the time of augmentation.

The periareolar approach is not an optimal choice for patients with smaller areolas (less than 3.5 cm diameter) when planned implant base width exceeds 13 cm for conventional gel implants or exceeds 12 cm for form stable gel implants. The approach is also not an optimal choice for patients with any history of parenchymal breast disease.

▓ THE UMBILICAL INCISION LOCATION—ADVANTAGES AND TRADEOFFS

The umbilical incision approach is the least used approach for breast augmentation. Its primary advantages are locating the scar off the visible aesthetic unit of the breast, no proximity to critical neurovascular structures, and the marketability of the incision approach to a segment of breast augmentation patients.

No other approach creates as much trauma to adjacent tissue as the umbilical approach that requires surgeons to create two tunnels through abdominal soft tissues from the umbilicus to each breast. Additional morbidity and complications relating to the blunt or sharp creation of the abdominal tunnels is clearly documented and detracts from the logic of this incision approach compared to other approaches.

Current techniques for umbilical augmentation use blunt, blind (no direct vision inside the pocket during dissection) dissection to create the pocket for the implant. Although proponents claim minimal bleeding and rapid recovery with the procedure, examination of the implant pocket with an endoscope following pocket creation uniformly shows markedly blood stained tissues with substantially more blood remaining in the tissues compared to peer reviewed and published dissection methods under direct vision.[1] Proponents of the umbilical approach claim equal facility creating submammary and partial retropectoral pockets, but published reports and observations during live surgery demonstrations of the techniques point out difficulties in predicting and assuring precise pocket locations.

The umbilical approach limits implant options to inflatable implants, and inflatable implants have a substantially higher device failure rate over time compared to latest generation form stable, silicone gel implants. No peer reviewed and published report of umbilical augmentation documents a recovery equal to the recovery reported with

---

Sidebar notes:

No other approach creates as much trauma to adjacent tissue as the umbilical approach that requires surgeons to create two tunnels through abdominal soft tissues from the umbilicus to each breast

Current techniques for umbilical augmentation use blunt, blind (no direct vision inside the pocket during dissection) dissection to create the pocket for the implant

The umbilical approach limits implant options to inflatable implants, and inflatable implants have a substantially higher device failure rate over time compared to latest generation form stable, silicone gel implants

Proponents of the umbilical approach claim equal facility creating submammary and partial retropectoral pockets, but published reports and observations during live surgery demonstrations of the techniques point out difficulties in predicting and assuring precise pocket locations

Table 9-1. Advantages and tradeoffs of incision approaches for primary breast augmentation

Incision approach	Potential advantages	Limitations and tradeoffs
Inframammary	Most widely used Best direct vision access Direct vision dissection all areas of pocket Best surgical control Applicable to all breast types Least traumatic to tissues for access Most versatile No immediately adjacent, critical neurovascular structures Requires no specialized instrumentation No additional incision required for secondary procedure Documented 24 hour return to normal activities via this approach[1] All pocket locations routinely accessible Applicable to all types of implant with maximal accuracy and options Most efficient of all approaches by documented operation times[1]	Scar located on the aesthetic unit of the breast For optimal location, requires that surgeons preoperatively plan the location of the postoperative inframammary fold
Axillary	Located off the aesthetic unit of the breast Documented 24 hour return to normal activities via this approach[1] All pocket locations routinely accessible Applicable to all types of implant, but requires special skills with shaped implants	Limited direct vision access Direct vision dissection requires endoscopic instrumentation in lower pocket Several adjacent critical neurovascular structures Requires specialized endoscopic instrumentation for optimal surgical techniques Morbidity can include axillary lymphadenopathy, axillary banding, difficulty shaving axilla Questions regarding potential effects on sentinel node mapping Requires additional incision for optimal control if reoperation required
Periareolar	Good direct vision access Direct vision dissection all areas of pocket Good surgical control Equidistant access to all areas of surgical pocket Few immediately adjacent, critical neurovascular structures Documented 24 hour return to normal activities via this approach[1] All pocket locations routinely accessible Applicable to all types of implant, but incision size may limit some options in shaped, form stable implants	Located on the most visible portion of the breast aesthetic unit Additional tissue trauma and bleeding required for access—must traverse breast parenchyma Increased implant exposure to endogenous bacteria in breast parenchyma Areolar size limits applicability for larger implants Limited field of view compared to inframammary Theoretically interrupts some innervation to nipple/areola Risks of areolar pigmentation abnormalities with intraareolar incisions in dark areolas Implant herniation through parenchymal tunnel Not ideal for patients with history of parenchymal breast disease
Umbilical	Located off the aesthetic unit of the breast Few immediately adjacent, critical neurovascular structures	No direct vision access Blunt, blind dissection techniques increase tissue trauma, decrease accuracy Traumatizes abdominal tissues for surgical access Limited to inflatable implants No documented recovery equal to other three approaches[1] Requires additional incision for optimal control if reoperations required

inframammary, axillary, and periareolar approaches.[1] Although reports of performing reoperations via the umbilicus exist, the approach does not provide optimal control for any reoperation except possibly exchange of a deflated implant that does not require any accurate capsule modification.

The umbilical approach is unlikely to become a mainstream approach for breast augmentation until surgeons can perform all dissection under direct endoscopic control and document recovery and outcomes comparable to the other incision approaches[1] and confirm comparable recovery and outcomes both in larger peer reviewed studies in indexed journals and in more live surgical demonstrations that show patient recovery in the days immediately following surgery. The approach will likely remain popular with surgeons who use it to successfully market breast augmentation.

Table 9-1 summarizes potential advantages, limitations, and tradeoffs of the four current incision locations for breast augmentation.

▦ REFERENCES

1. Tebbetts JB: Achieving a predictable 24 hour return to normal activities after breast augmentation Part II: Patient preparation, refined surgical techniques and instrumentation. *Plast Reconstr Surg* 109:293–305, 2002.

2. Tebbetts JB, Adams WP: Five critical decisions in breast augmentation using 5 measurements in 5 minutes: the high five system. *Plast Reconstr Surg* 116(7):2005–2016, 2005.

3. Tebbetts JB: Dual plane (DP) breast augmentation: optimizing implant–soft tissue relationships in a wide range of breast types. *Plast Reconstr Surg* 107:1255, 2001.

4. Tebbetts JB: Axillary endoscopic breast augmentation: processes derived from a 28-year experience to optimize outcomes. *Plast Reconstr Surg* 118(7S):53S–80S, 2006.

5. Tebbetts JB: Patient acceptance of adequately filled breast implants using the tilt test. *Plast Reconstr Surg* 106(1):139–147, 2000.

6. Food and Drug Administration. U.S. Food and Drug Administration. General and Plastic Surgery Devices Panel Meeting Transcript. Washington, D.C. October 14–15, 2003. Online. Available: http://www.fda.gov/ohrms/dockets/ac/03/transcripts/3989T1.htm.

7. Food and Drug Administration. U.S. Food and Drug Administration. General and Plastic Surgery Devices Panel Meeting Transcript. Washington, D.C. February 18, 1992.

8. Food and Drug Administration. U.S. Food and Drug Administration. General and Plastic Surgery Devices Panel Meeting Transcript. Washington, D.C. March 1–3, 2000. Online. Available: http://www.fda.gov/cdrh/gpsdp.html#030100.

Surgical Principles and Instrumentation

CHAPTER 10

Specific surgical principles are critical to optimize the patient experience and outcomes in breast augmentation, regardless of the incision approach, pocket location, or type of implant. Compulsively addressing seemingly minor technical issues can dramatically impact the patient experience, outcomes, and reoperation rates. Analyzing every aspect of surgical technique and continually improving efficiency and eliminating unnecessary and unproductive actions using process engineering principles[1,2] can dramatically impact short- and long-term outcomes. Optimally controlling surgical variables that impact outcomes requires that surgeons continually reassess established practices, avoid preconceptions, and demonstrate a willingness to implement proved processes.[1–4]

Rate of recovery is the single best indicator of the degree of surgical trauma a patient experiences during a breast augmentation. Surgical techniques determine the degree of tissue trauma and bleeding that directly impact levels of inflammation and wound healing response that subsequently define recovery, pain, medication requirements, capsule formation and contraction, risks of infection and resultant reoperation rates. Patients who recover and return to normal activities rapidly have undoubtedly experienced less tissue trauma and bleeding compared to patients who require longer recovery periods complicated by numerous adjunctive measures, devices, and pain medications. The surgical techniques that dramatically shorten and simplify patient recovery and reduce reoperation rates impact short- and long-term outcomes by reducing tissue trauma, reducing bleeding, and increasing accuracy.

Surgeons can ask a very simple set of questions regarding every surgical maneuver that can dramatically improve efficiency and patient outcomes:

Optimally controlling surgical variables that impact outcomes requires that surgeons continually reassess established practices, avoid preconceptions, and demonstrate a willingness to implement proved processes

Rate of recovery is the single best indicator of the degree of surgical trauma a patient experiences during a breast augmentation

- What does it really do?

- Is it really necessary?

- What is the objective, published evidence of its necessity and efficacy?

- Is there an alternative that causes less tissue trauma and bleeding?

- How can I implement it and improve it?

◼ IMPACT OF DECISION PROCESSES AND SURGICAL PLANNING

Surgical planning and the decision process define and limit the potential success of every surgical maneuver

Chapter 7 details principles and methodologies that optimize surgical planning. Surgical planning and the decision process define and limit the potential success of every surgical maneuver. Every suboptimal or unnecessary surgical maneuver increases bleeding and tissue trauma, increases operative time and costs, increases medication doses intraoperatively, decreases the predictability of the outcome, and increases risks of complications and reoperations. The key for surgeons is to identify and optimize surgical maneuvers that are proved to impact outcomes, and eliminate all maneuvers, techniques, and adjuncts that are unnecessary and unproductive.

Unnecessary and unproductive surgical maneuvers are not harmless, and while many alternative techniques allow surgeons to perform breast augmentation many different ways, defined sets of proved processes and techniques deliver optimal recovery and outcomes

Unnecessary and unproductive surgical maneuvers are not harmless, and while many alternative techniques allow surgeons to perform breast augmentation many different ways, defined sets of proved processes and techniques deliver optimal recovery and outcomes. Surgeons' willingness to continually reevaluate established practices, implement proved processes, and eliminate unnecessary and unproductive practices determines patient recovery, outcomes, and reoperation rates.

Every decision that a surgeon can make before entering the operating room positively impacts potential patient recovery and outcome. With current proved processes for operative planning and implant selection that are peer reviewed and published in the plastic surgery literature, operating times for an uncomplicated, primary breast augmentation should not exceed 45 minutes. The cost of making decisions in the operating room, especially decisions that could be made preoperatively, is substantial. Unnecessarily prolonging operative times may seem inconsequential to some surgeons, but lack of optimal planning and inefficiency during surgery are not inconsequential to patients who experience increased costs, increased doses of anesthetic and narcotic medications, and prolonged recovery with unnecessary morbidity.

Every decision that a surgeon can make before entering the operating room positively impacts potential patient recovery and outcome

Some of the most inefficient, time wasting practices intraoperatively relate to implant selection and the use of intraoperative sizer implants. Currently available systems and decision processes for preoperative implant selection[3,5] eliminate any need for sizer implants in routine primary augmentation, and reduce or eliminate the costly practice of surgeons ordering multiple sizes of implants for every breast augmentation. In addition to unnecessarily increasing operative times and costs, routine use of sizer implants increases risks of pocket contamination, may increase tissue trauma and bleeding, and has no proved necessity or efficacy in valid scientific studies.

Currently available systems and decision processes for preoperative implant selection[3,5] eliminate any need for sizer implants in routine primary augmentation, and reduce or eliminate the costly practice of surgeons ordering multiple sizes of implants for every breast augmentation

Operative planning is most productive and least prone to errors of omission when surgeons complete defined forms[3,5] that record objective measurement data and record decisions and operative plans, and then have these forms available in the operating room for every breast augmentation. Having standardized, preoperative photographs in the operating room is also helpful, but virtually every decision that a surgeon makes looking at photographs in the operating room could have been made preoperatively and recorded on the operative planning form, increasing efficiency and accuracy.

Virtually every decision that a surgeon makes looking at photographs in the operating room could have been made preoperatively and recorded on the operative planning form, increasing efficiency and accuracy

■ DIRECT VISION ACCESS AND POCKET DISSECTION TECHNIQUES

Blunt and blind (no direct vision inside the pocket) dissection techniques unquestionably increase tissue trauma and bleeding and decrease the accuracy of pocket dissection compared to techniques that perform pocket dissection under direct vision, with or without endoscopic assistance. While blunt dissection and blunt, blind dissection techniques remain in common use, no peer reviewed and published studies and no live surgery demonstrations have ever documented equivalent patient recovery and outcomes compared to more controlled, accurate, and efficient direct vision techniques.[1,2,6,7]

Inframammary and periareolar incision approaches allow surgeons to perform all areas of pocket dissection under direct vision control, but some surgeons continue to use digital or blunt instrument dissection techniques, citing the speed and efficiency of blunt dissection techniques. In reality, blunt dissection techniques cannot compare with optimal electrocautery dissection techniques with respect to efficiency, because the former produces bleeding which the surgeon must control, while the latter prevents bleeding before it occurs and routinely allows surgeons to develop an entire pocket via the inframammary approach in less than 4 minutes.[2,4,7] The author's experience with blunt dissection for axillary augmentation[8] and subsequent experience with optimal electrocautery dissection techniques[2,9] has produced conclusive evidence that blunt dissection techniques are more inefficient, prolong operating times, and significantly increase morbidity and prolong recovery compared to direct vision, electrocautery techniques.

Current endoscopic instrumentation enables surgeons to perform all areas of pocket dissection in axillary augmentation under direct vision control. For optimal recovery and outcomes, surgeons should avoid any blunt dissection whatever in axillary augmentation, and use optimal endoscopic instrumentation[9] to optimize control, minimize tissue trauma, and minimize bleeding.

Despite claims by its proponents that the umbilical approach for augmentation provides equivalent outcomes to direct vision approaches, current descriptions of surgical techniques for the umbilical approach do not allow surgeons direct vision control inside the pocket during pocket dissection. Dissection techniques are blunt and blind, and recovery data are not equivalent to techniques that use direct vision techniques.[2,7,9]

Incision Length

"Short scar" is a highly marketable term in breast augmentation, but certain facts are inarguable: a smaller incision decreases a surgeon's field of vision, makes many surgical maneuvers more difficult, and subjects prefilled implants to greater stresses during implant insertion. Obviously, no surgeon wants to create excessively long scars, but optimizing accuracy and minimizing damage to prefilled implants requires that surgeons prioritize adequate incision length over bragging rights and marketing concerns.

With inflatable implants, surgeons can reasonably limit incision length to 3.5 cm. Incisions less than 3.5 cm are largely illogical, even using endoscopic instrumentation, because shorter incisions increase risks of wound edge trauma, and compromised scars.

With state-of-the-art form stable, silicone gel implants such as the Allergan Style 410, incision lengths should be longer to facilitate exposure and implant insertion while avoiding damage to the implant. Implant dimensions and volume determine optimal decisions of incision length for form stable implants. When planning incision length for the form stable Allergan Style 410, to minimize risks of device damage and reoperations,[4] surgeons should plan a minimum incision length of 5.0–5.5 cm for Style 410 implants less than 300 grams, and 6.0–6.5 cm for implants larger than 300 grams. These guidelines

Sidebar notes:

For optimal recovery and outcomes, surgeons should avoid any blunt dissection whatever in axillary augmentation, and use optimal endoscopic instrumentation[9] to optimize control, minimize tissue trauma, and minimize bleeding

"Short scar" is a highly marketable term in breast augmentation, but certain facts are inarguable: a smaller incision decreases a surgeon's field of vision, makes many surgical maneuvers more difficult, and subjects prefilled implants to greater stresses during implant insertion

afforded a level of patient satisfaction and device safety that defined a zero percent reoperation rate in a consecutive premarket approval (PMA) series.

Surgical Instrumentation

Inframammary and periareolar approaches for breast augmentation are optimized by specific instrumentation that can improve efficiency and accuracy while decreasing tissue trauma. The author's breast instrument set (Figure 10-1) includes instruments for augmentation and all other types of breast surgery. Instruments in the set are listed in Table 10-1. Instruments in the set are designed or modified from other designs to optimize efficiency and accuracy. A limited number of these instruments are required to perform augmentation via the three main incision approaches, and the specific use of each instrument is detailed in respective chapters that address each incision approach.

Specialized instrumentation for axillary augmentation includes a right angled endoscope that moves the endoscope camera away from the single access port for the operation and a specialized, multipurpose electrocautery dissection instrument that are described in detail in Chapter 12.

Retractor design and specific techniques for positioning and repositioning retractors optimize exposure and minimize tissue trauma. The narrower a retractor blade, the narrower the surgeon's field of vision at the most distal extent of the surgical exposure area. Optimal retractor widths for inframammary, periareolar, and the upper pocket in axillary augmentation are at least 2.5–3 cm. Retractors narrower than 2.5 cm limit exposure. While surgeons can successfully perform augmentation with narrower retractors, during dissection the surgeon cannot visualize areas of the pocket adjacent to the immediate area of

Retractor design and specific techniques for positioning and repositioning retractors optimize exposure and minimize tissue trauma

Retractors narrower than 2.5 cm limit exposure

Figure 10-1.

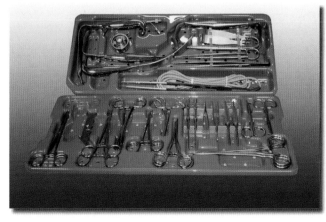

Table 10-1. Tebbetts™ instruments for breast augmentation, reduction, and mastopexy

Diagram Ref. #	Units	Instrument name	Manufacturer	Mfr stock no.
Bottom layer				
1	1	Tebbetts fiberoptic retractor 15 × 36 mm blade	Snowden Pencer	88-1088
2	2	Maxwell flap retractor	Snowden Pencer	88-1092
3	1	Mayo scissors, serrated	Snowden Pencer	32-5830
4	1	Bonney diamond point thumb forceps	Snowden Pencer	32-0518
5 & 6	2	Tebbetts double ended retractor	Snowden Pencer	88-1080
7	1	Skinner, micro 9" 1 × 2 forceps	W. Lorenz*	51-9869
8	1	Tebbetts spatula retractor	Snowden Pencer	88-1082
9	1	Olsen 9½" Potts-Smith monopolar forceps	Olsen Electrosurgical	120 tip E
10	1	Maxwell Marker 42 mm	Snowden Pencer	88-2347
Top layer				
11	2	Allis forceps	Snowden Pencer	88-0350
12	2	Towel clamps non-perforating	Snowden Pencer	88-0345
13	2	Kocher forceps	Snowden Pencer	32-0334
14	2	Lahey Vulsellum mass clamp	Snowden Pencer	88-0363
15	1	Tebbetts precision caliper	Snowden Pencer	88-7616
16	2	Halstead Mosquito forceps (one larger, one smaller)	Snowden Pencer	88-0303
17	2	Tebbetts ultra-delicate needle holder	Snowden Pencer	32-5406
18	2	Tebbetts delicate needle holder	Snowden Pencer	32-0409
19	2	Crile Wood needle holder 6", on top of a single fine tipped, curved tonsil clamp	Snowden Pencer	32-0430
20	1	Iris, curved serrated	Snowden Pencer	32-5705
21	1	Iris, straight	Snowden Pencer	32-0706
22 & 23	2	Tebbetts precision knife handle	Snowden Pencer	88-2012
24	1	Adson 1 × 2	Snowden Pencer	32-0501
25	1	Gorney–Adson 1 × 2	Snowden Pencer	32-5511
26 & 27	2	Tebbetts self-retaining single skin hook	Snowden Pencer	88-1542
28	1	Tonsil forceps	Snowden Pencer	88-0358

*Need a comparable Snowden Pencer substitute.

dissection as clearly, and surgeons are less likely to identify and control blood vessels before cutting them. This seemingly minor issue of retractor width can make a substantial difference in the accuracy and efficiency of pocket dissection.

When placing and moving retractors, surgeons frequently cause inadvertent trauma to rib periosteum and perichondrium in the subpectoral plane, producing small subperichondrial hematomas that can substantially increase postoperative pain. To avoid contacting periosteum and perichondrium during retractor insertion, surgeons should lift the soft tissues anteriorly before inserting and advancing the retractor tip immediately posterior to the soft tissues. When advancing a retractor tip, surgeons should directly visualize the tip of the retractor to avoid advancing the tip past the existing extent of dissection, causing blunt dissection by the retractor tip and increasing tissue trauma and risks of inadvertent bleeding. When exchanging one retractor for a previously placed retractor, surgeons can increase efficiency and minimize risks of traumatizing periosteum by placing the blade of the new retractor beneath the blade of the existing retractor while the soft tissues remain elevated, and then removing the original retractor. This simple maneuver prevents collapse of the soft tissues, reduces unnecessary movements, and avoids rib contact as the surgeon introduces the new retractor. Double ended retractors increase efficiency by allowing surgeons to use increasing length retractor blades without exchanging instruments.

> When advancing a retractor tip, surgeons should directly visualize the tip of the retractor to avoid advancing the tip past the existing extent of dissection, causing blunt dissection by the retractor tip and increasing tissue trauma and risks of inadvertent bleeding

> Double ended retractors increase efficiency by allowing surgeons to use increasing length retractor blades without exchanging instruments

Optimal electrocautery instrumentation is critical to state-of-the-art breast augmentation by any approach and for all pocket locations. Electrocautery dissection enables surgeons to apply principles of prospective hemostasis,[2] controlling blood vessels before cutting them, and preventing blood soaking into adjacent tissues where it causes increased inflammation and pain. All electrocautery instruments are not equal with respect to efficiency and efficacy, and specific techniques can increase the efficacy of each different type of electrocautery dissection instrument. Handswitching electrocautery pencils with blade type tips are effective for pocket dissection, but needlepoint tips on these instruments more effectively focuses electrical current, enabling the surgeon to dissect rapidly with lower electrocautery settings. A needle tip, handswitching electrocautery pencil is an optimal instrument for initial dissection with all approaches, but is not the optimal instrument for dissection after entering the plane of the pocket.

> Optimal electrocautery instrumentation is critical to state-of-the-art breast augmentation by any approach and for all pocket locations

237

Figure 10-2.

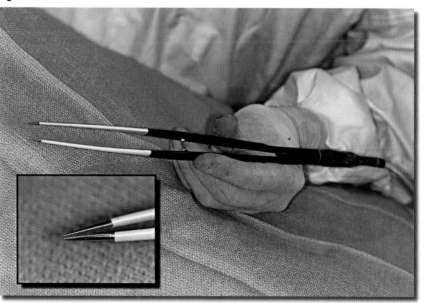

Handswitching, *monopolar*, needle tip electrocautery forceps (Figure 10-2) dramatically increase efficiency of dissecting submammary and subpectoral pockets. The goal of prospective hemostasis is to prevent bleeding before it starts, and prevent any blood from soaking into adjacent tissues. Handswitching, monopolar, needle tip electrocautery forceps enable surgeons to use a single instrument for dissection and hemostasis without ever having to change instruments to control bleeding after inadvertently cutting a vessel. In addition to increasing efficiency, this instrument significantly decreases the time from cutting a vessel to coagulating it, decreasing the amount of blood that can potentially soak into adjacent tissues. Incorporating a hand switch into the instrument that enables current flow when the surgeon closes the forceps tips avoids the inefficiency and clumsiness of locating and activating a foot switch. Very fine needle tips on the instrument focus current for optimal dissection when the surgeon closes the tips.

Three significant variables determine the efficiency of electrocautery instruments for dissection and hemostasis: (1) the cut and coagulation settings on the electrocautery generator, (2) the size of the surface area of the tip that contacts tissues, and (3) the electrical resistance of the specific tissue that the surgeon is cutting or coagulating. Electrocautery generator settings vary among manufacturers and models, and surgeons should experiment and adjust settings intraoperatively for optimal efficiency. A blend of cutting current with coagulation current enables surgeons to effectively dissect and control bleeding vessels with a single instrument. Optimal settings for the previously described handswitching, monopolar, needle tip electrocautery forceps using a Valleylab™ generator are cut 50, coagulation 50, and blend 3.

By reducing the surface area of the electrocautery tip that contacts the tissues, fine tips on forceps and needle tips for handswitching electrocautery pencils most effectively focus current for the most efficient and effective dissection. Electrical resistance of tissues varies with the type of tissue and with the presence of any kind of fluid or blood. With preferred general anesthesia, injection of any type of local anywhere except the incision line is unnecessary, and local anesthetic fluid in the tissues increases electrical resistance and decreases the efficacy of any type of electrocautery instrument. Fat has a higher electrical resistance compared to muscle tissue, so a needle tip on a handswitching electrocautery pencil is most effective when dissecting through subcutaneous fat compared to the handswitching electrocautery forceps. For optimal efficiency, surgeons should use the needle tip electrocautery pencil for dissection from the dermal level through fascia, and switch to the handswitching, monopolar, needle tip electrocautery forceps to complete the remainder of the pocket dissection in both submammary and subpectoral pockets. Extensive published data prove unequivocally that electrocautery dissection as described causes no more tissue trauma or inflammation from charring compared to any other type of dissection, and electrocautery dissection causes much less trauma and bleeding compared to any other method of pocket dissection.

Electrocautery instruments require specific care to avoid damage to insulation that can allow current leakage and cause burns. Electrocautery forceps should never contact other instruments during surgery or during cleaning and sterilization to avoid damage to insulation. Electrocautery forceps should be transported, cleaned, and sterilized either in a custom case or in a container away from other instruments. Surgeons should always keep the forceps either in the surgeon's hand or in an insulated holster, never allowing the forceps to lie on any surface in the operating field. When dissecting inside the pocket, surgeons should always be aware of the proximity of the switch on the forceps to skin edges and keep skin edges and adjacent surfaces dry to prevent inadvertent current leakage and skin burns. These simple principles enable surgeons to optimize safety with these valuable instruments.

Prospective Hemostasis

1:10

Prospective hemostasis[1] describes electrocautery pocket dissection techniques that emphasize prevention of bleeding before it occurs, in contrast to conventional methods of

---

Margin notes:

By reducing the surface area of the electrocautery tip that contacts the tissues, fine tips on forceps and needle tips for handswitching electrocautery pencils most effectively focus current for the most efficient and effective dissection

Local anesthetic fluid in the tissues increases electrical resistance and decreases the efficacy of any type of electrocautery instrument

Electrocautery forceps should never contact other instruments during surgery or during cleaning and sterilization to avoid damage to insulation

---

Figure 10-3.

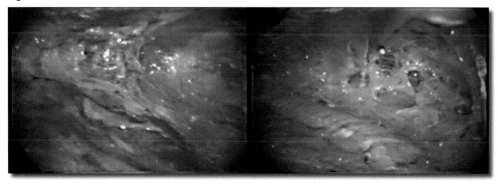

1:11
3:1:3-5
3:2:2-4

dissection that create and then control bleeding, leaving blood soaked into adjacent tissues and increasing inflammation and pain. Optimal prospective hemostasis requires that surgeons focus on vascular anatomy details, consciously anticipating the location of blood vessels as pocket dissection proceeds and controlling even the smallest vessels with the handswitching, monopolar, electrocautery forceps before cutting the vessels. Avoiding the necessity of changing instruments to control a bleeding vessel enables surgeons to prevent or dramatically reduce even minor bleeding that causes tissue staining and inflammation. An optimally dissected pocket via any incision approach should appear as dry as a fresh cadaver dissection (Figure 10-3), with the greatest amount of bleeding occurring at the dermal level of the initial incision.

> Avoiding the necessity of changing instruments to control a bleeding vessel enables surgeons to prevent or dramatically reduce even minor bleeding that causes tissue staining and inflammation

■ SEQUENCE OF POCKET DISSECTION

> Strictly adhering to a defined sequence of pocket dissection that establishes exposure before entering areas of known increased vascularity enables surgeons to have a wider, clearer field of view to identify and control vessels before inadvertently cutting them

Strictly adhering to a defined sequence of pocket dissection that establishes exposure before entering areas of known increased vascularity enables surgeons to have a wider, clearer field of view to identify and control vessels before inadvertently cutting them. Optimal sequences of pocket dissection are different for each incision approach and are described in Chapters 11, 12, and 13. Defining a sequence of dissection also allows surgeons to establish exposure peripheral to areas where perforating vessels are located so that in the event the surgeon inadvertently divides a larger perforator, the surgeon has already established exposure that allows the surgeon to rapidly control the bleeding.

■ POCKET DIMENSIONS AND LANDMARKS FOR ACCURATE DISSECTION

> With current implant technology, implant pockets that widely exceed the medial–lateral dimension or base width of the proposed implant are unnecessary and undesirable

With current implant technology, implant pockets that widely exceed the medial–lateral dimension or base width of the proposed implant are unnecessary and undesirable. During the past three decades, many surgeons have been taught to dissect excessively large pockets, believing that a pocket much larger than the implant, combined with implant displacement exercises, reduces the incidence of capsular contracture. Peer reviewed and published literature during the past decade has proved that for smooth or textured shell implants filled with either saline or silicone, dissecting excessively large pockets is unnecessary and undesirable.[1–7] Capsular contracture rates of less than 3% at up to 7 years with all types of implant devices listed previously, and implant malposition rates of 0.2% with both round and full height, form stable anatomic implants are now predictable by implementing proved processes in published literature.[1–7] With anatomic implants, especially reduced height anatomic implants, accurate pocket dissection is essential to minimize risks of implant malposition. With round implants, especially round, smooth shell implants, accurate, limited pocket dissection is the only means by which a surgeon has any control over distribution of fill and breast aesthetics. With smooth, round implants, accurate, limited pocket dissection does not increase risks of capsular contracture, and does not result in an excessively immobile breast postoperatively. Limiting pocket dissection in proportion to implant dimensions reduces wound surface area, thereby reducing trauma, bleeding, sensory loss, postoperative pain, and recovery time, while increasing control of breast shape by controlling distribution of fill in the breast.

Dissecting an adequate pocket is important to assure that the base footprint of the implant is not compressed and that overlying soft tissue mobility is adequate to permit optimal draping over the proposed implant. Creating a pocket of optimal vertical dimension is especially important when using any type of reduced height, anatomic or shaped implant. When using reduced height, shaped implants, the vertical dimension of the pocket should not exceed the vertical height of the implant more than approximately 2 cm to minimize risks of implant rotation. Full height, form stable anatomic implants, such as the Allergan Style 410 FM, have a vertical dimension that is greater than the base width of the implant. If the width of the pocket for full height, shaped, form stable implants does not exceed the base width by more than 1–2 cm, the device is highly unlikely to rotate because full height implants have a vertical dimension greater than their base width. This fact is proved by peer reviewed and published data that document a 0.1% implant malposition rate at up to 7 years using full height, shaped devices,[1,6,7] and a zero percent malposition rate at 3 years in a 50 consecutive case series from the Allergan Style 410 PMA study.[4]

To dissect optimally accurate pockets, surgeons must (a) define proposed implant base dimension, (b) initially stop lateral pocket dissection before the width of the pocket exceeds the base width of the implant, (c) insert the implant, and (d) incrementally adjust the size of the lateral pocket until it precisely accommodates the base width of the implant without any restriction or compression. When using reduced height, shaped implants, surgeons must also carefully control the vertical dimension of the pocket. Table 10-2

> Limiting pocket dissection in proportion to implant dimensions reduces wound surface area, thereby reducing trauma, bleeding, sensory loss, postoperative pain, and recovery time, while increasing control of breast shape by controlling distribution of fill in the breast

> If the width of the pocket for full height, shaped, form stable implants does not exceed the base width by more than 1–2 cm, the device is highly unlikely to rotate because full height implants have a vertical dimension greater than their base width

Table 10-2. Optimizing pocket size implant dimension relationships to avoid excessive pocket dissection.

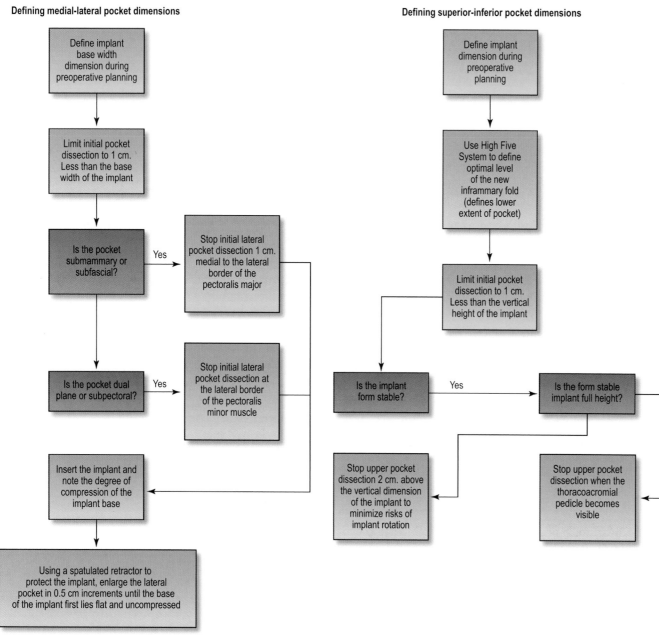

Defining medial-lateral pocket dimensions

Define implant base width dimension during preoperative planning

Limit initial pocket dissection to 1 cm. Less than the base width of the implant

Is the pocket submammary or subfascial? — Yes → Stop initial lateral pocket dissection 1 cm. medial to the lateral border of the pectoralis major

Is the pocket dual plane or subpectoral? — Yes → Stop initial lateral pocket dissection at the lateral border of the pectoralis minor muscle

Insert the implant and note the degree of compression of the implant base

Using a spatulated retractor to protect the implant, enlarge the lateral pocket in 0.5 cm increments until the base of the implant first lies flat and uncompressed

Defining superior-inferior pocket dimensions

Define implant dimension during preoperative planning

Use High Five System to define optimal level of the new inframmary fold (defines lower extent of pocket)

Limit initial pocket dissection to 1 cm. Less than the vertical height of the implant

Is the implant form stable? — Yes → Is the form stable implant full height?

Stop upper pocket dissection 2 cm. above the vertical dimension of the implant to minimize risks of implant rotation

Stop upper pocket dissection when the thoracoacromial pedicle becomes visible

outlines principles of optimizing pocket size–implant dimension relationships to avoid excessive pocket dissection that increases risks of implant malposition (shaped or round).

Surgeons can easily perform the steps for optimal pocket dissection through inframammary and periareolar approaches without removing the implant. By placing a spatula retractor to protect and retract the implant medially and a double ended retractor to retract the lateral soft tissues laterally, the surgeon can then incrementally enlarge the lateral pocket in 0.5 cm increments with the handswitching, monopolar, needle tip electrocautery forceps (Figure 10-4). Through axillary and umbilical approaches, the surgeon must remove the implant to incrementally enlarge the pocket for precise pocket dimensions. With increasing experience, surgeons can more accurately estimate and dissect pockets using inframammary, periareolar, and axillary approaches without first limiting pocket dissection, but overdissection of the lateral pocket is a very common occurrence that allows excessive lateral shift of the implant and widening of the intermammary distance. Topographic markings of implant dimensions on the skin preoperatively are of little use and can be misleading, because implant–soft tissue interactions and the implant lying on varying curvatures of the chest wall affect the fit of the implant to the pocket internally.

Figure 10-4. A spatula retractor protects the implant medially while a double ended retractor retracts the soft tissues laterally, exposing the lateral pocket. The surgeon adjusts or enlarges the lateral pocket in 0.5 cm increments until the pocket exactly fits the base dimension of the implant.

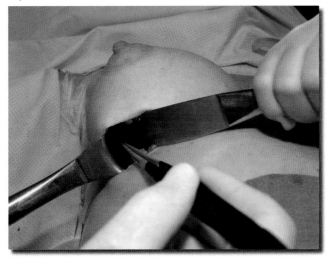

Identifying specific anatomic landmarks inside the pocket at which surgeons should stop lateral pocket dissection helps prevent inadvertent, excessive dissection laterally. In the submammary plane, surgeons can avoid excessive lateral pocket dissection by stopping lateral pocket dissection 1 cm medial to the lateral border of the pectoralis major muscle, and in the subpectoral plane by

Topographic markings of implant dimensions on the skin preoperatively are of little use and can be misleading, because implant–soft tissue interactions and the implant lying on varying curvatures of the chest wall affect the fit of the implant to the pocket internally

Identifying specific anatomic landmarks inside the pocket at which surgeons should stop lateral pocket dissection helps prevent inadvertent, excessive dissection laterally

stopping lateral pocket dissection at the lateral border of the pectoralis minor. After inserting the implant, the limited lateral pocket dissection holds the implant medially, producing an excessively projecting appearance with a limited lateral curvature (Figure 10-5, A). Using a spatula retractor to protect the implant, and a double ended retractor to retract the soft tissues laterally, the surgeon can then incrementally enlarge the lateral pocket in 0.5 cm increments to make the pocket precisely fit the base dimension of the implant. Incrementally enlarging the lateral pocket to fit decreases the excess projection and allows implant volume to distribute laterally and produce a more curved lateral profile line of the breast (Figure 10-5, B, C). More importantly, fitting the pocket to the implant avoids an excessively large lateral pocket that sacrifices control of implant position, distribution of fill in the breast, and control of breast shape.

Precise fitting of the implant to the pocket is desirable and necessary to reduce risks of malposition of shaped implants, but the principle also applies to round, smooth shell implants which can easily displace excessively laterally or inferiorly, causing widening of the intermammary distance or inferior malposition. Fitting the pocket to the implant does not detract from the naturalness of the result, because in the absence of grade 2 or greater capsular contracture, attachments at the capsule–soft tissue interface allow adequate movement of the implant to simulate movement of the normal breast.

> Fitting the pocket to the implant does not detract from the naturalness of the result, because in the absence of grade 2 or greater capsular contracture, attachments at the capsule–soft tissue interface allow adequate movement of the implant to simulate movement of the normal breast

Figure 10-5 A. Limited lateral pocket dissection prevents fill of the lateral breast, producing an excessively projecting appearance with limited curvature of the lateral breast profile.

Figure 10-5 B. Incremental enlargement of the lateral pocket to fit the base of the implant allows fill of the lateral breast with a rounding of the lateral breast profile.

Figure 10-5 C. Overlay of breast profile images before (black arrows) and after (white arrows) lateral pocket enlargement, demonstrating loss of excess projection and rounding of the lateral breast profile after precise, incremental lateral pocket enlargement to fit the base dimension of the implant.

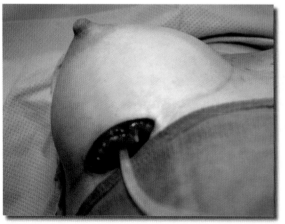
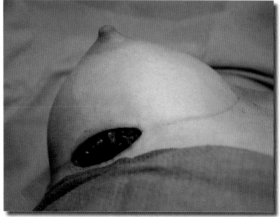
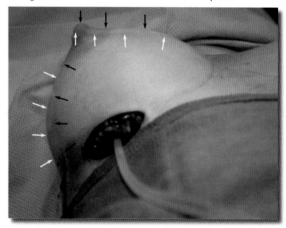

The location of the desired, postoperative inframammary fold is critical to establish optimal relationships of breast width to nipple-to-inframammary fold distance; therefore surgeons must plan and dissect the inferior aspect of the pocket accurately according to principles and methods discussed in Chapter 7. Surgeons can more accurately define the extent of inferior pocket dissection by using proved processes[3,5] instead of visually or subjectively estimating optimal inframammary fold level pre- or intraoperatively. Intraoperative assessments are much less accurate compared to planning based on implant dimensions because of the large number of positioning variables and tissue pressures that exist intraoperatively and limit accuracy of visual determinations.

Depending on the type of implant selected, surgeons have some flexibility in the extent of pocket dissection superiorly. With conventional round smooth and textured shell saline and silicone gel implants, pocket dissection that exceeds the height of the implant causes few problems, and can improve tissue draping over larger implants. With shaped implants that are full height such as the Allergan/Inamed Style 410, pocket dissection to the level of the thoracoacromial vessels in the subpectoral plane significantly improves soft tissue draping over the superior portion of the implant and does not increase risks of implant malposition. Full height, shaped, form stable implants are taller than they are wide. When medial–lateral pocket dissection fits the base width of full height, shaped implants, implant malposition does not occur unless tissue stretch significantly enlarges the medial–lateral dimension of the pocket.

With all other implants that purport to be form stable, and with all reduced height shaped implants including Inamed/Allergan's reduced height, shaped implants and Mentor Contour Profile® gel (CPG) implants, surgeons should consider limiting upper pocket dissection to minimize risks of rotational malposition, because reduced height implants are often wider than they are tall. In the absence of tissue adherence to the textured surface, especially with Mentor CPG® implants, rotational malposition is a higher risk and probably occurs at a higher rate than some surgeons recognize, because the dimensions of some of these implants can allow rotational malposition without the rotation being clinically apparent. Rotational malposition with the Allergan/Inamed Style 468 full height, anatomic saline implant with Biocell™ texturing is exceedingly rare, occurring in only 0.1% of 1662 reported cases with up to 7 year followup.[1,6,7] Rotational malposition did not occur in a consecutive 50 case series in the Food and Drug Administration (FDA) PMA study for the Allergan/Inamed Style 410 form stable, cohesive gel anatomic implant with Biocell™ texturing.[4]

Surgeons can more accurately define the extent of inferior pocket dissection by using proved processes[3,5] instead of visually or subjectively estimating optimal inframammary fold level pre- or intraoperatively

ANTIBIOTICS AND ANTIBIOTIC IRRIGATION

Preoperative antibiotics and antibiotic or antibacterial irrigation of the pocket prior to implant insertion are logical measures to limit risks of clinical infection or capsular contracture from skin contaminants or endogenous bacteria in the breast parenchyma. Agents and regimens vary among surgeons, but the studies of Adams et al.,[10-12] Netscher et al.,[13] and Shah et al.[14] present convincing data regarding the efficacy of antibacterial irrigation with respect to capsular contracture and the clinical relevance of positive periprosthetic cultures without overt infection. A previous classic randomized, controlled, double blinded clinical study using povidone-iodine irrigation (Burkhardt et al.[15,16]) demonstrated conclusive reduction of capsular contracture. Subsequent FDA mandates regarding the use of povidone-iodine force surgeons who want to use this tremendously effective agent to off label use that requires patient consent preoperatively. The FDA labeling requirements regarding use of povidone-iodine are based on laboratory studies done by Mentor Corporation that documented delamination of valve patches in implants containing intraluminal Betadine, but no damage when the same implants were immersed in full strength Betadine for 7 weeks. These studies have absolutely no relationship to the clinical use of diluted povidone-iodine solutions that only contact the outer surface of the implant briefly until the body absorbs the solution postoperatively. Hopefully the FDA will reconsider this labeling that ignores the results of one of the best clinical studies ever performed in breast augmentation patients and forces surgeons to off label use of the product. A subsequent, definitive in vitro study by Zambacos and colleagues[17] demonstrated no decrease in tensile strength of implant specimens incubated in various concentrations of povidone-iodine for 4 weeks.

IMPLANT HANDLING AND PREPARATION

1:16
3:1:5
3:2:5

Breast implants should be transferred to the sterile field in the inner thermoform packaging provided by the manufacturer. Inflatable implants should be leak tested by submersion in sterile saline solution prior to evacuating sterile air from within the implant using a closed system to prevent intraluminal contamination. While on the sterile field, all implants should remain in the thermoform packaging until the surgeon removes the implant to evacuate air from inflatable implants or to insert a prefilled implant. Surgeons should insist on proper handling techniques to prevent contact of the implant with any surface, instrument, or material in the operating field.

Some surgeons advocate glove changes and various "no-touch" techniques that ultimately cannot be "no touch" and still achieve implant insertion. The author does not perform glove changes, but uses gloves with no powder, wipes the gloved hands prior to touching the implant, and places antibacterial solution on the implant, glove fingers that touch the implant, and the skin surface surrounding the incision prior to inserting inflatable or prefilled implants. When inserting Allergan/Inamed Style 410 anatomic, form stable silicone gel implants, the author uses a polyethylene introducing sleeve that eliminates all contact of the implant with skin and subcutaneous tissue during insertion and distributes pressure more evenly over the implant surface during insertion to minimize risks of contamination and damage to the implant shell. Use of introducing sleeves could potentially reduce risks of skin contamination or device damage with all types of breast implants, but historically, surgeons have resisted the use of introducing sleeves as an unnecessary additional adjunct.

Adequate incision length should relate to the dimensions and filler material characteristics of the implant, and whether the implant is inflatable or prefilled. To minimize risks of damage to implants during insertion, longer incisions are always preferable to short incisions that subject the implant to much greater pressures during insertion. When inserting prefilled implants, surgeons should carefully avoid any focal digital pressure that could weaken or damage the implant shell. By focusing on maximizing surface area contact of the fingers in contact with the implant, and exercising patient vigilance to avoid focal pressure, surgeons can substantially reduce iatrogenic damage to implant devices. Similar principles apply when repositioning implants within the pocket.

Iatrogenic damage to implants is relatively common, and the damage may not be visually apparent at the time of surgery. Surgeons should exercise vigilant attention to detail when handling and inserting the implant and meticulous surgical closure techniques to eliminate risks of suture needle contact with the implant to minimize risks of damage to implants. During closure of inframammary incisions when the implant is in close proximity to the suture line, surgeons should lift the deep fascial edges and place them onto the suture needle with the point of the needle always directed anteriorly away from the implant (Figure 10-6). Similar methods to avoid arcing or sweeping a needle through tissue also help avoid implant damage when closing deeper tissue layers in periareolar augmentations.

■ ADJUNCTIVE MEASURES IN BREAST AUGMENTATION

Most adjunctive measures and devices for use postoperatively in breast augmentation have no scientifically validated evidence of efficacy. Anecdotal reports, expert opinions,

Use of introducing sleeves could potentially reduce risks of skin contamination or device damage with all types of breast implants, but historically, surgeons have resisted the use of introducing sleeves as an unnecessary additional adjunct

Iatrogenic damage to implants is relatively common, and the damage may not be visually apparent at the time of surgery

Most adjunctive measures and devices for use postoperatively in breast augmentation have no scientifically validated evidence of efficacy

Figure 10-6. The surgeon holds the tip of the suture needle in a static position and uses forceps to place the tissue edges on the static needle. Keeping the tip of the suture needle facing away from the implant and placing the tissue edges onto the needle tip using forceps prevents inadvertent needle damage to the implant.

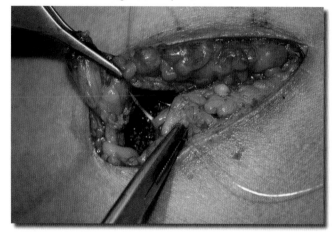

and manufacturer economic considerations promote the use of many adjunctive devices and methods that are totally unnecessary, and that increase costs and morbidity and complicate recovery.

In studies that document a 96% rate of return to normal activities within 24 hours and an overall reoperation rate of less than 3%, a seroma rate of zero, and an implant malposition rate of 0.1% in 1664 consecutive primary augmentations with submammary and subpectoral pocket locations via three incision approaches with up to 7 year followup, all of the following adjuncts were conclusively proved to be unnecessary: drains, pain pumps, special bras, bandages, implant positioning straps, compression garments, narcotic strength pain medications, intercostal blocks, and local anesthetic instilled into the pocket.[1,6,7]

By implementing proved processes,[1,3,4] surgeons can eliminate all of these unnecessary adjuncts and, dramatically simply, improve and shorten patient recovery while minimizing postoperative morbidity.

■ REFERENCES

1. Tebbetts JB: Achieving a predictable 24 hour return to normal activities after breast augmentation Part I: Refining practices using motion and time study principles. *Plast Reconstr Surg* 109:273–290, 2002.

2. Tebbetts JB: Achieving a predictable 24 hour return to normal activities after breast augmentation Part II: Patient preparation, refined surgical techniques and instrumentation. *Plast Reconstr Surg* 109:293–305, 2002.

3. Tebbetts JB, Adams WP: Five critical decisions in breast augmentation using 5 measurements in 5 minutes: the high five system. *Plast Reconstr Surg* 116(7):2005–2016, 2005.

4. Tebbetts JB: Achieving a zero percent reoperation rate at 3 years in a 50 consecutive case augmentation mammaplasty PMA study. *Plast Reconstr Surg* 118(6):1453–1457, 2006.

5.   Tebbetts JB: A system for breast implant selection based on patient tissue characteristics and implant–soft tissue dynamics. *Plast Reconstr Surg* 109(4):1396–1409, 2002.

6.   Tebbetts JB: Patient acceptance of adequately filled breast implants using the tilt test. *Plast Reconstr Surg* 106(1):139–147, 2000.

7.   Tebbetts JB: Dual plane (DP) breast augmentation: optimizing implant–soft tissue relationships in a wide range of breast types. *Plast Reconstr Surg* 107:1255, 2001.

8.   Tebbetts JB: Transaxillary subpectoral augmentation mammaplasty: long-term follow-up and refinement. *Plast Reconstr Surg* 74:636–647, 1984.

9.   Tebbetts JB: Axillary endoscopic breast augmentation: processes derived from a 28-year experience to optimize outcomes. *Plast Reconstr Surg* 118(7S):53S–80S, 2006.

10.   Adams WP, Jr, Conner WC, Barton FE, Jr, Rohrich RJ: Optimizing breast pocket irrigation: an in vitro study and clinical implications. *Plast Reconstr Surg* 105:334–338, discussion 339–343, 2000.

11.   Adams WP, Jr, Conner WC, Barton FE, Jr, Rohrich R J: Optimizing breast pocket irrigation: the post-Betadine era. *Plast Reconstr Surg* 107:1596–1601, 2001.

12.   Adams WP, Rios JL, Smith SJ: Enhancing patient outcomes in aesthetic and reconstructive breast surgery using triple antibiotic breast irrigation: six-year prospective clinical study. *Plast Reconstr Surg* 117:30–36, 2006.

13.   Netscher DT, Weizer G, Wigoda P, Walker LE, Thornby J, Bowen D: Clinical relevance of positive breast periprosthetic cultures without overt infection. *Plast Reconstr Surg* 96:1125–1129, 1995.

14.   Shah Z, Lehman JA, Tan J: Does infection play a role in breast capsular contracture? *Plast Reconstr Surg* 68:34–43, 1981.

15.   Burkhardt BR, Demas CP: The effect of Siltex texturing and povidone-iodine irrigation on capsular contracture around saline-inflatable breast implants. *Plast Reconstr Surg* 93:123–128, discussion 129–130, 1994.

16.   Burkhardt BR, Eades E: The effect of Biocell texturing and povidone-iodine irrigation on capsular contracture around saline-inflatable breast implants. *Plast Reconstr Surg* 96:1317–1325, 1995.

17.   Zambacos G, Nguyen D, Morris R: Effect of povidone iodine on silicone gel implants in vitro: implications for clinical practice. *Plast Reconstr Surg* 114(3):706–710, 2004.

The Inframammary Approach for Augmentation

The inframammary approach for breast augmentation is the most widely used incision location for breast augmentation. During the past three decades, more surgeons have learned this approach during residency compared to all other incision approaches combined, and more augmentations have been performed through the inframammary approach compared to all other incision approaches combined. Reasons for popularity of the inframammary approach include direct vision for optimal control, minimal tissue trauma, and minimal bleeding. Each of these reasons directly impacts patient outcome short- and long-term. As a result, the inframammary approach sets a standard based on logic that is currently unmatched by any other incision approach.

The inframammary approach is the most logical approach for breast augmentation if a surgeon prioritizes tissue trauma, bleeding, and accurate pocket dissection. Using the inframammary approach, a surgeon can gain access to the prosthetic pocket with minimal trauma to tissues between the incision and the pocket. Reducing tissue trauma reduces postoperative inflammation and pain, and facilitates a faster recovery with fewer potential wound healing tradeoffs. In most cases, the surgeon traverses less than 2 cm of normal tissue prior to entering the implant pocket, whether the pocket is submammary, subpectoral, or dual plane. Through the inframammary incision, all areas of the pocket are accessible to the surgeon under direct vision, allowing the highest level of control during dissection, and the most accurate pocket dimensions. Wide, direct visualization allows the surgeon to identify and control potential bleeding before it occurs (prospective hemostasis), preventing tissue staining from bleeding that occurs with conventional sharp

> The inframammary approach for breast augmentation is the most widely used incision location for breast augmentation

> The inframammary approach is the most logical approach for breast augmentation if a surgeon prioritizes tissue trauma, bleeding, and accurate pocket dissection

Avoiding any traces of blood in tissues reduces postoperative inflammation and discomfort that prolong patient recovery and return to normal activities, and reduces risks of capsular contracture postoperatively

or blunt dissection techniques that create bleeding that the surgeon must then control. Avoiding any traces of blood in tissues reduces postoperative inflammation and discomfort that prolong patient recovery and return to normal activities, and reduces risks of capsular contracture postoperatively. The inframammary approach requires very few instruments, increases efficiency and reduces operating times and doses of anesthetic medications that can unnecessarily prolong and complicate recovery.

■ INSTRUMENTATION FOR THE INFRAMAMMARY APPROACH

Optimal instrumentation is essential to reduce tissue trauma, increase efficiency, and execute the details of surgical technique that enable surgeons to deliver 24 hour recovery.[1,2] Minimizing total numbers of instruments optimizes efficiency and cost effectiveness. By consolidating and optimizing the instrument set, the surgeon can increase accuracy and control, save valuable time, and reduce morbidity.

Specific instrument design features effectively reduce tissue trauma

Specific instrument design features effectively reduce tissue trauma. Integrating instrument design features with specific surgical techniques improves outcomes.[1,2] For example, the ratio of retractor width to retractor length is critical to optimize exposure. Choosing narrower blade retractors in order to minimize incision length is shortsighted, because a narrower retractor blade substantially reduces exposure and peripheral visibility in the pocket, increasing risks of inadvertent bleeding if the surgeon is unable to identify larger perforating vessels before dividing them (Figure 11-1, A). Retractor blades that curve slightly downward at the lateral edges of the retractor minimize skin edge and deeper tissue trauma (Figure 11-1, B), and incorporating a smoke evacuation tube into retractor design minimizes smoke in the pocket during electrocautery dissection (Figure 11-1, C), improving visualization and accuracy. Substituting a headlight and eliminating the fiberoptic bundle on retractors (Figure 11-1, D) decreases risks of the bundle contacting periosteum and causing bleeding during retractor insertion and repositioning.

Figure 11-1 A. A narrow blade retractor significantly limits a surgeon's field of view (indicated by white lines and arrows) compared to a slightly wider blade retractor. A wider field of view enables the surgeon to exert more control over every surgical maneuver.

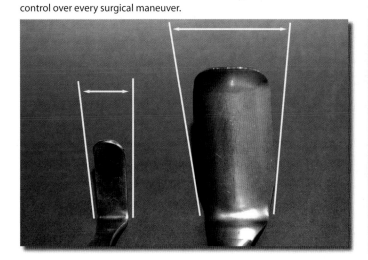

Figure 11-1 B. A downward curvature of retractor blades can help minimize trauma to skin edges and adjacent tissues.

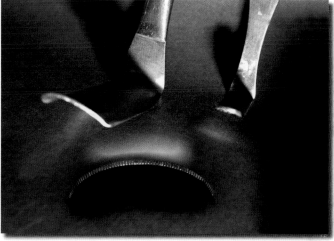

Figure 11-1 C. Smoke evacuation tubes incorporated into retractors with a fiberoptic bundle (right) and without a fiberoptic bundle (left).

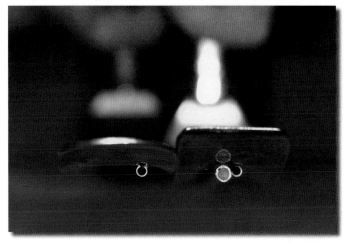

Figure 11-1 D. A fiberoptic headlight reduces the need for retractor fiberoptic bundles that frequently traumatize rib periosteum when dissecting pockets for breast implants.

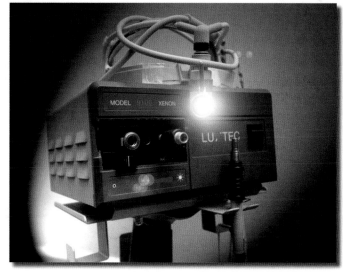

Figure 11-2. The rib periosteum and blood vessels on its surface are particularly susceptible to blunt trauma from retractors and fiberoptic bundles on retractors. Disrupting these small vessels causes subperiosteal and subperichondrial hematomas (inset) that increase postoperative pain and retard recovery.

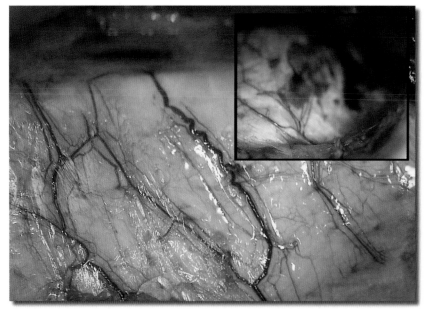

Minimizing retraction forces minimizes tissue trauma and bleeding. Surgeons can minimize tissue trauma and increase efficiency by following simple principles of retraction:

1. Use a strict no-touch approach to the periosteum and perichondrium during pocket dissection to avoid trauma to the small vessels on the surface of periosteum and perichondrium (Figure 11-2). Trauma to these vessels causes subperichondrial or subperiosteal hematomas that increase postoperative pain and morbidity. Before inserting or moving a retractor, lift the soft tissues with the monopolar forceps or another instrument to reduce risks of the retractor contacting periosteum. When replacing one retractor with another, leave the first retractor in place, insert a second retractor beneath the first, then remove the first retractor (Figure 11-3).

> Use a strict no-touch approach to the periosteum and perichondrium during pocket dissection to avoid trauma to the small vessels on the surface of periosteum and perichondrium

Figure 11-3.

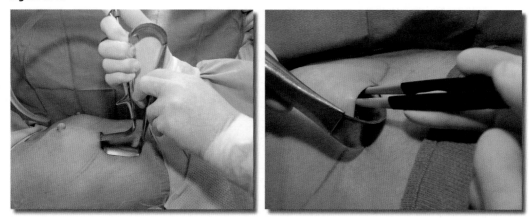

2. When inserting a retractor, never insert the tip past the current extent of pocket dissection. Advancing the retractor tip past the point of previous dissection avulses small or large perforating vessels and increases bleeding and residual blood in tissues.

3. Use short acting muscle relaxants such as Nimbex to reduce the tension of the pectoralis muscle, allowing optimal exposure while minimizing retractor forces that increase tissue trauma.

4. Eliminate teeth on the end of the retractor blade, and maintain position of the tip in the most distal portion of the pocket dissection by using the long, ring, and small fingers to keep tissues pulled onto the blade of the retractor.

A fiberoptic headlight optimizes visualization and efficiency by providing optimal illumination at all times without the necessity of fiberoptic bundles and cables on retractors, and without the necessity of manipulating operating room lights. After a short time using a high quality headlight, surgeons rapidly recognize how invaluable a headlight is compared to other illumination alternatives.

The Tebbetts™ breast set (Figure 11-4) includes the following instruments that are designed specifically to optimize efficiency and control when using the inframammary approach to augmentation:

Figure 11-4. The Tebbetts™ breast set includes instrumentation for all types of breast surgery.

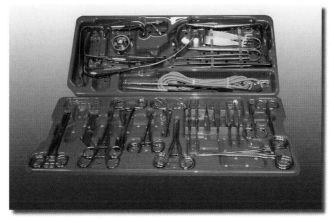

Figure 11-5. Double ended retractors, used singly or in pairs, are indispensable instruments for every approach to augmentation.

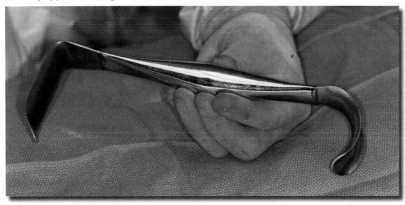

- Double ended retractor

- Handswitching, monopolar, needlepoint electrocautery forceps

- Fiberoptic retractor with smoke evacuation capability

- Spatula retractor.

The double ended retractor (Figure 11-5) is designed for multiple purposes, and is an important instrument for use with all incision approaches. The shorter blade of the retractor facilitates exposure and minimizes tissue trauma during initial stages of pocket dissection, while the longer blade provides optimal exposure as dissection proceeds more distal to the incision. By using two double ended retractors, the surgeon can insert the longer blade of a second retractor beneath the shorter blade of a retractor already in the pocket, then remove the shorter blade of the first retractor. This maneuver is far more efficient compared to completely removing, rotating, and reinserting a single retractor, reducing risks of the retractor contacting rib periosteum or perichondrium, saving time, and reducing tissue trauma and potential contamination.

To minimize tissue trauma, bleeding, and residual blood in tissues, surgeons should avoid any type of blunt dissection while developing the pocket for the implant, and also avoid any type of sharp scissor or scalpel dissection that causes bleeding. Any bleeding that occurs inevitably leaves more blood in the tissues surrounding the pocket and causes more pain, inflammation, prolonged recovery, and potential problems such as seroma and capsular contracture.

To minimize tissue trauma, bleeding, and residual blood in tissues, surgeons should avoid any type of blunt dissection while developing the pocket for the implant, and also avoid any type of sharp scissor or scalpel dissection that causes bleeding

Figure 11-6. A handswitching electrocautery pencil with needle tip is used with blended cut and coagulation current to incise dermis, and with coagulation current to dissect through subcutaneous fat to the level of the pectoralis fascia.

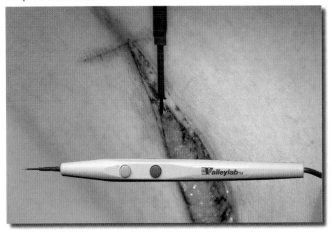

A standard scalpel incises the epidermis and superficial dermis, but avoids midlevel dermis to avoid excessive bleeding from the subdermal plexus. A needle tip electrocautery pencil with blended cut and coagulation current is ideal for incising through dermis (Figure 11-6), subcutaneous tissue, and for subpectoral and dual plane pocket locations, through pectoralis fascia. When the pectoralis muscle (or in the case of a retromammary pocket, the pectoralis fascia) becomes visible, the surgeon switches to the handswitching, monopolar, needlepoint electrocautery forceps (Figure 11-7), and performs the entire pocket development using only this one instrument for both dissection and hemostasis. Handswitching,

Handswitching, monopolar, needlepoint electrocautery forceps have revolutionized pocket dissection for augmentation, allowing surgeons to routinely develop the entire pocket for the implant with a single instrument, in less than 5 minutes, with virtually zero bleeding and minimal residual blood in tissues

Figure 11-7. After incising pectoralis fascia with the needlepoint electrocautery, when the pectoralis muscle becomes visible (white arrow), the surgeon switches to the handswitching, monopolar, needlepoint electrocautery forceps for dissection through pectoralis origins and for development of the dual plane or subpectoral pocket. For a submammary pocket, the surgeon dissects with the forceps immediately adjacent to pectoralis muscle.

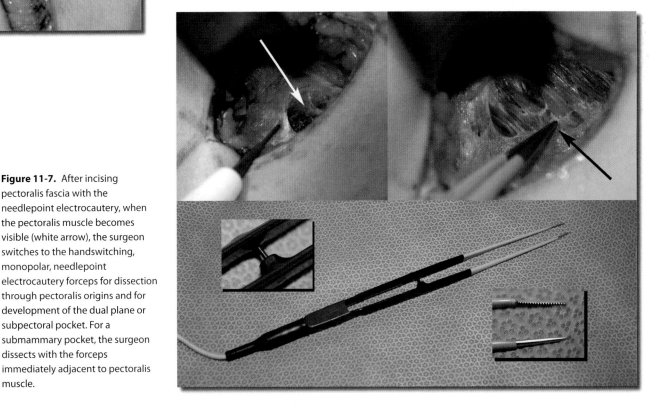

monopolar, needlepoint electrocautery forceps have revolutionized pocket dissection for augmentation, allowing surgeons to routinely develop the entire pocket for the implant with a single instrument, in less than 5 minutes, with virtually zero bleeding and minimal residual blood in tissues.

The spatula retractor (Figure 11-8) is a specialized, multifunctional instrument that is indispensable in inframammary augmentation and in open capsulectomy, especially when used in combination with a double ended retractor. Avoiding excessive lateral pocket dissection is critically important to avoid lateral implant displacement and widening of the intermammary distance. The most predictable method to avoid excessive lateral pocket development is for the surgeon to stop lateral dissection at the lateral border of the pectoralis minor muscle initially, insert the implant, and then incrementally enlarge the lateral pocket in 0.5 cm increments until the footprint of the implant lies flat and just fits the base of the pocket. After inserting the implant, the surgeon uses a double ended retractor to retract the lateral soft tissues laterally, and a spatula retractor to retract and protect the implant medially, then enlarges the pocket incrementally using the handswitching, monopolar, electrocautery forceps.

> The spatula retractor is a specialized, multifunctional instrument that is indispensable in inframammary augmentation and in open capsulectomy, especially when used in combination with a double ended retractor

Figure 11-8. The spatula retractor is frequently used in combination with a double ended retractor for exposure and precise adjustments of the lateral pocket for precise fit of the pocket to the implant. The spatula retractor protects the implant medially while the double ended retractor provides exposure laterally for incremental pocket enlargement.

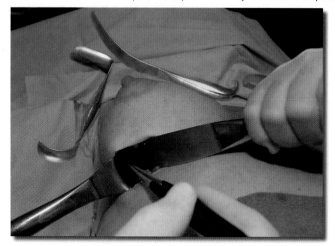

■ SURGICAL TECHNIQUES FOR THE INFRAMAMMARY APPROACH

Specific details of surgical technique enable surgeons to predictably assure over 90% of patients that they can return to full, normal, non-aerobic activities within 24 hours following either subpectoral or submammary augmentation for the first time in the history of breast augmentation.[1,2] This rapid recovery is remarkable, because it completely redefines the patient experience in modern augmentation mammaplasty, and is predictable using inframammary, periareolar, and axillary incision approaches. Rapid recovery and return to normal activities within 24 hours is impossible without dramatically reducing tissue trauma and bleeding. The following techniques, combined with optimal anesthetic management, predictably allow surgeons to deliver their patients a completely redefined experience in breast augmentation.

Specific details of surgical technique enable surgeons to predictably assure over 90% of patients that they can return to full, normal, non-aerobic activities within 24 hours following either subpectoral or submammary augmentation for the first time in the history of breast augmentation

Table 11-1 is a detailed script in tabular form that details surgeon and personnel subroutines for inframammary augmentation. This document details every step and every action for every person in the operating room, and derives from hundreds of hours of detailed videotape analysis, applying principles of motion and time studies.[1,2] Due to the length of this document, it is included in the Resources folder on the DVDs that accompany this book.

Principles of Prospective Hemostasis

Prospective hemostasis is a term that describes a process of avoiding bleeding by controlling vessels before bleeding occurs and manipulating instrumentation to prevent inadvertent disruption of small vessels. This simple concept requires a different mindset for the operation that follows rigid guidelines, and can be challenging for even the most experienced surgeons. Requirements for prospective hemostasis are as follows:

Prospective hemostasis is a term that describes a process of avoiding bleeding by controlling vessels before bleeding occurs and manipulating instrumentation to prevent inadvertent disruption of small vessels

1. Zero tolerance for even the most minor bleeding, and a goal of developing the entire pocket with less than 1 cc blood loss.

2. Detailed knowledge of vascular anatomy and variations, and a commitment to see every blood vessel of 0.5 mm and larger before dividing it. Locations for the most

common vessels encountered in the inframammary subpectoral pocket dissection are shown in Figure 11-9.

3. Optimal, accurate retractor placement and movement. By visualizing the location of all significant blood vessels distant to the current dissection, the surgeon must constantly place retractors to optimize visualization of those vessels before inadvertently cutting them. One of the most common errors that produces minor but significant bleeding occurs when a surgeon or assistant inadvertently advances the tip of a retractor past the point of established dissection.

4. Using a single instrument for dissection and hemostasis. When dissection and hemostasis functions occur simultaneously, no bleeding occurs that leaves blood in adjacent tissues. Sharp dissection instruments such as scissors or scalpel, and all blunt dissection instruments, produce bleeding that the surgeon must then control. The result is more residual blood in tissues that produces more inflammation, postoperative pain, and risks seroma and capsular contracture. Regardless of how rapidly a surgeon can develop a pocket using conventional sharp or blunt dissection

Figure 11-9. The approximate locations of the major blood vessels a surgeon encounters in the subpectoral and submammary planes in breast augmentation are marked by Xs. By anticipating the locations during dissection, the surgeon can control these vessels for prospective hemostasis and prevent blood staining of tissues in the pocket.

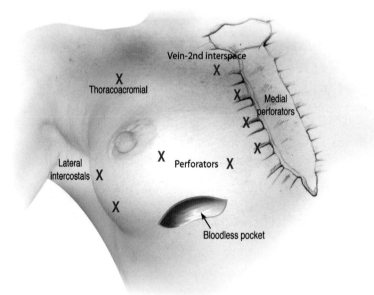

techniques, total times for pocket dissection and hemostasis using these outdated techniques can never match the 5 minutes or less total time to develop a pocket using techniques and instrumentation of prospective hemostasis.

5. Optimal electrocautery instrumentation and settings. A handswitching, monopolar, needle tip electrocautery forceps is the optimal instrument for pocket dissection using prospective hemostasis techniques, and has objectively proved its effectiveness in large peer reviewed clinical series.[1-4] A blended cut and coagulation current optimizes pocket development by providing efficient cutting with simultaneous coagulation and hemostasis while avoiding excessive current spread and tissue charring. The electrocautery generator and settings are also important for optimal prospective hemostasis. Using Valleylab™ electrosurgical generators, a setting of 50% cut and 50% coagulation currents, blended at a Blend 3 or similar setting produce optimal results.

6. A focused, prospective mindset during pocket dissection. The surgeon must constantly focus on the location of vessels, potential bleeding sites, and anatomic landmarks that lie well ahead of the current location of pocket dissection. This prospective mindset enables optimal prospective hemostasis and minimizes postoperative sequelae that detract from an optimal outcome.

Incision Location and Length

The optimal location for the inframammary incision is exactly in the deepest portion of the desired, new (established intraoperatively) inframammary fold. If the surgeon does not plan to lower the fold intraoperatively based on quantitative measurements, the incision will be in the existing (preoperative) inframammary fold. If the surgeon lowers the fold, the incision should be exactly at the new fold level. If the incision is located any higher on the breast (an outdated principle to "minimize visibility in a swimsuit"), greater tension by the implant on lower pole tissues tends to stretch and widen the scar. Tissue stretch always occurs postoperatively. Even when the surgeon places the incision exactly in the new fold, the inevitable stretch of lower pole skin postoperatively usually results in a scar location 0.5 cm above the new fold during the first 6 months postoperatively, provided inferior pocket closure or capsular contracture does not occur.

In patients with an established, well defined inframammary fold, the surgeon should place the incision in the deepest visual portion of the fold. In patients with poorly defined folds, or measured dimensions mandate lowering the fold onto chest skin, the surgeon should drop a perpendicular line from the medial border of the nipple to the inframammary fold,

The optimal location for the inframammary incision is exactly in the deepest portion of the desired, new (established intraoperatively) inframammary fold and then place 1–1.5 cm of the incision medial to the perpendicular line at the desired new fold level and the remainder lateral to the line (Figure 11-10).

Incision length must be adequate for optimal visualization, control, introduction of instruments, and implant insertion. When surgeons make incisions with inadequate length in order to market their short incision abilities and techniques, patients frequently suffer compromises. An excessively short incision limits visibility, limits control, limits the use of instrumentation that can provide optimal visibility and control, and increases trauma to the skin edges, resulting in a shorter but often a lower quality scar.

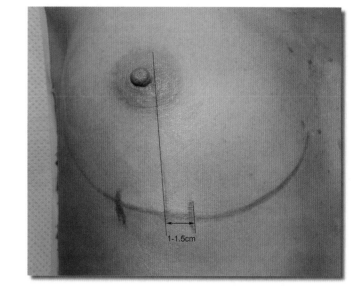

Figure 11-10. Surgeons can avoid placing inframammary incisions excessively laterally by drawing a perpendicular line from the medial nipple to the 6 o'clock position of the inframammary fold, and then placing 1–1.5 cm of the incision medial to the perpendicular line and the remainder lateral to the line.

The following guidelines for incision length have produced predictably high quality, low visibility scars in more than 2000 augmentations with long-term followup. ***An adequate length incision that minimizes trauma to skin edges is far more important compared to shortening the incision a centimeter or more simply for the sake of marketing a shorter incision to patients.*** Adequate incision length provides the surgeon excellent visibility and control for optimal results:

An adequate length incision that minimizes trauma to skin edges is far more important compared to shortening the incision a centimeter or more simply for the sake of marketing a shorter incision to patients

- For inflatable implants: 4.0–4.5 cm
- For conventional prefilled *non-cohesive* gel (older type of conventional gel) implants: 4.0–5.5 cm, depending on implant size
- For form stable, cohesive gel, full height, textured anatomic implants: 5.0–6.5 cm. For Allergan Style 410, full height implants (the most form stable implant currently

available in the United States), surgeons should use the following incision lengths to minimize risks of device damage during insertion: up to 250 grams, 5.0 cm; 250–350 grams, 5.5 cm; greater than 350 grams, 6.0 cm.

- For Style 410 implants smaller than 300 grams, surgeons may choose to decrease incision length to 5.0 cm, but an additional half centimeter of incision length is inconsequential to scar length, decreases trauma to skin edges, provides more optimal visibility and control, and minimizes potential damage to the implant during insertion.

Shortening incisions even 0.5 cm in many cases produces tradeoffs that outweigh a slightly longer scar of higher quality that affords the surgeon more control. In more than 2000 inframammary augmentations, the author has performed zero inframammary scar revisions, and cannot recall a patient complaining about the quality of her inframammary scar. When surgeons create a beautiful result in the breast, an inframammary scar is not an issue. *Additional incision length for placement of form stable implants is not an issue for optimally educated and informed patients.* Peer reviewed and published data and data from FDA PMA studies on form stable implants supports this fact.

Initial Incision and Dissection

The surgeon incises skin with the scalpel according to preoperative markings, and then lifts the tissues superior to the incision with the non-dominant hand to delineate the deep subcutaneous fascia and lift it away from the underlying fascia, reducing risks of inadvertently dissecting too deeply. Switching to the handswitching needlepoint electrocautery pencil, the surgeon dissects through subcutaneous tissue and deep subcutaneous fascia to expose pectoralis fascia (Figure 11-7, top left). For a retromammary pocket, the plane of dissection remains superficial to the pectoralis fascia. For subpectoral or dual plane pocket dissection, the surgeon incises the pectoralis fascia with the electrocautery pencil, and then switches to the handswitching, monopolar, needlepoint electrocautery forceps (Figure 11-7).

Chapter 9 detailed the relative advantages and tradeoffs of retromammary, subfascial, traditional partial retropectoral, and dual plane pocket techniques. Assuring adequate soft tissue coverage long-term is the highest priority in breast augmentation, because inadequate soft tissue coverage dramatically increases risks of complications and reoperations long-term. The development of the dual plane pocket for augmentation has largely eliminated the tradeoffs of traditional subpectoral pocket locations, and if pocket

Figure 11-11. When the surgeon visualizes fascia deep to the subcutaneous tissue, the surgeon should then lift firmly anteriorly on the double ended retractor. If the underlying muscle tents upward (white arrow), the muscle is pectoralis major and the surgeon can dissect parallel to the thoracic wall 1 cm anterior to the ribs through pectoralis to enter the subpectoral space. If the muscle does not tent, it is either intercostals or serratus, and the surgeon should continue dissecting superiorly to identify tenting pectoralis.

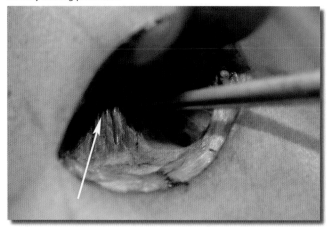

Figure 11-12. From the inframammary incision, the surgeon should dissect in a direction medial to the areola in the direction of the white arrow to enter the subpectoral space where the pectoralis is least adherent to adjacent and underlying structures.

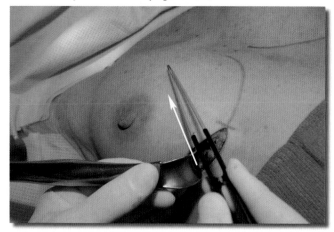

location is based on logic, the dual plane pocket has rendered submammary and subfascial pockets largely obsolete. The description of technical details of inframammary augmentation in this chapter details dual plane techniques.[3]

Entering the Subpectoral Space

Surgeons can avoid inadvertently dissecting through the intercostal or serratus muscles, potentially causing a pneumothorax by following a simple, straightforward technique. Inserting the shorter blade of a double ended retractor with the tip at the level of the pectoralis fascia, the surgeon lifts directly anteriorly. *If the underlying muscle layer tents upward (Figure 11-11), the muscle is pectoralis major. Intercostal or serratus muscles will never tent upward.* After assuring that the muscle layer tents, the surgeon checks topographical landmarks, and then aims dissection medial to the areola, in the area of the subpectoral pocket where the pectoralis is never adherent to either the serratus or pectoralis minor muscles (Figure 11-12).

Surgeons can avoid inadvertently dissecting through the intercostal or serratus muscles, potentially causing a pneumothorax by following a simple, straightforward technique

Figure 11-13. Large perforator artery and vein (white arrow), usually located inferomedial to the areola.

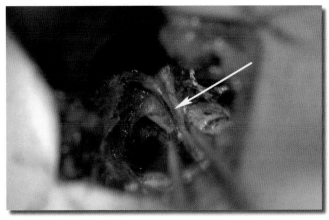

To enter the subpectoral space, the surgeon sweeps the closed needle tips of the handswitching, monopolar, electrocautery forceps back and forth over the tented pectoralis muscle, using a light, sweeping motion and dividing the pectoralis muscle at least 0.5 cm above the origins on the ribs. If the surgeon divides pectoralis origins immediately adjacent to the origin on the ribs, perforating vessels can retract and become very difficult to control without risking pneumothorax. Leaving small stumps of muscle origins on the ribs completely avoids this potential problem. Throughout this portion of the dissection, the surgeon maintains exposure using the short blade of the double ended retractor, repositioning it frequently to the most distal area of dissection to optimally define the dissection plane. As the surgeon dissects through the pectoralis origins to enter the pocket, a large perforator is usually located inferomedial to the areola (Figure 11-13). Thorough electrocoagulation with the forceps in two or three locations along the vessels before dividing them minimizes risks of bleeding from the cut stumps later in the procedure or postoperatively.

Sequence and Techniques of Pocket Dissection

Optimizing the sequence of pocket dissection is important to establish and maintain optimal exposure first in areas where natural tissue planes exist, and then extend dissection into areas that have more unpredictable anatomic variations and larger blood vessels.

In addition to the static photographs and illustrations in this chapter, endoscopic views of dissection landmarks inside the pocket are included on the DVDs that accompany this book.

Figure 11-14 illustrates an optimal sequence for pocket dissection through the inframammary incision. Establishing initial dissection in a direction medial to the areola avoids inadvertently dissecting deep to the pectoralis into serratus when attempting to enter the pocket lateral to the lateral border of the pectoralis. Having established the subpectoral plane, the surgeon next opens the medial pocket for exposure to divide inferior origins of the pectoralis.

Optimizing the sequence of pocket dissection is important to establish and maintain optimal exposure first in areas where natural tissue planes exist, and then extend dissection into areas that have more unpredictable anatomic variations and larger blood vessels

Figure 11-14. Optimal sequence for dissection of a retromammary, subpectoral, or dual plane pocket from the inframammary approach. This sequence enters areas of least adherence before proceeding to areas of greater tissue plane adherence, and maximizes exposure before dissecting along the medial sternal border where large perforators are located.

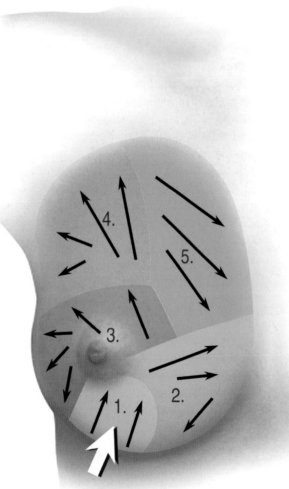

Pocket dissection sequence
via the inframammary approach

To develop a dual plane pocket, the surgeon next divides the inferior origins of the pectoralis major across the inframammary fold, stopping division of muscle origins at the point where the inframammary fold joins the sternum

To develop a dual plane pocket, the surgeon next divides the inferior origins of the pectoralis major across the inframammary fold, stopping division of muscle origins at the point where the inframammary fold joins the sternum (Figure 11-15). Maintaining exposure with the shorter blade of the double ended retractor, the surgeon divides the pectoralis origins along the fold from the undersurface of the muscle, from lateral to medial, using the handswitching, monopolar, electrocautery forceps. By incrementally dividing the muscle with light, sweeping strokes on its undersurface while maintaining tension on the muscle with gentle upward retraction, the surgeon can optimally identify and control intramuscular vessels to avoid bleeding and tissue staining. The surgeon should always divide the pectoralis origins at least 1 cm above the desired, new inframammary fold to avoid excessive inferior pocket dissection from a retractor. In addition, the surgeon should divide the pectoralis origins at least 0.5 cm off the origins' attachment to the ribs to avoid bleeding from retracting intramuscular vessels that can be difficult to control and can increase risks of pneumothorax when the surgeon attempts control.

As a final step after dividing the muscle origins along the fold, the surgeon should palpate the undersurface of the line of muscle division to assure complete release of all bands along the fold, and visually check the superior cut edge of the pectoralis for optimal hemostasis. When dividing muscle at the fold, the surgeon should not make any attempt to maintain the integrity of the deep subcutaneous fascia, because this fascia does not provide any meaningful, additional coverage, and risks blunting irregularities along the fold. *Inferior origins of the pectoralis should be left intact when pinch thickness of the skin, subcutaneous tissue, and muscle is less than 0.5 cm.* After establishing the subpectoral plane, opening the medial pocket, and dividing inferior pectoralis origins, the surgeon should exchange the longer end of a second double ended retractor for the short end of the retractor already in place, using the techniques described previously. Midpocket dissection (Figure 11-14, Step 3) is the next step in the dissection sequence.

Inferior origins of the pectoralis should be left intact when pinch thickness of the skin, subcutaneous tissue, and muscle is less than 0.5 cm

In some cases, the pectoralis minor can be adherent and difficult to distinguish from the pectoralis major. By establishing the plane of dissection medial to the pectoralis minor, then lifting and retracting laterally, the plane between the pectoralis major and minor becomes distinct and easy to enter, avoiding potential inadvertent dissection beneath the pectoralis minor. From the middle of the pocket, the surgeon uses the monopolar forceps to open the relatively avascular plane in the mid portion of the pocket by lifting and dissecting directly superiorly. After the middle portion of the pocket is open, the surgeon redirects the retractor to pull laterally over the mid portion of the pectoralis minor. By making the transition laterally higher over the pectoralis minor, the surgeon minimizes risks of inadvertent dissection into the serratus anterior muscle which is sometimes

By establishing the plane of dissection medial to the pectoralis minor, then lifting and retracting laterally, the plane between the pectoralis major and minor becomes distinct and easy to enter, avoiding potential inadvertent dissection beneath the pectoralis minor

Figure 11-15. Upper left: The surgeon divides origins across the inframammary fold, stopping exactly where the inframammary fold joins the sternum (white X). Upper right: Fresh cadaver dissection showing division of pectoralis origins across the inframammary fold (black line), dividing all origins at least 1–2 cm superior (purple line) to the desired inframammary fold (black line). Lower left: Using the double ended retractor for surgical exposure in the lower medial pocket (left), the surgeon divides the origins of the pectoralis across the inframammary fold from the undersurface of the muscle, 1 cm above the marked inframammary fold level (left, white arrows). Lower right: View medially along the undersurface of the inframammary fold. While viewing the topographic purple line of the inframammary fold on the skin, the surgeon uses monopolar needle tip electrocautery forceps to divide pectoralis origins (white arrows) along a line that corresponds to a line 1 cm above the desired inframammary fold (yellow arrow and dots). The surgeon proceeds medially from the incision, in the direction of the yellow arrow. Dividing pectoralis origins and fascia exposes the subcutaneous fat deep to the skin. Surgeons can choose to leave deep subcutaneous (pectoralis) fascia intact, but it is of no significance to long-term coverage or support.

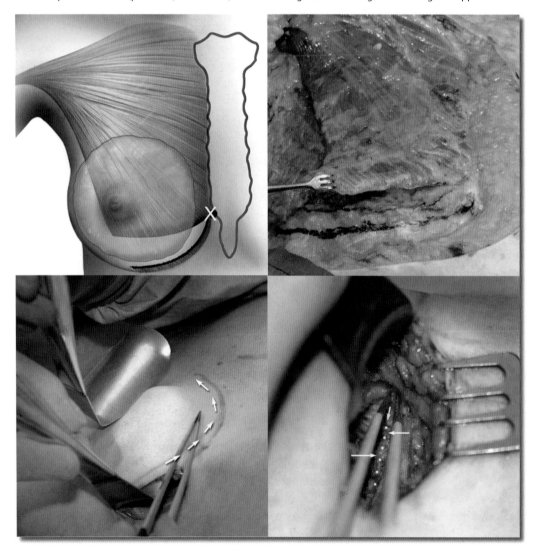

Figure 11-16. Endoscopic view from inferior to superior in the lateral pocket gutter. Surgeons should initially limit and stop dissection at the lateral border of the pectoralis minor (white arrows) to prevent overdissection of the lateral pocket. The thoracoacromial pedicle (blue arrow) is visible in the fat pad adjacent to the lifted pectoralis major muscle.

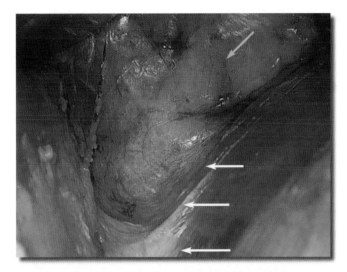

Figure 11-17. Endoscopic view in the upper pocket. Surgeons should enlarge the upper pocket until the thoracoacromial pedicle (white arrows) is clearly visible in the fat pad on the undersurface of the pectoralis major. This view provides a wide perspective of the pectoralis minor (green arrows) beneath. Surgeons should initially limit lateral pocket dissection to the lateral edge of the pectoralis minor.

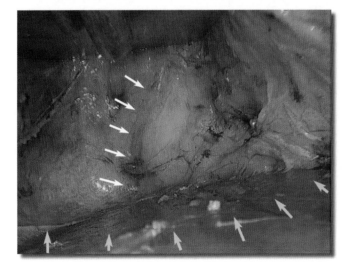

adherent to the pectoralis in the lower lateral pocket. After defining the plane into the lateral pocket gutter superiorly, the surgeon dissects the lateral pocket inferiorly, limiting dissection to the lateral border of the pectoralis minor (Figure 11-14). Exchanging the longer blade of the double ended retractor with a longer retractor (Figure 11-14, Step 4) with smoke evacuating capability, the surgeon dissects superiorly until the thoracoacromial pedicle is visible (Figure 11-17), then continues laterally slightly over the edge of the pectoralis minor.

The final step in pocket dissection is finalizing the medial pocket by dissecting medially from superior to inferior (Figure 11-14, Step 5). Moving the longer retractor to the most superomedial aspect of the pocket, the surgeon dissects from superior to inferior along the medial border of the pocket. At each increment of dissection, the surgeon should carefully check skin markings medially to avoid excessive medial pocket dissection. By carefully avoiding dissection medial to a line 1.5 cm lateral to the sternal midline, the surgeon will avoid inadvertently dividing large medial perforating vessels that can be very difficult to control.

Preserving all Medial Origins of the Pectoralis—a Critically Important Principle

Visible implant edges and visible traction rippling medially are almost totally preventable. To avoid visible implant edges and visible traction rippling deformities medially, the surgeon should preserve all medial origins of the pectoralis major along the sternum, from the sternal notch to the junction of the sternum with the inframammary fold. In some patients, white, tendinous origins of pectoralis are visible just lateral to the main body of the muscle along the sternum (Figure 11-18). The surgeon can safely divide these white, tendinous origins that are discrete origins located lateral to the main body of origins medially without compromising the integrity of the main body of muscle origins medially that are critical to optimal implant coverage medially. *Surgeons should never divide medial pectoralis origins that appear to be separate pinnate origins unless the surgeon can clearly see the intact main body of pectoralis origins medial to the pinnate origins.*

Visible implant edges and traction rippling deformities are caused by failing to assure optimal implant coverage medially. These deformities often do not become visible for many months postoperatively and are largely uncorrectable. Division of medial pectoralis origins in an attempt to

Figure 11-18. Left: Surgeons can safely divide individual, pinnate origins of pectoralis (red circles) that are located lateral to the main body of the pectoralis origins along the sternum (purple rectangle). Right, top: Cadaver dissections viewing from lateral to medial show large pinnate origins (large white arrow) with a yellow band marker behind the pinnate origins but in front of the main body of pectoralis origins along the sternum. Right, middle: Smaller black arrows define other pinnate origins with varying tissue characteristics. Right, bottom: After dividing the pinnate origins, the black arrows point out the tendinous appearance of some of the origins, and the main body of pectoralis origins remains intact medially along the sternum.

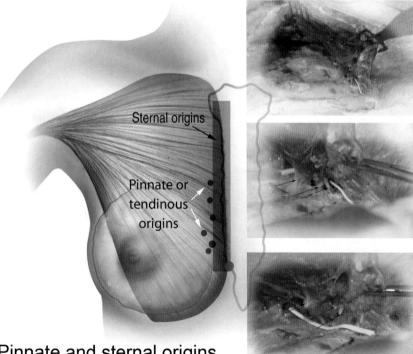

Sternal origins

Pinnate or tendinous origins

Pinnate and sternal origins of the pectoralis major muscle

To avoid visible implant edges and visible traction rippling deformities medially, the surgeon should preserve all medial origins of the pectoralis major along the sternum, from the sternal notch to the junction of the sternum with the inframammary fold

Division of medial pectoralis origins in an attempt to narrow the intermammary distance is illogical and unwarranted, because the potential uncorrectable deformities that can result are much more disastrous compared to a slightly wider intermammary distance

narrow the intermammary distance is illogical and unwarranted, because the potential uncorrectable deformities that can result are much more disastrous compared to a slightly wider intermammary distance, regardless of patient and surgeon desires for a narrower intermammary distance. If the patient desires a gluteal appearance of the cleavage area, the surgeon should encourage her to create that appearance with an appropriate push up brassiere, and avoid the temptation to create it surgically.

For dual plane techniques types 2 and 3 that are so effective in glandular ptotic breasts, constricted lower pole breasts, and tubular breasts, the surgeon completes pocket dissection as previously described, and then separates the inferior cut edge of the pectoralis from overlying parenchyma. Disrupting attachments at the parenchyma–muscle interface allows the muscle edge to rotate superomedially (Figure 11-19), and removes pectoralis pressure that impedes full expansion of the lower envelope by the implant. Removing pectoralis pressure that restricts anterior projection of the implant is essential to correct glandular ptosis and constricted lower pole deformities.

To separate the pectoralis from the overlying parenchyma, the surgeon exposes the inferior cut edge of the pectoralis using the short blade of a double ended retractor, and frees the muscle from the overlying parenchyma using short sweeping

Figure 11-19. With pectoralis origins released across the inframammary fold, the extent to which the surgeon separates attachments of parenchyma to underlying pectoralis determines the degree of superomedial muscle rotation (white arrow) for a dual plane 2 or 3 pocket.

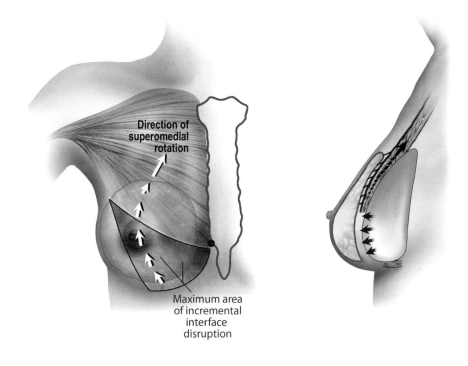

Direction of superomedial rotation

Maximum area of incremental interface disruption

For dual plane techniques types 2 and 3 that are so effective in glandular ptotic breasts, constricted lower pole breasts, and tubular breasts, the surgeon completes pocket dissection as previously described, and then separates the inferior cut edge of the pectoralis from overlying parenchyma

strokes with the handswitching, monopolar, needle tip forceps (Figure 11-20). In routine glandular ptotic breasts, the dual plane 2 techniques require freeing the pectoralis adequately to allow it to move upward to the lower border of the areola. Dual plane 3 techniques for constricted lower pole and tubular breasts require mobilization adequate to allow movement of the inferior edge of the pectoralis to the upper border of the areola. The surgeon separates the parenchyma–muscle interface in small increments, then inserts fingers into the pocket and pulls anteriorly to palpate the position of the inferior pectoralis cut edge to accurately confirm the position of the inferior muscle border.

Before irrigating the pocket and placing the implant, the surgeon should insert a finger and lift the skin envelope anteriorly to check for any residual restriction of anterior movement of the lower envelope (Figure 11-21). If any banding or restriction is palpable at the level of the inferior border of the pectoralis, it is important to separate the muscle from the overlying parenchyma in additional 1 cm increments with electrocautery forceps, stopping when palpation with fingers inside the pocket detects no remaining restrictions to full anterior expansion of the envelope.

Figure 11-20. Upward traction on the shorter, curved blade of a double ended retractor with the tip in the subcutaneous fat (black arrow) exposes and defines the parenchyma–muscle interface (white arrows). For dual plane 2 and 3 pockets, the surgeon separates parenchyma from muscle and detaches this interface with side-to-side sweeping motions of the closed tip forceps in the direction of the white arrows.

Figure 11-21. Anterior traction on the envelope by the surgeon's finger allows the surgeon to precisely determine the position of the inferior cut edge of pectoralis origins, and to assure unrestricted anterior expansion of the envelope by the implant. If restriction exists, further separation at the parenchyma–muscle interface is necessary to assure complete release laterally.

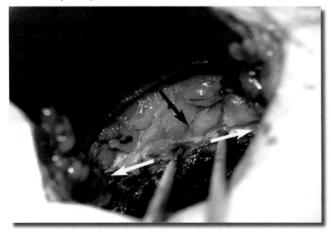

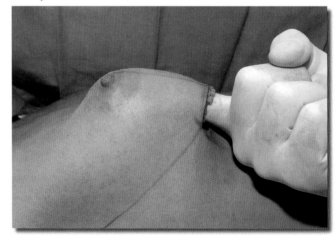

Reinspection and Pocket Irrigation

At the conclusion of pocket dissection, the surgeon should carefully reinspect all areas of the pocket for optimal hemostasis. Abrading any areas of the pocket with gauze sponges is unnecessary and undesirable, because sponge abrasion is traumatic to tissues and often causes bleeding from small vessels. Pocket irrigation with saline and antibiotic or topical solutions, removing all excess solution by suction, helps remove residual blood or loose tissue fragments from inner pocket surfaces, and provides potentially helpful reduction of bacterial contaminants that could increase risks of infection or capsular contracture.

Both pockets can be dissected from one side of the table, eliminating time waste and prolonged anesthesia, provided the operating table is capable of rotating adequately side-to-side. Few brands of operating tables match the functionality of Skytron tables in side-to-side movement. Following the specific processes and techniques described in this chapter, pocket dissection routinely requires no more than 4 minutes per side.

Both pockets can be dissected from one side of the table, eliminating time waste and prolonged anesthesia, provided the operating table is capable of rotating adequately side-to-side.

Implant Sizers in Primary Breast Augmentation

Implant sizers increase contamination risks, tissue trauma, time waste, and costs, and are totally unnecessary in primary breast augmentation, provided a surgeon is willing to quantitate tissue characteristics and use proved processes and systems such as the High Five™ System[5,6] during preoperative planning and implant selection. Many sizers do not accurately simulate the shape surface characteristics of the implant, and therefore do not accurately reflect the visual appearance that a similar volume implant may produce. Sizer surface characteristics seldom duplicate the surface characteristic of the implant, guaranteeing that distribution of fill in the breast with the sizer will not be the same as it will with the implant. Sizer use is addictive, and surgeons who insist on using sizers rarely learn to use quantitative systems that are much more accurate, reliable, and risk free.

Implant sizers increase contamination risks, tissue trauma, time waste, and costs, and are totally unnecessary in primary breast augmentation, provided a surgeon is willing to quantitate tissue characteristics and use proved processes and systems such as the High Five™ System[5,6] during preoperative planning and implant selection

Implant Preparation and Filling

All inflatable implants should be leak tested by submerging the implant in sterile saline, applying pressure to the implant, and checking the valve and all shell surfaces for air bubbles or leaks. Prefilled implants and inflatable implants can sustain shell damage from contact with other objects, so all implants should remain in their thermoform packaging until they are brought onto the operative field.

A simple sequence of techniques optimizes preparation of inflatable implants. The scrub nurse brings the implant to the operative field, where the surgeon removes the implant from its thermoform packaging, inverts the package, and places the implant filled with presterilized air on top of the inverted thermoform container (Figure 11-22, top). The surgeon or assistant inserts the fill tube (that is connected to a closed stopcock on the other end) into the implant, and uses closed suction to remove air from the implant while the surgeon simultaneously flattens the implant (Figure 11-22, middle). The surgeon can then easily roll the implant inward from both sides, placing the filler tube in the middle of the roll, and the implant is ready for insertion (Figure 11-22, bottom).

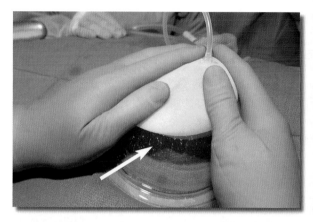

Use of an introducer sleeve, though cumbersome to many surgeons, offers protection for the implant when using prefilled implants. An introducing sleeve helps avoid focal pressures on the implant during insertion by distributing forces more evenly around the shell, and prevents the implant shell contacting skin or other surfaces during introduction, potentially reducing risks of pocket contamination by skin bacterial flora. The surgeon places a hand through the polyethylene sleeve (Figure 11-23, A), grasps the implant, pulls it into the sleeve, leaving approximately 2 cm of sleeve protruding above the implant (Figure 11-23, B), and then twists the sleeve closed beneath the implant (Figure 11-23, C). If desired, saline or other solutions can be placed into the sleeve with the implant to facilitate sleeve removal.

> An introducing sleeve helps avoid focal pressures on the implant during insertion by distributing forces more evenly around the shell, and prevents the implant shell contacting skin or other surfaces during introduction, potentially reducing risks of pocket contamination by skin bacterial flora

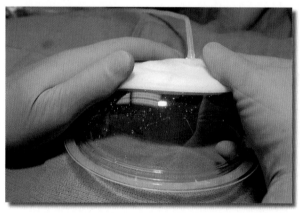

Holding the twisted rear sleeve between the ring and small fingers (Figure 11-23, D), the surgeon introduces the sleeve tip first, and then the first portion of the implant (Figure 11-23, E). Applying continuous gentle pressure to the sleeved rear of the implant outside the incision, the surgeon uses alternating index finger pressure and push to progressively insert the implant (Figure 11-23, F).

Figure 11-22. Top: Implant in place on top of thermoform packaging with fill tube connected to a closed suction system. The surgeon applies gentle, smoothing pressure on the implant as the assistant opens a stopcock to evacuate the sterile air from within the implant (middle). The surgeon then rolls the collapsed implant with the filler tube between the side rolls (bottom), and the implant is ready for insertion.

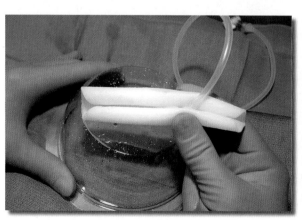

Figure 11-23 A. The surgeon inserts the hand through the polyethylene sleeve and grasps the implant.

Figure 11-23 B. No more than 2 cm of sleeve should protrude past the upper border of the implant.

Figure 11-23 C. Holding the implant and sleeve with one hand near the top of the implant, the surgeon twists the lower sleeve tightly to the 6 o'clock position of the implant and the assistant places a small amount of a 50% dilution of Betadine saline inside the sleeve to facilitate sleeve removal.

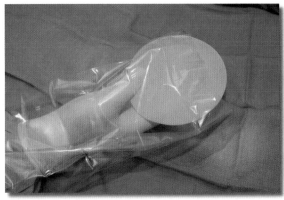

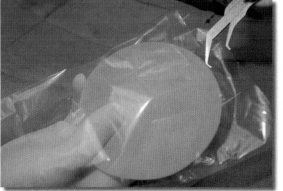

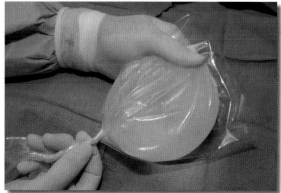

Figure 11-23 D. Holding the twisted sleeve between the ring and small fingers, the surgeon inserts the tip of the sleeve and implant.

Figure 11-23 E. Maintaining constant, even, gentle pressure on the posterior implant within the sleeve, the surgeon uses alternating index finger pressure and push to insert the implant in increments.

Figure 11-23 F. The sleeve prevents all contact of the implant with the skin, and evenly distributes pressure over the implant shell to minimize risks of focal pressure damage to the implant shell.

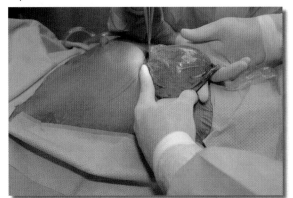

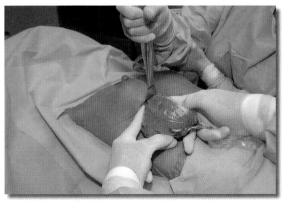

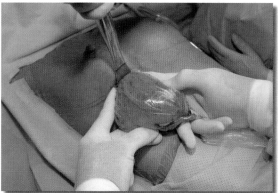

As the surgeon completes implant insertion (Figure 11-23, *G*), throughout the process the implant has remained oriented vertically due to alternating motion, so that when insertion is complete (Figure 11-23, *H*), the twisted portion of the sleeve at the 6 o'clock position of the implant exits the incision at the 6 o'clock position of the inframammary fold.

To remove the sleeve, the surgeon untwists the rear of the sleeve and inserts the index and long fingers inside the posterior sleeve, between the inside of the sleeve and the posterior surface of the implant (Figure 11-23, *I*). After advancing the fingers cephalad, the surgeon lifts the posterior wall of the implant anteriorly away from the sleeve, and with the other hand, slides the posterior sleeve out from behind the implant (Figure 11-23, *J*). By first removing the posterior sleeve, the anterior sleeve then slides easily off the anterior surface of the implant and out of the pocket (Figure 11-23, *K*).

To remove the sleeve without disturbing implant position, the surgeon inserts the index and long fingers between the posterior surface of the sleeve and the implant, lifts the implant anteriorly away from the sleeve, and then removes the posterior portion of the sleeve followed by the anterior portion of the sleeve. With minimal experience, use of an introducing sleeve requires less than 2 minutes of time intraoperatively.

With minimal experience, use of an introducing sleeve requires less than 2 minutes of time intraoperatively

Figure 11-23 G. By using equal and alternating pressure for insertion, the surgeon maintains orientation of the implant during insertion.

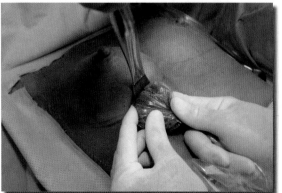

Figure 11-23 H. After the implant is inserted, if the surgeon has maintained optimal implant orientation, the twisted sleeve exits the 6 o'clock position of the inframammary fold.

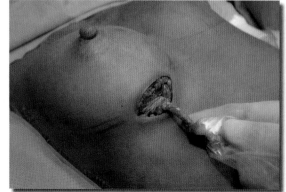

Figure 11-23 I. To remove the sleeve, the surgeon inserts two fingers inside the posterior sleeve, behind the implant, and then lifts the implant anteriorly away from the posterior sleeve to decrease friction while pulling the posterior sleeve out from behind the implant.

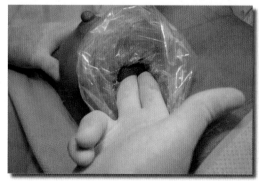

Figure 11-23 J. The surgeon first slides the posterior sleeve out with side-to-side inferiorly directed traction.

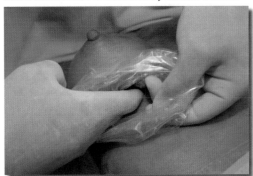

Figure 11-23 K. After the posterior sleeve is completely out of the incision, the anterior sleeve easily slides out with inferior traction to complete sleeve removal.

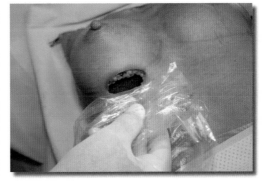

Implant Positioning

Round, smooth shell implants require no special positioning techniques, because they do not maintain position in the periprosthetic pocket. The only influences that a surgeon can exert over the position and fill distribution of round, smooth implants are to fill the implant adequately to prevent shell collapse, and to precisely control pocket dimensions and shape.

With shaped implants, especially full height anatomic implants such as the Allergan/Inamed Style 410 full height, textured, cohesive gel implant and the Style 468 full height textured, anatomic saline implant, surgeons can better control distribution of fill within the implant, and by controlling implant position, can better control distribution of fill and shape of the breast. *All anatomic or shaped implants require accurate pocket development and optimal positioning intraoperatively, but also enable surgeons to better control distribution of fill within the breast.*

The shape of full height, anatomic implants allows the implant to compensate for a wide range of skeletal and breast deformities, by placing fill more specifically where it is needed to fill deficient areas of a breast, by exerting more pressure on selected areas of the soft tissue envelope to correct constriction deformities, or by placing fill in selected areas to mask underlying skeletal deformities.

Contrary to the intuition of many surgeons, the optimal position of a full height, anatomic implant is rarely exactly vertical, from the 12 o'clock to the 6 o'clock position of the

Round, smooth shell implants require no special positioning techniques, because they do not maintain position in the periprosthetic pocket

The shape of full height, anatomic implants allows the implant to compensate for a wide range of skeletal and breast deformities, by placing fill more specifically where it is needed to fill deficient areas of a breast, by exerting more pressure on selected areas of the soft tissue envelope to correct constriction deformities, or by placing fill in selected areas to mask underlying skeletal deformities

All anatomic or shaped implants require accurate pocket development and optimal positioning intraoperatively, but also enable surgeons to better control distribution of fill within the breast

Contrary to the intuition of many surgeons, the optimal position of a full height, anatomic implant is rarely exactly vertical, from the 12 o'clock to the 6 o'clock position of the breast

breast. In most cases, slight rotation of the implant in one direction or the other off the vertical axis produces a more optimal and natural appearance of the breast and allows the surgeon to compensate for and minimize the visible effects of chest wall asymmetries. Another erroneous assumption is that aggressive texturing of the implant shell and adherence of the shell to the surrounding capsule are essential to maintain position of full height anatomic implants. When a full height anatomic implant is designed taller than it is wide, and the surgeon develops the pocket to fit the implant, the primary role of texturing is to provide friction, not necessarily adherence, as the capsule forms around the implant. When the capsule has formed, the capsule helps maintain implant position. Movement at the capsule–external tissue interface is adequate to allow enough implant mobility to satisfy patient desires regarding natural breast movement. These facts are proved by peer reviewed and published evidence in more than 3500 cases.[1-6]

Implant Malposition Risks

Implant malposition can occur with round, textured or smooth implants, and with anatomic shaped implants. One of the criticisms of anatomic implants that have been disseminated by surgeons who prefer round implants is that implant malposition or malrotation is more common with anatomic implants compared to round implants. *Scientifically valid data, however, do not support a higher incidence of malposition with full height anatomic implants.*[1-4] The largest currently reported series of round saline implants are the saline premarket approval (PMA) studies submitted to the Food and Drug Administration (FDA) by McGhan and Mentor Corporations.[7] At 3 year followup, in the combined series of 2165 patients, an average of 2% of patients underwent reoperation for implant malposition.[1-4] Of 1628 cases published in the journal *Plastic and Reconstructive Surgery* from January 2000 to January 2002 using full height Style 468 McGhan anatomic implants,[1-4] only 0.12% of patients had a reoperation for malposition, a difference of 1562%. *These data conclusively prove that a full height anatomic saline implant, used in conjunction with quantitative tissue criteria, the TEPID™ and High Five™ systems*[5,6] *of implant selection, and state-of-the-art surgical techniques*[1-4] *has as low (or lower) a rate of malposition compared to round implant.*

Implant malposition with *reduced* height anatomic implants has not yet been documented in large enough series to draw scientifically valid conclusions. Reduced height anatomic implants may be more prone to malposition, but in order to judge based on scientifically valid criteria, surgeons must carefully compare designs and types of texturing on the implant as well as patient tissue criteria and surgical implantation methods. Anecdotal

Implant malposition can occur with round, textured or smooth implants, and with anatomic shaped implants

Scientifically valid data do not support a higher incidence of malposition with full height anatomic implants

These data conclusively prove that a full height anatomic saline implant, used in conjunction with quantitative tissue criteria, the TEPID™ System[5] of implant selection, and state-of-the-art surgical techniques[1-4] has as low (or lower) a rate of malposition as any round implant

Implant malposition with *reduced* height anatomic implants has not yet been documented in large enough series to draw scientifically valid conclusions

reports of small series of Mentor Contour Profile® implants that raise concern over implant malposition[8] are not scientifically valid, because no information is published regarding the many tissue variables and surgeon variables[5] that could affect results, and the patient population or sample is not large enough to be scientifically valid. In addition, surgeons should not equate malposition risks of reduced height anatomic implants with less aggressive texturing such as the Mentor Contour Profile® saline implants or Mentor Contour Profile® gel implants to implants with more aggressive Biocell™ texturing such as the McGhan/Inamed Styles 363 saline, 410 MM gel, and other Biocell™ products. Other reports[7-9] of reduced height anatomic saline implants with more aggressive Biocell™ texturing such as the McGhan/Inamed Style 363 saline and McGhan/Inamed Style 410 MM indicate exceedingly low malposition rates,[9-11] so the type of texturing and other factors are key to minimizing malposition risks with reduced height saline implants.

When using full height, Biocell™ textured anatomic implants such as the McGhan/Inamed Style 468 saline and 410 FM, FF, and FL, the surgeon only needs to make the width of the pocket fit the width of the implant, because the full height anatomics are taller than they are wide, and if the width of the pocket fits the width of the implant, the height of the implant restricts risks of the implant malpositioning rotationally. In contrast, when using any reduced height anatomic or shaped implants, especially those with less aggressive texturing such as the Mentor Siltex™ and Mentor Contour Profile® gel products, the surgeon should carefully consider limiting upper pocket dissection as well as lateral pocket dissection to make the pocket fit the implant vertically as well as horizontally in order to minimize risks of malrotation.

> Visual decisions made intraoperatively with the patient sitting on the operating table can also be deceptive, unless the surgeon reconciles any visual findings with preoperative photographs taken with the patient standing

With all implants, the surgeon can often gain useful information by elevating the patient to as near a sitting position as possible on the operating table. Visual decisions made intraoperatively with the patient sitting on the operating table can also be deceptive, unless the surgeon reconciles any visual findings with preoperative photographs taken with the patient standing. On the operating table, soft tissue compression and forces occur that do not accurately simulate the forces on the breast with the patient standing, so the surgeon must be very careful and thorough when visually assessing the breasts with the patient sitting intraoperatively.

Incision Closures

Incision closure is a critically important step in augmentation. Achieving a watertight closure is much more predictable using continuous suture techniques instead of

> Achieving a watertight closure is much more predictable using continuous suture techniques instead of interrupted sutures. The most critical layer for watertight closure is the deep subcutaneous fascia, because if fluid escapes through this layer, fluid can accumulate immediately beneath the skin and promote thinning and disruption of the skin closure

interrupted sutures. The most critical layer for watertight closure is the deep subcutaneous fascia, because if fluid escapes through this layer, fluid can accumulate immediately beneath the skin and promote thinning and disruption of the skin closure.

Some surgeons prefer a three layer closure including deep subcutaneous fascia, deep dermis, and superficial dermis. A three layer closure leaves more foreign material in the deep dermis compared to a two layer closure of subcutaneous fascia and mid level dermis. Based on more than two decades of clinical experience, the three layer closure produces more inflammatory reaction in the wound that lasts significantly longer compared to a two level closure, and does not afford greater protection against fluid leak or scar widening compared to an optimal two layer closure.

Optimal suture materials handle and tie easily, provide predictable support of the tissues during the early stages of wound healing, and then absorb to leave less foreign material in the wound. No scientifically valid evidence supports a superiority of permanent compared to absorbable sutures, and suture removal is an unnecessary procedure that can be distasteful to patients, and uniformly wastes surgeon and personnel time without offering any scientifically documented advantages.

Optimal two layer incision closure begins with precise placement of a continuous, running 4-0 Monocryl suture in the subcutaneous fascia (Figure 11-24). Lifting a single hook placed in the corner of the incision optimally exposes the fascia in the corner of the incision for placement of the initial suture in the distal end of the incision. A minimum of four squared knots reduces risks of suture knot disruption postoperatively in this critically important layer. Maintaining upward tension on the hook in the corner of the wound, the assistant places gentle hand traction on the skin inferior to the wound edge, pulling

> Based on more than two decades of clinical experience, the three layer closure produces more inflammatory reaction in the wound that lasts significantly longer compared to a two level closure, and does not afford greater protection against fluid leak or scar widening compared to an optimal two layer closure

Figure 11-24. Continuous 4-0 Monocryl suture in the deep subcutaneous fascia.

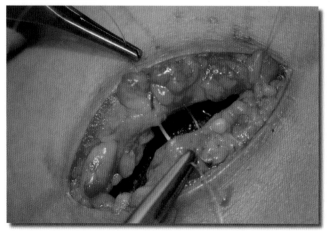

Figure 11-25. The surgeon holds the tip of the suture needle in a static position and uses forceps to place the tissue edges on the static needle. Keeping the tip of the suture needle facing away from the implant and placing the tissue edges onto the needle tip using forceps prevents inadvertent needle damage to the implant.

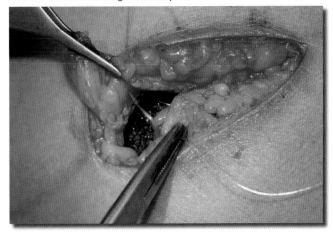

the skin downward and providing excellent exposure of the fascial layer for the surgeon. A simple technique helps prevent inadvertent contact of the needle tip with the implant. Instead of inserting the needle through both edges of the fascia using a typical arcing motion of the needle, the surgeon keeps the tip of the curved suture needle facing directly anteriorly away from the implant, then alternatively lifts each fascial edge with forceps and places the tissue onto the needle tip (Figure 11-25).

A simple technique helps prevent inadvertent contact of the needle tip with the implant. Instead of inserting the needle through both edges of the fascia using a typical arcing motion of the needle, the surgeon keeps the tip of the curved suture needle facing directly anteriorly away from the implant, then alternatively lifts each fascial edge with forceps and places the tissue onto the needle tip

The surgeon can place a minimum of three suture bites of fascia before pulling the suture through, saving time during the closure. The assistant must maintain constant traction on the suture, following the surgeon throughout the closure to avoid laxity in the suture which usually results in a loose closure and fluid leakage. At the completion of closure, the surgeon should carefully assure that the final suture is immediately adjacent to the corner of the wound, and must maintain tension on the continuous suture while placing at least four square knots. To protect the implant during placement of the final suture, the surgeon can insert the rear handle of the tissue forceps beneath the fascia to protect the implant. During closure of the deep subcutaneous fascia, the surgeon should try to avoid incorporating fat into the sutures, because strangulated fat undergoes fat necrosis, risking wound healing complications postoperatively.

A continuous suture of 5-0 Monocryl placed in the mid level dermis provides a rapid, optimal closure that predictably produces excellent scar results and does not require removal. Placement of a single hook outside the corner of the incision facilitates placement of this suture. The initial suture passes from superficial to deep 1–2 mm inside

A continuous suture of 5–0 Monocryl placed in the mid level dermis provides a rapid, optimal closure that predictably produces excellent scar results and does not require removal

Figure 11-26. Continuous subcuticular 5-0 Monocryl suture for skin closure.

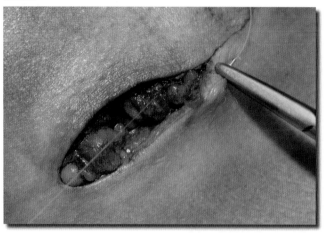

Figure 11-27. The only dressing, bandage, or postsurgical adjunct is a single piece of flesh colored Dermicel tape applied over Mastisol™ adherent.

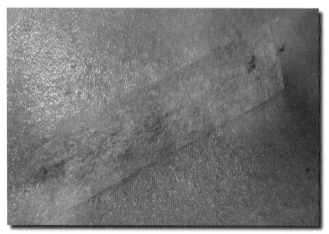

the corner of the wound. A minimum of three squared knots secures the suture. The suture needle then passes from deep to superficial, exactly in the corner of the wound which is not obscured by the hook which is outside the corner of the wound. The surgeon then continues a running subcuticular suturing technique to close the incision (Figure 11-26). The final suture passes from superficial to deep dermis, and the surgeon ties three squared knots, tying the single tag end of the suture to the doubled loop of suture material created by the previous suture. This closure technique places the knots on the deep surface of the dermis to minimize risks of knot extrusion postoperatively. Properly executed, this closure technique is highly predictable, producing watertight closures with excellent quality scar results.

Dressings, Drains, and Postoperative Care

The entire surgical dressing consists of a single layer of flesh colored Dermicel tape placed over Mastisol™ adherent solution applied to the incision skin edges (Figure 11-27). Drains

Drains are totally unnecessary and undesirable in primary augmentation.[1-4] Other adjuncts such as special bras or straps, indwelling catheters for injection of local anesthetics, pain pumps, narcotic strength pain medications, and implant motion exercises are likewise totally unnecessary and undesirable, because they unnecessarily complicate and prolong patient recovery

are totally unnecessary and undesirable in primary augmentation.[1-4] Other adjuncts such as special bras or straps, indwelling catheters for injection of local anesthetics, pain pumps, narcotic strength pain medications, and implant motion exercises are likewise totally unnecessary and undesirable, because they unnecessarily complicate and prolong patient recovery. Details of postoperative management using principles of 24 hour recovery are included in Chapters 20 and 21. Patients are instructed to shower 3–4 hours following return home, perform straight arm raising exercises, and to go out of the house for dinner or to shop the evening of surgery with ibuprofen as their only pain medication. Using this regimen, 96% of 627 patients returned to full normal (non-aerobic) activities within 24 hours following augmentation.[1,2]

Challenges and Potential Solutions

Every incision approach has potential challenges that can occur intraoperatively. Common challenges that occur with the inframammary approach with alternatives for avoidance or correction include the following:

1. Difficulty determining the optimal level of the inframammary fold and the optimal level for the inframammary incision:

   - Use the recommendations in the TEPID™ System, locating the volume of the implant planned for the procedure, then locating the desired nipple-to-fold distance recommendation below that volume in the table.

   - Remember to make all measurements under maximal skin stretch to simulate stretch that the implant will produce.

   - If leaving all inferior origins of the pectoralis major muscle intact along the inframammary fold (as opposed to dividing the origins for dual plane augmentations), lower the fold an additional 0.5 cm to compensate for the added pressure of the pectoralis on the lower pole of the implant.

2. Tendency to dissect the inferior pocket excessively, causing excessively low implant position and "bottoming":

   - When dissecting to enter the pocket, angle the dissection superiorly from the incision.

   - Avoid excessive upward traction on retractors during the operation, especially in thinner patients with more mobile chest skin, because retractor forces can separate

Use the recommendations in the TEPID™ System, locating the volume of the implant planned for the procedure, then locating the desired nipple-to-fold distance recommendation below that volume in the table

Avoid excessive upward traction on retractors during the operation, especially in thinner patients with more mobile chest skin, because retractor forces can separate the deep subcutaneous fascial attachments inferior to the incision edge to deeper structures, resulting in an excessively low inferior pocket border

the deep subcutaneous fascial attachments inferior to the incision edge to deeper structures, resulting in an excessively low inferior pocket border.

- When dividing pectoralis origins along the inframammary fold, constantly check topographic landmarks and preoperative markings to avoid dissection excessively inferiorly.

- Avoid excessively large implants that place excessive anterior traction on the skin envelope.

3. Risk of inadvertently entering the pleural space during electrocautery dissection:

- Always dissect parallel to the chest wall, dividing only those tissues that tent upward off the chest wall under retractor tension.

- Never cut any muscle tissue that does not tent upward off the chest wall under retractor tension.

- If desired, palpate a rib, and enter the subpectoral space directly over that rib.

- If pneumothorax occurs inadvertently, insert a small catheter through a pursestring suture in the intercostals or pleura, reinforce with a second layer of any adjacent tissue that is available, apply maximal suction to the catheter while providing positive pressure ventilation, and tie the pursestring suture. Obtain a chest x-ray in the recovery room to verify lung expansion, or alternatively, leave the catheter in place, exiting a separate stab incision, and provide water seal suction while seeking thoracic surgical consultation. Keep the patient under constant observation for at least 24 hours, and confirm lung expansion with another chest x-ray prior to discharge.

4. Difficulty controlling larger perforating vessels in the pocket:

- Coagulate all larger perforators in three locations with the handswitching, monopolar, electrocautery forceps prior to dividing the vessel.

- Divide all muscle origins at least 1 cm away from their origins on the ribs to avoid retraction of intramuscular vessels.

- Check all cut muscle edges and previously coagulated perforators prior to implant insertion.

- Do not perform pocket dissection with any type of sharp instrument, with blunt dissection, or even with needlepoint electrocautery pencil only.

> Never cut any muscle tissue that does not tent upward off the chest wall under retractor tension

> Coagulate all larger perforators in three locations with the handswitching, monopolar, electrocautery forceps prior to dividing the vessel

5. Excess lateral pocket dissection, risking lateral implant displacement and widening of the intermammary distance postoperatively:

- In the subpectoral plane, stop pocket dissection at the lateral border of the pectoralis minor, and after inserting the implant, incrementally enlarge the lateral pocket using double ended and spatula retractors until the footprint of the implant exactly fits the posterior surface of the pocket.

- In the submammary plane, stop initial lateral pocket dissection at the lateral border of the pectoralis major, or 2 cm inside the projected base width of the planned implant.

In the subpectoral plane, stop pocket dissection at the lateral border of the pectoralis minor, and after inserting the implant, incrementally enlarge the lateral pocket using double ended and spatula retractors until the footprint of the implant exactly fits the posterior surface of the pocket

6. Difficulty estimating or determining optimal pocket size compared to implant base dimensions:

- Always underdissect the lateral pocket, then incrementally enlarge it to fit the implant after the implant is in place.

- Avoid excessively large implants, especially in patients with thin soft tissue envelopes.

- Measure from the medial aspect of the pocket laterally intraoperatively using a sterile skin marking ruler or other instrument, and stop lateral pocket dissection at least 2 cm medial to the projected base width of the planned implant.

Always underdissect the lateral pocket, then incrementally enlarge it to fit the implant after the implant is in place

7. Excessive bleeding from inadvertent surgical trauma to the thoracoacromial pedicle or the larger perforator and vein at the second intercostal space:

- When dissecting superiorly, assure an adequate length retractor, and maintaining constant upward traction on the retractor, dissect parallel and close to the ribs, not upward toward the pectoralis muscle.

- Do not dissect within 2 cm of the second intercostal space medially, remaining at least 3 cm lateral to the sternum in the upper pocket where the large perforating vein and artery are located.

8. Excessive medial pocket dissection with excessive bleeding from medial perforating vessels:

- Mark at least a 3 cm wide intermammary distance preoperatively, and constantly check skin markings during medial pocket dissection to avoid dissecting medial to those markings.

Do not dissect within 2 cm of the second intercostal space medially, remaining at least 3 cm lateral to the sternum in the upper pocket where the large perforating vein and artery are located

Mark at least a 3 cm wide intermammary distance preoperatively, and constantly check skin markings during medial pocket dissection to avoid dissecting medial to those markings

- Remember that the most distal extent of the pocket is always distal to the tip of the retractor, so keep the retractor tip at least 1 cm inside pocket boundary skin markings at all times.

- When using the handswitching monopolar forceps, instead of dividing medial tissues with a sweeping motion, grasp and pinch each area of tissues to divide them in order to provide more effective coagulation.

9. Difficulty inserting a prefilled implant:

   - Enlarge the incision.

   - Reduce the size of the implant.

   - Use an introducing sleeve with techniques described in this chapter.

10. Difficulty achieving bilateral symmetry intraoperatively:

    - Remember that breast symmetry never exists in any patient pre- or postoperatively.

    - Recheck preoperative breast measurements, and remember that the smaller breast has quantitatively less skin, so an equivalent volume implant may produce more upper fullness compared to the larger skin envelope of the opposite breast.

    - Compare measurements very carefully to preoperative patient images. Note the amount, consistency, and distribution of parenchyma preoperatively, and reconcile that information with implant volume and shape, and with visible impressions intraoperatively.

    - Never attempt to put significantly more volume in the smaller envelope, as this practice is likely to produce an excessively bulging, globular appearing shape that differs significantly from shape in the opposite breast and is visibly apparent.

    - Remember that the human eye sees breast shape much more than breast size, and try to create similar shapes bilaterally instead of trying to force a match in size that is impossible.

11. Breast appears too full and globular intraoperatively:

    - Implant is too large for the dimensions and tissue characteristics of the patient's tissues.

    - Implant pocket is too small. Enlarge it in small increments laterally.

Enlarge the incision

Remember that the human eye sees breast shape much more than breast size, and try to create similar shapes bilaterally instead of trying to force a match in size that is impossible

Implant is too large for the dimensions and tissue characteristics of the patient's tissues

- Parenchyma is very firm and concentrated centrally. In severe circumstances, consider vertical radial scoring to splay out the parenchyma. This cause is very rare compared to the first two causes listed, and scoring should be a last resort.

12. Failure to achieve a watertight suture closure intraoperatively:

- Interrupted closure of deep subcutaneous fascia is not as watertight compared to a continuous suture closure.

- Maintain constant tension on the continuous sutures during closure and knot tying.

- Tie at least four squared knots in each end of the deep subcutaneous fascia closure and three squared knots in the dermal subcuticular suture.

- The surgeon may cut the knots more accurately compared to an assistant.

- Avoid incorporating excess fat in the deep subcutaneous fascia closure to avoid fat necrosis that often produces incision disruption.

13. Risk of suture needle puncture of the implant during suture closure:

- Keep the tip of the suture needle pointed anteriorly, away from the implant at all times, and use tissue forceps to place the fascial edges onto the needle.

- Use the rear of the tissue forceps beneath the fascial edge to protect the implant while placing a suture.

Maintain constant tension on the continuous sutures during closure and knot tying

Keep the tip of the suture needle pointed anteriorly, away from the implant at all times, and use tissue forceps to place the fascial edges onto the needle

▓ REFERENCES

1. Tebbetts JB: Achieving a predictable 24 hour return to normal activities after breast augmentation Part I: Refining practices using motion and time study principles. *Plast Reconstr Surg* 109:273–290, 2002.

2. Tebbetts JB: Achieving a predictable 24 hour return to normal activities after breast augmentation Part II: Patient preparation, refined surgical techniques and instrumentation. *Plast Reconstr Surg* 109:293–305, 2002.

3. Tebbetts JB: Dual plane (DP) breast augmentation: optimizing implant–soft tissue relationships in a wide range of breast types. *Plast Reconstr Surg* 107:1255, 2001.

4. Tebbetts JB: Patient acceptance of adequately filled breast implants using the tilt test. *Plast Reconstr Surg* 106(1):139–147, 2000.

5. Tebbetts JB: A system for breast implant selection based on patient tissue characteristics and implant–soft tissue dynamics. *Plast Reconstr Surg* 109(4):1396–1409, 2002.

6. Tebbetts JB, Adams WP: Five critical decisions in breast augmentation using 5 measurements in 5 minutes: the high five system. *Plast Reconstr Surg* 116(7):2005–2016, 2005.

7. Food and Drug Administration. U.S. Food and Drug Administration. Product labeling data for Mentor and Allergan/Inamed core studies of saline implants. Online. Available: http://www.fda.gov/cdrh/breastimplants/labeling/mentor_patient_labeling_5900.html.

8. Baeke JL: Breast deformity caused by anatomical or teardrop implant rotation. *Plast Reconstr Surg* 109(7):2555–2564, 2002.

9. Spear SL: Breast augmentation with reduced-height anatomic implants: the pros and cons. *Clin Plast Surg* 28(3):561–565, 2001.

10. Spear SL, Elmaraghy M, Hess C: Textured-surface saline-filled silicone breast implants for augmentation mammaplasty. *Plast Reconstr Surg* 105(4):1542–1552, 2000.

11. Heden P, Jernbeck J, Hober M: Breast augmentation with anatomical cohesive gel implants: the world's largest current experience. *Clin Plast Surg* 28(3):531–552, 2001.

The Axillary Approach for Augmentation

The axillary incision approach to breast augmentation was published by Hoehler in 1973. As a plastic surgery resident in 1977, after reading published studies available at the time,[1-5] the author performed a series of fresh cadaver dissections and operations to better define the pertinent surgical anatomy of the axillary approach.[7] The author performed his first axillary augmentation as a plastic surgery resident in 1977, and in 1984 reported early clinical experience in 90 cases with up to 5 year followup[7] in the journal *Plastic and Reconstructive Surgery*. From 1977 to 1993, all published reports of axillary augmentation used blunt, blind dissection techniques to create the implant pocket.[1-8] In 1991, the availability of endoscopic instrumentation enabled the author to dissect the entire submammary or subpectoral pocket with direct vision, electrocautery dissection instead of the previous blunt dissection techniques. Other reports of endoscopically assisted methods for pocket dissection continued to use blunt dissection in various areas of the pocket, causing tissue trauma and bleeding that precluded optimal control and predictably rapid patient recovery.[9,10] From 1992 to 2002, elimination of all blunt dissection, improved operative planning, improved instrumentation, and more precise and controlled surgical techniques enabled the author to predictably deliver 24 hour recovery and equivalent long-term outcomes via axillary subpectoral, dual plane, or submammary routes.[13]

A detailed knowledge of axillary and breast surgical anatomy is essential for surgeons to deliver predictably optimal outcomes with the axillary approach. Detailed knowledge of surgical anatomy enables surgeons to dissect adjacent to the axillary fat pad and enter the submammary or subpectoral space while minimizing risks of inadvertent injury to critical adjacent structures including intercostobrachial and medial brachial cutaneous nerves, the axillary artery and vein and their branches, and the brachial plexus.[7,8]

■ SURGICAL ANATOMY AND EVOLUTION OF TECHNIQUES

Early techniques of axillary augmentation accessed the implant pocket using scalpel and scissor dissection techniques.[1,2] A significant number of surgeons continue to use blunt, blind dissection techniques in some areas of the pocket for both retromammary and retropectoral pocket dissection, despite the availability of endoscopic instrumentation that can eliminate blunt dissection.[1-12] For the past 15 years, the author has completely eliminated all blunt dissection for submammary and subpectoral augmentations, significantly reducing bleeding and tissue trauma to improve patient recovery in axillary augmentation.

Surgical Anatomy for Axillary Augmentation

A detailed knowledge of the neurovascular anatomy of the axilla is essential to avoid damaging vasculature and the brachial plexus, to avoid damage to intercostobrachial and medial brachial cutaneous nerve branches in and near the axillary fat pad, and to preserve vascularity and innervation to the pectoralis musculature during surgical access for axillary retromammary, partial retropectoral, and dual plane augmentation.

The most important priorities for the surgeon during surgical access to the pocket are: (1) optimal incision location and length, (2) completely avoiding *any* dissection into the axillary fat to avoid damaging branches of the intercostobrachial and medial brachial cutaneous nerves, (3) locating the incision in the lateral pectoral fascia at 90 degrees to and anterior to the axillary skin incision, (4) avoiding bleeding from cutaneous branches of the posterior humeral circumflex artery and vein that course anteriorly over the lateral edge of the pectoralis major, (5) precisely defining the desired plane of pocket dissection before proceeding, and (6) entering the pocket (submammary or subpectoral) in an inferomedial direction to intersect the halfway point of a line between the midclavicular point and the nipple.

> More common sensory compromises in the axilla and upper arm occur when the surgeon dissects into the axillary fat, inadvertently damaging branches of the intercostobrachial or medial brachial cutaneous nerves, causing upper inner arm anesthesia or paresthesias

Figure 12-1, *A*, illustrates pertinent surgical anatomy of the axilla in a fresh cadaver dissection. Although the axillary artery, vein, and brachial plexus lie superior and deep to the access plane for axillary augmentation, suboptimal retractor positioning or inappropriate dissection into the fat of the axilla can damage any of these structures. More common sensory compromises in the axilla and upper arm occur when the surgeon dissects into the axillary fat, inadvertently damaging branches of the intercostobrachial or

Figure 12-1 A. Surgical anatomy of the right axilla. Branches of the intercostobrachial nerve (ICBN) and medial brachial cutaneous nerve (MBCN) course through the fat pad posterior to the tunnel for access that lies immediately posterior to the Army–Navy retractor at top. The brachial plexus (BR PLEX) and axillary artery and axillary vein (AX VEIN) course just deep and posterior to the tunnel. Surgeons should limit all dissection to the area of the small black dotted line rectangle at the top of the photo at far right.

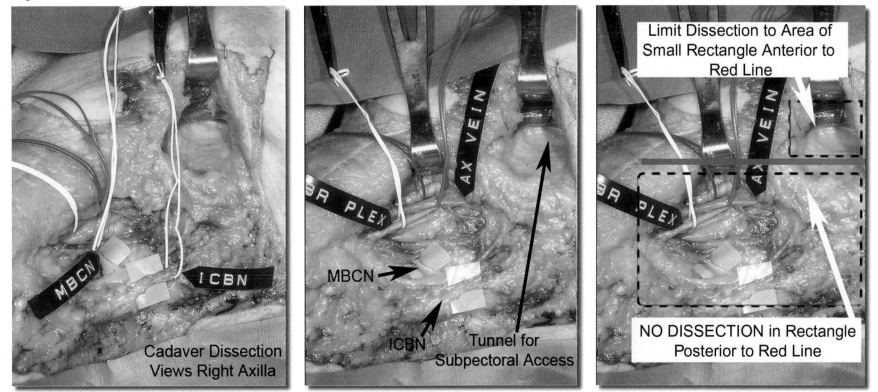

medial brachial cutaneous nerves (Figure 12-1 A, B), causing upper inner arm anesthesia or paresthesias. Chapter 4 presents additional, detailed descriptions and illustrations of surgical anatomy related to axillary augmentation.

Surgeons can completely avoid damage to neurovascular structures in the axilla by strictly adhering to specific landmarks and principles that are detailed later in the techniques section of this chapter. A key principle is to avoid any dissection whatever within the axillary fat pad, incising the lateral pectoral fascia or deep subcutaneous fascia directly over the lateral border of the pectoralis major, and entering a submammary, subfascial, or subpectoral pocket via a tunnel that is located anterior to all critical structures in the

A key principle is to avoid any dissection whatever within the axillary fat pad, incising the lateral pectoral fascia or deep subcutaneous fascia directly over the lateral border of the pectoralis major, and entering a submammary, subfascial, or subpectoral pocket via a tunnel that is located anterior to all critical structures in the axilla

Figures 12-1 B. Locations of the medial brachial cutaneous nerve and intercostobrachial nerves that pass through the axillary fat pad.

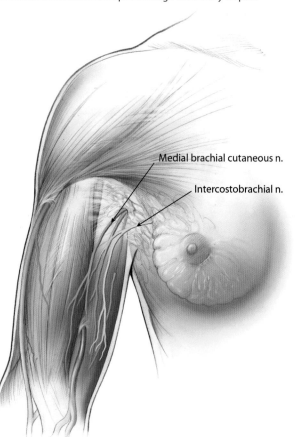

Medial brachial cutaneous n.

Intercostobrachial n.

axilla (Figure 12-1A). During preoperative marking, surgeons can replicate the red line in Figure 12-1A on the skin, 1 cm posterior to and parallel to the lateral border of the pectoralis. Keeping all *deep* dissection anterior to this line avoids damaging the structures described previously. Superficial skin edge undermining for access and mobility, described later in more detail, does not risk damage to key structures. Figure 12-1B illustrates the relational anatomy of the medial brachial cutaneous nerve and intercostobrachial nerves to the breast and axillary fat pad.

Figure 12-2 illustrates relational anatomy of the access tunnel to neurovasculature and musculature of the chest. In the tunnel for access, the dissection plane to enter the subpectoral space is immediately beneath the pectoralis muscle. Any dissection more posteriorly in the axillary fat risks damage to intercostobrachial nerve branches and branches of the lateral thoracic artery and vein that course in a superior–inferior direction in the fat on the floor of the tunnel. The optimal direction from the skin incision to enter the subpectoral pocket is in an inferomedial, not directly medial, direction to minimize risks of damage to branches of the thoracodorsal artery or vein.

Figure 12-2. Medial to lateral view of left chest wall with pectoralis major muscle retracted laterally. The gloved fingertip is visible in the tunnel for axillary access, and the green arrow indicates the direction in which the surgeon should first enter the subpectoral plane for pocket dissection. The intercostobrachial nerve (ICBN) is located immediately posterior to the tunnel, and the thoracodorsal artery and vein (TDA, V) are located in the fat pad on the undersurface of the pectoralis major muscle cephalad and anterior to the plane of the tunnel.

Figure 12-3. When bluntly dissecting a subpectoral pocket via the axillary approach, the dissector passes deep to the pectoralis major. As it sweeps from medial to lateral, at the lateral border of the rectus sheath, the dissector avulses the attachments of the deep subcutaneous fascia to the lateral border of the rectus sheath.

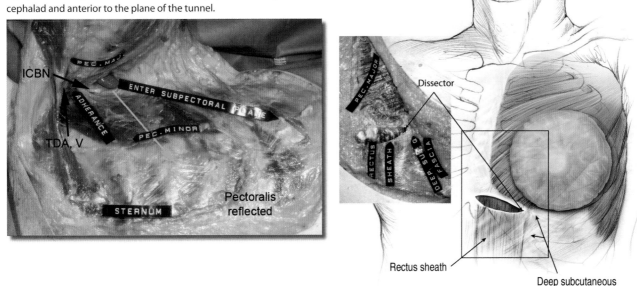

Figure 12-3 illustrates the musculofascial anatomy of the right chest with breast, skin, and subcutaneous tissue reflected. A blunt dissector beneath the pectoralis has been pushed inferiorly to demonstrate that subpectoral blunt dissection inferior to the pectoralis passes deep to the deep subcutaneous fascia lateral to the lateral border of the rectus sheath, detaching the deep subcutaneous fascia from its fusion with the lateral rectus sheath. Under direct endoscopic control, surgeons can divide origins of the pectoralis inferiorly to create a dual plane type 1 pocket, or leave the pectoralis origins intact for a partial retropectoral pocket. When relocating the inframammary fold inferiorly without dividing the pectoralis along the inframammary fold, dissection below the inframammary fold usually elevates the inferior-most origins of the pectoralis in continuity with deep subcutaneous fascia lateral to the rectus sheath.

Based on dissections after performing axillary augmentation in fresh cadavers,[7,8] the author's findings contradict findings of other surgeons who presented or reported that blunt dissection predictably divided the main medial origins of the pectoralis major muscle along the sternum and along the inframammary fold and that blunt dissection could predictably elevate the serratus muscle laterally.[9] Instead, the author found it virtually impossible to divide the main body of pectoralis origins medially with blunt dissectors, that inferiorly along the inframammary fold the blunt dissector divided pectoralis origins off the fourth and fifth ribs and passed deep to the deep subcutaneous fascia below the inframammary fold, and predictable blunt blind elevation of the serratus muscle intact and in continuity with the pectoralis via the axillary approach is impossible. These findings were further confirmed when endoscopes became available by examining a bluntly dissected pocket with an endoscope.

Predictable blunt blind elevation of the serratus muscle intact and in continuity with the pectoralis via the axillary approach is impossible

Evolution of Pocket Dissection Techniques

Prior to endoscopically assisted, electrocautery dissection, techniques for pocket dissection used various blunt dissecting instruments to develop submammary and subpectoral pockets.[1–8] Blunt dissection techniques, though successful, cause significant bleeding from vessels including the two large perforators in the inferior pocket of every subpectoral augmentation[10] and sometimes the medial perforators along the sternum. Absent direct visualization, surgeons controlled bleeding almost entirely with pressure over the dissected area for extended periods. Blunt dissection causes substantial tissue trauma and trauma to rib periosteum and perichondrium, contributing to postoperative pain and immobility that incapacitated these patients for a minimum of 7–10 days and often longer, usually required narcotic strength pain medications, and encouraged the use of adjuncts such as intercostals blocks, local anesthetic instillation into the pocket, and pain pumps. Although bleeding is usually controlled by pressure and clots are removed by irrigation, significant amounts of blood soak into and remain in adjacent tissues, increasing inflammation, prolonging recovery and healing, and contributing to a significant rate of capsular contracture despite motion exercises, intraluminal steroids, and other measures. As a result, *no published reports that use blunt dissection techniques can deliver as rapid recovery compared to published data on techniques that eliminate all blunt dissection.*[13]

Blunt dissection techniques, though successful, cause significant bleeding from vessels including the two large perforators in the inferior pocket of every subpectoral augmentation[10] and sometimes the medial perforators along the sternum

Blunt dissection causes substantial tissue trauma and trauma to rib periosteum and perichondrium, contributing to postoperative pain and immobility that incapacitated these patients for a minimum of 7–10 days and often longer

No published reports that use blunt dissection techniques can deliver as rapid recovery compared to published data on techniques that eliminate all blunt dissection

The development and refinement of endoscopic instrumentation and techniques[10–13] enabled surgeons to dramatically improve the accuracy of axillary augmentation by providing direct visualization during pocket dissection, and providing control that allows more precise modification of pectoralis origins. Further refinements in techniques described later in this chapter have totally eliminated blunt dissection, dramatically reduced or eliminated bleeding, and enabled surgeons to deliver 24 hour return to normal activities following axillary augmentation without narcotic strength pain medications, and without drains, special bras, special straps or positioning devices, intercostal blocks, pain pumps, motion exercises, or any other adjuncts.[13]

◼ CLINICAL EXPERIENCE

From 1977 to 2005, 690 patients aged 19 to 64 years (median age 31 years) chose the axillary augmentation approach for breast augmentation. Eighty-four patients had implants placed in the retromammary (RM) pocket location, 294 patients had partial retropectoral (PRP), and 312 patients had dual plane (DP) placement. From 1977 to 1992, blunt dissection was used to create partial retropectoral pockets (inframammary fold pectoralis origins left intact) and submammary pockets. From 1992 to 2005, all dissection was performed under direct visualization with endoscopic assistance using electrocautery dissection to create partial retropectoral pockets in 13 patients and to create dual plane 1 pockets (dividing origins of pectoralis along the inframammary fold) in 282 patients.

Beginning in 1994, a Snowden Pencer ROAM™ right angled endoscope and Ethicon Probe Plus II™ endoscopic dissector were used exclusively for pocket dissection, totally eliminating all blunt dissection in all cases.

Beginning in 1993, patients educated about all incision approaches could choose whatever incision approach they preferred according to staged, repetitive education and informed consent processes.[14] Based on more extensive surgical experience and followup with axillary augmentation, the surgeon and staff more specifically informed patients of all potential nuisances, surgical control factors, and potential tradeoffs of the axillary approach beginning in 1995. A much smaller percentage of patients subsequently chose the axillary approach, with a substantial majority of patients (more than 70%) having augmentation between 1995 and 2005 selecting an inframammary approach.

Preoperative planning and implant selection after 1993 utilized dimensional and tissue based processes published in *Plastic and Reconstructive Surgery*.[15,16] Beginning in 1997, all patients were encouraged to immediately resume full normal activities the evening of surgery. No drains, special bras or straps, intercostal blocks, pain pumps or narcotic strength pain medications were used in any patient after 1996.

CLINICAL ASSESSMENT, OPERATIVE PLANNING, AND IMPLANT SELECTION

Current preoperative clinical assessment and operative planning for axillary augmentation precisely follows the methods and processes of the High Five™ System[15] and the previous TEPID™ System of quantitative tissue assessment and implant selection[16] that is incorporated in the High Five™ System. Clinical assessment using this system prioritizes five critical decisions and uses five simple measurements that enable surgeons to complete all pertinent clinical assessment and operative planning decisions in 5 minutes or less. All decisions of pocket location, implant size, and inframammary fold position are based on defined, quantifiable tissue parameters individual to each patient.

Choice of implant pocket location determines soft tissue coverage for the patient's lifetime, is the most important decision in every breast augmentation, and is based on quantitative measurements of soft tissue thickness. If soft tissue pinch thickness superior to the breast parenchyma (STPTUP) is >2 cm, submammary or subfascial pocket locations are options. If STPTUP is <2 cm, pocket location options to optimize long-term soft tissue coverage are limited to dual plane[10] or traditional subpectoral pocket locations, in both cases preserving intact all medial origins of the pectoralis major along the sternum to the inframammary fold junction in every case. Measurement of soft tissue pinch thickness at the inframammary fold (STPTIMF) provides quantitative criteria on which to base a decision of whether to preserve all pectoralis origins intact along the inframammary fold to assure optimal coverage. If STPTIMF is <0.5 cm, surgeons should preserve the inferior origins of the pectoralis intact along the inframammary fold, and create a traditional retropectoral pocket. When STPTIMF is >0.5 cm at the IMF, coverage is adequate to allow surgeons to divide origins of pectoralis along the fold to create a dual plane pocket. These criteria and processes resulted in zero incidence of visible traction rippling or visible implant edges in 1664 reported cases with up to 7 year followup via axillary, inframammary, and periareolar approaches.[10,12,17]

If the patient requests the surgeon's input in selecting an implant that is safest for the patient's tissues long-term with the lowest risk of reoperation, implant selection is based on the High Five™ System[15] that estimates an approximate implant volume based on quantitative measurements of individual patient tissue characteristics. This approximate implant volume is based on quantitated, measured, individual patient tissue characteristics, derived from the base width measurement of the patient's existing breast parenchyma (BW), the stretch characteristics of the envelope (anterior pull skin stretch measurement or APSS), and assessment of the contribution of the patient's existing breast parenchyma to stretched envelope fill (percent contribution to stretched envelope fill or PCSEF). If the patient has a specific implant size request based on a specific number of cc's or grams, the patient must individually assume all responsibility for that decision in detailed, written, line-item informed consent documents,[14] and the surgeon then considers whether that request is acceptable given the patient's tissue characteristics and breast dimensions.

The third decision in planning is the specific type and dimensions of the implant (implant volume was determined as the second step of the High Five™ process). All current saline filled implants and all current silicone gel filled implants up to approximately 350 cc volumes can be safely and predictably inserted via the axillary approach. Larger gel implants, cohesive gel, and larger, round form stable cohesive gel implants can also be inserted via the axillary approach, but require larger incisions that extend more posteriorly where they may be more visible, require more surgical experience and skill for insertion, and entail a greater risk of implant device damage during insertion.

The fourth step in preoperative planning is defining desired nipple-to-inframammary fold distance (N:IMF) to create intraoperatively. The desired, new intraoperative position of the inframammary fold was determined subjectively by intraoperative visualization in cases prior to 1996 when the TEPID™ System[16] provided a much more accurate, objective method of defining optimal fold position relative to the implant selected for augmentation. The TEPID™ System is integrated into the High Five™ System as the fourth critical decision in every breast augmentation. Specific methodology is detailed in the TEPID™ and High Five™ papers.[15,16]

■ IMPLANT TYPES

Table 12-1 summarizes implant types and sizes in the series.

Table 12-1. Implant types and sizes

	1977–1992	1992–2005
Implant types		
Round, smooth shell, double lumen gel-saline (20 cc methylprednisolone in 20 cc saline in outer lumen)	307	0
Smooth, round gel	24	0
Round, textured saline	0	6
Round, smooth saline	0	5
McGhan/Inamed Style 468 full height textured saline		348
Implant size range/(average)	180–400 cc/(273 cc)	195–400 cc/(286 cc)

Despite recent reports of inserting form stable, cohesive, anatomic gel implants (Inamed Style 410) via the axilla,[17] no implants of this type were placed via the axilla by the author in the 410 premarket approval (PMA) study in the United States[18] because the author feels that the axillary approach does not provide the most optimal control for insertion and consistent, predictable positioning of these devices, and adds additional risks of implant damage during insertion. Since 1992, the patient, not the surgeon, chooses implant type (except in complicated cases) using our previously described patient education and informed consent process.[14]

▓ PREOPERATIVE MARKING

Axillary incision location is critically important to minimize scar visibility. Optimal incision location is in the hairbearing skin of the deepest apical portion of the axillary hollow, with the anterior-most extent of the incision posterior to the lateral border of the pectoralis (Figure 12-4). Incision length can vary from 2 to 6 cm to accommodate varying instrumentation and implants. Axillary scar quality and minimizing damage to implants during insertion are far more important than incision length. Average ideal incision

> Axillary incision location is critically important to minimize scar visibility

Figure 12-4. Left: The surgeon places a dot in the apex of the axillary hollow and outlines the lateral border of the pectoralis major muscle. Middle: The surgeon then draws a line through the dot from anterior to posterior, keeping the incision line high in the axillary hollow, not necessarily paralleling or within an axillary crease line. Right: With the patient's hand on her hip, no portion of a properly located incision line is visible.

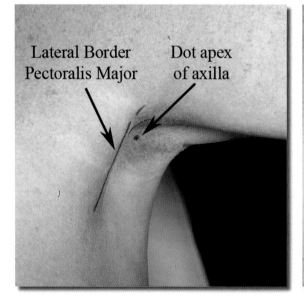

Lateral Border Pectoralis Major

Dot apex of axilla

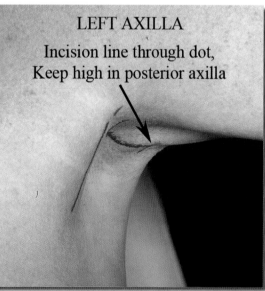

LEFT AXILLA

Incision line through dot, Keep high in posterior axilla

Incision line not visible with hand on hip

lengths of 4–5 cm minimize instrument trauma to skin edges and damage to implants from excessively short incisions. Although it is technically possible to insert inflatable implants through axillary incisions as short as 1.5 cm, incision lengths of 4–5 cm provide increased control and decreased skin edge trauma for surgeons who use state-of-the-art instrumentation and techniques. Scar visibility relates far more to scar quality compared to scar length, and an additional centimeter of incision length can dramatically improve control while minimizing trauma to skin edges and damage to the implant shell. Scar location (determined by incision placement) is the factor that most affects axillary scar visibility.

With the patient standing with her hands on her hips and flexing the pectoralis to define its superolateral border and deepen the axilla, the surgeon marks a line vertically over the middle of the lateral protruding border of the pectoralis (Figure 12-4, left), and places a dot in the apex of the hairbearing skin of the axillary hollow. Beginning at least 1 cm posterior to the lateral border of the pectoralis, the surgeon marks the incision line coursing superiorly and posteriorly through the dot in the apical hairbearing skin of the axilla. Paralleling skin creases in the axilla is not necessary, but it is important to keep the posterior part of the incision high in the axilla to minimize visibility. The objective is to create at least a 4 cm incision that begins posterior to the lateral border of the pectoralis and remains in the axillary apical hollow. Although shorter incisions are technically possible, they limit retractor width and visualization and encourage skin edge trauma that compromises scar quality.

After placing a dot at the sternal notch and xiphoid, and connecting the two with a series of vertical dots to define a visual midline of the sternum, the surgeon then places additional dots 1.5 cm lateral to each of the midline dots to define the maximal medial extent of pocket dissection that prevents inadvertently disrupting medial perforators that are usually located 1 cm lateral to the midline. Maintaining at least a 3 cm intermammary distance in all cases minimizes risks of medial perforator disruption, compromised medial soft tissue coverage, visible implant edges medially, visible medial traction rippling, and synmastia.

After marking the existing inframammary fold, the surgeon places the tip of a tape measure at the nipple, lifts the nipple maximally superiorly to maximally stretch the skin of the breast lower pole, and then at the 6 o'clock position, marks the desired, new nipple-to-inframammary fold distance recommended by the TEPID™/High Five™ System by placing a dot. If the desired new fold level is below the existing fold, the surgeon outlines the desired, new inframammary fold below the existing fold, and in the process, corrects any fold contour irregularities.

Scar visibility relates far more to scar quality compared to scar length, and an additional centimeter of incision length can dramatically improve control while minimizing trauma to skin edges. Scar location (determined by incision placement) is the factor that most affects axillary scar visibility

Additional topographic markings can include the desired lateral border of the implant pocket, taking into account the desired base width of the implant selected, its base imprint over the curvature of the chest wall, the compliance of the patient's soft tissue envelope, and the projection of the implant. All of these variables make defining a lateral pocket border nothing more than an estimate that should always be conservative in a medial direction to avoid overdissection of the lateral pocket.

■ ANESTHESIA AND LOCAL ANESTHETIC INSTILLATION

Optimal, state-of-the-art breast augmentation and optimal recovery require general anesthesia and muscle relaxants

Chapter 14 is devoted to preoperative care, anesthesia, and postoperative care. Optimal, state-of-the-art breast augmentation and optimal recovery require general anesthesia and muscle relaxants. General anesthesia can reduce the amount of intraoperative sedative and narcotic drugs a patient requires while enabling surgeons to perform a more accurate, controlled operation and dramatically reducing patient recovery times, enabling axillary augmentation patients who have had a general anesthetic to leave the surgical facility with an ASPAN score of 10 within 45 minutes of their transfer to recovery following the procedure.[13] Instillation of a vasoconstrictive agent along the incision line may reduce dermal bleeding, but instillation of local anesthetic into any other area of the breast or pocket is unnecessary and has the following potential risks: (1) multiple small hematomas within the breast parenchyma, (2) increased electrical resistance in all infiltrated tissues that decrease the efficacy of electrocautery dissection, and (3) increased risks of pneumothorax with deeper infiltration or intercostal blocks. Intercostal blocks, instillation of local anesthetic agents into the pocket, and pain pumps are totally unnecessary for patient comfort postoperatively if surgeons apply proved processes that predictably deliver 24 hour recovery.[1]

■ SURGICAL TECHNIQUES AND SURGICAL SCRIPTS FOR THE AXILLARY APPROACH

Specific details of surgical technique enable surgeons to predictably assure over 90% of patients that they can return to full, normal, non-aerobic activities within 24 hours following either axillary subpectoral or submammary augmentation for the first time in the history of breast augmentation

Specific details of surgical technique enable surgeons to predictably assure over 90% of patients that they can return to full, normal, non-aerobic activities within 24 hours following either axillary subpectoral or submammary augmentation for the first time in the history of breast augmentation.[3] This rapid recovery is remarkable, because it completely redefines the patient experience in modern augmentation mammaplasty, and this level of recovery is predictable using inframammary, periareolar, and axillary incision approaches. Rapid recovery and return to normal activities within 24 hours is impossible without dramatically reducing tissue trauma and bleeding. The following techniques, combined with optimal anesthetic management, predictably allow surgeons to deliver their patients a completely redefined experience in breast augmentation.

Table 12-2 is a detailed script for inframammary augmentation derived from process engineering principles analysis[1] that defines virtually every essential movement of every person in the operating room. Pilots, astronauts, and many business and industrial personnel routinely use defined processes and derived scripts or checklists for training and to optimize performance of numerous processes. Electronic files of this script are available in the Resources folder on the DVDs that accompany this book. After distributing this script to operating room personnel for review, surgeons can place these documents on a laptop computer in the operating room and have a designated person read steps of the operation in sequence. This simple process can dramatically reduce unnecessary and time wasting maneuvers, dramatically reducing operating times and patient recovery times.[1] This script is also a valuable learning tool for plastic surgery residents.

▓ PREMEDICATIONS AND ANESTHESIA

The preanesthetic and anesthetic regimens and printed protocols that allow patients to be out to dinner the evening of surgery and resume full normal activities within 24 hours are available in a previous publication[13] and in the Resources folder on the DVDs that accompany this book. All axillary augmentation patients follow exactly the same postoperative management regimen as inframammary and periareolar approach patients. Minimizing sedative and narcotic medications pre-, intra-, and postoperatively is critical to early return to full activities, and requires that the surgeon minimize surgical trauma and bleeding. Total narcotic doses intraoperatively average 2–4 cc of fentanyl. In recovery and stepdown, total narcotic doses are 25 mg of Demerol in two divided doses preceded by 6.25 mg of Phenergan administered 3–4 minutes prior to the Demerol. Using this regimen, nausea and vomiting have been virtually non-existent. Details of dosing and timing of doses are included in the previously referenced publication.[13]

All patients have general endotracheal anesthesia with muscle relaxants intraoperatively to minimize retraction forces and trauma to the pectoralis muscle while relaxing the pectoralis to allow optimal visualization and control.

▓ SURGICAL INSTRUMENTATION

Endoscopic visualization and dissection substantially increase control and accuracy in axillary augmentation and render blind, blunt dissection techniques unnecessarily

Endoscopic visualization and dissection substantially increase control and accuracy in axillary augmentation and render blind, blunt dissection techniques unnecessarily traumatic and obsolete

traumatic and obsolete. A variety of effective endoscopic instrumentation is available to surgeons. Instrumentation optimizes flexibility, accuracy, control, and efficiency when a minimum number of instruments and minimum number of instrument changes and moves provide maximum exposure and control. After using all instrumentation that was available in the 1990s, the author integrated available instrumentation that was most effective with new designs that better optimized flexibility, accuracy, and control.

Most surgeons perform axillary endoscopic dissection through a single port. Conventional, straight endoscopes with a camera mounted in line with the endoscope partially obstruct optimal access for dissecting instrumentation that the surgeon introduces alongside the endoscope. The ROAM™ right angled endoscope–retractor system (Figure 12-5) was designed to (1) alleviate obstruction of the single axillary port by an in-line camera, and (2) allow rapid, omnidirectional endoscope movement independent of a retractor that provides exposure while allowing the surgeon to clamp the endoscope into the retractor when desired to free both hands for hemostatic control or delicate dissection. The ROAM™ right angled endoscope system is designed to function as surgeons are trained—establish exposure with appropriate retraction, then allow the eye (in this case, the endoscope) to roam the dissection field with a wider field of vision, constantly moving to visualize and anticipate anatomic details and neurovasculature for maximal control.

One of the most functionally important design considerations for endoscopic equipment for axillary augmentation is assuring that the surgeon can move the endoscope independent of the retractor. When the endoscope is attached to a retractor, every move of the endoscope

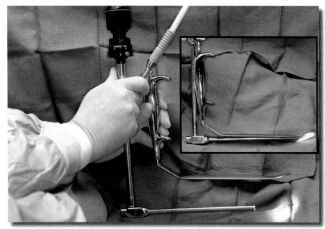

Figure 12-5. The ROAM™ right angled endoscope–retractor system consists of a specially designed retractor that incorporates smoke evacuation, and a right angled endoscope that the surgeon can manipulate independently of the retractor for bimanual visualization and dissection. The retractor also has a groove (inset photo) that allows the surgeon to attach the endoscope to the retractor if desired. This right angled endoscopic system eliminates obstruction of the single operative port by the camera and adapter that are mounted on the endoscope.

The ROAM™ right angled endoscope system is designed to function as surgeons are trained—establish exposure with appropriate retraction, then allow the eye (in this case, the endoscope) to roam the dissection field with a wider field of vision, constantly moving to visualize and anticipate anatomic details and neurovasculature for maximal control

One of the most functionally important design considerations for endoscopic equipment for axillary augmentation is assuring that the surgeon can move the endoscope independent of the retractor

to optimize visualization incorporates a move of the retractor which increases trauma to overlying pectoralis and underlying rib periosteum and perichondrium, and often increases bleeding and blood staining of tissues. Establishing retraction in a minimum number of positions with an adequate width retractor minimizes these negatives. Holding the endoscope in one hand and the dissecting instrument in the other, the surgeon can move the endoscope freely in all directions, "zooming" views by moving in or out of the pocket to recheck previously dissected and adjacent areas for vessels or bleeding. The freely moving endoscope and dissector increase accuracy, control, and efficiency while minimizing tissue trauma and bleeding. Any system that allows free movement of the endoscope independent of a retractor accomplishes these goals.

The width of a retractor blade at its tip determines the angle of view accessible to the surgeon, and narrower retractors provide less exposure at their tips compared to wider retractors. Optimizing prospective hemostasis requires that surgeons see and control vessels before inadvertently dividing them, and the greater the field of vision at the furthest extent of dissection, the greater accuracy and control is available to the surgeon. Excessively narrow retractors used through very small incisions may sound enticing to uninformed patients and surgeons, but offer distinctly less visualization and control compared to moderate width retractors through 4 cm incisions.

> The width of a retractor blade at its tip determines the angle of view accessible to the surgeon, hence narrower retractors provide less exposure at their tips compared to wider retractors

Figure 12-6. Ethicon Probe Plus II™ endoscopic, electrocautery dissector with retractable insulating sleeve, needle tip, cut and coagulation switches (rocker switch on top of handle) and suction and irrigation controls (square buttons on oblique back of handle).

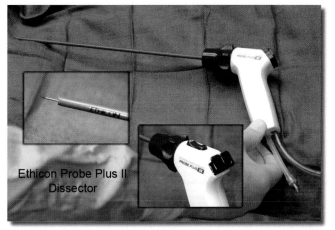

Ethicon Probe Plus II Dissector

Many designs of right and left endoscopic dissectors exist, but a single, straight, endoscopic dissecting device functions equally or better and eliminates excess instrumentation. Originally designed for endoscopic cholecystectomy, the Ethicon Probe Plus II™ endoscopic, electrocautery dissector (Figure 12-6) is superior to all other dissecting instruments the author has used. This instrument integrates handswitching cut and coagulation needlepoint with suction and irrigation in a single instrument that provides superior functionality and efficiency for axillary endoscopic augmentation. A retractable sleeve over the electrode needle tip allows the surgeon to easily introduce the dissector with the sleeve over the sharp tip to prevent penetrating tissues. Retracting the sleeve while grasping the pistol grip of the dissector allows the surgeon to use a 50:50 blend of cut and coagulation current controlled by the coagulation switch on the instrument for dissection and hemostasis.

A needle tip dissector focuses current and optimizes visualization more effectively compared to blade or wider tip dissectors. The greater the surface area of the tip of the dissector, the more coagulum adheres to the tip during dissection, decreasing the instrument's efficacy and accuracy.

> A needle tip dissector focuses current and optimizes visualization more effectively compared to blade or wider tip dissectors

■ ANESTHESIA

General endotracheal anesthesia using short acting muscle relaxants provides optimal control and precision to predictably deliver 24 hour return to normal activities following dual plane and subpectoral axillary augmentation. Detailed descriptions and protocols for pre- and perioperative anesthesia are included in a previous publication.[13] Key to rapid recovery is the principle of minimizing preoperative, intraoperative, and postoperative narcotics.

> General endotracheal anesthesia using short acting muscle relaxants provides optimal control and precision to predictably deliver 24 hour return to normal activities following dual plane and subpectoral axillary augmentation

For optimal hemostasis at the incision line, the surgeon injects a maximum of 2 cc of xylocaine or saline with epinephrine (adrenaline) in the immediate subcutaneous plane only. No other injection of any type of local anesthetic is necessary or desirable in any other area, because fluid in the tissues increases electrical resistance that decreases the efficacy of the electrocautery dissecting instruments.

■ SURGICAL TECHNIQUES

The following surgical techniques evolved and improved primarily as a result of (a) extensive fresh cadaver dissections to define and understand key surgical anatomy,[7,8] and (b) analysis and refinement of surgical techniques to better define processes using principles of process engineering and motion and time studies.[13] Details, not generalities, of surgical technique processes define differences between optimal and average or suboptimal outcomes. A video of the High Five™ assessment process[15] and another of the surgical techniques for axillary augmentation are available on the accompanying DVDs.

Details, not generalities, of surgical technique processes define differences between optimal and average or suboptimal outcomes. This fact is especially true with more technically demanding procedures such as axillary endoscopic augmentation. The following detailed descriptions of technique and logic are purposefully detailed to minimize the learning curve for surgeons who wish to perform axillary endoscopic breast augmentation.

Details, not generalities, of surgical technique processes define differences between optimal and average or suboptimal outcomes

Patient Positioning and Draping

Optimal patient positioning is essential for optimal axillary exposure while minimizing risks of arm hyperextension that can produce brachial plexus injury. When placing the arms on movable arm boards, the surgeon is responsible for informing and reminding anesthesia and surgery facility personnel to *never at any time raise the arm to a position greater than 90 degrees to the torso.* Arm boards should be heavily padded and the arms should be stabilized with two sterile towels of 6–8″ width overwrapped with 3″ tape or wide (6″ or greater) Velcro arm stabilizing bands.

Creating and maintaining a sterile field in the axillary area requires precise draping techniques using carefully applied adherent drapes. Using a sponge stick, the surgical assistant applies a stripe of Mastisol™ adherent along the lateral thorax, continuing across the posterior axilla onto the posterior upper arm, and then curving across the upper arm and across the clavicles. The surgeon or assistant blots the adherent and then applies adherent edged Steri-drapes to the Mastisol™ line, carefully placing the posterior axillary skin under tension when applying the drape to assure a watertight seal in all areas. A second layer of adherent edge final drapes assures a sterile field.

Creating and maintaining a sterile field in the axillary area requires precise draping techniques using carefully applied adherent drapes

Incision and Access to the Implant Pocket

Before making the initial incision, the surgeon places two or three small crosshatch marks at intervals perpendicular to the preoperatively marked incision line (Figure 12-7, left). These marks assist the surgeon with precise realignment of skin edges at closure. The initial incision with the scalpel is only to midlevel dermis to minimize bleeding. Using a needlepoint electrocautery pencil with blended cut and coagulation current (approximately 50 : 50), the surgeon deepens the incision only another 2 mm, until axillary fat is visible. Placing the skin edges under tension and lifting to define the

Figure 12-7. Left: Light cross marks perpendicular to the incision line facilitate exact realignment of skin edges at closure. Right: A small rake retractor places the skin under tension as the surgeon undermines for 1 cm adjacent to the incision line with a needle tip electrocautery pencil.

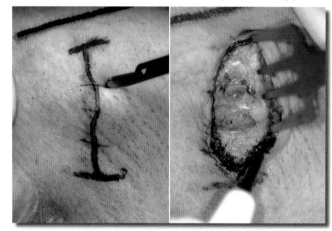

Figure 12-8. Incision in lateral pectoral fascia. Left: After completing the very superficial undermining of the skin incision (white arrow), the surgeon visualizes a line (yellow) overlying the most lateral surface on the lateral border of the pectoralis. Center: Incision with blended cut and coagulation current and a needle tip cautery through the lateral pectoral fascia (white arrow) exposes the lateral border of the pectoralis major muscle (white arrow). Right: The incision in the lateral pectoral fascia (yellow line) is perpendicular to the skin incision (red line). The surgeon carefully avoids any type of dissection in the axillary fat pad (area within the white triangle).

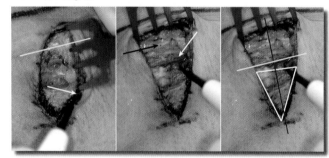

dissection plane, the surgeon undermines the incision edges in the immediate subdermal plane for 3–5 mm in all directions (Figure 12-7, right). A 1 cm undermining of skin edges immediately adjacent to the incision substantially increases the mobility of the skin edges to minimize skin edge trauma from retractors while facilitating retractor and instrument placement and movement.

While the skin incision is oriented in an anterior–posterior direction, the incision in the lateral pectoral fascia should lie exactly over the posterolateral edge of the pectoralis in the axilla, in a superior–inferior direction. This bidirectional, overlapping orientation of the superficial and deep incisions reduces risks of linear, superficial to deep scar retraction that can occur in the axillary fat from a single direction incision and tunnel.

Using a toothed retractor or skin hooks to expose the subcutaneous fat and palpating the lateral border of the pectoralis, the surgeon makes a 4 cm long incision through the subcutaneous fat and through the superficial pectoral fascia overlying the lateral border of the pectoralis in a superior–inferior direction (Figure

A 1 cm undermining of skin edges immediately adjacent to the incision substantially increases the mobility of the skin edges to minimize skin edge trauma from retractors while facilitating retractor and instrument placement and movement

Surgeons should avoid making the fascial incision over the lateral pectoralis excessively cephalad and entering the subpectoral plane excessively cephalad because of risk of interrupting cutaneous branches of the posterior humeral circumflex artery and vein that course anteriorly over the lateral border of the pectoralis

12-8). Surgeons should avoid making the fascial incision over the lateral pectoralis excessively cephalad and entering the subpectoral plane excessively cephalad because of risk of interrupting cutaneous branches of the posterior humeral circumflex artery and vein that course anteriorly over the lateral border of the pectoralis. The fascial incision exposes the muscle of the lateral border of the pectoralis. At this point, the surgeon can elect to continue dissection anterior to the pectoralis in a subfascial or submammary plane, or elect to create a subpectoral or dual plane pocket by dissecting posterior to the pectoralis major. In either case, to facilitate pocket entry and minimize surgical trauma to adjacent structures, *the surgeon should create the tunnel in a plane immediately adjacent to the pectoralis muscle.* This discussion will focus on dissecting a dual plane type 1 subpectoral pocket, but the principles are similar for dissecting a submammary or subfascial pocket.

Figure 12-9 graphically demonstrates the stages of pocket dissection for subpectoral, dual plane, and retromammary pockets from the surgeon's perspective on

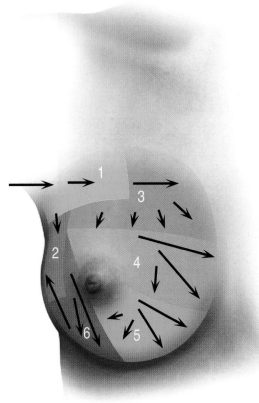

Figure 12-9. Optimal entry and dissection sequence for axillary subpectoral augmentation in the right breast. Numbered and color coded segments indicate the optimal sequence of pocket dissection. Direction and size of the black arrows in each area indicate the desired direction and extent of dissection before transitioning to the next zone.

Pocket dissection sequence via the axillary approach

A systematic dissection sequence establishes visualization in zones of minimal vascularity before proceeding to areas where more vessels are located

the right breast. A systematic dissection sequence establishes visualization in zones of minimal vascularity before proceeding to areas where more vessels are located. If the surgeon then inadvertently divides a vessel, exposure already exists for optimal visualization and control. Zone 1 dissection extends from the skin incision into the subpectoral pocket.

The optimal direction to enter the subpectoral plane from the incision location is to aim for a point approximately halfway between the nipple and the clavicle, in a direction inferior to the incision. The key is to avoid dissecting directly medially from the incision in an area that usually contains more blood vessels including branches of the posterior humeral circumflex artery and vein coursing anteriorly and branches of the thoracoacromial artery and vein on the posterior surface of the pectoralis superiorly.

The optimal direction to enter the subpectoral plane from the incision location is to aim for a point approximately halfway between the nipple and the clavicle, in a direction inferior to the incision

To enter the subpectoral plane, many surgeons insert a finger and bluntly dissect posterior to the pectoralis and push medially beneath the pectoralis. While this maneuver is effective, it often causes unnecessary bleeding that the surgeon then must control quickly to avoid blood staining in the pocket that obscures optimal visualization. Instead, the surgeon should insert the smaller end of a double ended retractor immediately beneath the muscle, and establish the subpectoral plane under direct vision using handswitching, monopolar, needlepoint electrocautery forceps (Figure 12-10). Surgeons should use these forceps to dissect the entire upper half of a subpectoral pocket under direct vision using a fiberoptic retractor. Cutaneous branches of the posterior humeral circumflex artery and vein usually course from posterior to anterior over the lateral border of the pectoralis near the fascial incision. If these vessels are visible, the surgeon should carefully electrocoagulate them in two locations with the forceps and then divide them to avoid inadvertent division by instrumentation later in the procedure.

Figure 12-10. Handswitching, monopolar, needlepoint electrocautery forceps. This instrument optimizes efficient, bloodless dissection of the upper pocket under direct vision using a fiberoptic retractor for exposure.

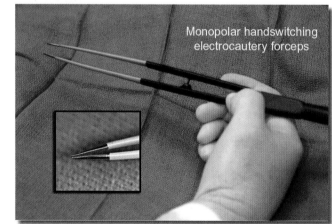

Monopolar handswitching electrocautery forceps

With the subpectoral plane established, the surgeon places the smaller blade of a second double ended retractor beneath the retractor blade already in place, and then rotates the second blade inferiorly and pulls laterally, handing the second retractor to an assistant who will hold the retractor at precise positions during pocket dissection (Figure 12-11). This maneuver, combined with minimal forceps dissection laterally, exposes the lateral border of the pectoralis minor muscle. Dissecting laterally to, but not past, the lateral border of the pectoralis minor at this stage establishes the lateral border of the pectoralis minor as an important landmark later in pocket dissection when connecting lateral pocket dissection to superior pocket dissection.

To increase exposure subpectorally, the surgeon places a longer blade of a fiberoptic retractor beneath the blade of the first double ended retractor that is lifting the pectoralis

Figure 12-11. Left: A double ended retractor lifting anteriorly provides exposure for initial upper pocket dissection inferomedially under direct vision with the electrocautery forceps. Right: A second double ended retractor pulling inferiorly and laterally allows dissection to expose the lateral border of the pectoralis minor under direct vision, before the surgeon proceeds with dissection of the other areas of the pocket. Dissection in Zone 2 utilizes only the electrocautery forceps. Zone 6 of the endoscopically assisted dissection later connects with the inferior-most portion of Zone 2.

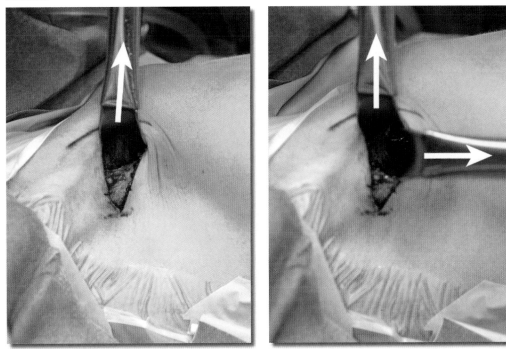

anteriorly, and then removes the double ended retractor. Placing a second retractor beneath a first, then removing the first, facilitates retractor exchange while minimizing tissue trauma, rib trauma, and bleeding that occurs more often when the surgeon removes one retractor completely and then inserts another. To avoid a retractor becoming a blunt dissector that causes unnecessary bleeding, the surgeon should insert longer retractors only as far as established pocket dissection, and then dissect ahead of the retractor with the electrocautery forceps.

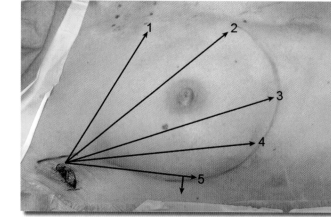

Figure 12-12. Retractor positions for pocket dissection. Precise retractor positioning and minimal retractor movements minimize tissue trauma and bleeding while optimizing control.

During endoscopically assisted pocket dissection, retractor positioning and tension are critical. Figure 12-12 illustrates five specific retractor positions for pocket dissection. For optimal control, the surgeon never holds the retractor except when reexamining areas of the pocket for hemostasis. The surgeon positions the retractor, and an assistant on the opposite side of the table holds it in position while the surgeon holds the endoscope in the non-dominant hand and the dissecting instrument in the dominant hand. If the endoscope is integrated into the retractor, the surgeon must move the retractor frequently, increasing tissue trauma and bleeding. Holding the endoscope in the nondominant hand and the dissecting instrument in the dominant hand dramatically increases accuracy and control by enabling the surgeon to move the endoscope while dissecting without moving the retractor.

Upper and Middle Pocket Dissection

In Zone 1 of pocket dissection, the surgeon first dissects under direct vision with the handswitching, monopolar, needlepoint electrocautery forceps. Techniques of prospective hemostasis[13] encourage surgeons to anticipate, visualize, and electrocoagulate all vessels before dividing them to avoid blood tissue staining that obscures visualization of anatomic details and increases postoperative inflammation and discomfort. The monopolar electrocautery forceps greatly facilitate these techniques by enabling the surgeon to use a single instrument for dissection and hemostasis, avoiding changing instruments to control a bleeding vessel and allowing blood to stain adjacent tissues. Superiorly, Zone 2 dissection continues only a few centimeters, stopping when the surgeon can visualize the fat pad on the undersurface of the pectoralis that contains the thoracoacromial pedicle. This extent of superior pocket dissection is adequate for the vertical dimensions of full height, form stable implants and for all round implants, regardless of filler material.

To define the medial pocket border in Zone 2 dissection, the surgeon places a longer, endoscopic retractor beneath the previous fiberoptic retractor and directs the tip of the retractor toward retractor position 1, approximately halfway between the sternal notch and the junction of the sternum with the inframammary fold (Figure 12-13, upper left).

Figure 12-13. Endoscopic dissection in the medial pocket. Upper left: Retractor position 1. Upper right: The surgeon increases visualization of the medial pectoralis origins (white arrow) by dissecting laterally and inferiorly (black arrow). Lower left: The pinnate, tendinous, white origins of the pectoralis major (black arrow) often arise lateral to the main body of muscle origins medially (white arrow). Lower right: Surgeons can safely divide individual pinnate origins that are located lateral to the main body of the muscle (black arrow). Surgeons should avoid any partial or complete division of the main body of the pectoralis along the sternum (white arrow) to optimize coverage and prevent banding and "windowshading" of the pectoralis.

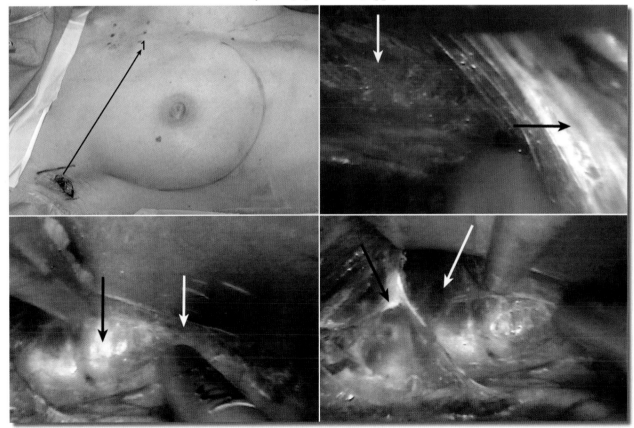

The surgeon transfers the retractor to an assistant on the opposite side of the operating table, then inserts the Probe Plus II™ dissector and uses a blend of cut and coagulation current in light, sweeping strokes to divide *only separate, pinnate origins of the pectoralis that arise lateral to the main body of muscle origins along the sternum, carefully avoiding dissection into the body of the muscle medially* (Figures 12-13 and 12-14). By frequently checking extent of dissection relative to the medial skin markings, the surgeon can avoid inadvertently dividing medial perforating vessels which can be very difficult to control. Excessive medial dissection to narrow the intermammary distance to less than 3 cm is never worth the tradeoffs. These tradeoffs include bleeding, loss of soft tissue coverage medially, and risks of synmastia.

Figure 12-14. Red dots identify common locations of individual, pinnate origins of the pectoralis muscle that are lateral to the main body of the muscle. The surgeon can safely divide these pinnate origins, *but the surgeon should never even partially divide any of the main body of pectoralis origins along the sternum.*

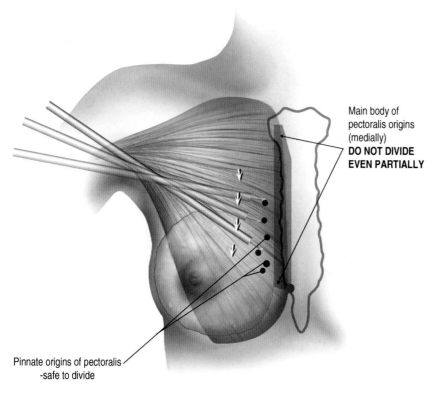

Main body of
pectoralis origins
(medially)
**DO NOT DIVIDE
EVEN PARTIALLY**

Pinnate origins of pectoralis
-safe to divide

When inferior visualization in this visual field decreases, the surgeon repositions the retractor to retractor position 2 exactly where the inframammary fold joins the sternum (see Figure 12-16, upper left). When repositioning the retractor, the surgeon keeps the tip of the retractor under direct visualization on the endoscope display and concentrates on avoiding contact with rib periosteum and perichondrium to reduce bleeding and subperichondrial hematomas.

As the surgeon dissects from superior to inferior along the medial pocket border, pinnate origins of the pectoralis that are located lateral to the main body of pectoralis origins along the sternum are *safe to divide, provided the surgeon never even partially divides any of the main body of pectoralis origins along the sternum* (Figures 12-13 and 12-14).

Precisely defining a sequence of zones of pocket dissection with precise retractor positioning points minimizes excessive retractor movements that cause tissue trauma and bleeding, optimizing exposure, control, and efficiency. With the retractor tip at the junction of the inframammary fold and sternum, the surgeon first enlarges the pocket medial and lateral to the body of the retractor by withdrawing the endoscope and dissector and dissecting side to side in light, sweeping strokes to enlarge the middle pocket. Slow, deliberate division of pectoralis origins on the third and fourth ribs in the midportion of the pocket optimizes coagulation hemostasis during muscle divisions. By dividing muscle origins at least 0.5 cm off the surface of the ribs, the surgeon avoids potential difficulty in controlling intramuscular or adjacent vessels that can retract into the intercostal musculature when dividing muscle origins flush with the ribs.

> By dividing muscle origins at least 0.5 cm off the surface of the ribs, the surgeon avoids potential difficulty in controlling intramuscular or adjacent vessels that can retract into the intercostal musculature when dividing muscle origins flush with the ribs.

Continuing to open the midportion of the pocket, the surgeon will encounter at least one large perforating artery and vein that is usually located 3–4 cm above the inframammary fold. A second large perforator is often located in the inferomedial portion of the pocket, 3–4 cm lateral to the sternal border. Locations of these vessels are illustrated in previous papers.[10,13] If the surgeon visualizes these vessels before cutting them with the dissecting instrument, the surgeon can activate the coagulation current of the endoscopic dissector and move it anterior and posterior while barely touching the outer wall of the perforator to very effectively coagulate before dividing the vessels. This technique avoids time wasting maneuvers of changing instruments to clamp and coagulate vessels with an endoscopic grasper.

> At each change of retractor position, the surgeon should stop and deliberately reexamine all previously dissected areas of the pocket for hemostasis, minimizing retractor movement by moving the endoscope instead of the retractor whenever possible

At each change of retractor position, the surgeon should stop and deliberately reexamine all previously dissected areas of the pocket for hemostasis, minimizing retractor movement by moving the endoscope instead of the retractor whenever possible. Incremental reexamination of the pocket allows the surgeon to identify and control even minor areas of bleeding that can stain the pocket and stain tissues, obscuring visualization of anatomic details and neurovascular structures.

Pectoralis Division along the Inframammary Fold

Having established visualization in the upper, medial, and mid pocket, the surgeon can begin dividing pectoralis origins along the inframammary fold to establish a dual plane pocket (if STPTIMF is >0.5 cm) or to define the inferior pocket without dividing pectoralis origins for a traditional subpectoral pocket (if STPTIMF is <0.5 cm). *It is critically important for long-term coverage and to avoid excessive superior retraction of the pectoralis, that surgeons not divide any medial origins of the pectoralis along the*

> It is critically important for long-term coverage and to avoid excessive superior retraction of the pectoralis, that surgeons not divide any medial origins of the pectoralis along the sternum superior to the junction of the sternum with the inframammary fold

sternum superior to the junction of the sternum with the inframammary fold (Figure 12-14). Even tiny increments of pectoralis release medially and superiorly along the lateral border of the sternum allow uncontrolled and unpredictable cephalad retraction of the pectoralis that can cause banding and windowshading. Additionally, pectoralis division medially along the sternum sacrifices invaluable soft tissue coverage and risks long-term implant edge visibility and traction rippling that are often uncorrectable.

Prior to beginning muscle division along the inframammary fold, two important maneuvers minimize uncorrectable surgical errors. The first is precisely identifying the junction of inframammary fold with sternum on the internal surface of the pocket (Figure 12-15), and the second is establishing a precise position of the retractor tip relative to the desired, new inframammary fold. The surgeon first repositions the retractor to retractor position 2 (Figure 12-16, upper left). Using the tip of the dissector with the needlepoint retracted, the surgeon identifies the precise junction of the inframammary fold by pressing internally with the tip of the dissector and observing the point relative to the preoperative skin markings, and coagulates a dot on the undersurface of the pectoralis major to mark the point internally (Figure 12-16, upper right). *Throughout the dissection along the inframammary fold, regardless of pocket location, the tip of the retractor should always*

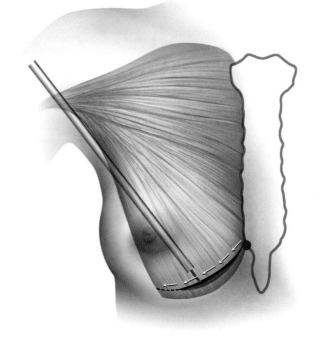

Figure 12-15. Before beginning any division of pectoralis origins along the inframammary fold, the surgeon uses the dissector tip, with sleeve extended to cover the tip, to identify the precise point where the inframammary fold meets the sternum (blue dot). The surgeon then divides pectoralis origins lateral to this point across the inframammary fold, and never divides any origins medial or superior to this point.

Figure 12-16. Endoscopic dissection at the junction of the inframammary fold with the sternum. Upper left: Retractor position 2. Upper right: Marking the junction of the inframammary fold with the sternum internally with the dissector (white arrow). Lower left: Dividing the pectoralis major origins (long white arrow) 1 cm above the desired new inframammary fold. Dissection proceeds through the pectoralis fascia (short black arrow) to expose the subcutaneous fat (long black arrow), leaving cut muscle stumps (short white arrow) anteriorly. Lower right: Dividing muscle origins at least 0.5 cm anterior to the rib surfaces (white arrow) off the fifth rib (black arrow) minimizes the risks of intramuscular vessels retracting and producing prolonged bleeding.

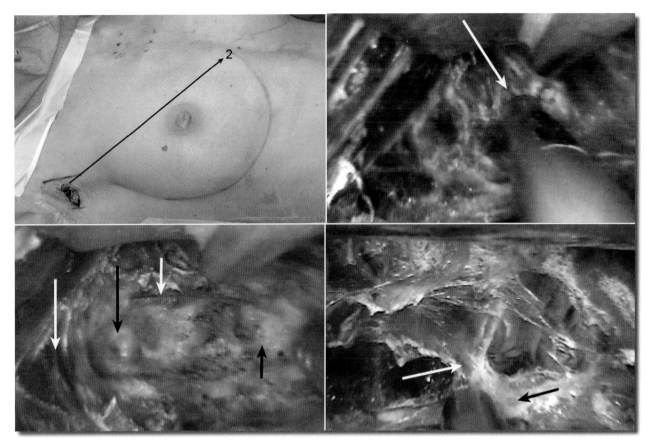

remain at least 1 cm cephalad to the desired, new inframammary fold marked on the skin. As the retractor lifts, it always separates overlying from underlying tissues to a point past the tip of the retractor, so if the surgeon dissects to the tip of the retractor, the actual pocket will extend past the point of dissection, risking implant malposition inferiorly and an excessively low inframammary fold. This common surgical technical error is one of the most common causes of inframammary fold malposition through the axillary and periareolar approaches.

The surgeon precisely positions the retractor centered on the previously marked point internally at retractor position 2 (Figure 12-16, upper left), then hands the retractor to an assistant, freeing the surgeon's hands for the endoscope in one hand and the Probe Plus II™ dissector in the other. To divide pectoralis origins along the inframammary fold, the

As the retractor lifts, it always separates overlying from underlying tissues to a point past the tip of the retractor, so if the surgeon dissects to the tip of the retractor, the actual pocket will extend past the point of dissection, risking implant malposition inferiorly and an excessively low inframammary fold

surgeon begins at the previous point marked internally on the posterior surface of the pectoralis at the junction of the inframammary fold with the sternum. Retracting the sleeve to expose the needle tip of the dissector, the surgeon uses very light, sweeping motions that barely contact the posterior surface of visible origins, progressing laterally from the initial point (Figure 12-16, lower left). Precise upward retraction with precise positioning of the retractor tip by an assistant is essential for optimal accuracy and to place muscle origins under slight tension prior to division. Depth of division of pectoralis origins proceeds until the surgeon sees superficial pectoral fascia or subcutaneous fat. Leaving superficial pectoralis fascia that is less than 1 mm thick intact does not add meaningful soft tissue coverage long-term, and does not reduce risks of ptosis or implant malposition by any scientifically valid, published data. Nevertheless, this fascia can serve as a very useful landmark during muscle division to avoid excessive, inadvertent dissection superficially into the fat and to prevent skin burns by the electrocautery dissector. Dissection proceeds laterally until visualization decreases or the muscle origins are no longer under adequate tension. At that point, the surgeon withdraws the retractor slightly, and divides pectoralis origins from the fourth and fifth ribs to open the middle pocket (Figure 12-16, lower right).

With the tip of the retractor under endoscopic visualization, the surgeon moves the retractor to retractor position 3 at the midpoint of the inframammary fold and positions the tip of the retractor 1 cm above the desired, new fold level while referring to the topographic skin markings (Figure 12-17). Division of pectoralis origins continues laterally

Figure 12-17. Inferior pocket dissection. Left: Retractor position 3. Right: Division of the pectoralis origins across the inframammary fold. Dissection through the pectoralis major (white arrow) and through the superficial pectoral fascia (short black arrow) exposes subcutaneous fat (long black arrow).

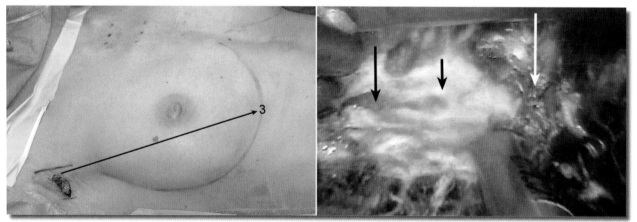

to the 7 o'clock position of the inframammary fold, or until visualization becomes suboptimal without moving the retractor. *After dividing inferior pectoralis origins along each segment of the inframammary fold, the surgeon should ask the assistant to slightly withdraw the retractor tip in a cephalad direction to expose the stumps of cut muscle and allow the surgeon to check for and control any intramuscular bleeders before they cause pocket staining.* Similarly, the surgeon should check inferior cut muscle stumps for hemostasis before proceeding to the next retractor position.

At this point, the surgeon should again stop and deliberately reexamine all previously dissected areas of the pocket for hemostasis.

Transition to the Lateral Pocket

With the retractor repositioned to position 4 (Figure 12-18, left), the surgeon completes division of the remaining pectoralis major muscle origins across the inferolateral inframammary fold. As dissection proceeds laterally, the assistant twists the tip of the retractor laterally to maintain optimal tension on remaining muscle origins, and the surgeon focuses on visualizing the inferolateral border of the pectoralis minor.

To avoid excessively lowering the inframammary fold in the inferolateral portion of the pocket, the surgeon constantly rechecks internal landmarks against external topographic

Figure 12-18. Inferolateral pocket dissection. Left: Retractor position 4. Right: Endoscopic view of the retractor at position 4 where the surgeon divides the final origins of the pectoralis major to the right (lateral to) the retractor. Subcutaneous fat (black arrow) should be exposed exactly at the level of the desired inframammary fold. The surgeon checks this level by pressing the dissector from the undersurface toward the skin and checking topographic markings on the skin. Before proceeding, at each step the surgeon should carefully recheck and coagulate all cut muscle stumps for intramuscular vessels (white arrow).

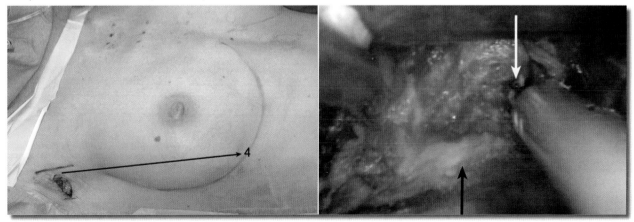

markings on the skin by covering the dissecting tip with the retractable sleeve, and pushing at points internally in the pocket to visualize corresponding points on the skin (Figure 12-18, right). When the lateral border of the pectoralis minor becomes visible, the surgeon establishes a plane of dissection immediately adjacent to the border of the pectoralis minor, and then repositions the retractor for lateral pocket dissection.

Lateral Pocket Dissection

Proper retractor positioning is essential to accurate lateral pocket dissection. While visualizing the tip of the retractor endoscopically, the surgeon moves the retractor tip to retractor position 5 (Figure 12-19, left) laterally and hands the retractor to the assistant. In the lateral pocket, in addition to the usual lifting motion on the retractor, the assistant lifts and simultaneously torques or twists the retractor tip laterally. This maneuver places tension on lateral pocket soft tissues to best define the junction of subcutaneous tissue with serratus and pectoralis minor along the lateral pocket and prevent inadvertent dissection into these muscles. Pectoralis origins tent upward anteriorly with tension; serratus and pectoralis minor origins do not tent upward regardless of retractor tension. This important distinction can prevent inadvertent dissection into serratus, regardless of the incision approach.

The straight dissecting tip of the Probe Plus II™ can easily reach all areas of the lateral pocket if retractor position and direction of retraction are correct. The surgeon can move

> In the lateral pocket, in addition to the usual lifting motion on the retractor, the assistant lifts and simultaneously torques or twists the retractor tip laterally

> The straight dissecting tip of the Probe Plus II™ can easily reach all areas of the lateral pocket if retractor position and direction of retraction are correct

Figure 12-19. Lateral pocket dissection. Left: Retractor position 5, with retractor twisting laterally. Right: A lifting and twisting (double ended white arrow) force on the retractor exposes the lateral border of the pectoralis minor (short white arrow) and places the lateral tissues containing the lateral intercostal nerve branches (black arrow) under tension. The dissector sweeps parallel to the lateral border of the pectoralis minor (long white arrow) to incrementally enlarge the lateral pocket.

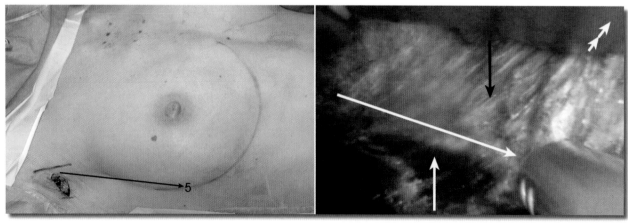

to a position cephalad to the arm board for this portion of the dissection, or remain below the arm board if comfortable in that position. Overdissection of the lateral pocket is a common surgical error that surgeons can avoid by stopping dissection at the lateral border of the pectoralis minor for implants with a base width of 11 cm or less, and stopping dissection 1 cm lateral to the lateral border of the pectoralis minor for implants with a base width between 11 and 13 cm. The surgeon then continues dissection laterally in light, incremental, inferior to superior sweeps of the needlepoint dissector (Figure 12-19, right). For smooth, accurate, and rapid connection to the upper lateral pocket, the surgeon constantly looks for the inferior-most extent of initial dissection that exposed the lateral border of the pectoralis minor at the beginning of pocket dissection, then connects the lateral dissection with the previous superolateral dissection. Sliding the retractor tip cephalad optimizes exposure to complete lateral pocket dissection.

At the conclusion of pocket dissection, prior to irrigation, the surgeon should meticulously reinspect all areas of the pocket and eliminate even the most minor bleeding points, and carefully recheck the entire inframammary fold for accuracy and lack of focal restrictions caused by incomplete division of muscle origins or incomplete dissection. The surgeon then places the endoscopic retractor at the 6 o'clock position of the inframammary fold, and using a Toomey syringe placed into the incision with a tonsil suction in the upper lateral pocket (eliminating the need for slower fill bulb syringes and irrigation catheters), the surgeon irrigates the pocket with sterile saline which should return completely clear, followed by antibiotic or povidone-iodine irrigation of the surgeon's choice (Figure 12-20). By irrigating in increments while allowing the suction to remove excess solution, the surgeon can prevent fluid egress from the incision that can wet and detach drapes in the axilla, contaminating the

Figure 12-20. Set-up for pocket irrigation. The surgeon places the tip of a tonsil suction in the upper lateral pocket, and then irrigates with a Toomey syringe in increments to prevent fluid egress from the incision.

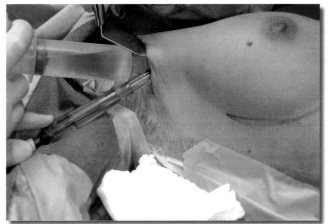

At the conclusion of pocket dissection, prior to irrigation, the surgeon should meticulously reinspect all areas of the pocket and eliminate even the most minor bleeding points, and carefully recheck the entire inframammary fold for accuracy and lack of focal restrictions caused by incomplete division of muscle origins or incomplete dissection

sterile field. If the surgeon has used optimal dissection techniques, no trace of blood is present in the aspirated irrigation solution.

Implant Insertion and Positioning

Currently available, peer reviewed and published processes eliminate the need for implant sizers in primary breast augmentation,[10,13,15,16,18] reducing risks of additional tissue trauma, bleeding, pocket contamination, and additional time waste and expense

Currently available, peer reviewed and published processes eliminate the need for implant sizers in primary breast augmentation,[10,13,15,16,18] reducing risks of additional tissue trauma, bleeding, pocket contamination, and additional time waste and expense.

Surgeons can expeditiously remove air from inflatable implants by placing the implant on the inverted molded plastic thermoform packaging and connecting the fill tube to a closed suction system with a valve attached to the implant fill tube. As the assistant opens the valve, the surgeon can rapidly flatten and inwardly roll the implant edges, creating a cylindrical roll for implant insertion. Full height, anatomic or shaped implants require attention to orientation during air evacuation so that the filler tube exits the *superior* edge of the rolled implant.

Figure 12-21, *A–F*, illustrates insertion and positioning of a full height, textured, anatomic, saline filled implant. With the retractor at the 6 o'clock position of the inframammary fold (retractor position 3), the surgeon wets the implant and the skin around the incision with antibiotic or povidone-iodine solution, and inserts the rolled implant directly beneath the retractor, pushing the roll inferiorly toward the retractor tip using the index finger while simultaneously keeping the rolled implant directly under the retractor with the opposite hand pinching from the skin surface to create a restricted tunnel. Depending on the surgeon's finger length, the tip of the rolled implant may or may not reach the inframammary fold at this point.

With full height, anatomic implants, the surgeon then displaces the cephalad edge of the rolled implant to the 12 o'clock (or slightly canted depending on the clinical situation) position of the pocket. Grasping the rolled implant through the skin with the hand on the skin surface to hold it in position, the surgeon slides the retractor out while maintaining implant position. As implant filling proceeds with at least two observers documenting fill increments, the surgeon can easily move the implant inferiorly to the precise new inframammary fold level with finger pressure on the upper pole when the implant is approximately two-thirds full. Precise positioning of textured shell implants is easier at two-thirds to three-fourths fill, before friction and pressure at full fill restrict movement of the device. It is not necessary (and often not desirable) to position anatomic implants

Figure 12-21.

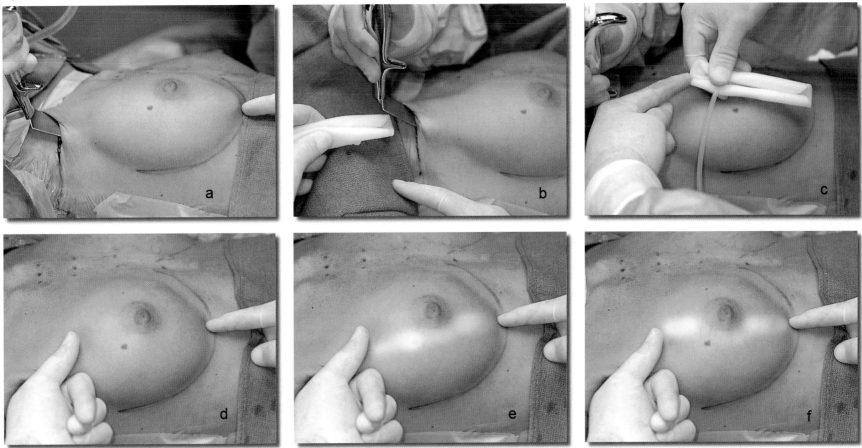

directly vertically. By orienting the upper pole of the implant slightly more medially or laterally, the surgeon can more precisely adjust upper pole fill and contour, while camouflaging upper chest wall asymmetries.

An adequate length incision and optimal implant insertion techniques are critical to avoid damage to implants during insertion. If any type of suspected damage occurs during implant insertion, including gel fracture or gel–shell separation in form stable devices, the surgeon should remove the suspect or damaged implant and replace it. Even if a surgeon only suspects any type of damage, the surgeon should replace the implant immediately.

Incision Closure

Failure to precisely realign and close anatomic layers in the axilla sacrifices control and invites inaccuracies and deformities that can result from secondary healing of wound edges, surfaces, and voids. At the conclusion of the procedure, the axillary fat pad falls posteriorly away from the posterolateral edge of the pectoralis. Approximating the anterior cut edge of the superficial pectoral fascia to its posterior counterpart can be technically demanding, but this closure restores normal layer relationships and prevents adherence of subcutaneous tissue to the lateral border of the pectoralis. After incision, this layer shears in a superior–inferior direction, and if closed without correcting the shear, can create banding. Grasping the posterior cut edge of the superficial pectoral fascia that is attached to the axillary fat pad, the surgeon moves the mass superiorly and inferiorly until it realigns with even length edges to the anterior cut edge, and then places a 5–0 Vicryl or Monocryl suture to align the edges (Figure 12-22). Surgeons should align and place this

Figure 12-22. Closure of the lateral pectoral fascia. Left: The white arrows define the incised edges of the lateral pectoral fascia for pocket access. Right: Reapproximation of the lateral pectoral fascial edges (white arrows) at closure restores fascial and subcutaneous tissue coverage of the lateral pectoralis and minimizes risks of skin adherence to the muscle.

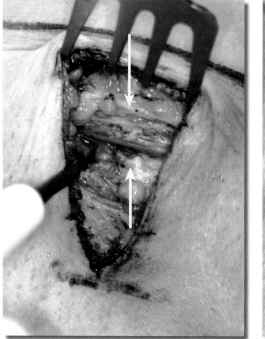 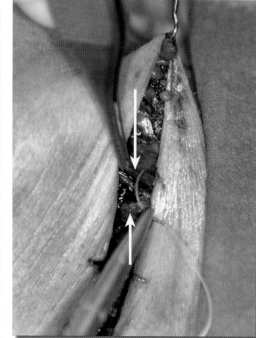

suture without a retractor in place because retraction exacerbates the shear effect on this layer and encourages misalignment. After placing the first suture, an assistant can hold a small retractor or skin hook to facilitate the surgeon placing two or three additional sutures to complete closure of this layer.

For skin closure, the assistant holds a single skin hook placed just outside the skin edges at the anterior-most extent of the skin incision. Tension on this hook should align the crosshatch marks placed prior to incision. At each crosshatch mark, placement of a single 5–0 Vicryl or Monocryl suture in the deep dermis reduces tension and reapproximates the skin edges while the surgeon completes final skin closure with a subcuticular 5–0 Monocryl suture. Precisely aligning skin edges in both planes and precise suture placement depth avoid skin dimpling while assuring a perfect, smooth closure and optimal healing. Everting skin edges in the axillary closure is neither necessary nor desirable, because it does not improve scar quality and impedes early shaving of the axilla. A subcuticular closure without external sutures simplifies and optimizes postoperative management.

Dressings and Adjunctive Measures

Dressings consist only of a single 4″ × 4″ gauze sponge and a very small piece of Microfoam™ tape to absorb any drainage in the first 2 hours following the procedure—there are no drains, special bras, implant positioning straps, instillation of local anesthetic in the pocket, intercostal blocks, or pain pumps. Patients remove the dressing 2 hours after returning home, and are instructed to shower and go out to dinner the evening of surgery after performing arm raising exercises following the postoperative regimen described in a previous publication.[13] Pain medication consists solely of ibuprofen 800 mg every 6 hours as needed for discomfort. Early motion and ibuprofen do not cause an increased incidence of hematoma. The efficacy of this regimen and the exceedingly low hematoma rate of 0.2% in 1664 patients with up to 7 year followup are documented in previously published studies.[10,13,17]

▪ RESULTS

Figures 12-23, 12-24, and 12-25 illustrate postoperative results in axillary augmentation in a range of breast types at the 2 year followup visit.

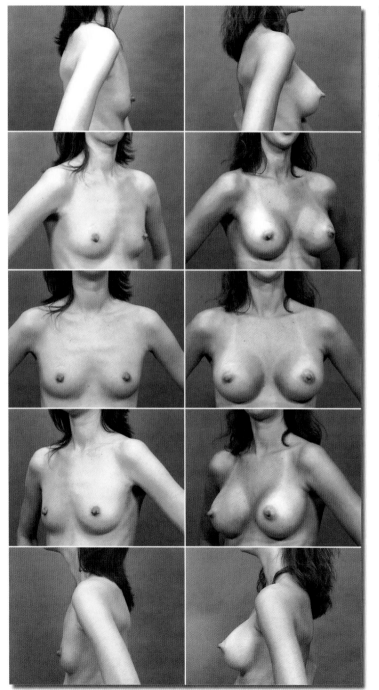

Figure 12-23. Gravida 1, para 1 patient. Base width, 11.5 cm (High Five™ volume recommendation: 275 cc); soft tissue pinch thickness upper pole, 0.7 cm; dual plane, 1; anterior pull skin stretch, 2.7 (High Five™/TEPID™ recommendation: add no volume); total High Five™ recommended volume, 275 cc; implant, Inamed Style 468, 270–285 cc, filled to 275 cc.

Figure 12-24. Gravida 4, para 3 patient. Base width, 11.0 cm (High Five™ volume recommendation: 250 cc); soft tissue pinch thickness upper pole, 0.7 cm; dual plane, 1; anterior pull skin stretch, 3.7 (High Five™/TEPID™ recommendation: add 30 cc); total High Five™ recommended volume, 280 cc; implant, Inamed Style 468, 270–285 cc, filled to 280 cc. Use of a wider implant in an attempt to narrow this patient's intermammary distance would place inadequate soft tissue coverage over the medial portions of the implants and result in implant edge visibility and visible traction rippling mid to long-term. The patient was informed of potential tradeoffs and elected the result shown.

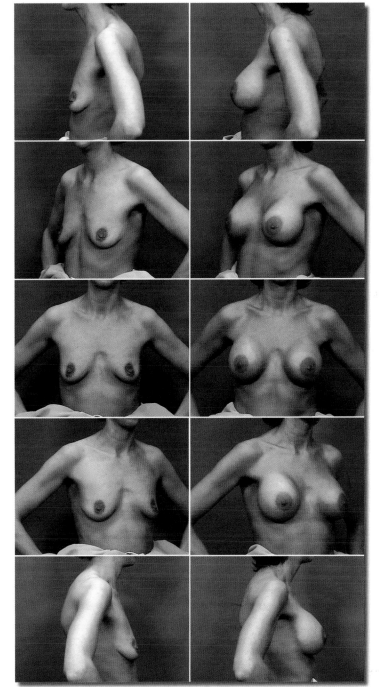

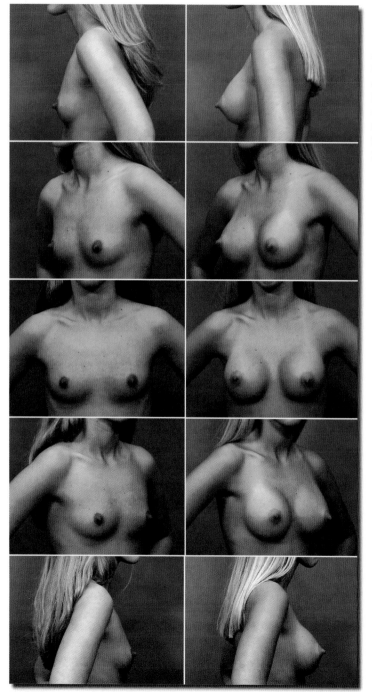

Figure 12-25. Gravida 0, para 0 patient. Base width, 12.0 cm (High Five™ volume recommendation: 300 cc); soft tissue pinch thickness upper pole, 0.14 cm; dual plane, 1; anterior pull skin stretch, 2.3 (High Five™/TEPID™ recommendation: add no volume); total High Five™ recommended volume, 300 cc; implant, Inamed Style 468, 300–315 cc, filled to 300 cc.

Table 12-3. Axillary augmentation clinical experience

Axillary augmentations 1977–2005 n = 690	Pre 1992 n = 331 Submammary n = 22 Subpectoral n = 309	Post 1992 n = 359 Submammary n = 64 Subpectoral n = 13 Dual plane n = 282

*In 1992, all blunt, blind dissection was eliminated, all pocket dissection completed under direct and endoscopic visualization with needlepoint electrocautery and Ethicon Probe Plus II™ electrocautery dissector. Data below reflect updated followup since 1988[8] publication.

Event	N = /% patients pre 1992 with blind blunt dissection	N = /% patients post 1992, no blind blunt dissection
Capsular contracture 3–4 (all had reoperations)	14/4.2% (16 breasts, 2.4% of breasts)	5/1.3% (6 breasts, 0.8% of breasts)
Hematoma	0/0%	1/0.2%
Seroma	0/0%	0/0%
Infection	0/0%	0/0%
Inframammary fold level or contour irregularity	11/3.6% (5 reoperations)	4/1.1% (1 reoperation)
Transient arm sensory changes	10/3%	2/0.5%
Transient lymphadenopathy or lymphatic banding	32/10.3%	8/2.2%
Localized axillary fluid collection	6/1.8%	2/0.5%
Size exchange reoperations	3/0.9%	0/0%
Implant malposition reoperations	6/1.8%	1/0.2%
Deflation replacement	9/2.7%	4/1.1%
Reoperations for all causes	31/9.3%	12/3.3%

Table 12-3 summarizes the clinical experience in this series, and reports pocket locations and adverse events in total and divided into timeframes prior to and after cessation of all blunt and blind dissection techniques.

■ DISCUSSION

Incision location in breast augmentation is not as important to optimal long-term outcomes as quantitative preoperative planning, the degree of tissue trauma and bleeding, the degree of intraoperative control and accuracy, and the predictability of delivering an optimal result in a specific clinical setting.

Incision location in breast augmentation is not as important to optimal long-term outcomes as quantitative preoperative planning, the degree of tissue trauma and bleeding, the degree of intraoperative control and accuracy, and the predictability of delivering an optimal result in a specific clinical setting

The axillary incision approach for breast augmentation is an important alternative for surgeons and patients for one reason: it is the most logical incision approach if patient and surgeon prioritize locating the incision off the breast. The umbilical incision approach traumatizes significant subcutaneous soft tissue before accessing the pocket and creates pocket dissection using blind, blunt techniques which, with current instrumentation, provide no control of pocket dissection under direct vision. In contrast, the axillary approach with endoscopic assistance and no blunt dissection allows surgeons equal control of pocket dissection under direct vision compared to inframammary and periareolar approaches, but requires more specialized instrumentation and more time intraoperatively to deliver equal control.

The inframammary incision approach remains the standard to which surgeons must compare all other incision approaches. Not only does it provide the ultimate visualization and control, but it also requires the least soft tissue trauma for access, and involves the least potential nuisances and morbidity for the patient postoperatively. While surgeons can deliver predictable 24 hour return to normal activity via the axillary approach,[13] postoperative nuisances (not necessarily complications) are greater with the axillary approach and anesthesia and operative times are longer compared to the inframammary approach. Using the techniques described in this paper, same surgeon overall reoperation rates are comparable to the inframammary approach.[13]

Alternative instrumentation and surgical techniques now exist that obsolete subjective planning, blunt dissection, unnecessary postoperative adjuncts, prolonged recovery, and high reoperation rates.[10,13,15,16,18]

Preoperatively defining desired inframammary fold position is particularly important with the axillary approach to eliminate risks and tradeoffs of adjusting the inframammary fold position intraoperatively after the implant is in place. Inserting any type of dissecting instrument after the implant is in place risks damage to the implant, risks creating bleeding which is difficult to control with the implant in place, and is less accurate compared to adjustments under direct endoscopic visualization. Optimal, accurate adjustment of fold position without bleeding or potential implant damage requires removal and replacement of the implant which adds an additional set of tradeoffs including additional tissue trauma, and risks of implant contamination or implant damage. Since 1992, three factors have contributed to reducing reoperations for inframammary fold level or contour irregularities: (1) quantitative breast measurements integrated into a system to define desired nipple to inframammary fold distance to set intraoperatively (the desired, new level of the

Alternative instrumentation and surgical techniques now exist that obsolete subjective planning, blunt dissection, unnecessary postoperative adjuncts, prolonged recovery, and high reoperation rates

Preoperatively defining desired inframammary fold position is particularly important with the axillary approach to eliminate risks and tradeoffs of adjusting the inframammary fold position intraoperatively after the implant is in place

inframammary fold) determined by the base width/volume of the implant selected,[15,16] (2) dual plane techniques that divide pectoralis origins along the inframammary fold, and (3) more precise electrocautery dissection under endoscopic control (compared to blunt, blind dissection).

Indications, Potential Benefits and Tradeoffs of the Axillary Approach

The primary indication for the axillary incision approach is patient choice. Surgeons often use the axillary approach as a marketing tool to differentiate themselves from competitors, encouraging patients to avoid a scar on the breast that is visible and "often unsightly". Experienced surgeons who use multiple incision approaches know that philosophy to be untrue based on facts, because skilled surgeons routinely deliver excellent scar results via any incision approach. Patients with optimal aesthetic outcomes without complications and reoperations virtually never complain about an incision line under the breast or in any other location.

Based on 30 years' experience with all incision approaches, patient choice of incision approach largely depends on the accuracy and completeness of the information the surgeon supplies the patient. Patients who are thoroughly informed about the potential benefits and tradeoffs of all incision approaches, especially the degree of surgical control and potential adjacent tissue trauma of each approach, overwhelmingly choose the inframammary approach. In some geographic areas, in some cultures, and especially if a friend has had a specific incision location with good results, patients will prefer and choose periareolar, axillary, or umbilical incision locations. Provided patients fully understand and accept responsibility for their choices in informed consent documents, surgeons with expanded skill sets can deliver equivalent accuracy, recovery, and results through at least three incision locations.

From a totally objective perspective, the only clear advantage of the axillary approach is scar location off the aesthetic unit of the breast. Dissection in the axilla, even when expert, causes tissue trauma in that area that although rare, can cause minor or major sensory denervation, enlarged lymph nodes, fluid collections, soft tissue banding, transient lymphatic obstruction, transient difficulty in shaving the axilla, and transient limitation of arm motion. Although each of these occurrences is rare, each occurs and impacts patient recovery when it occurs. As a result, patients considering axillary augmentation should be thoroughly informed of each of these occurrences and that each can vary from being a transient nuisance to a significant problem. Though exceedingly rare with the axillary

> The primary indication for the axillary incision approach is patient choice

> Dissection in the axilla, even when expert, causes tissue trauma in that area that although rare, can cause minor or major sensory denervation, enlarged lymph nodes, fluid collections, soft tissue banding, transient lymphatic obstruction, transient difficulty in shaving the axilla, and transient limitation of arm motion. Although each of these occurrences is rare, each occurs and impacts patient recovery when it occurs

approach, patient positioning, retractor or surgical trauma can even permanently damage brachial plexus structures. Surgeons must be aware that axillary augmentation demands more knowledge of critical neurovascular anatomy in the axilla and more attention to detail in operative planning and execution compared to other approaches in order to deliver predictably optimal outcomes.

Recent reports[19,20] describing techniques for subfascial augmentation and placement of soft, cohesive silicone gel implants via the axilla demonstrate new technical capabilities for surgeons. The question, however, is whether long-term patient outcomes and reoperation rates will be improved by subfascial compared to dual plane pocket location and for placement of cohesive, shaped implants via axillary as compared to inframammary and periareolar approaches. Surgeons should remain aware that in terms of optimal patient outcomes and minimal reoperation rates, decisions of operative planning and technique selections should be based on long-term followup and documented recovery and outcomes in peer reviewed and published studies in indexed professional journals. Subfascial implant placement, regardless of the incision approach, does not add meaningful additional, long-term soft tissue coverage in any area. The maximum thickness of the superficial pectoral fascia is less than 1 mm, and no published data exist that documents recovery and outcomes comparable to data with up to 7 year followup that document 24 hour recovery and less than 3% overall reoperation rates with dual plane pocket location.[10,13,15,18]

> Subfascial implant placement, regardless of the incision approach, does not add meaningful additional, long-term soft tissue coverage in any area

Surgeons have placed full height, anatomic, cohesive gel implants via the axilla for more than a decade, and a recent report[19] is encouraging, but the axillary approach unquestionably adds variables and reduces surgeon direct visualization, control, and efficiency compared to the inframammary approach. Data in the latter half of this study document results, recovery, low implant malposition rates, and 3% overall reoperation rates that are comparable to the most state-of-the-art inframammary techniques, using full height, textured, anatomic saline implants.[13] When placing any type of implant via the axilla, surgeons should first have considerable experience placing that same type of implant via the inframammary approach if the goal is optimizing long-term patient outcomes and reducing reoperation rates.

▓ CONCLUSIONS

The axillary incision approach is a valid incision approach for augmentation mammaplasty, provided the surgeon has a thorough knowledge of the applicable surgical anatomy and utilizes surgical instrumentation and techniques that enable patients who choose this approach to expect similar results to patients who choose other incision approaches.[13] The axillary, endoscopic approach has evolved significantly and, optimally applied, can deliver comparable results and outcomes to the inframammary approach, acknowledging a larger number of variables, longer operative times, and greater technical demands on surgeons.[13] To achieve comparable accuracy, recovery, outcomes, and reoperation rates to the inframammary approach, surgeons choosing the axillary approach must be able to deliver the operation with comparable accuracy and control, while minimizing tissue trauma and bleeding. All comparisons of the axillary approach to other incision and pocket alternatives should be based strictly on peer reviewed and published, long-term data, not purely on subjective surgeon preferences and considerations. Absent comparable long-term outcomes data to the inframammary approach, the axillary approach will remain more of a marketing alternative and "off the breast" incision alternative that by peer reviewed and published data does not offer any real, substantive improvements in patient outcomes.

The author does not recommend the axillary approach in glandular ptotic or ptotic breasts, constricted lower pole breasts, or for any type of reoperation procedure where better alternatives exist that deliver more predictable patient outcomes.

> The author does not recommend the axillary approach in glandular ptotic or ptotic breasts, constricted lower pole breasts, or for any type of reoperation procedure where better alternatives exist that deliver more predictable patient outcomes

■ REFERENCES

1. Hoehler H: Breast augmentation: the axillary approach. *Br J Plast Surg* 26:272–276, 1973.

2. Eiseman G: Augmentation mammaplasty by the axillary approach. *Plast Reconstr Surg* 57:229–232, 1974.

3. Agris J, Dingman RO, Wilensky RJ: A dissector for the transaxillary approach in augmentation mammaplasty. *Plast Reconstr Surg* 57(1):10–13, 1976.

4. Wright JH, Bevin AG: Augmentation mammaplasty by the transaxillary approach. *Plast Reconstr Surg* 58(4):429–433, 1976.

5. Hoehler H: Further progress in the axillary approach in augmentation mammaplasty. Prevention of encapsulation. *Aesthetic Plast Surg* 1:107–113, 1977.

6. Watanabe K, Tsurukiyi K, Fugii Y: Subpectoral transaxillary method of breast augmentation in orientals. *Aesthetic Plast Surg* 6(4):231–236, 1982.

7. Tebbetts JB: Transaxillary subpectoral augmentation mammaplasty: long-term follow up and refinements. *Plast Reconstr Surg* 74(5):636–649, 1984.

8. Tebbetts JB: Transaxillary subpectoral augmentation mammaplasty: a 9-year experience. *Clin Plast Surg* 15(4):557–568, 1988.

9. Troilius C: Total muscle coverage of a breast implant is possible through the transaxillary approach. *Plast Reconstr Surg* 95(3):509–512, 1995.

10. Tebbetts JB: Dual plane (DP) breast augmentation: optimizing implant–soft tissue relationships in a wide range of breast types. *Plast Reconstr Surg* 107:1255, 2001.

11. Ho LC: Endoscopic assisted transaxillary augmentation mammaplasty. *Br J Plast Surg* 46(4):332–336, 1993.

12. Price CI, Eaves FF, Nahai F, Jones G, Bostwick J 3rd. Endoscopic transaxillary subpectoral breast augmentation. *Plast Reconstr Surg* 94:612–619, 1994.

13. Tebbetts JB: Achieving a predictable 24 hour return to normal activities after breast augmentation Part II: Patient preparation, refined surgical techniques and instrumentation. *Plast Reconstr Surg* 109:293–305, 2002.

14. Tebbetts JB: An approach that integrates patient education and informed consent in breast augmentation. *Plast Reconstr Surg* 110(3):971–978, 2002.

15. Tebbetts JB, Adams WP: Five critical decisions in breast augmentation using 5 measurements in 5 minutes: the high five system. *Plast Reconstr Surg* 116(7):2005–2016, 2005.

16. Tebbetts JB: A system for breast implant selection based on patient tissue characteristics and implant–soft tissue dynamics. *Plast Reconstr Surg* 109(4):1396–1409, 2002.

17. Tebbetts JB: Patient acceptance of adequately filled breast implants using the tilt test. *Plast Reconstr Surg* 106(1):139–147, 2000.

18. Tebbetts JB: Achieving a zero percent reoperation rate at 3 years in a 50 consecutive case augmentation mammaplasty PMA study. *Plast Reconstr Surg* 118(6):1453–1457, 2006.

19. Graf RM, Bernardes A, Auersvald A, Damasio RC: Subfascial endoscopic transaxillary augmentation mammaplasty. *Aesthetic Plast Surg* 24(3):216–229, 2000.

20. Serra-Renom J, Garrido MF, Yoon T: Augmentation mammaplasty with anatomic, soft, cohesive silicone gel implants using the transaxillary approach at a subfascial level with endoscopic assistance. *Plast Reconstr Surg* 116(2):640–645, 2005.

The Periareolar Approach for Augmentation

The periareolar incision approach to breast augmentation is a realistic option for patients who request the incision approach and for surgeons who prefer it. Chapter 9 details the relative advantages and tradeoffs of the periareolar approach compared to other incision approaches. Proponents of the periareolar approach emphasize the superior scar qualities of periareolar scars compared to inframammary scars, and although there is no valid scientific evidence in comparative cohorts to validate the claim, this approach is very popular in some areas of Europe and South America. Surgeons can place implants in all pocket locations via the periareolar approach. However, accuracy and control of dual plane techniques is limited because precise control of the degree of detachment at the parenchyma-pectoralis interface is not as accurate compared to the inframammary approach. Dual plane 1 procedures via the periareolar approach are often inadvertently dual plane 2 or 3 procedures and risks of pectoralis banding, windowshading, or animation deformities are greater when surgeons develop a dual plane pocket via a periareolar approach.

▓ INDICATIONS AND CONTRAINDICATIONS

The strongest indications are excessive areolar size, asymmetry, or pseudoherniation deformities that require correction at the time of breast augmentation, or surgeon or patient preference for the periareolar approach and scar location. The approach is relatively contraindicated in patients with areolar diameter of less than 3 cm due to limited surgical exposure and control, skin edge trauma at the incision site, and necessity of extending incisions off the areola or areolar border.

▓ INSTRUMENTATION

Surgeons can perform periareolar augmentation with a wide variety of instruments. Specific instruments increase control and accuracy in the operation, and facilitate implant

Figure 13-1. Rake retractors stabilize the skin edges and place tension on skin flaps to define and maintain optimal planes of dissection.

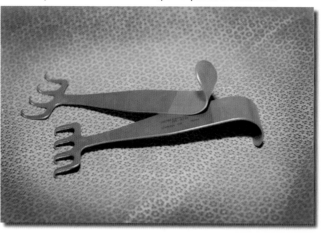

2:1:4
3:2:1-8

Figure 13-2. Double ended retractors, often used in pairs, provide optimal exposure for a wide variety of incision approaches to breast augmentation. The blades on these retractors provide much wider exposure compared to Army–Navy or other narrower retractors.

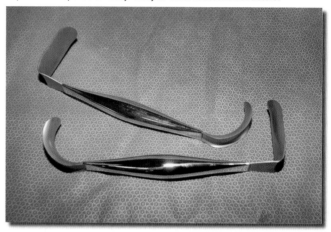

insertion and positioning. Rake retractors (Figure 13-1) lift and stabilize the skin edges after the initial incision and enable the surgeon to accurately tunnel through or around breast parenchyma to the level of the desired pocket. A pair of double ended retractors, each with a shorter and a longer blade, is indispensable for opposing retraction during mid depth dissection, initial dissection of the pocket plane, and to provide optimal access for implant insertion (Figure 13-2). The most effective dissecting instrument for initial dissection through dermis, subcutaneous tissue, and breast parenchyma is a handswitching, needlepoint, electrocautery pencil (Figure 13-3, upper). For dissection of a submammary, partial retropectoral or dual plane pocket and for hemostatic control in all areas, a handswitching, monopolar, needlepoint electrocautery forceps is the most effective instrument, enabling surgeons to dissect and control bleeders with a single instrument (Figure 13-3, lower).

Figure 13-3. Upper: Handswitching electrocautery pencil with needle tip, cut and coagulation switches. Lower: Handswitching, monopolar, needle tip electrocautery forceps used for dissection and electrocoagulation.

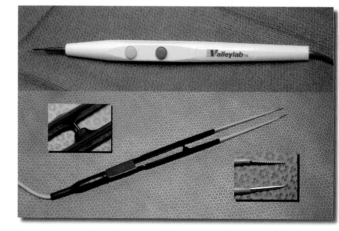

A fiberoptic retractor with a blade length of 10–15 cm and a blade width of 2.5–3 cm provides optimal exposure in more distal areas of the pocket and facilitates dissection in breasts with considerable thickness of breast parenchyma (Figure 13-4). Long forceps with teeth and tungsten carbide inserts and a pair of Lahey clamps (Figure 13-5) enable the surgeon to grasp the pectoralis for initial incision access to the subpectoral plane and for subsequent initial pocket dissection.

Figure 13-4. Fiberoptic retractor with smoke evacuation capability for dissection in distal areas of the pocket.

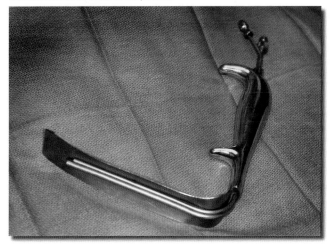

Figure 13-5. Long forceps with tungsten inserts and teeth and Lahey clamps for control of the pectoralis muscle when entering a dual plane or subpectoral pocket via the periareolar approach.

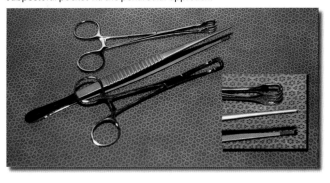

■ INCISION LOCATION AND LENGTH

The most practical location for the periareolar incision is at the lower border of the areola from the 3 o'clock to the 9 o'clock position. Placing the incision barely inside the pigmented border of the areola prevents disrupting the natural, fading pigmentation at the areola border, but this location is most logical for patients with lighter pigmented areolas. In darker pigmented areolas, a depigmented scar in an intraareolar location is much more noticeable compared to a scar exactly at the border of the areola.

Incision length is largely determined by the diameter of the areola, and surgeons should consider alternative incision locations when areola diameter is less than 3 cm. Although

3:2:2

Incision length is largely determined by the diameter of the areola, and surgeons should consider alternative incision locations when areola diameter is less than 3 cm

With full height, anatomic, form stable silicone gel implants, surgeons should carefully consider alternative incision approaches when planning to use implants with greater than a 12 cm base width or in patients with an areolar diameter of 4 cm or less

surgeons have reported various extensions of a periareolar incision onto the skin in patients with small areolas, the potential compromise in the resulting scar on the most prominent portion of the breast is illogical compared to choosing an alternative incision location. With full height, anatomic, form stable silicone gel implants, surgeons should carefully consider alternative incision approaches when planning to use implants with greater than a 12 cm base width or in patients with an areolar diameter of 4 cm or less. Placing this type of implant with these dimensions through a smaller periareolar incision poses illogical risks of damage to the implant and excessive trauma to the skin edges.

If surgeons frequently need to trim the skin edges of the areola or adjacent skin prior to skin closure, they should consider whether their selection of incision location, implant dimensions, instrumentation, and surgical techniques are optimal. Alternative incision approaches of adequate length for the planned operation and implant are available, and eliminate the likelihood of excessive skin edge trauma that requires debridement in a primary, aesthetic operation.

■ PREOPERATIVE MARKINGS

To define the level of the desired, postoperative inframammary fold, the surgeon places the tip of a flexible tape measure at the level of the nipple, maximally lifts the nipple upward to stretch the lower pole skin of the breast, and places a dot at or beneath the existing inframammary fold to define the desired, new nipple-to-inframammary fold distance (Figure 13-6)

Preoperative markings begin by placing a dot at the sternal notch and xiphoid and aligning a row of dots between these two points to define a visual midline. Placing a row of dots 1.5 cm lateral to the midline row defines a 3 cm intermammary distance and defines the maximal extent of safe medial pocket dissection to avoid medial perforating vessels and risking optimal soft tissue coverage in this critical area. The surgeon then outlines the existing inframammary fold, and depending on the base width of the proposed implant, defines the level of the new, desired inframammary fold using the High Five™ process and measurements detailed in Chapter 7. To define the level of the desired, postoperative inframammary fold, the surgeon places the tip of a flexible tape measure at the level of the nipple, maximally lifts the nipple upward to stretch the lower pole skin of the breast, and places a dot at or beneath the existing inframammary fold to define the desired, new nipple-to-inframammary fold distance (Figure 13-6). As a final step, the surgeon marks the periareolar incision line.

Although it is possible for surgeons to adjust the level of the inframammary fold intraoperatively via the periareolar approach, visual intraoperative judgments of optimal fold level are subject to many variables of patient positioning that make visual judgments less accurate compared to objective, quantitative, planned measurements. Surgeons can always check fold levels visually, but absent quantitative tissue measurements and

Figure 13-6. Setting the level of the desired, new inframammary fold. Using the N:IMF calculated using the High Five™ System, the surgeon places the tip of a flexible tape measure at the nipple, lifts to put the skin of the lower pole under maximal stretch, and then places a dot to define the desired N:IMF for the base width of the implant. Using this dot to define the level of the new inframammary fold, the surgeon draws the new fold in or below the existing fold, adjusting fold curvature for optimal aesthetics.

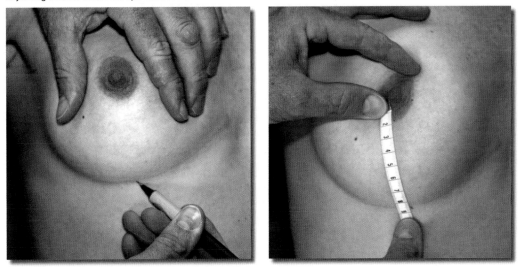

planning preoperatively, the check is always a subjective opinion compared to an objective, planned measurement.

■ ANESTHESIA AND LOCAL ANESTHETIC INSTILLATION

Chapter 15 is devoted to preoperative care, anesthesia, and postoperative care. Optimal, state-of-the-art breast augmentation and optimal recovery require general anesthesia and muscle relaxants. General anesthesia can reduce the amount of intraoperative sedative and narcotic drugs a patient requires while enabling surgeons to perform a more accurate, controlled operation and dramatically reducing patient recovery times.[1] Instillation of a vasoconstrictive agent along the incision line may reduce dermal bleeding, but instillation of local anesthetic into any other area of the breast or pocket is unnecessary and has the following potential risks: (1) multiple small hematomas within the breast parenchyma, (2) increased electrical resistance in all infiltrated tissues that decrease the efficacy of electrocautery dissection, (3) increased risks of pneumothorax with deeper infiltration or intercostal blocks, and (4) delayed bleeding postoperatively as the effects of vasoconstrictors decrease. Intercostal blocks, instillation of local anesthetic agents into the pocket, and pain pumps are totally unnecessary for patient comfort postoperatively if surgeons apply proved processes that predictably deliver 24 hour recovery.[1]

■ INITIAL INCISION AND TUNNEL ALTERNATIVES

After making the initial skin incision, the surgeon places two rake retractors on the opposing skin edges and the assistant lifts and keeps the soft tissues under tension as the surgeon deepens the dissection with the needlepoint electrocautery pencil (Figure 13-7). The surgeon has three basic alternatives for access to the submammary, subfascial, or subpectoral spaces: (1) dissect superficially in a deep subcutaneous plane inferiorly and around the breast parenchyma inferiorly, (2) dissect directly posteriorly through breast parenchyma to the surface of the pectoralis major muscle, or (3) dissect obliquely from the incision to a level inferiorly that is approximately 2 cm above or superior to the desired, postoperative inframammary fold (Figure 13-8). While dissection superficially in a deep subcutaneous plane inferiorly and around the breast parenchyma inferiorly may seem logical to avoid dissection through breast parenchyma, this approach has several distinct tradeoffs that include increased postoperative ecchymosis or fluid accumulations in the subcutaneous tunnel, possible surface contour irregularities postoperatively, maldistribution of breast parenchyma over the implant, and greater technical difficulty in larger breasts.

Figure 13-7.

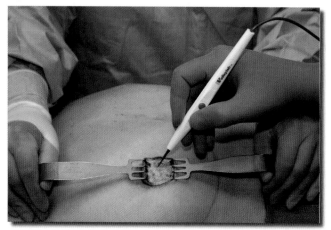

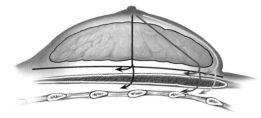

Figure 13-8. Approaches to pocket locations via periareolar incision. Direct posterior approach (red arrows); oblique approach (blue arrows); superficial tunnel approach (aqua arrows).

If a surgeon plans a submammary or subfascial pocket location, the surgeon should select either a straight posterior or oblique approach through the parenchyma (Figure 13-9). For a partial retropectoral pocket, if the surgeon plans a muscle splitting or lateral approach to the subpectoral space, a directly posterior dissection is most logical (Figure 13-10). If, however, the surgeon plans a dual plane pocket, the most logical approach is obliquely through the parenchyma on a line from the incision to a level inferiorly that is approximately 2 cm above or superior to the desired, postoperative inframammary fold (Figure 13-11). For a dual plane pocket, this is the level at which the surgeon should divide inferior origins of the pectoralis across the inframammary fold for access to the subpectoral space.

Figure 13-9. Approaches for submammary or subfascial pockets via periareolar incision. A direct posterior approach (red arrows) or oblique approach (blue arrows) is most logical.

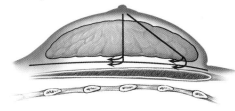

Figure 13-10. Direct posterior approach to subpectoral space (red arrow) if surgeon plans to split the pectoralis or enter the subpectoral space laterally.

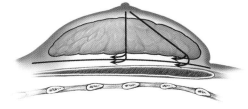

Figure 13-11. Approach for a dual plane pocket. An oblique approach (blue arrow) is most logical, directing the tunnel from the incision toward a point 2 cm above the desired, new inframammary fold.

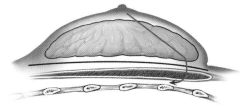

■ ENTERING THE SUBMAMMARY OR SUBFASCIAL SPACES

The surgeon can dissect either directly posteriorly or obliquely through breast parenchyma to access the submammary or subfascial spaces, using the handswitching, needlepoint electrocautery pencil with a blended cut and coagulation current that optimizes hemostasis. To minimize postoperative morbidity, surgeons should control bleeding very meticulously during tunnel creation through parenchyma. As the dissection deepens to 3–4 cm, the surgeon places opposing double ended retractors for deeper exposure, and then removes the rake retractors

3:2:2

As the dissection deepens to 3–4 cm, the surgeon places opposing double ended retractors for deeper exposure, and then removes the rake retractors (Figure 13-12)

339

Figure 13-12. Two double ended retractors enable the surgeon to establish opposing retraction for optimal exposure while developing the tunnel from the incision to the pocket plane.

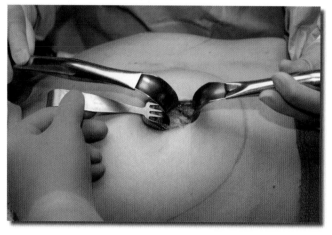

(Figure 13-12). As discussed in Chapter 8, the pectoralis fascia is less than 0.2 mm thick in most patients, so a subfascial pocket does not add any meaningful coverage over any type of breast implant, and has not been shown in scientifically valid, comparative cohorts to have any proved advantage over a submammary pocket. Nevertheless, surgeons can elect to dissect superficial or deep to the pectoralis fascia for access to submammary or subfascial pocket locations. At the level of the pectoralis fascia or to increase exposure at any time, the surgeon switches from the shorter blade to the longer blade of the opposing double ended retractors.

ENTERING THE RETROPECTORAL SPACE AND DUAL PLANE ALTERNATIVES

To enter the partial retropectoral pocket location (leaving origins of the pectoralis major muscle intact inferiorly across the inframammary fold), the surgeon can dissect directly posteriorly through parenchyma to the pectoralis major muscle and then split the muscle for access to the subpectoral space. Splitting the pectoralis, however, risks causing more bleeding compared to accessing the pocket laterally by lifting the lateral border of the pectoralis. If the surgeon chooses a lateral approach, the parenchymal tunnel can angle slightly laterally from the incision toward the lateral border of the pectoralis.

3:2:2
3:2:3

A dual plane approach and pocket best addresses the widest range of breast types and breast deformities while optimizing the number one priority in breast augmentation—long-term soft tissue coverage of the implant medially and superiorly. The remainder of this chapter focuses on the description of surgical techniques for a periareolar, dual plane pocket location.

When a surgeon plans a dual plane pocket location via the periareolar approach, the parenchymal tunnel should angle obliquely inferior from the incision to a level 2 cm above the desired, new inframammary fold level defined by the High Five™ System (Figure 13-13)

3:2:2-4

When a surgeon plans a dual plane pocket location via the periareolar approach, the parenchymal tunnel should angle obliquely inferior from the incision to a level 2 cm above the desired, new inframammary fold level defined by the High Five™ System (Figure 13-13). At this level, the surgeon next dissects medially and laterally to expose a band of lower pectoralis major muscle 2–3 cm wide transversely, carefully avoiding any dissection inferiorly past a level at least 2–3 cm above the desired, new inframammary fold. By aiming above the desired, new fold level, the surgeon avoids the retractor tip inadvertently lifting the inferior tissues and dissecting the pocket border excessively inferiorly. After dividing pectoralis major muscle origins across the inframammary fold, the surgeon can incrementally lower the pocket border and fold to the precise, desired level.

Depending on the thickness of the overlying breast parenchyma, the surgeon can use either the long blade of the double ended retractor, or switch to the fiberoptic retractor to expose the lower pectoralis major origins across the inframammary fold. Before dividing any of these origins, the surgeon should carefully check the proposed level of pectoralis muscle origin division and assure that the level of muscle division *is at least 1–2 cm superior to the desired new inframammary fold level marked externally on the skin.* Passing a 25 gauge, 1½ inch needle through the skin and subcutaneous tissue 1 cm above the desired or new inframammary fold level can help visually confirm that division of pectoralis origins occurs 1 cm above the desired fold level.

To facilitate retraction of the pectoralis for dissection of the subpectoral pocket, surgeons should avoid excessive initial separation of breast parenchyma from the anterior surface of the pectoralis major superior to the desired level of division of pectoralis origins, even if the surgeon is planning a dual plane 2 or 3 pocket. *Surgeons should always develop the subpectoral portion of the pocket superiorly first, before performing any separation of parenchyma off the pectoralis,* to leave parenchyma–muscle attachments intact and prevent excessive upward movement and banding of the inferior cut border of the pectoralis. Surgeons should also avoid dividing inferior pectoralis origins more than 2 cm

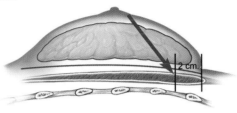

Figure 13-13. Approach for dual plane pocket via periareolar incision. The oblique tunnel from the incision should aim for a level approximately 2 cm above the desired new inframammary fold for the surgeon to divide pectoralis origins across the IMF and enter the subpectoral space.

off the rib origins to avoid excessive bleeding from intramuscular vessels that increase in caliber more superiorly. The ideal level to divide pectoralis muscle origins is 1–2 cm off their rib origins to prevent retraction of cut vessels into the intercostal musculature and prolong bleeding or risk pneumothorax while trying to achieve hemostasis.

■ SEQUENCE AND TECHNIQUES OF POCKET DISSECTION

While performing pectoralis muscle division across the inframammary fold (IMF), placing the ring or small finger of the non-dominant hand that is holding the retractor precisely on the point of the junction of the IMF with the sternum prevents inadvertently incising or releasing any pectoralis major muscle origins along the lateral border of the sternum

Switching from the handswitching electrocautery pencil to the handswitching, monopolar, needlepoint forceps, the surgeon incises the pectoralis fascia and pectoralis muscle origins across the inframammary fold, 1–2 cm above the level of the desired, new fold and from the lateral-most extent of pectoralis major origins medially to the point at which the inframammary fold joins the sternum. While performing pectoralis muscle division across the inframammary fold (IMF), placing the ring or small finger of the non-dominant hand that is holding the retractor precisely on the point of the junction of the IMF with the sternum prevents inadvertently incising or releasing any pectoralis major muscle origins along the lateral border of the sternum. The surgeon should lift the pectoralis by lifting the retractors to tent the pectoralis away from the chest wall or, alternatively, lift the muscle origins with a long forceps, dividing the muscle with light, sweeping strokes of the handswitching forceps to avoid inadvertently entering the pleural space.

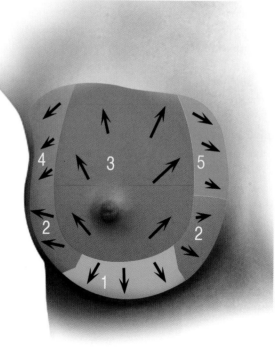

Figure 13-14. Sequence of pocket dissection for periareolar dual plane or subpectoral pockets.

Figure 13-14 demonstrates an optimal sequence for pocket dissection in the subpectoral plane via the periareolar approach. Compared to inframammary and axillary approaches, the dissection via the periareolar approach is more extensive and involves greater tissue surface areas, because it requires creating a transparenchymal tunnel in addition to a dual plane dissection that does not traverse breast parenchyma. Zone 1 of the dissection is the transparenchymal tunnel and transverse dissection 2–3 cm above the new IMF described previously. Zone 2 dissection then opens the pocket medially and laterally to increase exposure. Following Zone 2 dissection, the surgeon incrementally divides origins of the pectoralis major muscle across the inframammary fold, always stopping where the fold meets the lateral border of the sternum. Before dividing any origins, the surgeon should assure that muscle division is no more than 2 cm above the desired, new inframammary fold, and that muscle origins are divided at least 1 cm anterior to any rib attachments to prevent retraction of intramuscular vessels that can be difficult to control.

When division of pectoralis origins across the inframammary fold is complete, the surgeon grasps and lifts the cephalad cut edge of the pectoralis muscle with long forceps or Lahey clamps, and rotates the retractor from an inferior to superior direction just medial to the nipple toward the middle of the pocket to begin dissection in Zone 3. Zone 3 is an area where the surgeon is least likely to encounter adherence of the pectoralis to deeper layers. By establishing the definitive tissue plane in Zone 3 and then sweeping the retractor laterally to develop Zone 4, the surgeon avoids inadvertently entering the serratus muscle laterally or the pectoralis minor muscle deep to the pectoralis. Serratus and pectoralis minor can be quite adherent to the pectoralis major in some cases, and this simple detail of establishing the correct plane in Zone 3 superiorly over the body of the pectoralis minor muscle, and then sweeping laterally into Zone 4 completely eliminates risks of dissecting into adjacent muscles. Zone 4 dissection continues laterally to the lateral border of the pectoralis minor.

Redirecting the long blade of the double ended retractor or fiberoptic retractor directly superiorly, the surgeon dissects directly cephalad in the mid portion of the pocket in Zone 3, stopping when the fat pad or vessels of the thoracoacromial pedicle are visible on the undersurface of the pectoralis major. From this point, the surgeon dissects laterally, slightly past the lateral edge of the pectoralis minor at its superolateral border, to complete dissection in Zone 4.

With the entire pocket developed except the medial edge along the sternum, the surgeon dissects from superior to inferior to establish Zone 5. Deferring this dissection until all other tissues are mobile provides additional exposure in Zone 5 to improve visualization, decreases risks of inadvertently dividing medial perforator vessels, and facilitates rapid control of bleeding should inadvertent division occur. When dissecting the medial portion of every subpectoral or dual plane pocket, the surgeon must be aware of which pectoralis origins are safe to divide and landmarks to assure that the surgeon preserves all of the main body of origins along the sternum for optimal, long-term coverage. Details of this anatomy are included in Chapter 4.

Final dissection in Zone 5 continues from superior to inferior and lateral to medial to define the lower pocket border exactly at the level of the desired, postoperative inframammary fold. This dissection is critical to maximize accuracy of IMF position. While defining the lower pocket border, the surgeon should constantly check the skin markings for the desired inframammary fold against the visual level of the inferior border within the pocket, and carefully avoid overdissection of the inferior pocket. In addition, the surgeon must carefully position the retractor inferiorly and warn the assistant to avoid excess traction on the retractor that can lift the deep subcutaneous fascia away from underlying fascia and muscle and cause an excessively low inframammary fold.

◼ PRESERVING ALL MEDIAL ORIGINS OF THE PECTORALIS— A CRITICALLY IMPORTANT PRINCIPLE

In some patients, discrete, sometimes tendinous origins of pectoralis are visible just lateral to the main body of the muscle along the sternum

Visible implant edges and visible traction rippling medially are almost totally preventable. To avoid visible implant edges and visible traction rippling deformities medially, the surgeon should preserve all medial origins of the pectoralis major along the sternum, from the sternal notch to the junction of the sternum with the inframammary fold. In some patients, discrete, sometimes tendinous origins of pectoralis are visible just lateral to the main body of the muscle along the sternum. The surgeon can safely divide these white, tendinous origins that are discrete origins located lateral to the main body of origins medially without compromising the integrity of the main body of muscle origins medially that are critical to optimal implant coverage medially. Figure 13-15, *A–D*, illustrates these types of origins in a fresh cadaver dissection.

Visible implant edges and traction rippling deformities are caused by failing to assure optimal implant coverage medially. These deformities often do not become visible for many months postoperatively and are largely uncorrectable. Division of medial pectoralis origins in an attempt to narrow the intermammary distance is illogical and unwarranted, because the potential uncorrectable deformities that can result are much more disastrous compared to a slightly wider intermammary distance, regardless of patient and surgeon desires for a narrower intermammary distance. If the patient desires a gluteal appearance of the cleavage area, the surgeon should encourage her to create that appearance with an appropriate push up brassiere, and avoid the temptation to create it surgically.

Figure 13-15. (*A, B*) Pinnate origins of the pectoralis major medially along the sternum lie lateral to the main body of the muscle and are shown lateral to the yellow band in the cadaver dissection. (*C, D*) Closeup views demonstrate the white, tendinous tissue (black arrows) in many of the pinnate origins that distinguishes them from the main body of the pectoralis that attaches to the sternum medially.

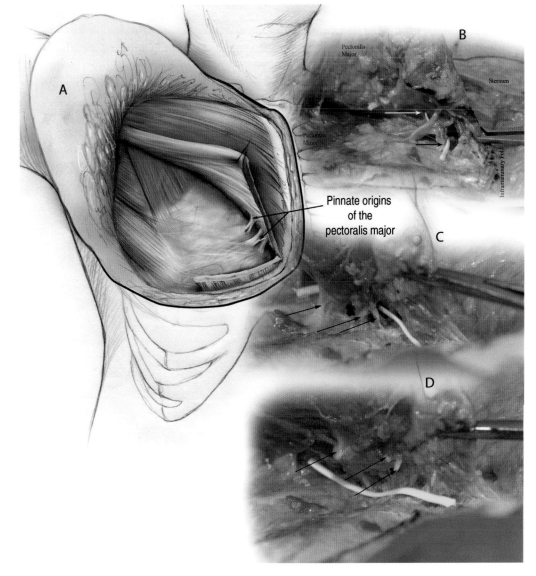

Pinnate origins
of the
pectoralis major

■ ADDITIONAL DISSECTION FOR DUAL PLANE 2 AND 3 POCKETS

For dual plane 2 and 3 techniques that are so effective in glandular ptotic breasts, constricted lower pole breasts, and tubular breasts, the surgeon completes pocket dissection as previously described, and then separates the inferior cut edge of the pectoralis from overlying parenchyma. Disrupting attachments at the parenchyma–muscle interface allows the muscle edge to rotate superomedially (Figure 13-16), and removes pectoralis pressure that impedes full expansion of the lower envelope by the implant. Removing pectoralis pressure that restricts anterior projection of the implant is

Figure 13-16. After dividing pectoralis origins across the inframammary fold, the surgeon incrementally separates the inferior edge of the pectoralis major from its interface attachments to the overlying parenchyma. 1 cm increments of separation allow the muscle edge to move superiorly to create a dual plane 2 or 3 pocket.

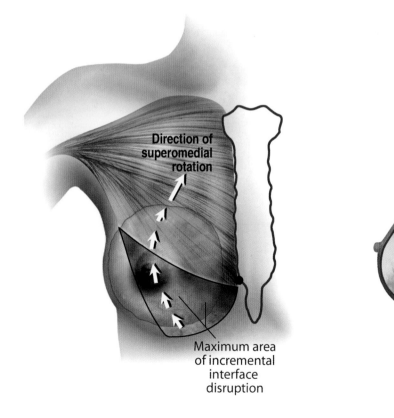
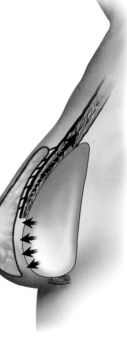

essential to correct glandular ptosis and constricted lower pole deformities. To separate the pectoralis from the overlying parenchyma via the periareolar approach, the assistant maintains directly inferior traction on the cut edge of the pectoralis muscle while the surgeon frees the muscle from the overlying parenchyma using short sweeping strokes with the handswitching, monopolar, needle tip forceps. In routine glandular ptotic breasts, the

Figure 13-17.

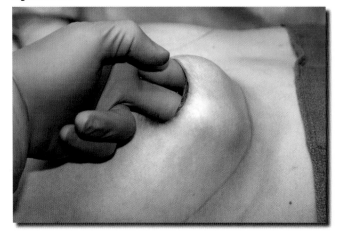

dual plane 2 techniques require freeing the pectoralis adequately to allow it to move upward to the lower border of the areola. Dual plane 3 techniques for constricted lower pole and tubular breasts require mobilization adequate to allow movement of the inferior edge of the pectoralis to the upper border of the areola. The surgeon separates the parenchyma–muscle interface in small increments, and then inserts fingers into the pocket and pulls anteriorly to palpate the position of the inferior pectoralis cut edge to accurately confirm the position of the inferior muscle border.

Before irrigating the pocket and placing the implant, the surgeon should insert one or two fingers into the periareolar incision and lift the skin envelope anteriorly to check for any residual restriction of anterior movement of the lower envelope (Figure 13-17). If any banding or restriction is palpable at the level of the inferior border of the pectoralis, it is important to separate the muscle from the overlying parenchyma in additional 1 cm increments with electrocautery forceps, stopping when palpation with fingers inside the pocket detects no remaining restrictions to full anterior expansion of the envelope.

Before irrigating the pocket and placing the implant, the surgeon should insert one or two fingers into the periareolar incision and lift the skin envelope anteriorly to check for any residual restriction of anterior movement of the lower envelope (Figure 13-17)

■ REINSPECTION AND POCKET IRRIGATION

At the conclusion of pocket dissection, the surgeon should carefully reinspect all areas of the pocket for optimal hemostasis. Abrading any areas of the pocket with gauze sponges is

unnecessary and undesirable, because sponge abrasion is traumatic to tissues and often causes bleeding from small vessels. The surgeon then irrigates the pocket with saline and antibiotic or topical solutions using a Toomey syringe, removing all excess solution by suction, removing residual blood or loose tissue fragments from inner pocket surfaces, and reducing potential bacterial contaminants that could increase risks of infection or capsular contracture.

Both pockets can be dissected from one side of the table, eliminating time waste and prolonged anesthesia, provided the operating table is capable of rotating adequately side-to-side. Few brands of operating tables match the functionality of Skytron tables in side-to-side movement.

IMPLANT SIZERS

Implant sizers increase contamination risks, tissue trauma, time waste, and costs, and are totally unnecessary in primary breast augmentation, provided a surgeon is willing to quantitate tissue characteristics and use systems such as the High Five™ System[2,3] that includes the TEPID™ measurement system during preoperative planning and implant selection. Many sizers do not accurately simulate the shape surface characteristics of the implant, and therefore do not accurately reflect the visual appearance that a similar volume implant may produce. Sizer use is addictive, and surgeons who insist on using sizers rarely learn to use quantitative systems that are much more accurate, reliable, and risk free.

IMPLANT PREPARATION, FILLING, AND INSERTION

All inflatable implants should be leak tested by submerging the implant in sterile saline, applying pressure to the implant, and checking the valve and all shell surfaces for air bubbles or leaks. Prefilled implants and inflatable implants can sustain shell damage from contact with other objects, so all implants should remain in their thermoform packaging until they are brought onto the operative field.

3:2:5

Preparation and insertion of implants via the periareolar approach is similar to insertion via the inframammary approach. Chapter 11 describes and illustrates these techniques in detail. For implant insertion via the periareolar approach, the surgeon places the longer blades of two double ended retractors into the incision, assuring that the more cephalad retractor blade captures and lifts the entire pectoralis major. The assistant holds both

The assistant holds both retractors while the surgeon inserts the implant (Figure 13-18)

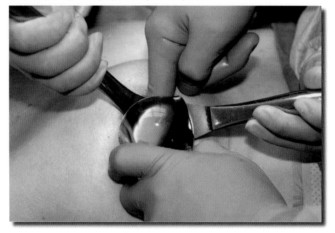

Figure 13-18. Opposing double ended retractors held by the assistant to open the pocket for implant insertion. These retractors should lift anteriorly to optimally open the pocket space.

retractors while the surgeon inserts the implant (Figure 13-18). When inserting inflatable or prefilled implants, especially form stable, cohesive gel implants, the surgeon should insert the upper portion of the implant beneath the pectoralis first, and then push the implant cephalad as much as possible before inserting the lower portion of the implant. With all prefilled implants, avoiding focal digital pressure on any area of the implant at any time, and maximizing surface area contact of the fingers with the implant, using alternating pressure movements, decreases risks of damage to the implant shell.

An adequate length incision and optimal implant insertion techniques are critical to avoid damage to implants during insertion. If any type of suspected damage occurs during implant insertion, including gel fracture or gel–shell separation in form stable devices, the surgeon should remove the suspect or damaged implant and replace it. Even if a surgeon only suspects any type of damage, the surgeon should replace the implant immediately.

■ IMPLANT POSITIONING

Round, smooth shell implants require no special positioning techniques, because they do not maintain position in the periprosthetic pocket. The only influences that a surgeon can exert over the position and fill distribution of round, smooth implants are to fill the implant adequately to prevent shell collapse, and to precisely control pocket dimensions and shape.

With shaped implants, especially full height, form stable, textured anatomic implants such as the Allergan Style 410 full height, textured, form stable gel implant and the Style 468 full height textured, anatomic saline implant, surgeons can better control distribution

of fill within the implant and, by controlling implant position, can better control distribution of fill and shape of the breast. All anatomic or shaped implants require accurate pocket development and optimal positioning intraoperatively, but also enable surgeons to better control distribution of fill within the breast.

The shape of full height, form stable, anatomic implants allows the implant to compensate for a wide range of skeletal and breast deformities, by placing fill more specifically where it is needed to fill deficient areas of a breast, by exerting more pressure on selected areas of the soft tissue envelope to correct constriction deformities, or by placing fill in selected areas to mask underlying skeletal deformities.

> The shape of full height, anatomic implants allows the implant to compensate for a wide range of skeletal and breast deformities, by placing fill more specifically where it is needed to fill deficient areas of a breast, by exerting more pressure on selected areas of the soft tissue envelope to correct constriction deformities, or by placing fill in selected areas to mask underlying skeletal deformities

Contrary to the intuition of many surgeons, the optimal position of a full height, form stable, anatomic implant is rarely exactly vertical, from the 12 o'clock to the 6 o'clock position of the breast. In most cases, slight rotation of the implant in one direction or the other off the vertical axis produces a more optimal and natural appearance of the breast and enables the surgeon to compensate for chest wall asymmetries. Another erroneous assumption is that aggressive texturing of the implant shell and adherence of the shell to the surrounding capsule are essential to maintain position of full height anatomic implants. When a full height, form stable, anatomic implant is designed taller than it is wide, and the surgeon develops the pocket to fit the implant, the primary role of texturing is to provide friction, not necessarily adherence, as the capsule forms around the implant. Once the capsule has formed, the implant maintains its position, yet moves adequately at the capsule–external tissue interface to satisfy patient desires regarding natural breast movement. These facts are proved by peer reviewed and published evidence in more than 2500 cases.[2,4,5]

■ TAILORING THE LATERAL POCKET TO FIT THE IMPLANT

Overdissection of the lateral pocket is a common error in breast augmentation that occurs with all incision locations and pocket locations. Excessive lateral pocket dissection increases wound surface area unnecessarily, and allows lateral shift of implants that causes widening of the intermammary distance. Most patients despise an excessively wide intermammary distance, and are willing to limit lateral shift when they are supine for naturalness in order to avoid an excessively wide intermammary distance.

> Overdissection of the lateral pocket is a common error in breast augmentation that occurs with all incision locations and pocket locations

Avoiding overdissection of the lateral pocket requires that surgeons stop lateral pocket dissection at the lateral border of the pectoralis major in the submammary and subfascial planes, and stop dissection at the lateral border of the pectoralis minor in partial

retropectoral and dual plane pockets. Chapter 10 emphasizes additional details of these principles. After inserting the implant, the surgeon should see slight flattening of the lateral border of the breast as the underdissected pocket soft tissues compress the lateral, curved border of the implant.

The surgeon can then insert a spatula retractor to protect and retract the lateral border of the implant medially, place a double ended retractor to retract the lateral pocket tissues laterally, and then incrementally enlarge the lateral pocket in 0.5 cm increments as described in Chapter 10 to precisely fit the pocket to the base dimension of the implant, allowing the footprint of the implant to lie uncompressed, and rounding the lateral profile contour of the breast.

■ INCISION CLOSURES

3:2:7
3:2:8

Incision closure is a critically important step in periareolar augmentation. If closure of the parenchyma, deep subcutaneous fascia, and skin do not produce a completely watertight closure, small amounts of serum can accumulate and leak through the closure to the skin and allow skin bacterial flora to contaminate the implant pocket.

Achieving a watertight closure is much more predictable using continuous suture techniques in the more superficial layers instead of interrupted sutures. The most critical layer for watertight closure is the deep subcutaneous fascia, because if fluid escapes through this layer, fluid can accumulate immediately beneath the skin and promote thinning and disruption of the skin closure.

Some surgeons do not close the breast parenchyma tunnel, but this practice increases dead space in the wound, risks protrusion of portions of the implant into the residual defect, and risks postoperative pseudoherniation of the implant that can produce visible and palpable deformities. Deep closure begins with placement of interrupted 4-0 Monocryl or Vicryl sutures to approximate the breast parenchyma over the implant. When placing the deepest sutures adjacent to the implant, the surgeon should keep the tip of the suture needle directed away from the implant at all times, lifting and placing the tissue onto the tip of the needle and never arcing the needle toward the implant. In fatty breasts, surgeons should place deep sutures into the most fibrous or dense tissues available, and avoid incorporating large bites of fat into the sutures to avoid focal areas of fat necrosis postoperatively.

Incision closure is a critically important step in periareolar augmentation

Achieving a watertight closure is much more predictable using continuous suture techniques in the more superficial layers instead of interrupted sutures

A second layer of continuous 4-0 or 5-0 Monocryl or Vicryl sutures approximates the deep subcutaneous fascia, and final closure consists of a layer of continuous, subcuticular 5-0 Monocryl.

Optimal suture materials handle and tie easily, provide predictable support of the tissues during the early stages of wound healing, and then absorb to leave less foreign material in the wound. No scientifically valid evidence supports a superiority of permanent skin suture that requires removal compared to absorbable suture, and suture removal is an unnecessary procedure that can be distasteful to patients, and uniformly wastes surgeon and personnel time without offering any scientifically documented advantages.

■ DRESSINGS, DRAINS, AND POSTOPERATIVE CARE

The entire surgical dressing consists of a single layer of flesh colored Dermicel tape placed over Mastisol™ adherent solution applied to the incision skin edges (Figure 13-19). Drains are totally unnecessary and undesirable in primary augmentation.[1-5] Other adjuncts such as special bras or straps, indwelling catheters for injection of local anesthetics, pain pumps, intercostal blocks, instillation of local anesthetic into the pocket, narcotic strength pain medications, and implant motion exercises are likewise totally unnecessary and undesirable, because they unnecessarily complicate and prolong patient recovery. Details of postoperative management using principles of 24 hour recovery are included in Chapters 16 and 17. Patients are instructed to shower 3–4 hours following return home, perform straight arm raising exercises, and to go out of the house for dinner or to shop the evening of surgery with ibuprofen as

Figure 13-19. Flesh colored Dermicel tape applied over the incision closure is the only postoperative dressing. No additional bandages, bras, or other adjuncts are necessary or desirable.

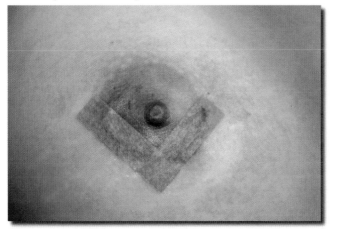

their only pain medication. Using this regimen, 96% of 627 patients returned to full, normal (non-aerobic) activities within 24 hours following augmentation.[1]

■ CHALLENGES AND POTENTIAL SOLUTIONS

Every incision approach has potential challenges that can occur intraoperatively. Common challenges that occur with the periareolar approach with alternatives for avoidance or correction include the following:

1. Difficulty determining the optimal level of the inframammary fold and the optimal level for the inframammary incision:

   - Use the recommendations in the TEPID[TM,3] and High Five[TM,2] systems, locating the volume of the implant planned for the procedure, then locating the desired nipple-to-fold distance recommendation below that volume in the table.

   - Remember to make all measurements under maximal skin stretch to simulate stretch that the implant will produce.

   - If leaving all inferior origins of the pectoralis major muscle intact along the inframammary fold (as opposed to dividing the origins for dual plane augmentations), lower the fold an additional 0.5 cm to compensate for the added pressure of the pectoralis on the lower pole of the implant.

2. Tendency to dissect the inferior pocket excessively, causing excessively low implant position and "bottoming":

   - When dissecting via the transparenchymal route, stop initial dissection at least 2–3 cm above the level of the desired postoperative inframammary fold.

   - Avoid excessive upward traction on retractors during the operation, especially in thinner patients with more mobile chest skin, because retractor forces can separate the deep subcutaneous fascial attachments inferior to the incision edge to deeper structures, resulting in an excessively low inferior pocket border.

   - When dividing pectoralis origins along the inframammary fold, constantly check topographic landmarks and preoperative markings to avoid dissection excessively inferiorly.

   - Avoid excessively large implants that place excessive anterior traction on the skin envelope.

3. Risk of inadvertently entering the pleural space during electrocautery dissection:

   - Always dissect parallel to the chest wall, dividing only those tissues that tent upward off the chest wall under retractor tension.

   - Never cut any muscle tissue that does not tent upward off the chest wall under retractor or forceps tension.

   - If desired, palpate a rib, and enter the subpectoral space directly over that rib.

   - If pneumothorax occurs inadvertently, insert a small catheter through a pursestring suture in the intercostals or pleura, reinforce with a second layer of any adjacent tissue that is available, apply maximal suction to the catheter while providing positive pressure ventilation, and tie the pursestring suture. Obtain a chest x-ray in the recovery room to verify lung expansion, or alternatively, leave the catheter in place, exiting a separate stab incision, and provide water seal suction while seeking thoracic surgical consultation. Keep the patient under constant observation for at least 24 hours, and confirm lung expansion with another chest x-ray prior to discharge.

4. Difficulty controlling larger perforating vessels in the pocket:

   - Coagulate all larger perforators in three locations with the handswitching, monopolar, electrocautery forceps prior to dividing the vessel.

   - Divide all muscle origins at least 1 cm away from their origins on the ribs to avoid retraction of intramuscular vessels.

   - Check all cut muscle edges and previously coagulated perforators prior to implant insertion.

   - Do not perform pocket dissection with any type of sharp instrument, with blunt dissection, or even with needlepoint electrocautery pencil only.

5. Excess lateral pocket dissection, risking lateral implant displacement and widening of the intermammary distance postoperatively:

   - In the subpectoral plane, stop pocket dissection at the lateral border of the pectoralis minor and after inserting the implant, incrementally enlarge the lateral pocket using double ended and spatula retractors until the footprint of the implant exactly fits the posterior surface of the pocket.

- In the submammary plane, stop initial lateral pocket dissection at the lateral border of the pectoralis major, or 2 cm inside the projected base width of the planned implant.

6. Difficulty estimating or determining optimal pocket size compared to implant base dimensions:

- Always underdissect the lateral pocket, and then incrementally enlarge it to fit the implant after the implant is in place.

- Avoid excessively large implants, especially in patients with thin soft tissue envelopes.

- Measure from the medial aspect of the pocket laterally intraoperatively using a sterile skin marking ruler or other instrument, and stop lateral pocket dissection at least 2 cm medial to the projected base width of the planned implant.

7. Excessive bleeding from inadvertent surgical trauma to the thoracoacromial pedicle or the larger perforator and vein at the second intercostal space:

- When dissecting superiorly, assure an adequate length retractor, and maintaining constant upward traction on the retractor, dissect parallel and close to the ribs, not upward toward the pectoralis muscle.

- Do not dissect within 2 cm of the second intercostal space medially, remaining at least 3 cm lateral to the sternum in the upper pocket where the large perforating vein and artery are located.

- Avoid dissection that extends medially more than 1.5 cm lateral to the midline.

8. Excessive medial pocket dissection with excessive bleeding from medial perforating vessels:

- Mark at least a 3 cm wide intermammary distance preoperatively, and constantly check skin markings during medial pocket dissection to avoid dissecting medial to those markings.

- Remember that the most distal extent of the pocket is always distal to the tip of the retractor, so keep the retractor tip at least 1 cm inside pocket boundary skin markings at all times.

- When using the handswitching monopolar forceps, instead of dividing medial tissues with a sweeping motion, grasp and pinch each area of tissues to divide them in order to provide more effective coagulation.

9. Difficulty inserting a prefilled implant:

   - Enlarge the incision.

   - Reduce the size of the implant.

   - Use an introducing sleeve with techniques described in Chapter 11.

10. Difficulty achieving bilateral symmetry intraoperatively:

    - Remember that breast symmetry never exists in any patient pre- or postoperatively and assure that every patient understands that fact preoperatively.

    - Recheck preoperative breast measurements, and remember that the smaller breast has quantitatively less skin, so an equivalent volume implant may produce more upper fullness compared to the larger skin envelope of the opposite breast. Attempting to put more volume in a smaller breast envelope to attempt to "match" a larger breast is illogical when the human eye distinguishes differences in breast shape to a much greater degree compared to differences in size that exist in every woman.

    - Compare measurements very carefully to preoperative patient images. Note the amount, consistency, and distribution of parenchyma preoperatively, and reconcile that information with implant volume and shape, and with visible impressions intraoperatively.

    - Never attempt to put significantly more volume in the smaller envelope, as this practice is likely to produce an excessively bulging, globular appearing shape with a more bulging upper breast that differs significantly from shape in the opposite breast and is visibly apparent.

    - Remember that the human eye sees breast shape much more than breast size, and try to create similar shapes bilaterally instead of trying to force a match in size that is impossible.

11. Breast appears too full and globular intraoperatively:

    - Implant is too large for the dimensions and tissue characteristics of the patient's tissues.

    - Implant pocket is too small. Enlarge it in small increments laterally.

- Parenchyma is very firm and concentrated centrally. In severe circumstances, consider vertical radial scoring to splay out the parenchyma. This cause is very rare compared to the first two causes listed, and scoring should be a last resort.

12. Failure to achieve a watertight suture closure intraoperatively:

- Interrupted closure of deep subcutaneous fascia is not as watertight compared to a continuous suture closure.

- Maintain constant tension on the continuous sutures during closure and knot tying.

- Tie at least four squared knots in each end of the deep subcutaneous fascia closure and three squared knots in the dermal subcuticular suture.

- The surgeon may cut the knots more accurately compared to an assistant.

- Avoid incorporating excess fat in the deep subcutaneous fascia closure to avoid fat necrosis that often produces incision disruption.

13. Risk of suture needle puncture of the implant during suture closure:

- Keep the tip of the suture needle pointed anteriorly, away from the implant at all times, and use tissue forceps to place the tissue edges onto the needle.

- Use the rear of the tissue forceps beneath the tissue edge to protect the implant while placing a suture.

■ REFERENCES

1. Tebbetts JB: Achieving a predictable 24 hour return to normal activities after breast augmentation Part II: Patient preparation, refined surgical techniques and instrumentation. *Plast Reconstr Surg* 109:293–305, 2002.

2. Tebbetts JB, Adams WP: Five critical decisions in breast augmentation using 5 measurements in 5 minutes: the high five system. *Plast Reconstr Surg* 116(7):2005–2016, 2005.

3. Tebbetts JB: A system for breast implant selection based on patient tissue characteristics and implant–soft tissue dynamics. *Plast Reconstr Surg* 109(4):1396–1409, 2002.

4. Tebbetts JB: Patient acceptance of adequately filled breast implants using the tilt test. *Plast Reconstr Surg* 106(1):139–147, 2000.

5. Tebbetts JB: Dual plane (DP) breast augmentation: optimizing implant–soft tissue relationships in a wide range of breast types. *Plast Reconstr Surg* 107:1255, 2001.

Preoperative Care, Anesthesia, and Postoperative Care

Assuming optimal decisions and planning, the patient's entire experience with breast augmentation is largely determined by the level of preoperative care, anesthesia, surgical and postoperative care that she receives. A surgeon's performance is limited by the surgical environment. Optimally, a surgeon creates an optimal environment for patient care, but this process may take years, and requires a strong commitment to learning, training personnel, allocating necessary resources, and continually reassessing and improving the processes that define care levels and outcomes. The details of processes and integration of processes determine success. A surgeon can implement 90% of required processes, but the 10% of proved processes that the surgeon cannot or will not implement will detract from an optimal, state-of-the-art patient experience, recovery, and outcome.

> Optimally, a surgeon creates an optimal environment for patient care, but this process may take years, and requires a strong commitment to learning, training personnel, allocating necessary resources, and continually reassessing and improving the processes that define care levels and outcomes

■ CREATING AN OPTIMAL PERIOPERATIVE ENVIRONMENT

Optimal perioperative care begins by creating and controlling an environment where optimally trained and motivated personnel will interface with and treat the patient the day of her augmentation. The quality and outcome of the entire patient experience begin with the surgeon. If the surgeon can perform at an optimal level, i.e. increase efficiency to do more operations in a day and enable patients to have a more rapid recovery, the surgeon will likely have much more success asking surgical facility management and anesthesia and surgery center personnel to work with the surgeon to develop and follow protocols that deliver a redefined level of care. If the surgeon does not have the motivation, resources, and commitment to expand the surgeon skill set and implement proved processes in order to be able to deliver a higher level of care, the other people in the surgical environment will not be optimally motivated and cooperative, and redefining the patient experience will be much more difficult or impossible.

> Optimal perioperative care begins by creating and controlling an environment where optimally trained and motivated personnel will interface with and treat the patient the day of her augmentation

Surgeon control of the surgery center environment and surgeon control of anesthesia are essential to optimize the patient experience and outcome, assuming the surgeon has first optimized the surgeon skill set. To reasonably expect to predictably deliver 24 hour recovery levels of care, the surgeon must do the following:

> Surgeon control of the surgery center environment and surgeon control of anesthesia are essential to optimize the patient experience and outcome, assuming the surgeon has first optimized the surgeon skill set

1. Develop surgeon skills to perform an augmentation mammaplasty in 45 minutes or less—this includes developing planning skills that optimize preoperative decisions, minimize decisions in the operating room, improve efficiency by decreasing operating times and narcotic drug requirement, and minimize unnecessary and unproductive practices.

2. Develop influence and control that allows the surgeon to implement specific surgical, anesthesia and perioperative care protocols.

3. Develop a relationship with surgical facility management that enables the surgeon to work with consistent personnel when performing augmentations, and to have paid personnel time allocated to train these personnel.

4. Develop a relationship with anesthesia personnel that allows the surgeon to provide specific protocols that the anesthesia personnel make every attempt to implement before modifying the protocols to their personal preferences.

5. Develop a relationship with postanesthesia care personnel that allows the surgeon to implement specific protocols to speed patient recovery.

6. Perform breast augmentation under general anesthesia, preferably general endotracheal anesthesia, and use muscle relaxants.

7. Have all patients arrive so that all can be marked by the surgeon before the surgeon enters the operating room. When doing more than eight cases per day, it may be necessary to have other patients arrive at a later time, depending on the capacity of the facility.

> Surgeons and the surgical facility can increase efficiency, profitability, and improve patient recovery by allocating two operating rooms for a single surgeon during a specific period

When surgeons can accomplish the requirements listed above, both the surgeons and the surgical facility can increase efficiency, profitability, and improve patient recovery by allocating two operating rooms for a single surgeon during a specific period (Figure 14-1). This system minimizes surgeon and personnel downtime, maximizes the surgical facility's return on investment of personnel resources and facility resources, and encourages all team members to perform at a higher level. This system is only logical if surgeons have a reasonable case load of augmentations, and if the surgeon and surgeon's personnel learn to manipulate patient scheduling to assure a minimum of three augmentations on any

Figure 14-1. (*A*) Room 1 in author's surgical facility. (*B*) Hallway that joins adjacent operating rooms. (*C*) Room 2 in author's surgical facility. Allocating two adjacent operating rooms for one surgeon dramatically increases surgeon and facility efficiency, provided the surgeon performs a minimum of three augmentations when the rooms are scheduled, with an operating time of less than 45 minutes per case.

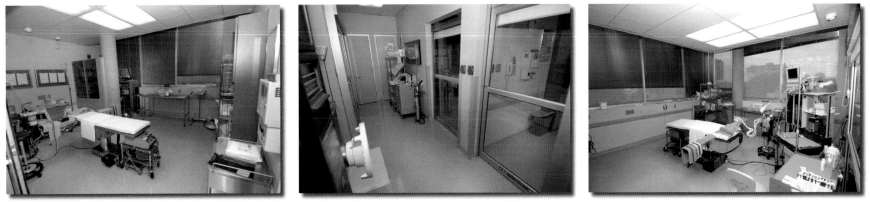

surgery day. The system fails miserably when surgeons want to perform one or two augmentations on a day, or during a block time.

Surgeons and surgery facility management personnel that have visited the author have successfully implemented this type of system, but implementation requires a commitment of time and resources by all parties. Key to the success of our system of two operating rooms for a single surgeon are: (1) strict scheduling requirements that require surgeons to post at least three cases in order to schedule, and (2) surgeon commitment to expanding the surgeon skill set, discarding preconceptions, and implementing proved processes.

Key to the success of our system of two operating rooms for a single surgeon are: (1) strict scheduling requirements that require surgeons to post at least three cases in order to schedule, and (2) surgeon commitment to expanding the surgeon skill set, discarding preconceptions, and implementing proved processes

■ PREOPERATIVE CARE

Preoperative Preparations

When a patient schedules surgery, the surgeon's personnel should begin to prepare the patient for surgery by providing detailed, consistent information about each of the following:

- Date of surgery
- Location of surgery facility

- Time to arrive

- Preoperative laboratory tests—where and when they will be performed

- Arrangement requirements for a driver and overnight caregiver

- What to expect the day of surgery—in detail

- Anesthesia information and arrangements for a preoperative anesthesia consult by phone

- FDA information and implant manufacturer warranty information

- Necessity of completing all required informed consent documents

- Drugs and herbal preparations to avoid preoperatively

- Necessity of no oral intake for 8 hours minimum prior to surgery.

All of this information should be included in printed information to the patient and on a checklist that is immediately accessible to all surgeon personnel who might interact with the patient. A specific surgeon employee should be responsible for providing this information and placing a preoperative checklist (Table 14-1) on the front of the patient's chart that provides instant information to all other personnel that interact with the patient. This document is available in the Resources folder on the DVDs that accompany this book.

Providing a consistent message in an efficient and comprehensive manner is essential to developing optimal patient confidence. Patient confidence is essential to an optimal perioperative experience

Providing a consistent message in an efficient and comprehensive manner is essential to developing optimal patient confidence. Patient confidence is essential to an optimal perioperative experience. Patients forget, lose confidence, and become fearful when they hear different answers to questions, so the surgeon should build a system that: (a) rechecks to assure that the patient received all of the information listed above, (b) someone calls the patient at intervals to assure that preoperative arrangements are on schedule, and (c) everyone who is in a position to answer patient questions delivers a prompt, consistent answer.

Patients must understand the critical importance of each of the following:

- Providing comprehensive and accurate medical history information

- Divulging all types of drugs or herbal medications

- Strict adherence to all surgeon instructions

Table 14-1. Surgical and postsurgical arrangements.

Surgical and
Postsurgical Arrangements

John B. Tebbetts, M.D., P.A.
Plastic and Reconstructive Surgery

SURGERY SCHEDULING

Patient Name _____ Spouse _____

DOB _____ Age _____ SS# _____

Home Telephone ( ) _____ Work Telephone ( ) _____

Cell Phone _____ State _____

Procedure _____ Physician John B. Tebbetts, M.D.

_____

_____

_____

Date _____ Surgery ❏ Posted

Case # _____ Hours _____ Admit Time _____

Facility ❏ LASC ❏ _____ Anesthesia ❏ L.T. ❏ K.T.

❏ T.L. ❏ _____

❏ Consent forms

❏ Surgery Scheduled on NexTech ❏ Routine Lab Work ❏ HIV ❏ PT, PTT, Platelets

❏ Will Anyone Else Part 1/Part 2 ❏ EKG

❏ Special Implant Consent ❏ Mammogram and report checked ❏ NA

❏ Confirmation Package ❏ Implants _____

❏ Photographs

❏ Post-op Instruction Sheet o Allergies _____

❏ Rhino Packet __/__/__

❏ Pharmacy # _____

  ❏ Called __/__/__ ❏ Insurance _____

❏ H & P Confirmed __/__/__ Surgical Fee _____ Implants _____

Dep Amount _____ Bal Amount _____

❏ PreOp Acc: _____ Dep Pd __/__/__ Bal Pd __/__/__

Date __/__/__ ph: _____ LASC _____

❏ PostOp Acc: _____ Anesthesia _____

Date __/__/__ ph: _____ EKG Fee _____ Bal pd. __/__/__

AFTER SURGERY CHECKLIST

❏ Flowers Sent ❏ Surgery In Computer

❏ Op Note In Chart ❏ Patient Financing Confirmed

Comments _____

_____

_____

- No oral intake for 8 hours minimum prior to surgery

- Necessity to arrange for transportation and 24 hour caregiver

- Availability to speak with anesthesia personnel at a specific time

- Arriving at the surgery facility promptly at the designated time

- Complying totally with all perioperative and postoperative instructions.

A phone call 48 hours prior to surgery from the surgeon office should reconfirm the patient's understanding and compliance with each of the above, and the personnel making the phone call must be responsible for documenting the contents of the call in the patient chart.

Arrival and Transfer to Surgical Holding

When the patient arrives at the surgery facility, personnel (ideally, personnel who know the patient) should be available to meet the patient and caregiver, and immediately accompany the patient to an area where the patient can change into a surgical gown (Figures 14-2, 14-3). All of the patient's valuables should remain with the patient's caregiver, and personnel should get a cell phone number for the caregiver or accompany the caregiver to an appropriate waiting area. Personnel should plan to have the caregiver

Personnel should plan to have the caregiver available at the surgery center when the patient first enters the recovery room, so that personnel can review postoperative instructions with the caregiver and review them with the patient within the hour after the patient's operation

Figure 14-3. Preoperative room where patient changes and can relax with caregiver prior to surgery. These rooms also function as stepdown rooms after the patient leaves recovery, prior to discharge.

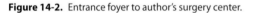

Figure 14-2. Entrance foyer to author's surgery center.

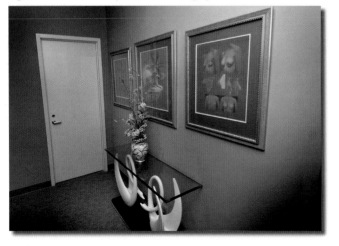

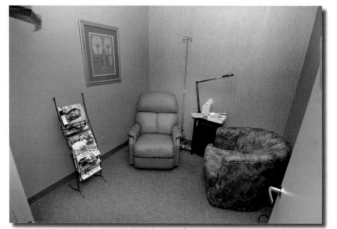

available at the surgery center when the patient first enters the recovery room, so that personnel can review postoperative instructions with the caregiver and review them with the patient within the hour after the patient's operation. In a 627 consecutive patient series of augmentation patients,[1,2] using management protocols and surgical techniques included in this chapter, the average time from the start of the patient's breast augmentation under general anesthesia to discharge with an ASPAN[3] score of 10 was 78 minutes. Continuing to monitor and improve proved processes has further reduced perioperative recovery times and time to discharge from the surgery facility, always with an ASPAN score of 10.

Surgery Facility Personnel Responsibilities and Patient Interactions

A member of the surgeon's staff who knows the patient should ideally accompany the patient and introduce the patient to the surgery center personnel who will care for her initially. Surgery center personnel who will interact with the patient should be familiar with the surgeon's protocols for care and be able to answer basic questions, but should refrain from extraneous discussions with the patient. If the patient asks the surgery center specific questions about her surgery, personnel should answer in general terms, avoid discussion of details of the operation, implants, or other areas which they should refer to the surgeon. If any patient approaches surgery center personnel about making last minute changes to the surgical approach, the operation listed on the operative permit previously signed by the patient, implant type or size, or any other aspect of the surgery, the personnel should immediately inform the surgeon. In most cases, patients who make these last minute requests for changes should be cancelled and repeat the education and informed consent steps defined in Chapter 3 that should have precluded any requests for last minute changes.

Most importantly, surgery center personnel should refrain from discussing or imposing any personal opinions on patients, regardless of the topic. The role of personnel is to support and care for the patient, not enter into discussions of personal opinions, even if they are meant to compliment the surgeon.

Surgery center personnel should carefully take a medical history, complete all forms in the surgery facility chart, assure that all laboratory data are available in the chart and that all operative consent forms are for the operation listed on the chart and are signed by the patient and witnessed. Personnel should recheck medical history, drug history, and drug reactions information they elicited to the same information provided by the surgeon's

A member of the surgeon's staff who knows the patient should ideally accompany the patient and introduce the patient to the surgery center personnel who will care for her initially

If any patient approaches surgery center personnel about making last minute changes to the surgical approach, the operation listed on the operative permit previously signed by the patient, implant type or size, or any other aspect of the surgery, the personnel should immediately inform the surgeon

Most importantly, surgery center personnel should refrain from discussing or imposing any personal opinions on patients, regardless of the topic

office. If differences exist in any of the information, personnel should notify the surgeon prior to administering any medications.

Anesthesia personnel (ideally, the same person that spoke with the patient preoperatively by phone) should greet the patient, reaffirm key items of the anesthesia and medical history discussed in a previous phone call, and give the patient a reassuring overview of what to expect in the operating room and recovery room.

Preoperative Medications

Patients should not receive preoperative medications in most cases until the surgeon has completed preoperative markings and had an opportunity to say hello to the patient and answer any last minute questions. Designated surgery center personnel should then insert an intravenous line, and according to defined protocols, administer preoperative medications. After the patient receives preoperative medications, personnel should make the patient comfortable and check on her frequently until time for her transfer to the operating room. If family or caregiver have been allowed to sit with the patient, they should be accompanied to a waiting area.

Table 14-2 is an integrated preoperative, anesthesia, and postanesthesia stepdown protocol used in the author's practice. Despite constant monitoring of trials with alternative medication and inhalation agents for more than a decade, the regimen in Table 14-2 continues to be the gold standard, and has consistently delivered the shortest times to discharge and most optimal recovery and outcomes. This document is included in the Resources folder on the DVDs that accompany this book for surgeon use and tailoring to suit practice preferences.

> The number one priority pharmacologically to optimize recovery following breast augmentation is to minimize doses of narcotic and sedative medications to enable patients to rapidly resume activity without nausea, vomiting, drowsiness, and lack of motivation

Premedications for breast augmentation should be minimal in order to minimize doses of sedative or other medications that could potentiate narcotics and narcotic side effects. The number one priority pharmacologically to optimize recovery following breast augmentation is to minimize doses of narcotic and sedative medications to enable patients to rapidly resume activity without nausea, vomiting, drowsiness, and lack of motivation.

In the author's practice, after preoperative marking, patients receive Versed 2 mg IV or less (start with 1 mg and if patient is comfortable do not increase the dose), Claforan (or other cephalosporin antibiotic) 1 gram IV, and if (and only if) the patient has a strong history of previous nausea and vomiting with anesthesia, Zofran 4–8 mg IV. No other premedications are necessary or desirable to achieve predictable 24 hour recovery.[1,2]

Table 14-2. **Integrated Anesthesia, PACU ð Stepdown Summary Protocol**

John B. Tebbetts, M.D.

*Integrated anesthesia, PACU and stepdown protocols for augmentation mammaplasty. Copyright John B. Tebbetts, M.D., 2004, surgeons may use with permission for their individual practices. For other reproduction purposes, contact Dr. Tebbetts.

Premeds

Versed 2 mg—minimize for more rapid recovery
Zofan 4–8 mg—only in patients with previous history of severe nausea post anesthesia
Claforan 1 gram IV (or other antibiotic per surgeon preference)

Induction

*See complete detailed anesthesia script in separate document "Anesthesia for Augmentation Mammaplasty"

►1	**INDUCTION**	Reglan	10 mg, 2 cc	Forehead strip—no esophageal temp probe
►		Inapsine	0.6 mg, 0.25 cc	Tape head in place—table moves side to side
►		Robinul	0.2 mg, 1 cc	
►		Fentanyl	50 µg/cc, 2 cc	
►5		Lidocaine Propofol 1–2.5 mg/kg Nimbex	20 mg IV, 2 cc 20 cc 4–6 mg	If incision is made within 10 minutes, will usually not require reversal **Timing is critical for optimal pectoralis relaxation and to obviate reversal
►		Decadron	4 mg	
►		Forane	2%	Connect upper op field suction to anesthesia suction
►		Oxygen		Hook up fill tube from field to bag of saline for implant filling
►				Connect surgeon's fiberoptic light source
10	Left pocket dissection complete			
►		Forane	1.5 or 1%	Reduce Forane concentration
►	**RETURN TO SUPINE, ROLL**	Off ventilator Reduce Forane	0.5–0.75%	**ROLL TABLE TOWARD SURGEON** for closure of left incision
►20–30	CLOSURE BEGINS			* If pocket adjustments necessary, surgeon may ask to reposition table as needed.

*The times in the left column decrease incrementally with increase in surgeon and team skills and efficiency.

PACU

Principles:
Vigorous, constant stimulation
Minimize narcotics
No narcotics without Phenergan first, never simultaneous

Table 14-2. **Integrated Anesthesia, PACU and Stepdown Summary Protocol—cont'd**

▶1	PACU			Stimulate on arrival, when respond to voice commands:
5		Phenergan	6.25 mg IV	Wait 3 minutes, then administer Demerol
▶		Demerol	12.5 mg IV	
▶				
▶15		Phenergan	6.25 mg IM	When patient can answer questions, administer these IM meds
▶		Demerol	12.5 mg IM	
17				Dress patient on PACU stretcher
20		(Repeat above ×1 maximum prn)		Transfer to stepdown

Times listed in the left column of this table decrease incrementally as surgeon and team skills and efficiency improve.

STEPDOWN
Reclining chair
Stimulation q 5 minutes × 2
Caregiver to room
Instructions to caregiver and patient
Arm raising demonstrated set of 5
Discharge home

■ ANESTHESIA

General endotracheal anesthesia provides maximal safety and an optimal surgical environment for surgeons who want to deliver state-of-the-art breast augmentation and 24 hour return to normal activity. Any type of local anesthesia with sedation requires more sedative and narcotic medications compared to the protocol described in this chapter, and these additional medications prolong and complicate recovery and contribute significantly to unnecessary potential morbidity. No current studies exist in the anesthesia or plastic surgery literature that document as rapid a recovery and as minimal side effects with anesthesia for breast augmentation compared to the author's 24 hour recovery publications.[1,2] Without administering muscle relaxants, surgeons are either more prone to perform submammary or subfascial augmentations and risk suboptimal long-term soft tissue cover of the implant, or they perform dual plane or submuscular augmentations that cause more trauma to the pectoralis with additional morbidity and prolonged recovery.

General endotracheal anesthesia provides maximal safety and an optimal surgical environment for surgeons who want to deliver state-of-the-art breast augmentation and 24 hour return to normal activity

No current studies exist in the anesthesia or plastic surgery literature that document as rapid a recovery and as minimal side effects with anesthesia for breast augmentation compared to the author's 24 hour recovery publications[1,2]

Some surgeons and anesthesia personnel prefer laryngeal airways instead of endotracheal tubes in order to avoid throat irritation that can result from an endotracheal tube. A properly sized and inserted endotracheal tube caused sore throat symptoms in less than 25% of the previously mentioned series of 627 patients, and all symptoms uniformly resolved spontaneously in 8 hours or less. This small amount of morbidity, in the author's opinion, is preferable to assure the utmost protection from aspiration, one of the deadliest of anesthetic complications. Should aspiration occur, surgeons and anesthesia personnel who use laryngeal airways may anticipate answering the obvious question: Why didn't you use an endotracheal tube? They might also anticipate answering whether the patient might be in a better situation with a sore throat compared to aspiration pneumonitis.

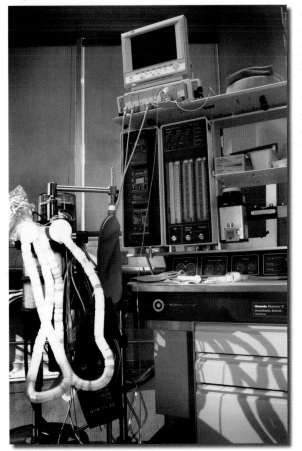

Figure 14-4. Anesthesia machine and monitoring equipment for general anesthesia.

State-of-the-art anesthesia equipment and monitoring equipment for general anesthesia is essential for patient safety and certification of the surgical facility (Figure 14-4). Rigid scheduled checks and maintenance assure predictable performance of this equipment.

Table 14-2 is an anesthesia script detail for inframammary dual plane augmentation that correlates drug administration with surgical events, and Table 14-3 is a flowchart

Table 14-3. Anesthesia protocol flowchart for inframammary augmentation.

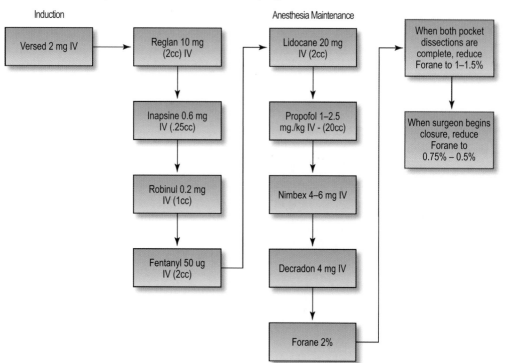

representation of the anesthesia protocol. These documents are available in the Resources folder on the DVDs that accompany this book.

In the operating room, patients should be positioned supine on the operating table with the arms extended and supported on movable arm boards (Figure 14-5). The patient should be supported on the operating table by Velcro strap supports that allow table rotation side-to-side with optimal safety and tape fixation for the head and endotracheal tube to prevent tube displacement. Forehead strips for temperature monitoring obviate the need for esophageal temperature probes.

On induction of anesthesia, the patient receives the following IV medications: Reglan 10 mg (2 cc), Inapsine 0.6 mg (0.25 cc), Robinul 0.2 mg (1 cc), Fentanyl 50 µg/cc

Figure 14-5.

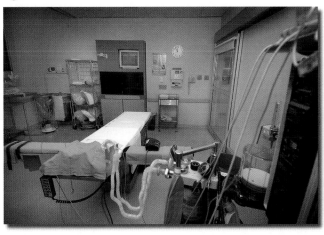

(maximum 2 cc), Lidocaine 20 mg (2 cc), Propofol 1–2.5 mg/kg (usually 20 cc), Nimbex 4–6 mg for muscle relaxation, and Decadron 4 mg for its antiemetic effects. Inhalation agents are limited to Forane 2% and oxygen.

The goal during surgery is for the surgeon to perform bilateral pocket dissections before the single dose of Nimbex loses its muscle relaxing effects on the pectoralis muscle in 20–35 minutes, so the surgeon needs to be available and ready to start the procedure immediately after induction of anesthesia and prep and drape. Another goal is to limit total dose of narcotics to 2 cc of Fentanyl, so the surgeon needs to limit surgical trauma and operative time. Table 14-2 details additional tasks performed by the anesthesiologist or anesthetist during the procedure. Times listed in the left column are average times for a surgeon who has practiced with the surgical scripts for this approach that accompany Chapter 11. When the surgeon completes pocket dissection on the second side, anesthesia reduces Forane concentrations to 1–1.5 %, and when the surgeon begins incision closures, anesthesia further reduces Forane concentrations to 0.5–0.75%.

When surgeon efficiency is suboptimal or operative times for other approaches exceed 40–45 minutes, anesthesia must administer additional doses of muscle relaxant that may require reversal at the conclusion of the procedure. All reversing agents potentiate narcotics and narcotic side effects, prolonging recovery and increasing morbidity. Building skills to most efficiently perform augmentation minimizes recovery times and morbidity.

■ POSTOPERATIVE CARE

Postoperative care begins preoperatively with information that educates the patient and helps the patient know what to expect postoperatively. Any surprise postoperatively is a

The goal during surgery is for the surgeon to perform bilateral pocket dissections before the single dose of Nimbex loses its muscle relaxing effects on the pectoralis muscle in 20–35 minutes

Another goal is to limit total dose of narcotics to 2 cc of Fentanyl, so the surgeon needs to limit surgical trauma and operative time

Postoperative care begins preoperatively with information that educates the patient and helps the patient know what to expect postoperatively. Any surprise postoperatively is a potential problem

potential problem. The perioperative care that the patient receives at the surgical facility sets the stage for a smooth, rapid, predictable recovery when the patient returns home.

Postanesthesia Recovery Care

At the conclusion of the procedure, the patient is transferred to a two bed recovery area (Figure 14-6) immediately adjacent to the operating rooms. Using the optimized, proved processes discussed in this chapter, the author routinely performs up to 10 primary breast augmentations in a 5–6 hour period, using only two recovery beds and three stepdown beds. All patients attain an ASPAN score of 10 prior to discharge from the surgery facility. In order to optimize efficiency and space utilization, this postanesthesia care unit operates according to strict protocols that minimize narcotics, constantly stimulate the patient, and assure an ASPAN (American Society of PeriAnesthesia Nurses) score of 10 for every patient before transfer to a step down room.

Specific goals in the postanesthetic care unit (PACU) and stepdown care include: (1) minimizing narcotics, (2) stimulating the patient continuously, (3) rapidly achieving an ASPAN score of 10, and (4) assuring full extended arm movements above the head in a jumping jack manner in the presence of the caregiver before the patient is discharged home.

In order to accomplish these objectives, PACU personnel must discard many typical preconceptions and follow the protocol in this chapter exactly. Most of all, personnel must avoid the preconception that more and newer medications make patients more comfortable compared to the drugs in this protocol, and understand that no protocol using newer or more medications documents recovery results equal to the protocol[1,2] presented in Table 14-1. Before surmising that additional drugs or different drugs are necessary and changing this protocol, surgeons should implement the protocol, establish a record of results, then change one drug at a time and record objective data that prove other drugs or regimens superior. The current

Figure 14-6.

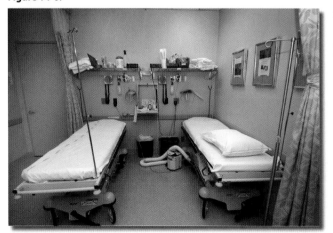

> Specific goals in the postanesthetic care unit (PACU) and stepdown care include: (1) minimizing narcotics, (2) stimulating the patient continuously, (3) rapidly achieving an ASPAN score of 10, and (4) assuring full extended arm movements above the head in a jumping jack manner in the presence of the caregiver before the patient is discharged home

protocol was developed in this manner,[1] recording recovery times to the second and performing extensive database analysis of several different drug regimens before simplifying and reducing drugs to produce the documented results in these studies.[1,2] Continual reevaluation of processes and evaluation of newer drugs for the past decade according to process engineering principles has continued to generate data that confirms the superior efficacy of the protocols in this chapter.

Table 14-4. Postanesthesia care unit (PACU) management protocol flowchart.

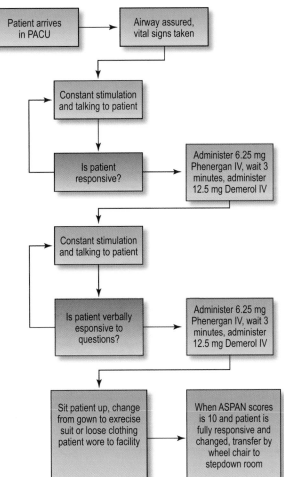

Table 14-4 is a flowchart that details management in the PACU, and this flowchart is available in the Resources folder on the DVDs that accompany this book.

Immediately on arrival in the PACU, the patient receives 6.25 mg of Phenergan IV. Personnel then wait 3 minutes for circulation time before administering Demerol 12.5 mg IV. With constant stimulation, when the patient is verbally responsive, personnel administer equivalent doses of these two medications IM, begin dressing the patient in an exercise suit on the stretcher, and sit her up as soon as possible. As soon as she can sit up and is totally responsive with an ASPAN score of 9–10, personnel transfer her to a wheelchair and transport her to a reclining chair in a stepdown room. In the stepdown room, personnel continue to continually stimulate her and bring her caregiver into the room to help keep her stimulated and awake.

Stimulation is essential during this period. Leaving a patient unattended and unstimulated to doze is unacceptable and unnecessarily prolongs recovery.

While the patient has been in PACU, surgeon personnel have reviewed Table 14-5, the Recipe for Recovery instructions, with the caregiver. This document is provided in the Resources folder on the DVDs that accompany this book for surgeon use and tailoring to suit practice preferences.

These instructions are printed on bright pink paper so that the patient can easily identify and locate them and so that personnel can refer to the "pink paper" during postoperative phone calls. When the caregiver arrives in the patient's room in stepdown, personnel instruct the patient and caregiver in arm raising exercises that require the patient to raise her fully straight arms out to the side and up over her head to touch the backs of her hands in a "jumping jack" manner. The patient repeats these movements at least five times prior to discharge, and repeats a set of five every hour after returning home. This protocol assures that patient and caregiver are on the same wavelength about what is required for optimal recovery, and assures that personnel can hold them accountable for their responsibilities during postoperative care at home.

> When the caregiver arrives in the patient's room in stepdown, personnel instruct the patient and caregiver in arm raising exercises that require the patient to raise her fully straight arms out to the side and up over her head to touch the backs of her hands in a "jumping jack" manner

Office personnel record the time the patient leaves the surgical facility, and depending on the time required for the patient to return home and take a 2 hour nap, personnel should call the patient $2-2\frac{1}{2}$ hours after the patient leaves the surgical facility to assure that she is up, has had something to eat, and is having a shower and washing her hair to get her arms over her head. When out of the shower, she repeats her arm raising exercises in a set of five, and then stays up and resumes normal activities until she goes out shopping or out to dinner. If child care precludes going out, the patient should resume normal activities at home as described in the Recipe for Recovery. The surgeon or surgeon personnel make a second call to the patient prior to bedtime to assure compliance with instructions and answer questions.

One of the most rewarding aspects of delivering rapid recovery for surgeons and surgeon personnel is hearing the enthusiastic voice of a patient who is out shopping, out to dinner, or caring for her children the evening of surgery. Representative examples of postoperative calls to patients are included as audio files in the Resources folder on the DVDs that accompany this book.

> The first 8 postoperative hours determine whether a patient will return to full normal activities within 24 hours

The first 8 postoperative hours determine whether a patient will return to full normal activities within 24 hours. If the patient is not up, moving, and following instructions during that period, chances are that she will become stiff, more apprehensive, and not

Table 14-5. **Recipe for Recovery**

Instructions to Our Patient and Her Caregiver
From John and Terrye Tebbetts

* Instructions for patients following inframammary, periareolar, or axillary breast augmentation. Copyright John B. Tebbetts, M.D., 2005, surgeons may use with permission for their individual practices. For other reproduction purposes, contact Dr. Tebbetts.

Terrye or a patient educator reviews this sheet in detail with the caregiver while the patient is in surgery. The same person who reviews these instructions with the caregiver calls the patient and caregiver 2 hours after she leaves the surgical facility to assure compliance with the instructions, and calls a second time before bedtime to further provide support. Finally, we print these instructions on bright pink colored paper, and constantly refer to the "Pink Recipe for Recovery".

The patient can go home and take a 2 hour nap. Two hours—that is all. Wake her up and get her moving! No more sleeping today. She can sit down and rest, but no more napping until bed time.

Next, make sure she eats something substantial. Crackers are simply not enough.

If she were going to get sick from the anesthesia, it would have already happened. That generally occurs with in the first 3–4 hours after surgery, which she has now peacefully slept through!

If she feels nauseous it is usually either because she took her medicine on an empty stomach or she is not drinking enough fluids and is becoming dehydrated. Make sure she eats something real— whatever she is craving. Make sure that she is doing more than taking a sip of something here and there. If she normally drinks a diet coke, make her drink a real coke—or something with sugar. We need to jump start her system.

As soon as she has eaten, give her an 800 mg ibuprofen, wait 30 minutes.

Then I want her arms above her head in slow jumping jack type motion. She will need to do a set of 5, every hour on the hour until bedtime. Try to keep her up until at least 10:00pm.

Encourage her to do normal things around the house. Unload the dishwasher, make dinner, read to the kids, for example. Better yet, get her out of the house and take her shopping or to dinner.

Remember, she cannot hurt herself through normal movement. We have NO incentive to tell you to do something that would send her back to the operating room! By moving, she will feel better faster and reduce her risk of capsular contracture and another operation! She knows all of this. It is important that you know and understand and help her get moving!

As soon as she feels comfortable moving, encourage her to shower and wash and blow dry her hair. Take her out to shop and walk around the mall. Take her out to dinner. I expect her to close her own car doors and put on her seat belt. A change of scenery is a wonderful thing!

She must lie on her breasts for 15 minutes before bed tonight and every night until it is simply not an issue any more—probably 8–12 weeks.

When it comes to lying down, it is the getting down there and getting up that is hard. Please don't let her cheat! It is important to put pressure on the breasts immediately. To get up, simply roll to the side and sit up.

Around 10:00pm, make sure she takes another 800 mg ibuprofen with food and the little pink pill—this is Benadryl and will help her sleep.

She can do anything she wants to make herself comfortable. That may mean a shower, or more arm movements or lying on her breasts more than once or wearing a bra.

Recipe for tomorrow morning

Get up, eat breakfast and take an 800 mg ibuprofen. Give it 30 minutes and get in a nice warm shower. That is when I want her arms above her head for the first time. It is hard to just pop out of bed and get your arms up—use the recipe and she will do great. The shower was optional last night. It is mandatory this morning!

Use the momentum she has built to get out and go do something. Walk around the mall, run errands, drive a car. I don't expect her to stop in the mall and start doing her arm exercises. But I do expect her to close her own car door, put on her own seat belt, carry a couple of shopping bags. Normal movement is essential.

Expect her to run out of energy around mid-day. The anesthesia will take approximately 48 hours to work itself out of her system. So plan your day so that she can stop and rest for a while. But after her nap, get her up and moving again.

You will find that the more she moves the better she feels. Help her treat this like a pulled muscle. Yes, you feel it, but it only gets better with movement.

Expect her to feel tighter, more swollen, at the end of the day. That is normal and temporary.

Expect her to begin to complain of soreness in the ribs and lower back around then end of day one or day two. This is simply fluid moving through the tissue. She will urinate it all out and loose the bloated feeling within 5–7 days.

If she complains of soreness in her upper back, she is tensing her shoulders. Patients often hold their shoulders in an unnatural position producing this complaint. Remind her to stretch her shoulders forward and back—relax!

Medication Schedule

We would like for her to take one 800 mg ibuprofen at breakfast, one around lunch and one at bedtime. If she needs additional relief around dinner-time, she can take two 200 mg Advil.

She can take the Benadryl if she likes, but it is not mandatory.

Please call the office some time during your day and let us know how she is doing.

comply with instructions. Personnel who speak with the patient on the phone are critical to aid with rapid recovery, and must encourage the slow patient by becoming increasingly assertive to assure compliance with instructions. Active participation by well trained surgeon personnel is essential to predictably deliver 24 hour recovery.

Surgeon willingness to prescribe narcotic strength pain medications in lieu of implementing proved processes that make these medications unnecessary deprives patients of the opportunity for the most rapid recovery with the least morbidity. A large percentage of patients might prefer a jar of narcotics and a bed, but nausea, constipation, stiffness, increased pain, more time off normal activities, and a more morbid recovery period are the tradeoffs for more and stronger medications. Early mobilization is unquestionably effective in redefining recovery in breast augmentation. Most importantly, more rapid recovery is the best indicator of minimal surgical trauma and bleeding, and rapid recovery correlates directly with superior long-term outcomes.

> Surgeon willingness to prescribe narcotic strength pain medications in lieu of implementing proved processes that make these medications unnecessary deprives patients of the opportunity for the most rapid recovery with the least morbidity

■ REFERENCES

1. Tebbetts JB: Achieving a predictable 24 hour return to normal activities after breast augmentation Part I: Refining practices using motion and time study principles. *Plast Reconstr Surg* 109:273–290, 2002.

2. Tebbetts JB: Achieving a predictable 24 hour return to normal activities after breast augmentation Part II: Patient preparation, refined surgical techniques and instrumentation. *Plast Reconstr Surg* 109:293–305, 2002.

3. Miller K, Sullivan E, Saufl N, et al. *Standards of peri-anesthesia nursing practice.* Cherry Hill, NJ: American Society of PeriAnesthesia Nurses, 1999, pp 32–35.

Essentials to Achieve 24 Hour Recovery

CHAPTER 15

Most informed patients considering breast augmentation want an optimal result with the shortest, most carefree recovery and the least risk of problems, reoperations, and costs in the future. Surgeons and breast implant manufacturers serve the patient and prioritize a commitment to continually deliver the best for the patient. The patient experience encompasses all aspects of education, perioperative care, and long-term outcome. An optimal patient experience requires surgeon commitment to continually optimize decisions and processes that determine outcomes.

Most plastic surgeons can develop a skill set to predictably deliver 24 hour return to normal activities following breast augmentation, provided they are willing and able to commit time and resources. Surgeons less than 5 years in practice have developed all of the necessary skills discussed in this chapter, and by implementing the processes detailed in this chapter and this book, predictably deliver 24 hour recovery. The same decision processes and surgical techniques that deliver 24 hour recovery also deliver optimal long-term outcomes with low complication and reoperation rates.[1–6] In 1664 reported consecutive augmentations using inframammary, axillary, and periareolar incision approaches and submammary, partial retropectoral, and dual plane pockets, patients experienced an overall reoperation rate of less than 3% with up to 7 year followup.[4,6,7] The incidence of other untoward occurrences in these combined series includes: capsular contracture Grades 3 and 4—0.7%, hematoma—0.2%, seroma—0.1%, infection—0.3%, implant deflations—0.8%, reoperations for implant malposition with anatomic implants—0.1%, and reoperations for size exchange—0.2%. The occurrence of visible wrinkling with the patient upright was zero by prioritizing tissue coverage based on quantitative

Most informed patients considering breast augmentation want an optimal result with the shortest, most carefree recovery and the least risk of problems, reoperations, and costs in the future

Most plastic surgeons can develop a skill set to predictably deliver 24 hour return to normal activities following breast augmentation, provided they are willing and able to commit time and resources

The same decision processes and surgical techniques that deliver 24 hour recovery also deliver optimal long-term outcomes with low complication and reoperation rates[1–6]

tissue parameters[2,3] and optimal surgical techniques.[4,6] These data prove that the same factors that enable 24 hour recovery also optimize long-term outcomes by minimizing complications and reoperations.

This chapter summarizes and codifies essential information that is included in other chapters, and focuses on specific requirements to deliver a redefined level of care and recovery. These processes are derived from a 15 year focus on breast augmentation, using process engineering principles to analyze and refine processes in each of the following areas: patient education and informed consent;[1] objective, quantitative preoperative tissue based assessment;[2] defined decision making priorities and processes;[3] surgical techniques and instrumentation;[4-6] perioperative care and anesthesia; and postoperative care.[5,6]

The methodologies and processes that allow surgeons to deliver a redefined level of care are complementary. Seemingly insignificant aspects of one process contribute significantly to the efficacy of other processes. Other alternatives and processes may predictably enable over 85% of patients to be out to dinner the evening of surgery and 96% to return to full, normal activities within 24 hours,[5,6] but other alternatives are not currently peer reviewed and published. Process engineering principles, motion and time study principles, and cause and effect analyses have provided invaluable tools that encouraged analysis and refinement of surgical processes from a perspective that is different compared to the "solution for problem" surgeon thought process that surgeons learn in an apprenticeship residency setting. Achieving 24 hour recovery is an excellent benchmark for the entire patient experience, because recovery is objective, and not subject to varying interpretations. Optimal recovery correlates directly with minimal complications, minimal reoperations, and optimal long-term outcomes.[1-6]

> Achieving 24 hour recovery is an excellent benchmark for the entire patient experience, because recovery is objective, and not subject to varying interpretations. Optimal recovery correlates directly with minimal complications, minimal reoperations, and optimal long-term outcomes[1-6]

Other chapters in this book present the details of the processes that deliver 24 hour recovery and optimal long-term outcomes. This chapter summarizes the key elements that determine optimal recovery and outcomes. Table 15-1 summarizes the six key defined process categories and the individual processes in each category that are essential for surgeons to predictably deliver this level of patient recovery and outcome.

Table 15-1. Essential processes to achieve 24 hour recovery and optimal outcomes.

Defined processes categories*

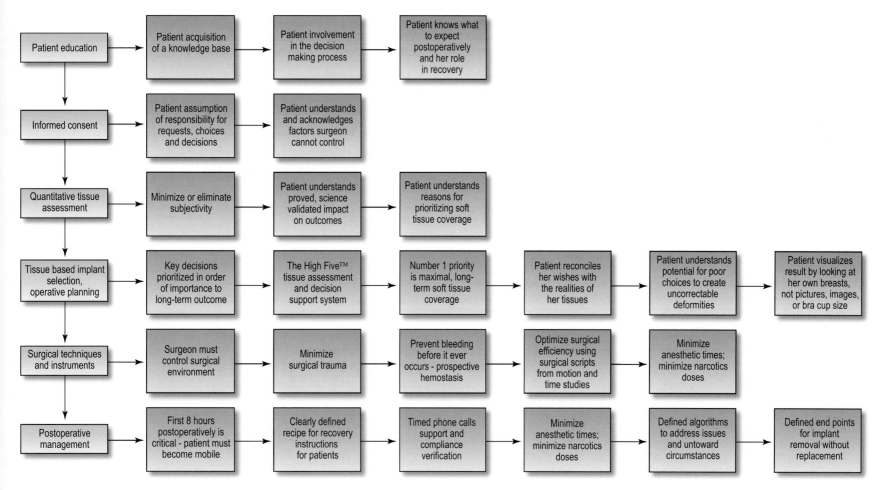

* All key processes are currently peer reviewed and published. See references at end of chapter

▥ PATIENT EDUCATION AND INFORMED CONSENT

Legally valid informed consent requires that patients make decisions. Optimal decisions require knowledge and decision support that provide patients factual information about all alternatives, and base patient and surgeon choices on proved decision processes.[1,3] Optimal patient education is staged and repetitive,[1] supports the patient in making decision, but requires that the patient ultimately makes choices and assumes documented responsibility for those choices.

> Patients who acquire more knowledge make better decisions. Patients who experience a more thorough, organized approach to education and decision making approach surgery more objectively and with more confidence

Patients who acquire more knowledge make better decisions. Patients who experience a more thorough, organized approach to education and decision making approach surgery more objectively and with more confidence. Actively participating in the decision process, understanding the factors that really determine long-term outcomes, and realizing that personal responsibility for choices is inherent to the process helps patients make better choices and develop a more realistic perspective about outcomes. Knowing preoperatively what will be done should suboptimal outcomes or problems occur helps patients and surgeons deal with untoward events and additional costs and risks.

Clearly defining what the patient and the surgeon cannot control is critically important during the patient education and informed consent process. Patients and surgeons cannot control two specific areas that can potentially produce untoward events or results postoperatively: wound healing (infection, capsular contracture), and tissue stretch (tissue stretch, thinning, and the resultant deformities). Understanding the decision parameters that minimize risks in these areas helps patients make better preoperative decisions, but patients must understand, accept, and take responsibility for the reality that neither patient nor surgeon can control the body's mechanisms in these two areas. Methods and documentation to assure patient understanding of these important limitations are detailed in Chapter 3.

> Clearly defining what the patient and the surgeon cannot control is critically important during the patient education and informed consent process

> To predictably deliver 24 hour recovery, surgeons must ensure preoperatively that patients know what is possible, why it is possible, and what decisions are required to make it possible

To predictably deliver 24 hour recovery, surgeons must ensure preoperatively that patients know what is possible, why it is possible, and what decisions are required to make it possible. Additionally, they must understand that optimal outcomes are a team effort where surgeon and patient contribute equally. That team effort begins with team education and team decisions, and continues throughout the patient experience.

■ QUANTITATIVE TISSUE ASSESSMENT AND PLANNING

Patients cannot realistically assume responsibility for subjective decisions, because decisions based on subjective opinions instead of objective data allow wide ranges of interpretation about cause if untoward events occur. When patients learn that optimal outcomes result from defined decision processes based on objective criteria instead of subjective opinions, they begin to understand that their individual tissue characteristics determine and limit choices if the goal is an optimal long-term outcome.

Surgeons who base decisions on objective data applied in defined, proved decision processes add another dimension to informed consent and are in a much better position to defend decisions and actions should untoward events occur. When untoward events occur, patients ask "Why me?" and question decisions and the decision process. Having data and defined decision processes documented preoperatively allows surgeons to answer with the following:

Our approach to caring for you has not changed. Here is what we based our decisions on—hard data about your tissues and what we have to work with; these are the choices we presented you with and the potential benefits, tradeoffs, and risks of those choices based on your individual tissue characteristics; here are the choices you made. You knew and know that untoward events are possible. Our choices were based on the best information and processes that are available, so we can deal with what has occurred knowing that we did everything right and that what has occurred did not result from anything we didn't do.

Applying the TEPID^{TM,2} system for quantitative tissue assessment integrated into the High Five^{TM,3} decision priority and support system is dramatically different compared to making random decisions based on subjective opinions and personal preferences. A surgeon can deliver only what a patient's tissues allow the surgeon to deliver. When a surgeon, however well meaning, does not recognize and prioritize the importance of maximizing long-term soft tissue coverage of implants, and does not recognize patient tissue characteristics that limit and define options, the surgeon is almost certain to make suboptimal decisions based on subjective, personal preferences that will detract from short- and long-term outcomes. During the clinical examination and consultation, the surgeon must reconcile the patient's wishes with her tissues, using techniques detailed in Chapter 7. Surgeons must also accept responsibility for operating on patients who insist on making suboptimal choices that conflict with tissue limitations, and understand that

Surgeons who base decisions on objective data applied in defined, proved decision processes add another dimension to informed consent and are in a much better position to defend decisions and actions should untoward events occur short-term economic considerations can create much greater long-term liabilities for patient and surgeon.

The High Five™,3 decision priority and support system detailed in Chapter 7 bases selection of implant weight, dimensions, and volume on quantified, objective, individual patient tissue characteristics. All surgeons have personal opinions and preferences, but having a defined decision process and priorities based on objective parameters helps surgeons temper subjective opinions within a defined decision process framework. The result is a better outcome for the patient and for the surgeon. This simple but powerful system requires less than 5 minutes of surgeon time preoperatively, and provides invaluable decision support and data based operative planning.

> All surgeons have personal opinions and preferences, but having a defined decision process and priorities based on objective parameters helps surgeons temper subjective opinions within a defined decision process framework

Surgeons should finalize as many decisions as possible before entering the operating room to optimize surgical efficiency, minimize unnecessarily prolonged operation times, and minimize drug dosages that can add morbidity and prolong recovery. Using the High Five™,3 system to define implant size and type preoperatively eliminates the use of sizer implants intraoperatively that unnecessarily add significant time, costs, and risks. Reviewing surgical scripts and practicing with surgery facility personnel using the scripts detailed in Chapters 11 and 12 dramatically reduces operating times and allows the surgeon to focus on factors that deliver a better result while simultaneously optimizing recovery and outcomes.

> Surgeons should finalize as many decisions as possible before entering the operating room to optimize surgical efficiency, minimize unnecessarily prolonged operation times, and minimize drug dosages that can add morbidity and prolong recovery

■ SURGICAL TECHNIQUES AND INSTRUMENTATION

Surgical instrumentation for breast augmentation can be relatively simple, but specific instrumentation allows surgeons to dramatically reduce bleeding and soft tissue trauma, two key determinants of recovery and outcomes. The degree of surgical trauma and bleeding, even if the surgeon achieves hemostasis after the bleeding occurs, dramatically impacts recovery. Extent of dissection, tissue trauma, and bleeding also define the wound surface area and degree of inflammation that, in turn, determines the wound healing response that can produce areas of pocket closure and capsular contracture, and that impact incidence of hematoma, seroma, and potential infection.

> The degree of surgical trauma and bleeding, even if the surgeon achieves hemostasis after the bleeding occurs, dramatically impacts recovery

A handswitching, monopolar, needlepoint electrocautery forceps is an indispensable instrument that allows surgeons to perform dissection, apply prospective hemostasis principles, and control bleeders that occur using a single instrument. This functionality, detailed in Chapter 11, provides an impressive increase in efficiency and routinely allows surgeons to dissect a retromammary, partial retropectoral, or dual plane pocket in less than 4 minutes. Specialized instrumentation for axillary endoscopically assisted augmentation detailed in Chapter 12 enables surgeons to eliminate all blunt dissection and have direct vision control of electrocautery dissection in all areas of the pocket.

General anesthesia that allows surgeons to use short acting muscle relaxants is critical to optimizing recovery. No currently published technique for local anesthesia with sedation for augmentation compares with the exceedingly rapid recovery and discharge from the surgical facility that is peer reviewed, published,[5,6] and detailed in Chapter 14. Muscle relaxants enable subpectoral dissection with minimal retraction pressure that decreases stretch and tissue trauma to the pectoralis, increasing surgeon visualization and accuracy of dissection, and minimizing postoperative discomfort.

> General anesthesia that allows surgeons to use short acting muscle relaxants is critical to optimizing recovery

Blunt dissection of any portion of a breast augmentation pocket unnecessarily increases soft tissue trauma, bleeding, and postoperative pain. Techniques of electrocautery dissection with specific instrumentation described in Chapters 11–13 enable surgeons to completely eliminate blunt dissection in all areas of the pocket through inframammary, axillary, and periareolar incision approaches.

> Blunt dissection of any portion of a breast augmentation pocket unnecessarily increases soft tissue trauma, bleeding, and postoperative pain

Implementing prospective hemostasis[5,6] techniques described in Chapter 11, combined with use of the handswitching, monopolar, needlepoint electrocautery forceps are two key elements to minimize even minor bleeding that can soak into adjacent tissues and increase inflammation, pain, and the inflammatory response. Adopting strict, no-touch techniques for rib periosteum or perichondrium prevents trauma to highly innervated periosteum and perichondrium, and prevents subperichondrial hematomas that substantially increase postoperative pain.

■ PERIOPERATIVE AND POSTOPERATIVE CARE

Unnecessary surgical adjuncts increase postoperative morbidity, increase costs, and convey an undisputable message to patients that they are injured, diverting the patient from a focus on early mobility and rapid return to normal activities. Current peer reviewed and published studies[2–6] prove that the following adjuncts are totally unnecessary for any pocket location in inframammary, axillary, and periareolar augmentation when surgeons implement proved techniques and decision processes: drains, bandages, special bras or straps, intercostal blocks, local instillation into the pocket, pain pumps, narcotic strength pain medications, and muscle relaxants.

> Unnecessary surgical adjuncts increase postoperative morbidity, increase costs, and convey an undisputable message to patients that they are injured, diverting the patient from a focus on early mobility and rapid return to normal activities

Minimizing doses of narcotics pre-, intra-, and postoperatively is essential to optimize recovery

Minimizing doses of narcotics pre-, intra-, and postoperatively is essential to optimize recovery. Minimizing narcotics requires that surgeons optimize surgical efficiency to limit operation times and minimize surgical trauma that increases anesthetic requirements. A maximum dose of 2 cc of Fentanyl intraoperatively and split 12.5 mg doses of Demerol during recovery are the maximum doses required for subpectoral and dual plane augmentation, allowing an average time under 80 minutes from the start of their augmentation to discharge from the surgical facility[5] and a 96% rate of return to normal activities within 24 hours.[5,6]

To optimize recovery and patient care, surgeons should define a simple, straightforward postoperative care regimen such as the Recipe for Recovery detailed in Chapter 14, and provide structured, scheduled telephone contact and support postoperatively. Achieving complete mobilization and resumption of normal activities, away from a bed, within the first 8 postoperative hours is critical to predictably delivering 24 hour recovery. Specific methods and documents are included in Chapter 14.

One of the most rewarding aspects of delivering rapid recovery for surgeons and surgeon personnel is hearing the enthusiastic voice of a patient who is out shopping, out to dinner, or caring for her children the evening of surgery. Representative examples of postoperative calls to patients are included as audio files in the Resources folder on the DVDs that accompany this book.

■ LONG-TERM CARE

Longer term, optimal outcomes require that surgeons provide follow up, a defined, rapid response to untoward events, and implement defined "out points" for implant removal without replacement. Chapter 16 addresses the difficult decision process when optimal patient long-term interests are best served by implant removal without replacement.[8] Chapter 18 provides detailed, comprehensive information and management algorithms for complications and issues in breast augmentation that were defined by the Food and Drug Administration and patient advocate groups.[9]

■ REFERENCES

1. Tebbetts JB: An approach that integrates patient education and informed consent in breast augmentation. *Plast Reconstr Surg* 110(3):971–978, 2002.

2. Tebbetts JB: A system for breast implant selection based on patient tissue characteristics and implant–soft tissue dynamics. *Plast Reconstr Surg* 109(4):1396–1409, 2002.

3. Tebbetts JB, Adams WP: Five critical decisions in breast augmentation using 5 measurements in 5 minutes: the high five system. *Plast Reconstr Surg* 116(7):2005–2016, 2005.

4. Tebbetts JB: Dual plane (DP) breast augmentation: optimizing implant–soft tissue relationships in a wide range of breast types. *Plast Reconstr Surg* 107:1255, 2001.

5. Tebbetts JB: Achieving a predictable 24 hour return to normal activities after breast augmentation Part I: Refining practices using motion and time study principles. *Plast Reconstr Surg* 109:273–290, 2002.

6. Tebbetts JB: Achieving a predictable 24 hour return to normal activities after breast augmentation Part II: Patient preparation, refined surgical techniques and instrumentation. *Plast Reconstr Surg* 109:293–305, 2002.

7. Tebbetts JB: Patient acceptance of adequately filled breast implants using the tilt test. *Plast Reconstr Surg* 106(1):139–147, 2000.

8. Tebbetts JB: Out points criteria for breast implant removal without replacement and criteria to minimize reoperations following breast augmentation. *Plast Reconstr Surg* 114(5):1258–1262, 2004.

9. Adams WP, Bengtson BP, Glicksman CA, et al. Decision and management algorithms to address patient and Food and Drug Administration concerns regarding augmentation and implants. *Plast Reconstr Surg* 114(5):1252–1257, 2004.

Defining Difficult Decisions and Out Points

Breast augmentation is a totally elective cosmetic surgical procedure. When a patient chooses to have a breast augmentation, the patient is choosing to place a medical device into the body—a device that is not medically necessary.

Each medical device has potential benefits, but every device also has potential risks, tradeoffs, and costs. Each medical device can potentially produce positive effects, but can also produce negative effects or undesired outcomes. Every patient who chooses to have breast augmentation should understand and accept that if certain problems or clinical situations arise, their surgeon will recommend removal of both implants without replacement. Every surgeon's first responsibility is the welfare of the patient, not the implant, and implant removal without replacement is sometimes the best option to minimize additional reoperations, risks, costs, and chances of developing uncorrectable deformities.

Most patients, in the author's practice experience, want to keep their implants regardless of the untoward events that occur. Most surgeons want to please their patients. Removing and not replacing breast implants is one of the most difficult decisions for surgeons and patients. Patients that are thoroughly informed preoperatively of specific events or conditions in which implant removal without replacement is in their best interests, and patients that document their acceptance of those conditions preoperatively are more likely to make the best decisions postoperatively. Explaining why implant removal without replacement is the safest and best option is exceedingly difficult postoperatively when the patient has not heard and acknowledged the explanation and reasons preoperatively.

> Every surgeon's first responsibility is the welfare of the patient, not the implant, and implant removal without replacement is sometimes the best option to minimize additional reoperations, risks, costs, and chances of developing uncorrectable deformities

■ FACTORS THAT AFFECT RESPONSES TO A BREAST IMPLANT

Every medical device implanted into the human body is placed in an environment where certain factors cannot be predicted or controlled by the surgeon or the patient, especially factors related to a patient's individual wound healing characteristics and the genetic characteristics of each individual patient's tissues.

Short- and long-term effects of a breast implant in the body depend on three different sets of factors: device related factors, surgically related factors, and patient wound healing and genetic tissue characteristics factors

A breast implant has a range of effects when placed into the body, effects that continue for the entire time the device is implanted. Short- and long-term effects of a breast implant in the body depend on three different sets of factors: *device related* factors, *surgically related* factors, and patient *wound healing and genetic tissue characteristic* factors. Surgeons and patients have some level of control over device related and surgically related factors, including selection of the type and size of implant, decisions to maximize soft tissue coverage over the implant, and optimizing surgical techniques to minimize tissue trauma and bleeding. Neither surgeons nor patients, however, can predict or control patient wound healing and genetic tissue characteristic factors. Table 16-1 summarizes factors that determine the effects of a breast implant in the body.

Table 16-1. Factors that determine the effects of a breast implant in the body

Implant device related factors	Surgical decision and technique related factors	Patient wound healing and genetic tissue characteristic factors
Implant size	Patient requests and patient's ability to reconcile wishes with tissue characteristics	Tendency to develop thicker, tighter capsule around implant
Implant shape and projection	Implant size	Tendency to produce more fluid around implant
Implant filler material	Implant match to tissue characteristics	Quantity and types of bacteria in breast tissue
Implant shell characteristics	Implant projection and shape	Body ability to resist infection
Implant shell durability	Implant fill volume	Ability of tissues to support implant weight
Implant fill volume	Degree of soft tissue coverage	Ability of tissues to tolerate implant weight and projection without excessive stretch or soft tissue atrophy
Other implant design factors	Implant pocket location Degree of surgical tissue trauma Amount of bleeding Patient compliance with instructions	Tissue response to previous pregnancies and nursing

When surgeons and patients prioritize wishes over the realities and limitations of an individual patient's tissues, compromised outcomes and negative tissue compromises over time are more likely to occur. Surgeons and patients can impact device related factors by choosing implants based on their proved track record and data in Food and Drug Administration (FDA) studies and peer reviewed and published data in indexed medical journals instead of choosing implants based on subjective preferences or marketing hype. Surgeons can definitely impact surgically related factors by implementing quantitative tissue assessment and proved processes for implant selection, by optimizing surgical processes and efficiency that are proved in peer reviewed and published studies, and by implementing techniques that preclude the necessity of unnecessary postoperative adjuncts. Surgeons and patients cannot, however, significantly impact certain wound healing and genetic tissue characteristic factors that can affect outcomes.

When surgeons and patients prioritize wishes over the realities and limitations of an individual patient's tissues, compromised outcomes and negative tissue compromises over time are likely

◼ FACTORS THAT NO SURGEON OR PATIENT CAN PREDICT OR CONTROL

No surgeon and no patient can predict or control a patient's wound healing characteristics or a patient's genetic tissue characteristics that can affect outcomes following breast augmentation. Each patient has unique, individual wound healing characteristics and unique, genetic tissue characteristics that influence the interaction between a breast implant and the surrounding tissues. Individual wound healing characteristics influence the characteristics of the capsule or lining that forms around every breast implant, and affect the degree to which that capsule tightens or contracts which in turn determines whether capsular contracture will cause excessive firmness of the breast or other deformities. Patient wound healing characteristics may also affect the quality of incision scars, risks of infection or fluid production around an implant, and other factors that can affect the aesthetic result. Genetic and hormonal effects of pregnancy and nursing vary from patient to patient, and can affect aesthetic results and outcomes.

No surgeon and no patient can predict or control a patient's wound healing characteristics or a patient's genetic tissue characteristics that can affect outcomes following breast augmentation

A patient's genetically determined tissue characteristics can affect the response of the patient's tissue to the implant, including how much the skin will stretch and thin in response to a specific size implant, and how the breast tissue overlying the implant will respond. Selecting excessively large implants is avoidable by surgeons and patients, but even an appropriate size implant for a patient's visible tissue characteristics may cause excessive stretch of the breast skin envelope in patients whose tissues do not adequately support the weight. Unfortunately, surgeons have no tests available to predict a patient's wound healing or tissue characteristic responses to a breast implant. As a result, no surgeon can predict or control the occurrence or severity of capsular contracture,

A patient's genetically determined tissue characteristics can affect the response of the patient's tissue to the implant, including how much the skin will stretch and thin in response to a specific size implant, and how the breast tissue overlying the implant will respond

infection, tissue stretch deformities, or other conditions relating to patient wound healing and tissue characteristics.

■ REOPERATIONS—THE RISKS, THE TRADEOFFS, AND THE LOGIC

Every additional reoperation that is required following placement of breast implants imposes additional risks, costs, and tradeoffs to the patient. Some reoperations are medically necessary, but others are not. Severe capsular contracture, infection, and fluid accumulation around an implant are medical reasons to perform an additional operation. A patient's request for a size change to a larger or smaller implant, though desirable to the patient, is not medically necessary, and imposes risks and costs that may not be logical medically. For example, although the risk of infection with implant exchange is small, it is not zero, and for the patient who experiences such a complication, the incidence is 100% and may require implant removal without replacement or produce an uncorrectable deformity. Surgeons can virtually eliminate reoperations for size exchange by implementing optimal patient education and informed consent processes preoperatively in which the patient documents her acceptance that her surgeon will only perform a size exchange if medical indications exist for a size exchange.[1]

Every reoperation causes additional surgical trauma and bleeding, and healing after each additional surgery produces more scar tissue, the effects of which are uncontrollable. Seemingly simple operations such as a minor revision for implant malposition or excessive stretch, though usually safe, invoke healing mechanisms that are uncontrollable and can result in exchanging one deformity for another. Logically, reoperations should not be performed for reasons that have no medical necessity, or to address relatively mild aesthetic conditions where the risks and effects of the surgery might possibly produce a change that is worse or different compared to the existing condition.

Implant Removal Without Replacement—The Logic

Breast implants are not medically necessary devices. Regardless of the efforts and costs to place breast implants, if certain conditions or complications occur, continuing to attempt to salvage the implants or leave implants in place can cause permanent damage to a patient's tissues, producing deformities that are uncorrectable.

Once a patient has breast implants, virtually every surgeon and patient want to keep the implants in place. The positive effects of implants make some patients unwilling to even

---

Surgeons can virtually eliminate reoperations for size exchange by implementing optimal patient education and informed consent processes preoperatively in which the patient documents her acceptance that her surgeon will only perform a size exchange if medical indications exist for a size exchange[1]

Logically, reoperations should not be performed for reasons that have no medical necessity, or to address relatively mild aesthetic conditions where the risks and effects of the surgery might possibly produce a change that is worse or different compared to the existing condition

The positive effects of implants make some patients unwilling to even consider removal without replacement under any circumstances

consider removal without replacement under any circumstances. Removal without replacement must be a joint decision of the patient and surgeon, recognizing and acknowledging that the aesthetic consequences of removing implants may be far preferable to possible permanent, uncorrectable deformities and additional reoperations with additional costs and risks if the implants are left in place. Surgeons and patients should define criteria for removal without replacement *before* the patient has a breast augmentation, and the patient should understand and document her acceptance of these conditions in informed consent documents. Surgeons' willingness to adhere to stringent criteria for reoperations determines reoperation rates, risks, tradeoffs, and costs to the patient.

Unilateral Versus Bilateral Implant Removal

Unilateral implant removal encourages patients and surgeons to prioritize implant replacement, often sooner than replacement is medically optimal

When a condition requiring implant removal occurs unilaterally, removing one implant creates a deformity (asymmetry) that virtually guarantees at least one reoperation to replace the implant. Unilateral implant removal encourages patients and surgeons to prioritize implant replacement, often sooner than replacement is medically optimal. Unilateral implant removal can compromise future decisions and the timing of those decisions. When removal is indicated, bilateral implant removal totally avoids these compromises and eliminates a demand for reoperation based on asymmetry.

When removal is indicated, bilateral implant removal totally avoids these compromises and eliminates a demand for reoperation based on asymmetry

Implant Removal Without Replacement—The Criteria

Every surgeon must define personal criteria for implant removal without replacement, based on clinical experience and medical indications, and logic. Based on more than three decades of experience, the author recommends breast implant removal without replacement for the following clinical conditions or situations, and requires that every patient accept and acknowledge these criteria in informed consent documents *before the primary augmentation*:

- Recurrence of capsular contracture after having performed a complete capsulectomy and implant replacement with a new implant for a first capsular contracture of Grade 3 or 4 (limits total reoperations for capsular contracture to two).

- Recurrence of stretch deformity (bottoming, lateral malposition) after a previous attempt at correction of a stretch deformity or excessive tissue thinning, including previous exchange to a smaller implant (limits total reoperations for stretch to two).

- Traction rippling or visible implant edges medially when there is no additional tissue coverage available locally (e.g. conversion of submammary to subpectoral), or when pectoralis coverage has been previously compromised by division of medial pectoralis origins.

- Culture documented contamination or infection of the periprosthetic pocket, regardless of implant type or pocket location (any occurrence of documented infection). Bilateral implant removal without replacement when infection is documented by cultures optimizes rapid resolution and minimizes inflammatory effects on tissues that occur with prolonged salvage efforts, effects that may produce significant and sometimes uncorrectable tissue deformities over time. Further, this approach minimizes risks and costs of future reoperations attempting reimplantation, and eliminates reoperations for recurrent infection or capsular contracture that can occur after attempted reimplantation. Virtually every tissue compromise and uncorrectable deformity that occurs as a result of attempted implant salvage or reimplantation following infection is potentially totally preventable by removal without replacement.

- Recurrent seroma, regardless of negative cultures, after treatment of an initial seroma with exploration, capsulectomy (if indicated), and prolonged drainage.

- Inadequate soft tissue coverage, when pinch thickness of tissues covering any area of the implant is less than 0.5 cm (except when coverage deficit is medial or superior and can be improved by dual plane or retropectoral implant placement).

- In any situation where two previous reoperations have been performed, for any reason (limits reoperations to three, including removal without replacement).

■ CRITERIA TO LIMIT REOPERATIONS

The following criteria have evolved over more than two decades to limit reoperations with their inevitable risks, tradeoffs, and costs:

- No reoperations for implant size exchange if not medically necessary (e.g. a slightly larger implant after performing a capsulectomy, provided adequate soft tissue coverage is available).

- No reoperations for Grade 2 capsular contracture.

- No reoperations for minor stretch deformities (<3 cm additional widening of the intermammary distance due to lateral envelope stretch), <2 cm elongation of nipple-to-inframammary fold distance (bottoming) 6 months or more postoperatively regardless of emptying of upper breast or slight excess volume in lower breast.

- No reoperations to adjust nipple-areola position if sternal notch to nipple distances are within 1.5 cm bilaterally (for either primary or secondary procedures).

- No implant replacement if patient has previously required bilateral implant removal for any condition or suspected condition, including replacement of saline filled implants following removal of silicone gel filled implants to address concerns of connective tissue disease or other undefined symptom complexes or psychological conditions.

- No reoperations if patient is unwilling to sign detailed informed consent documents acknowledging that she understands and accepts that every reoperation involves additional risks, tradeoffs, and costs, that correction of any condition by reoperation is not guaranteed, and that with any reoperation, we may exchange one set of problems or compromises for a different and not necessarily better set of conditions.

■ CLINICAL DATA

Applying the criteria described previously combined with implant selection based on quantifiable tissue characteristics[2] and more detailed patient education and informed consent[1] in 1662 reported cases using textured, saline filled breast implants with up to 7 year followup resulted in an overall reoperation rate of 3%.[3–5] Acknowledging the limitations of comparing the studies, this 3% overall reoperation rate up to 7 years compares favorably to the overall reoperation rates of 13 and 21% at 3 years in the saline premarket approval (PMA) studies of Mentor[6] and McGhan,[7] and to the 20% reoperation rate at 2 years in a silicone gel PMA submission by Inamed Corporation.[8]

Factors including surgeon experience, surgeon technical skill, and categories of reasons for reoperations (device related versus surgically related) and other factors preclude direct, scientifically valid comparisons of our reoperation rates with the PMA reoperation rates. Nevertheless, the large clinical experience with long-term followup reported in our studies[3–5] includes every reoperation for any reason, similar to the PMA study results. In the PMA study, capsular contracture was categorized as a device related reason for reoperation, when in fact surgical tissue trauma and bleeding are significant, if not major stimuli for capsular contracture. A reoperation is a reoperation, regardless of whether the

A reoperation is a reoperation, regardless of whether the patient requests it for size change or an improvement in aesthetics. Selective categorizing and analysis to shade interpretation of results and causes is largely non-productive, if reducing reoperation rates is a goal

Applying the criteria described previously combined with implant selection based on quantifiable tissue characteristics[2] and more detailed patient education and informed consent[1] in 1662 reported cases using textured, saline filled breast implants with up to 7 year followup resulted in an overall reoperation rate of 3%[3–5]

patient requests it for size change or an improvement in aesthetics. Selective categorizing and analysis to shade interpretation of results and causes is largely non-productive, if reducing reoperation rates and optimizing long-term patient outcomes is a goal. Defining and implementing out points and decision and management algorithms have dramatically reduced reoperation rates in our practice over the past two decades.

Reducing reoperation rates with their inevitable risks, tradeoffs, and costs to patients, and reducing the incidence of tissue compromising deformities resulting from multiple reoperations, requires that surgeons define strict criteria for reoperations following breast augmentation and criteria for bilateral implant removal without replacement

■ CONCLUSION

Reducing reoperation rates with their inevitable risks, tradeoffs, and costs to patients, and reducing the incidence of tissue compromising deformities resulting from multiple reoperations, requires that surgeons define strict criteria for reoperations following breast augmentation and criteria for bilateral implant removal without replacement. The criteria described in this paper resulted in overall reoperation rates that are substantially lower compared to overall reoperation rates in recent large PMA submissions to the FDA. Each surgeon must define criteria according to individual surgical experience and practice characteristics, but current FDA rulings and guidance suggest that continued availability of breast implant devices for patients demands that patients experience lower reoperation rates.

■ REFERENCES

1. Tebbetts JB: An approach that integrates patient education and informed consent in breast augmentation. *Plast Reconstr Surg* 110(3):971–978, 2002.

2. Tebbetts JB: A system for breast implant selection based on patient tissue characteristics and implant–soft tissue dynamics. *Plast Reconstr Surg* 109(4):1396–1409, 2002.

3. Tebbetts JB: Patient acceptance of adequately filled breast implants using the tilt test. *Plast Reconstr Surg* 106(1):139–147, 2000.

4. Tebbetts JB: Dual plane (DP) breast augmentation: optimizing implant–soft tissue relationships in a wide range of breast types. *Plast Reconstr Surg* 107:1255, 2001.

5. Tebbetts JB: Achieving a predictable 24 hour return to normal activities after breast augmentation Part II: Patient preparation, refined surgical techniques and instrumentation. *Plast Reconstr Surg* 109:293–305, 2002.

6. Mentor Corporation. *Saline-filled breast implant surgery: making an informed decision.* Santa Barbara: Mentor Corporation, 2000, pp 11–19.

7. McGhan Medical Corporation. *Saline-filled breast implant surgery: making an informed decision*, Santa Barbara: McGhan Medical Corporation, 2000, pp 11–19.

8. Food and Drug Administration. U.S. Food and Drug Administration. General and Plastic Surgery Devices Panel Meeting Transcript. Washington, D.C. October 14–15, 2003. Online. Available: http://www.fda.gov/ohrms/dockets/ac/03/transcripts/3989T1.htm.

Managing Problems and Patient and FDA Concerns

During the United States Food and Drug Administration (FDA) Advisory Panel hearings on October 14 and 15, 2003,[1] the FDA panel members and patient advocate organization representatives voiced concerns about four specific areas regarding breast augmentation and breast implant devices:

1. Reoperation rates in primary breast augmentation
2. Levels, depth, and methods of patient education and informed consent
3. Modes, frequency, and management of silicone gel implant device failures, including management of "silent" ruptures
4. Methods of monitoring and management of symptoms or symptom complexes that may or may not be associated with connective tissue disease or other undefined symptom complexes.

These four concerns and the rates of reoperation that accompany primary breast augmentation in the augmentation core studies (averaging 20% within just 3 years) have remained largely unchanged for more than a decade,[2,3] are independent of the specific type of breast implant, and largely focus on surgeon related issues more than device related issues. Comparing reoperation rates and panel concerns from the 1990 FDA Advisory Panel hearings to the 2000 and 2003 reoperation rates and concerns reveals that while implant devices may have changed (e.g. saline versus silicone), overall reoperation rates for primary augmentation have not changed appreciably. Understandably, scientists on the panel and patient advocacy representatives question why devices, reoperation rates, and outcomes have not improved substantially over the

> Four concerns and the rates of reoperation that accompany primary breast augmentation in the augmentation core studies (averaging 20% within just 3 years) have remained largely unchanged for more than a decade,[2,3] are independent of the specific type of breast implant, and largely focus on surgeon related issues more than device related issues

past decade. Interestingly, when FDA Advisory Panel members questioned surgeons and manufacturer representatives about management of specific clinical entities that concerned the panel, clearly defined management solutions were not readily available. Testimony during the October 2003 panel hearings clearly defined a need for decision and management algorithms for clinical entities that concerned the FDA panel members.

For decades, the world's most successful businesses have understood and implemented the concept of "best practices"—"best" ways to perform business processes, derived from processes that have proved effective in use[4]

For decades, the world's most successful businesses have understood and implemented the concept of "best practices"—"best" ways to perform business processes, derived from processes that have proved effective in use.[4] A "best practice" does not necessarily mean that the process is literally "best"; instead, it suggests that a business practice or process "solution" is a method that has been implemented and has delivered consistently positive results. A wide range of medical specialties are currently deriving best practices for specific clinical situations using evidence based medicine principles integrated with process engineering principles that define proved processes and best practices.

This chapter, derived from a paper published in the October 2004 issue of *Plastic and Reconstructive Surgery*,[5] presents decision and management algorithms that have been implemented for over 5 years in a busy augmentation practice and further expanded and refined by a group of surgeons with a wide range of experience and expertise. The author is grateful to each of the coauthors of this paper for their effort and time to define these important algorithms, and to the editor of the journal for permission to reprint them in this chapter.

◼ A NEED FOR "BEST PRACTICES"

We realized that when faced with an issue or a difficult clinical situation or problem, if we had carefully prospectively defined and documented a process of addressing and managing the problem, management was much easier, more refined, less costly, and more comfortable to us, our patients, and their families

More than 12 years ago, as we (John B. Tebbetts, Terrye Tebbetts—J.B.T., T.T.) focused on expanding and refining our patient education and informed consent practices,[6] we adopted a "best practices" approach to help us and our personnel address specific clinical issues or problems. Problems or situations that arise rarely can often be the most challenging for patients, surgeons, and surgeons' personnel, because patient interaction, management, and clinical "solutions" are less defined compared to everyday clinical situations and issues. We realized that when faced with an issue or a difficult clinical situation or problem, if we had carefully prospectively defined and documented a process of addressing and managing the problem, management was much easier, more refined, less costly, and more comfortable to us, our patients, and their families. Predefined management templates (decision and management algorithms) also allow surgeons to focus on more sophisticated concerns and innovative solutions instead of having to rethink an entire process each time a problem occurs.

■ DECISION AND MANAGEMENT ALGORITHM FLOWCHARTS

As a first step to develop a "best practices" approach to managing issues and problems, we developed decision and management algorithms for specific clinical problems or issues that we have encountered over the past two decades. Developing decision and management algorithms is a stimulating and challenging process. Despite the fact that alternative approaches to every clinical problem or issue exist, a flowcharted, algorithmic approach demands a "solution" compared to a list of alternatives that stimulate endless debate. A decision algorithm flowchart is a visible template that depicts one process that has proved clinically useful and can be easily changed or adjusted when new facts or data become available. Graphically representing thought processes, decisions, and actions stimulates alternative thinking about problems or issues. A graphic algorithm flowchart helps surgeons define the sequence of decisions, and the logic of management alternatives. In addition, the process stimulates surgeons to reexamine sacrosanct "answers" and develop even better solutions.

When issues or problems occur, the patient usually speaks first with a surgeon's personnel, and the information they receive in response to their problem, concern, or issue can have a critical impact on the patient's comfort and confidence as the surgeon and the surgeon's staff address the problem. Decision and management algorithms are invaluable to train personnel—not necessarily to deliver definitive answers, but to develop a basic knowledge of how we will approach problems when they arise. Consistency in decision making and management processes builds confidence in a surgeon's personnel, and that confidence transmits directly to patients when they most need confidence to deal with issues and adversity.

Defined processes to manage issues and problems are most effective when patients are aware of how an issue or problem will be managed *before* the issue or problem arises. As we (J.B.T., T.T.) implemented our decision and management algorithms, we learned that their value increased exponentially when we used them to help educate our patients *preoperatively* about how we would manage each issue or problem postoperatively, offering them alternatives of management and an opportunity to help make sometimes difficult decisions.

A decision algorithm flowchart is a visible template that depicts one process that has proved clinically useful and can be easily changed or adjusted when new facts or data become available

Decision and management algorithms are invaluable to train personnel—not necessarily to deliver definitive answers, but to develop a basic knowledge of how we will approach problems when they arise

Defined processes to manage issues and problems are most effective when patients are aware of how an issue or problem will be managed *before* the issue or problem arises

■ PATIENT EDUCATION AND INFORMED CONSENT

When a clinical situation or problem arises postoperatively, the more a patient knows from preoperative education about the problem, how it will be handled, who is responsible for costs, and the chances for correction, the more comfortably the patient can face the challenges. Preoperative informed consent materials and documents addressing the most common potential postoperative problems are available online from a previous publication,[6] and are also included in the Resources folder on the DVDs that accompany this book. When a reoperation may be necessary, patients are often more stressed and face additional costs and risks compared to the primary operation. Before undertaking any reoperation procedure, detailed information and informed consent documentation are arguably more critical and more challenging compared to the primary operation. Detailed decision and management algorithms—which contain essential summary information of potential benefits and risks to help clarify the realistic choices or alternatives, and contain spaces for the patient to document her understanding and acceptance of choices at each decision making stage—are invaluable to assure optimal informed consent and guarantee the patient's involvement in the decision making process. According to Mark Gorney, M.D., "It is the prerogative of the patient and not the physician to determine the direction in which it is believed his or her best interests lie",[7] emphasizing that informed consent law mandates that patients be involved in the decision making process. An integrated document that defines alternatives, provides potential risk and benefit information, and documents the patient's choices and decisions helps surgeons assure optimal informed consent before a reoperation. More importantly, the documents can sometimes prevent unnecessary reoperations such as implant size exchange by providing patients more definitive information about the risks and tradeoffs they may incur. By demanding that the patient accept responsibility for her decisions, optimal informed consent documents sometimes encourage patients to reconsider their requests and decisions.

> According to Mark Gorney, M.D., "It is the prerogative of the patient and not the physician to determine the direction in which it is believed his or her best interests lie",[7] emphasizing that informed consent law mandates that patients be involved in the decision making process

■ PRACTICAL CLINICAL INTEGRATION AND IMPLEMENTATION

Currently in our practice (J.B.T., T.T.), each decision and management algorithm integrates with (a) information provided the patient in preoperative patient education and informed consent documents, and (b) more detailed information and alternatives contained in additional education and informed consent documents when an issue or problem occurs. After providing the patient with detailed information addressing a specific clinical situation or problem, a patient educator and the surgeon review the information with the patient in detail. After discussion and answering the patient's questions, the patient then re-reads and signs the informed consent document and defines her choices on the decision and management flowchart to verify her understanding and acceptance of the information and the choices she makes.

Reality sometimes demands difficult choices, none of which may seem ideal

Reality sometimes demands difficult choices, none of which may seem ideal. One of the most difficult challenges in managing issues and problems is defining choices—translating a myriad of grey areas, unknowns, questions, wishes, and fears into realistic alternatives from which a patient may choose. A second challenge is helping the patient understand that there is no perfect choice—not at the primary operation, and certainly not at a reoperation for an issue or problem—there are only different sets of tradeoffs, benefits, risks, and costs for each alternative. A clearly defined approach to management of each issue or problem, and a practical, efficient system to optimize patient education and informed consent, are invaluable. On first review, decision and management algorithms may seem complex, but they are only as complex as required to define the alternatives available to the patient according to informed consent law.

One of the most difficult challenges in managing issues and problems is defining choices

■ MANAGEMENT AND DECISION ALGORITHM FLOWCHARTS— OBJECTIVES AND LOGIC

Each of the following flowcharts addresses a specific clinical problem or issue. None is intended to be definitive. No "best practice" is ever definitive. Instead, each algorithm is simply an snapshot in time of an process that has proved clinically useful and effective—a template alternative that surgeons can examine, modify and individualize according to surgeon and patient preferences and specific clinical situations. Each algorithm flowchart is a continuous work in progress that provides a basic set of alternatives from which to evolve better solutions.

For efficiency and to provide as much summary information as possible while outlining choices in flowchart form to help the patient make decisions, each decision and management flowchart incorporates two additional components: (1) a summary of potential benefits and tradeoffs associated with each decision, and (2) a space for the patient to specifically accept or decline alternatives at each stage of the decision making process, documented in writing by the patient's initials.

Each algorithm flowchart has six specific objectives that coincide with concerns expressed by patients and the FDA

Each algorithm flowchart has six specific objectives that coincide with concerns expressed by patients and the FDA: (1) minimize reoperations, (2) prioritize alternatives that are most likely to reduce reoperations, (3) define realistic choices for surgeon and patient,

(4) involve the patient in the decision making process, (5) define "out" points for removal without replacement in specific clinical situations, and (6) provide thorough documentation of choices and assumption of responsibility for the choices. When examining any decision or management suggestion in the algorithm flowcharts, surgeons should carefully consider these priorities. In each flowchart, decisions and management alternatives are prioritized in a specific order to prevent additional reoperations with their inevitable risks and costs.

Every reoperation increases costs and risks. Reoperation rates approximating 20% are, at the least, highly questionable for medically necessary operations, and are logically unjustifiable for any totally elective, primary cosmetic surgical procedure. Implant size change, a common reoperation which may be a totally elective patient preference, increases risks and costs. If preoperative patient education and informed consent are optimal, and implant size choice is based on quantifiable tissue characteristics, reoperations for size change can be virtually eliminated.[6,8–10] A reoperation is a reoperation, regardless of whether it is medically necessary or requested by the patient for aesthetic or personal reasons. Reoperations inarguably increase costs and risks that would not be present if the reoperation did not occur. While patients have a right to request operations they choose, limiting medically unnecessary reoperations and reducing overall reoperation rates require that surgeons define and enforce strict indications for reoperations.

Implant removal without replacement is an alternative available to every surgeon and every patient before performing any reoperation following breast augmentation, and is the most certain alternative to minimize additional risks, costs of reoperations, and potentially uncorrectable deformities. If implant size choice was based on quantifiable tissue dimensions and characteristics preoperatively, implant removal without replacement (in the absence of infection or severe inflammation) usually allows the breast to return to a form that approximates the effects of a pregnancy on the breast. Few patients or surgeons ever want to remove breast implants after the patient has experienced their benefits. In specific situations (e.g. multiple reoperations for capsular contracture, multiple attempts to salvage contaminated or infected implants, or severe stretching or thinning of overlying tissues with traction rippling or visible implant edges), implant removal without replacement is medically the best and most logical solution.

Genetic characteristics of patients' tissues that allow excessive stretching with even small implants, wound healing predispositions that produce recurrent capsular contractures,

---

Sidebar notes:

Reoperation rates approximating 20% are, at the least, highly questionable for medically necessary operations, and are logically unjustifiable for any totally elective, primary cosmetic surgical procedure

Genetic characteristics of patients' tissues that allow excessive stretching with even small implants, wound healing predispositions that produce recurrent capsular contractures, and inflammatory processes around an implant are all factors that surgeons cannot predict or control

If preoperative patient education and informed consent are optimal, and implant size choice is based on quantifiable tissue characteristics, reoperations for size change can be virtually eliminated[6,8,9,10]

In specific situations (e.g. multiple reoperations for capsular contracture, multiple attempts to salvage contaminated or infected implants, or severe stretching or thinning of overlying tissues with traction rippling or visible implant edges), implant removal without replacement is medically the best and most logical solution

and inflammatory processes around an implant are all factors that surgeons cannot predict or control. Patients should understand and document their acceptance of those facts before the primary augmentation. When any of those events occur, surgeons and patients need predefined "out" points discussed and agreed upon preoperatively before the primary augmentation. These "out" points are criteria defined and accepted before the primary augmentation for bilateral implant removal without replacement.[11] When patients or surgeons choose to not define these "out" points, or choose not to remove and not replace implants when irreversible tissue consequences are present, both patient and surgeon assume responsibility for risks of deformities which may be uncorrectable.

■ DECISION AND MANAGEMENT ALGORITHMS

The following six decision and management algorithm flowcharts address the following clinical issues or problems: implant size exchange, capsular contracture grades 3–4, infection, stretch deformities (implant bottoming or displacement), silent rupture of gel implants, and patients presenting with undefined symptom complexes that may be associated with connective tissue disease (CTD) or other undefined problems. Each of these algorithms has evolved in our (J.B.T., T.T.) clinical practice over the past 5 years and has been effective in helping us address these issues, resulting in an overall reoperation rate of 3%, deflation or implant failure rate of 0.78%, and a reoperation rate of 0.24% for size adjustment or exchange in 1662 cases reported in the journal *Plastic and Reconstructive Surgery* with up to 7 year followup.[8–10] The same processes in these algorithms also resulted in a zero percent reoperation rate at 3 years in a consecutive series of 50 patients in the FDA premarket approval (PMA) study for the Allergan Style 410 implant.[12] Each algorithm presented in this paper addresses a specific clinical situation of concern to the FDA Advisory Panel of 2003.

■ REFINING THE DECISION AND MANAGEMENT ALGORITHMS— A SURGEONS FOR PATIENTS INITIATIVE

Additional input from surgeons with a wide range of experience and expertise could undoubtedly refine and improve the decision and management algorithms derived in a single practice. Ethical issues, medicolegal issues, variations in practice orientation and management, and issues addressing standards of practice could best be addressed by seeking input from other surgeons with expertise in each of these areas. Variations in practice occur as practices evolve. Fresh, innovative ideas and approaches from surgeons earlier in their practice careers are essential for solutions to be applicable to the widest possible range of practices.

To further improve and widen the scope of the decision and management algorithms, we (J.B.T., T.T.) sought the input and expertise of the other authors of the paper on this topic in the journal *Plastic and Reconstructive Surgery*.[5] To address patient and FDA concerns, the Breast Augmentation Surgeons for Patients Initiative (BASPI) focused on a single objective—reducing reoperation rates in breast augmentation. The participants who coauthor this paper each prepared extensively by developing and submitting alternative decision and management solutions for each topic listed previously. During 2 days of intensive workgroup sessions and followup communications to verify revisions, key points from all participants' solutions were integrated to derive the final algorithms presented in this paper.

The effort by this joint workgroup of plastic surgeons with diverse backgrounds and experience was to develop decision and management algorithms to assist in reducing reoperation rates in breast augmentation and improve patient outcomes. All templates are optional, additional resources for surgeons to consider when addressing the specific clinical topics listed previously.

BASPI materials and solutions are designed to codify and present information and alternatives to make repetitive decision making processes more efficient by defining templates for management that have proved effective in long-term clinical experience. Basic management templates allow surgeons to focus on more detailed specifics of each clinical situation to hopefully improve reoperation rates and outcomes. BASPI provides defined solutions that prove to patients, the FDA, and patient advocate groups that defined alternatives and solutions exist to address their areas of concern regarding causes of reoperations.

Materials and solutions from BASPI are not intended to define standards of practice. Rather, the templates are intended to delineate a set of options to patients and surgeons, not define or limit surgeon or patient choices. No component of any algorithm is intended to supplant any area of surgeon clinical decision making. These decision and management algorithms cannot and do not address all of the variables that may exist in any clinical situation and, in every situation, must be adjusted by the surgeon to fit the clinical issues.

■ CONCLUSION

Defined management algorithms have proved invaluable to a wide range of businesses and professionals to optimize business practices and address issues and problems. The decision and management algorithms presented in this chapter (Tables 17-1 to 17-5) have

> BASPI materials and solutions are designed to codify and present information and alternatives to make repetitive decision making processes more efficient by defining templates for management that have proved effective in long-term clinical experience

> Defined management algorithms have proved invaluable to a wide range of businesses and professionals to optimize business practices and address issues and problems

Table 17-1. Decision support flowchart for implant size exchange.

Implant Size Exchange to Larger Implants Alternatives for
John B. Tebbetts, M.D.
Copyright 2000

**The larger a patients' breasts, augmented or not, the worse the breasts are likely to look over time. Also, the larger the breasts following a breast augmentation, the greater the risks of additional operations, additional risks costs to the patient, and additional risks of permanent, uncorrectable deformities.

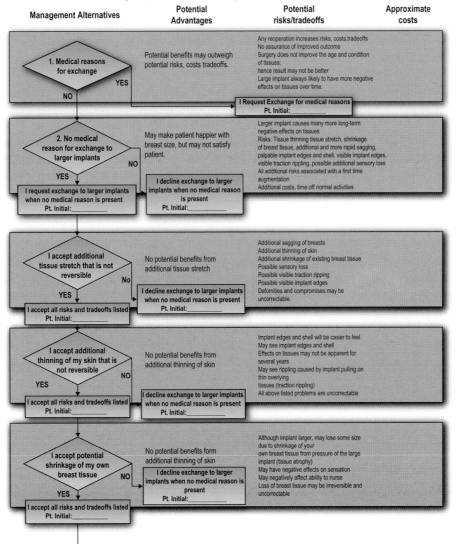

Management Alternatives	Potential Advantages	Potential risks/tradeoffs	Approximate costs

1. Medical reasons for exchange — YES / NO

Potential benefits may outweigh potential risks, costs tradeoffs.

Any reoperation increases risks, costs,tradeoffs
No assurance of improved outcome
Surgery does not improve the age and condition of tissues;
hence result may not be better
Large implant always likely to have more negative effects on tissues over time.

I Request Exchange for medical reasons
Pt. Initial:_____

2. No medical reason for exchange to larger implants — YES / NO

May make patient happier with breast size, but may not satisfy patient.

Larger implant causes many more long-term negative effects on tissues
Risks: Tissue thinning tissue stretch, shrinkage of breast tissue, additional and more rapid sagging, palpable implant edges and shell, visible implant edges, visible traction rippling, possible additional sensory loss
All additional risks associated with a first time augmentation
Additional costs, time off normal activities

I request exchange to larger implants when no medical reason is present
Pt. Initial:_____

I decline exchange to larger implants when no medical reason is present
Pt. Initial:_____

I accept additional tissue stretch that is not reversible — YES / No

No potential benefits from additional tissue stretch

Additional sagging of breasts
Additional thinning of skin
Additional shrinkage of existing breast tissue
Possible sensory loss
Possible visible traction ripping
Possible visible implant edges
Deformities and compromises may be uncorrectable.

I accept all risks and tradeoffs listed
Pt. Initial:_____

I decline exchange to larger implants when no medical reason is present
Pt. Initial:_____

I accept additional thinning of my skin that is not reversible — YES / NO

No potential benefits from additional thinning of skin

Implant edges and shell will be easier to feel
May see implant edges and shell
Effects on tissues may not be apparent for several years
May see rippling caused by implant pulling on thin overlying tissues (traction rippling)
All above listed problems are uncorrectable

I accept all risks and tradeoffs listed
Pt. Initial:_____

I decline exchange to larger implants when no medical reason is present
Pt. Initial:_____

I accept potential shrinkage of my own breast tissue — YES / NO

No potential benefits form additional thinning of skin

Although implant larger, may lose some size due to shrinkage of your own breast tissue from pressure of the large implant (tissue atrophy)
May have negative effects on sensation
May negatively affect ability to nurse
Loss of breast tissue may be irreversible and uncorrectable

I decline exchange to larger implants when no medical reason is present
Pt. Initial:_____

I accept all risks and tradeoffs listed
Pt. Initial:_____

Table 17-1. Decision support flowchart for implant size exchange.—cont'd

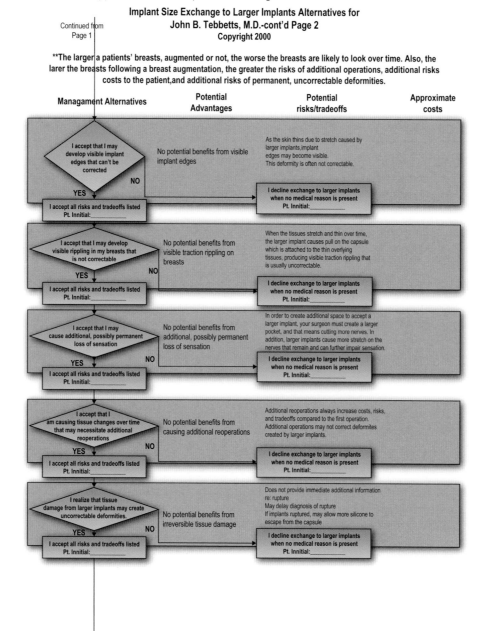

Implant Size Exchange to Larger Implants Alternatives for
John B. Tebbetts, M.D.-cont'd Page 2
Copyright 2000

Table 17-1. Decision support flowchart for implant size exchange.—cont'd

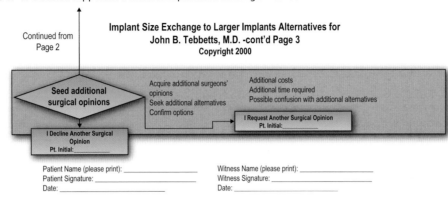

been used successfully for 5 years in a busy breast augmentation practice, and further expanded and refined by surgeons with a wide range of experience and expertise to address the following issues and concerns that have been expressed by patients and the FDA: implant size exchange, capsular contracture grades 3–4, infection, stretch deformities (implant bottoming or displacement), silent rupture of gel implants, and patients presenting with undefined symptom complexes (CTD or other).

Text continued on p. 415

Table 17-2. Decision support flowchart for management of capsular contracture.

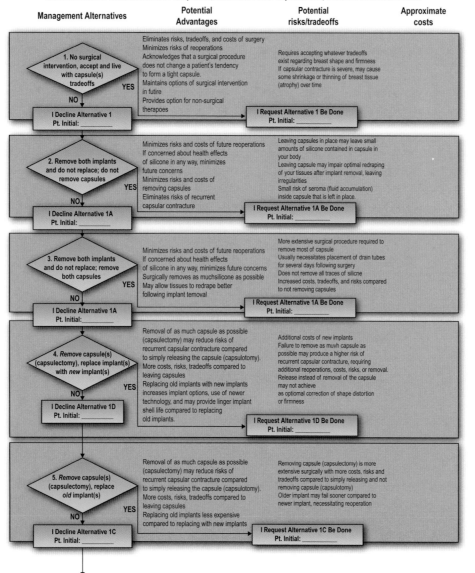

Alternatives for Management of Capsular Contracture
John B.Tebbetts, M.D.
Copyright 2000

Management Alternatives — Potential Advantages — Potential risks/tradeoffs — Approximate costs

1. No surgical intervention, accept and live with capsule(s) tradeoffs

Potential Advantages: Eliminates risks, tradeoffs, and costs of surgery. Minimizes risks of reoperations. Acknowledges that a surgical procedure does not change a patient's tendency to form a tight capsule. Maintains options of surgical intervention in future. Provides option for non-surgical therapoes

Potential risks/tradeoffs: Requires accepting whatever tradeoffs exist regarding breast shape and firmness. If capsular contracture is severe, may cause some shrinkage or thinning of breast tissue (atrophy) over time

YES → I Request Alternative 1 Be Done / Pt. Initial: ___

NO → I Decline Alternative 1 / Pt. Initial: ___

2. Remove both implants and do not replace; do not remove capsules

Potential Advantages: Minimizes risks and costs of future reoperations. If concerned about health effects of silicone in any way, minimizes future concerns. Minimizes risks and costs of removing capsules. Eliminates risks of recurrent capsular contracture

Potential risks/tradeoffs: Leaving capsules in place may leave small amounts of silicone contained in capsule in your body. Leaving capsule may impair optimal redraping of your tissues after implant removal, leaving irregularities. Small risk of seroma (fluid accumulation) inside capsule that is left in place.

YES → I Request Alternative 1A Be Done / Pt. Initial: ___

NO → I Decline Alternative 1A / Pt. Initial: ___

3. Remove both implants and do not replace; remove both capsules

Potential Advantages: Minimizes risks and costs of future reoperations. If concerned about health effects of silicone in any way, minimizes future concerns. Surgically removes as muchsilicone as possible. May allow tissues to redrape better following implant temoval

Potential risks/tradeoffs: More extensive surgical procedure required to remove most of capsule. Usually necessitates placement of drain tubes for several days following surgery. Does not remove all traces of silicone. Increased costs, tradeoffs, and risks compared to not removing capsules

YES → I Request Alternative 1A Be Done / Pt. Initial: ___

NO → I Decline Alternative 1A / Pt. Initial: ___

4. *Remove* capsule(s) (capsulectomy), replace implant(s) with *new* implant(s)

Potential Advantages: Removal of as much capsule as possible (capsulectomy) may reduce risks of recurrent capsular contracture compared to simply releasing the capsule (capsulotomy). More costs, risks, tradeoffs compared to leaving capsules. Replacing old implants with new implants increases implant options, use of newer technology, and may provide linger implant shell life compared to replacing old implants.

Potential risks/tradeoffs: Additional costs of new implants. Failure to remove as muvh capsule as possible may produce a higher risk of recurrent capsular contracture, requiring additional reoperations, costs, risks, or removal. Release instead of removal of the capsule may not achieve as optimal correction of shape distortion or firmness

YES → I Request Alternative 1D Be Done / Pt. Initial: ___

NO → I Decline Alternative 1D / Pt. Initial: ___

5. *Remove* capsule(s) (capsulectomy), replace *old* implant(s)

Potential Advantages: Removal of as much capsule as possible (capsulectomy) may reduce risks of recurrent capsular contracture compared to simply releasing the capsule (capsulotomy). More costs, risks, tradeoffs compared to leaving capsules. Replacing old implants less expensive compared to replacing with new implants

Potential risks/tradeoffs: Removing capsule (capsulectomy) is more extensive surgically with more costs, risks and tradeoffs compared to simply releasing and not removing capsule (capsulotomy). Older implant may fail sooner compared to newer implant, necessitating reoperation

YES → I Request Alternative 1C Be Done / Pt. Initial: ___

NO → I Decline Alternative 1C / Pt. Initial: ___

**Management alternatives are listed prioritizing alternatives most likely to reduce risks of additional operations, reduce additional risks and costs to the patient, and reduce risks of permanent, uncorrectable deformities.

Table 17-2. Decision support flowchart for management of capsular contracture.—cont'd

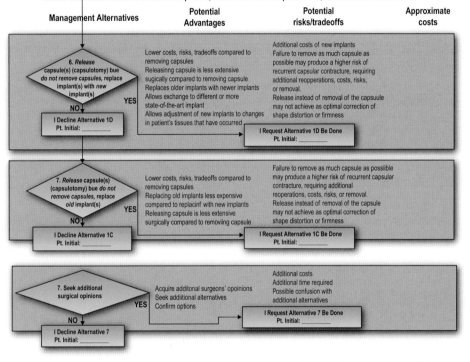

Continued from
Page 1

Alternatives for Management of Capsular Contracture
Continued from Page 1

**Management alternatives are listed prioritizing alternatives most likely to reduce risks of additional operations, reduce additional risks and costs to the patient, and reduce risks of permanent, uncorrectable deformities.

Management Alternatives	Potential Advantages	Potential risks/tradeoffs	Approximate costs

6. *Release* capsule(s) (capsulotomy) bue *do not remove capsules,* replace implant(s) with *new* implant(s)

YES

NO
I Decline Alternative 1D
Pt. Initial: _____

Lower costs, risks, tradeoffs compared to removing capsules
Releasinng capsule is less extensive sugically compared to removing capsule
Replaces older implants with newer implants
Allows exchange to different or more state-of-the-art implant
Allows adjustment of new implants to changes in patient's tissues that have occurred

Additional costs of new implants
Failure to remove as much capsule as possible may produce a higher risk of recurrent capsular contracture, requiring additional reopperations, costs, risks, or removal.
Release instead of removal of the capsule may not achieve as optimal correction of shape distortion or firmness

I Request Alternative 1D Be Done
Pt. Initial: _____

7. *Release* capsule(s) (capsulotomy) bue *do not remove capsules,* replace *old* implant(s)

YES

NO
I Decline Alternative 1C
Pt. Initial: _____

Lower costs, risks, tradeoffs compared to removing capsules
Replacing old implants less expensive compared to replacinf with new implants
Releasing capsule is less extensive surgically compared to removiling capsule

Failure to remove as much capsule as possiible may produce a higher risk of recurrent capsular contracture, requiring additional reoperations, costs, risks, or removal.
Release instead of removal of the capsule may not achieve as optimal correction of shape distortion or firmness

I Request Alternative 1C Be Done
Pt. Initial: _____

7. Seek additional surgical opinions

YES

NO
I Decline Alternative 7
Pt. Initial: _____

Acquire additonal surgeons' opoinions
Seek addiitional alternatives
Confirm options

Additional costs
Additional time required
Possible confusion with additional alternatives

I Request Alternative 7 Be Done
Pt. Initial: _____

**If patient, surgeon, or patient's family are concerned about any aspect of silicone causing symptoms or possible associated conditions, see additional information and flowchart alternatives entitled "If Patient Has Symptoms or Concerens Related to Silicone"

Patient Name (please print): _____   Witness Name (please print): _____
Patient Signature: _____   Witness Signature: _____
Date: _____   Date: _____

Table 17-3. Decision support flowchart for management of possible periprosthetic space infection.

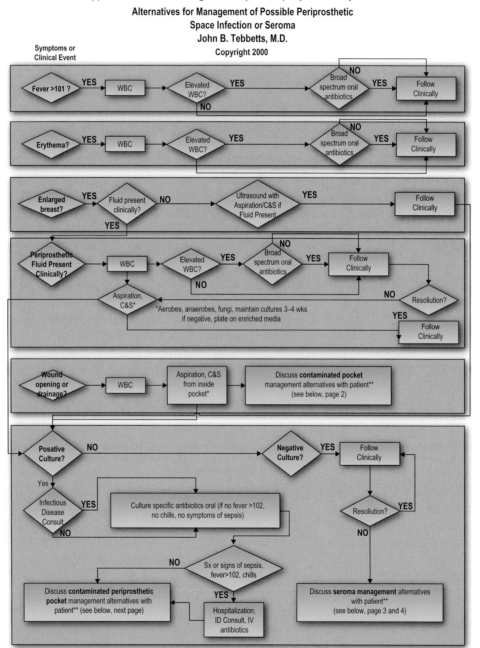

Alternatives for Management of Possible Periprosthetic
Space Infection or Seroma
John B. Tebbetts, M.D.
Copyright 2000

Table 17-3. Decision support flowchart for management of possible periprosthetic space infection.—cont'd

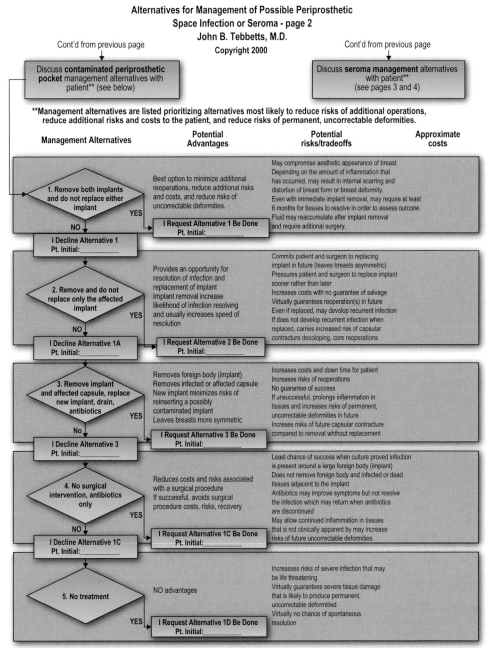

Alternatives for Management of Possible Periprosthetic Space Infection or Seroma - page 2
John B. Tebbetts, M.D.
Copyright 2000

Cont'd from previous page

Cont'd from previous page

Discuss **contaminated periprosthetic pocket** management alternatives with patient** (see below)

Discuss **seroma management** alternatives with patient** (see pages 3 and 4)

Management alternatives are listed prioritizing alternatives most likely to reduce risks of additional operations, reduce additional risks and costs to the patient, and reduce risks of permanent, uncorrectable deformities.

Management Alternatives	Potential Advantages	Potential risks/tradeoffs	Approximate costs
1. Remove both implants and do not replace either implant YES / NO — I Decline Alternative 1 Pt. Initial:_____ / I Request Alternative 1 Be Done Pt. Initial:_____	Best option to minimize additional reoperations, reduce additional risks and costs, and reduce risks of uncorrectable deformities.	May compromise aesthetic appearance of breast Depending on the amount of inflammation that has occurred, may result in internal scarring and distortion of breast form or breast deformity. Even with immediate implant removal, may require at least 6 months for tissues to resolve in order to assess outcone. Fluid may reaccumulate after implant removal and require aditional surgery.	
2. Remove and do not replace only the affected implant YES / NO — I Decline Alternative 1A Pt. Initial:_____ / I Request Alternative 2 Be Done Pt. Initial:_____	Provides an opportunity for resolution of infection and replacement of implant Implant removal increase likelihood of infection resolving and usually increases speed of resolution	Commits patient and surgeon to replacing implant in future (leaves breasts asymmetric) Pressures patient and surgeon to replace implant sooner rather than later Increases costs with no guarantee of salvage Virtually guarantees reoperation(s) in future Even if replaced, may devolop recurrent infection If does not develop recurrent infection when replaced, carries increased risk of capsular contracture decoloping, core reoperations	
3. Remove implant and affected capsule, replace new implant, drain, antibiotics YES / No — I Decline Alternative 3 Pt. Initial:_____ / I Request Alternative 3 Be Done Pt. Initial:_____	Removes foreign body (implant) Removes infected or affected capsule New implant minimizes risks of reinserting a possibly contaminated implant Leaves breasts more symmetric	Increases costs and down time for patient Increases risks of reoperations No guarantee of success If unsuccessful, prolongs inflammation in tissues and increases risks of permanent, uncorrectable deformities in future Increase risks of future capsular contracture compared to removal whthout replacement	
4. No surgical intervention, antibiotics only YES / NO — I Decline Alternative 1C Pt. Initial:_____ / I Request Alternative 1C Be Done Pt. Initial:_____	Reduces costs and risks associated with a surgical procedure If successful, avoids surgical procedure costs, risks, recovery	Least chance of success when culture proved infection is present around a large foreign body (implant) Does not remove foreign body and infected or dead tissues adjacent to the implant Antibiotics may improve symptoms but not resolve the infection which may return when antibiotics are discontinued May allow continued inflammation in tissues that is not clinically apparent by may increase risks of future uncorrectable deformities.	
5. No treatment YES — I Request Alternative 1D Be Done Pt. Initial:_____	NO advantages	Increases risks of severe infection that may be life threatening Virtually guarantees severe tissue damage that is likely to produce permanent, uncorrectable deformitied Virtually no chance of spontaneous resolution	

409

Table 17-3. Decision support flowchart for management of possible periprosthetic space infection.—cont'd

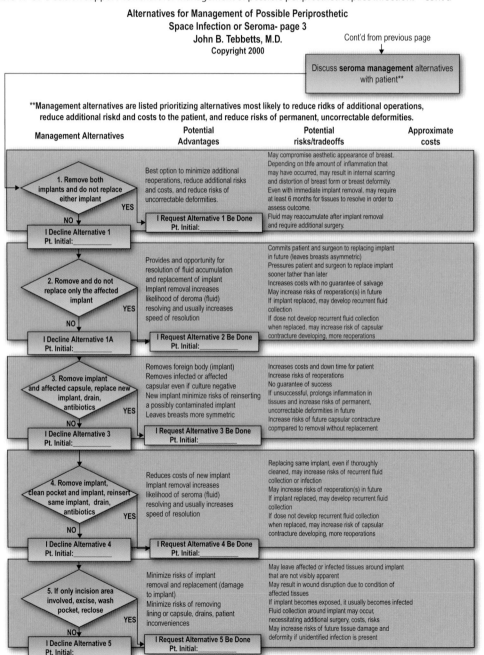

Alternatives for Management of Possible Periprosthetic
Space Infection or Seroma- page 3
John B. Tebbetts, M.D.
Copyright 2000

Cont'd from previous page

Discuss **seroma management** alternatives with patient**

**Management alternatives are listed prioritizing alternatives most likely to reduce ridks of additional operations, reduce additional riskd and costs to the patient, and reduce risks of permanent, uncorrectable deformities.

Management Alternatives	Potential Advantages	Potential risks/tradeoffs	Approximate costs
1. Remove both implants and do not replace either implant — YES	Best option to minimize additional reoperations, reduce additional risks and costs, and reduce risks of uncorrectable deformities.	May compromise aesthetic appearance of breast. Depending on thfe amount of inflammation that may have occurred, may result in internal scarring and distortion of breast form or breast deformity. Even with immediate implant removal, may require at least 6 months for tissues to resolve in order to assess outcome. Fluid may reaccumulate after implant removal and require additional surgery.	
NO → I Decline Alternative 1 Pt. Initial:___	I Request Alternative 1 Be Done Pt. Initial:___		
2. Romove and do not replace only the affected implant — YES	Provides and opportunity for resolution of fluid accumulation and replacement of implant Implant removal increases likelihood of deroma (fluid) resolving and usually increases speed of resolution	Commits patient and surgeon to replacing implant in future (leaves breasts asymmetric) Pressures patient and surgeon to replace implant sooner tather than later Increases costs with no guarantee of salvage May increase risks of reoperation(s) in future If implant replaced, may develop recurrent fluid collection If dose not develop recurrent fluid collection when replaced, may increase risk of capsular contracture developing, more reoperations	
NO → I Decline Alternative 1A Pt. Initial:___	I Request Alternative 2 Be Done Pt. Initial:___		
3. Romove implant and affected capsule, replace new implant, drain, antibiotics — YES	Removes foreign body (implant) Removes infected or affected capsular even if culture negative New implant minimize risks of reinserting a possibly contaminated implant Leaves breasts more symmetric	Increases costs and down time for patient Increase risks of reoperations No guarantee of success If unsuccessful, prolongs inflammation in tissues and increase risks of permanent, uncorrectable deformities in future Increase risks of future capsular contracture copmpared to removal without replacement	
NO → I Decline Alternative 3 Pt. Initial:___	I Request Alternative 3 Be Done Pt. Initial:___		
4. Romove implant, clean pocket and implant, reinsert same implant, drain, antibiotics — YES	Reduces costs of new implant Implant removal increases likelihood of seroma (fluid) resolving and usually increases speed of resolution	Replacing same implant, even if thoroughly cleaned, may increase risks of recurrent fluid collection or infection May increase risks of reoperation(s) in future If implant replaced, may develop recurrent fluid collection If dose not develop recurrent fluid collection when replaced, may increase risk of capsular contracture developing, more reoperations	
NO → I Decline Alternative 4 Pt. Initial:___	I Request Alternative 4 Be Done Pt. Initial:___		
5. If only incision area involved, excise, wash pocket, reclose — YES	Minimize risks of implant removal and replacement (damage to implant) Minimize risks of removing lining or capsule, drains, patient inconveniences	May leave affected or infected tissues around implant that are not visibly apparent May result in wound disruption due to condition of affected tissues If implant becomes exposed, it usually becomes infected Fluid collection around implant may occur, necessitating additional surgery, costs, risks May increase risks of future tissue damage and deformity if unidentified infection is present	
NO → I Decline Alternative 5 Pt. Initial:___	I Request Alternative 5 Be Done Pt. Initial:___		

Table 17-3. Decision support flowchart for management of possible periprosthetic space infection.—cont'd

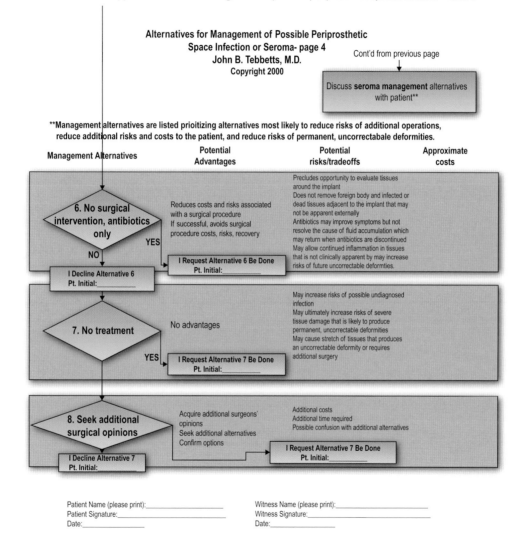

**Alternatives for Management of Possible Periprosthetic
Space Infection or Seroma- page 4**
John B. Tebbetts, M.D.
Copyright 2000

Cont'd from previous page

Discuss **seroma management** alternatives with patient**

**Management alternatives are listed prioitizing alternatives most likely to reduce risks of additional operations, reduce additional risks and costs to the patient, and reduce risks of permanent, uncorrectabale deformities.

Management Alternatives	Potential Advantages	Potential risks/tradeoffs	Approximate costs

6. No surgical intervention, antibiotics only

Reduces costs and risks associated with a surgical procedure
If successful, avoids surgical procedure costs, risks, recovery

Precludes opportunity to evaluate tissues around the implant
Does not remove foreign body and infected or dead tissues adjacent to the implant that may not be apparent externally
Antibiotics may improve symptoms but not resolve the cause of fluid accumulation which may return when antibiotics are discontinued
May allow continued inflammation in tissues that is not clinically apparent by may increase risks of future uncorrectable deformties.

YES

NO

I Request Alternative 6 Be Done
Pt. Initial:_____

I Decline Alternative 6
Pt. Initial:_____

7. No treatment

No advantages

May increase risks of possible undiagnosed infection
May ultimately increase risks of severe tissue damage that is likely to produce permanent, uncorrectable deformities
May cause stretch of tissues that produces an uncorrectable deformity or requires additional surgery

YES

I Request Alternative 7 Be Done
Pt. Initial:_____

8. Seek additional surgical opinions

Acquire additional surgeons' opinions
Seek additional alternatives
Confirm options

Additional costs
Additional time required
Possible confusion with additional alternatives

I Request Alternative 7 Be Done
Pt. Initial:_____

I Decline Alternative 7
Pt. Initial:

Patient Name (please print):_____
Patient Signature:_____
Date:_____

Witness Name (please print):_____
Witness Signature:_____
Date:_____

Table 17-4. Decision support flowchart for management of stretch deformities of the breast.

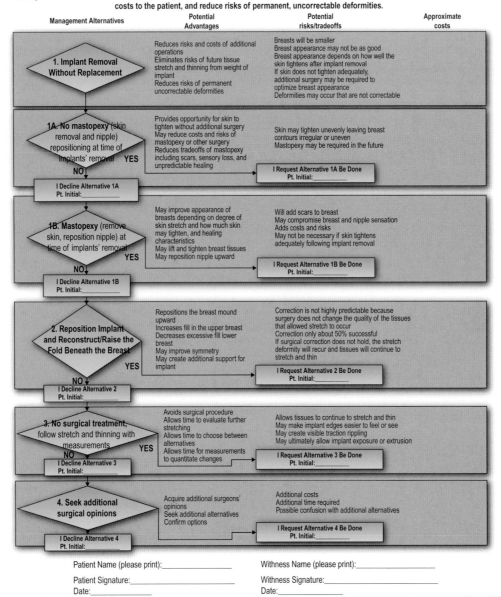

Stretch Deformities of the Breast
John B. Tebbetts, M.D
Copyright 2000

**Management alternatives are listed prioritizing alternatives most likely to reduce risks of additional operations, reduce additional risks and costs to the patient, and reduce risks of permanent, uncorrectable deformities.

Management Alternatives	Potential Advantages	Potential risks/tradeoffs	Approximate costs
1. Implant Removal Without Replacement	Reduces risks and costs of additional operations Eliminates risks of future tissue stretch and thinning from weight of implant Reduces risks of permanent uncorrectable deformities	Breasts will be smaller Breast appearance may not be as good Breast appearance depends on how well the skin tightens after implant removal If skin does not tighten adequately, additional surgery may be required to optimize breast appearance Deformities may occur that are not correctable	
1A. No mastopexy (skin removal and nipple) repositioning at time of implants' removal **YES** / **NO**	Provides opportunity for skin to tighten without additional surgery May reduce costs and risks of mastopexy or other surgery Reduces tradeoffs of mastopexy including scars, sensory loss, and unpredictable healing	Skin may tighten unevenly leaving breast contours irregular or uneven Mastopexy may be required in the future I Request Alternative 1A Be Done Pt. Initial:_____	
I Decline Alternative 1A Pt. Initial:_____			
1B. Mastopexy (remove skin, reposition nipple) at time of implants' removal **YES** / **NO**	May improve appearance of breasts depending on degree of skin stretch and how much skin may tighten, and healing characteristics May lift and tighten breast tissues May reposition nipple upward	Will add scars to breast May compromise breast and nipple sensation Adds costs and risks May not be necessary if skin tightens adequately following implant removal I Request Alternative 1B Be Done Pt. Initial:_____	
I Decline Alternative 1B Pt. Initial:_____			
2. Reposition Implant and Reconstruct/Raise the Fold Beneath the Breast **YES** / **NO**	Repositions the breast mound upward Increases fill in the upper breast Decreases excessive fill lower breast May improve symmetry May create additional support for implant	Correction is not highly predictable because surgery does not change the quality of the tissues that allowed stretch to occur Correction only about 50% successful If surgical correction does not hold, the stretch deformity will recur and tissues will continue to stretch and thin I Request Alternative 2 Be Done Pt. Initial:_____	
I Decline Alternative 2 Pt. Initial:_____			
3. No surgical treatment, follow stretch and thinning with measurements **YES** / **NO**	Avoids surgical procedure Allows time to evaluate further stretching Allows time to choose between alternatives Allows time for measurements to quantitate changes	Allows tissues to continue to stretch and thin May make implant edges easier to feel or see May create visible traction rippling May ultimately allow implant exposure or extrusion I Request Alternative 3 Be Done Pt. Initial:_____	
I Decline Alternative 3 Pt. Initial:_____			
4. Seek additional surgical opinions	Acquire additional surgeons' opinions Seek additional alternatives Confirm options	Additional costs Additional time required Possible confusion with additional alternatives I Request Alternative 4 Be Done Pt. Initial:_____	
I Decline Alternative 4 Pt. Initial:_____			

Patient Name (please print):_____ Witness Name (please print):_____

Patient Signature:_____ Witness Signature:_____

Date:_____ Date:_____

Table 17-5. Decision support flowchart for management of concerns of rupture of silicone gel implant.

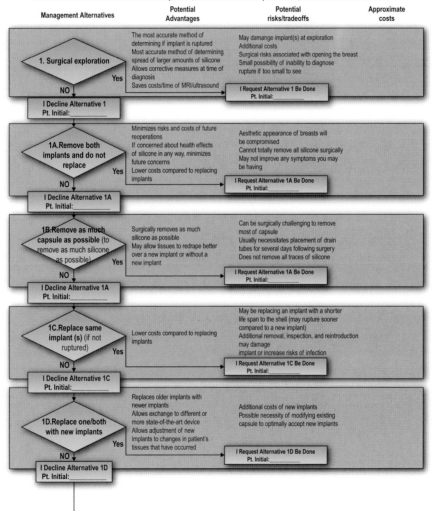

Concern Regarding Rupture of Silicone Gel Implant
John B. Tebbetts, M.D.
Copyright 2000

**Management alternatives are listed prioritizing alternatives most likely to reduce risks of additional operations, reduce additional risks and costs to the patient, and reduce risks of permanent, uncorrectable deformities.

Table 17-5. Decision support flowchart for management of concerns of rupture of silicone gel implant.—cont'd

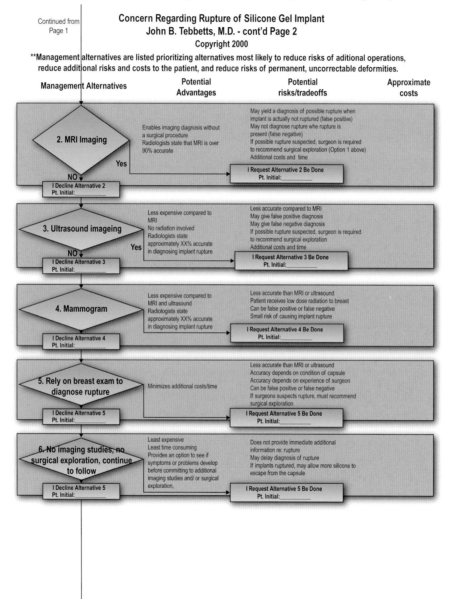

Table 17-5. Decision support flowchart for management of concerns of rupture of silicone gel implant.—cont'd

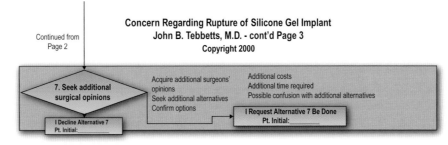

Concern Regarding Rupture of Silicone Gel Implant
John B. Tebbetts, M.D. - cont'd Page 3
Copyright 2000

Continued from Page 2

7. Seek additional surgical opinions

Acquire additional surgeons' opinions
Seek additional alternatives
Confirm options

Additional costs
Additional time required
Possible confusion with additional alternatives

I Decline Alternative 7
Pt. Initial:_____

I Request Alternative 7 Be Done
Pt. Initial:_____

**If patient, surgeon, or patient's family are concerned about any aspect of silicone causing symptoms or possible associated conditions, see additional information and flowchart alternatives entitled "If Patient Has Symptoms or Concerns Related to Silicone"

Patient Name (please print):_____   Witness Name (please print):_____

Patient Signature:_____   Witness Signature:_____
Date:_____   Date:_____

■ REFERENCES

1. Food and Drug Administration. U.S. Food and Drug Administration. General and Plastic Surgery Devices Panel Meeting Transcript. Washington, D.C. October 14–15, 2003. Online. Available: http://www.fda.gov/ohrms/dockets/ac/03/transcripts/3989T1.htm.

2. Food and Drug Administration. U.S. Food and Drug Administration. General and Plastic Surgery Devices Panel Meeting Transcript. Washington, D.C. February 18, 1992.

3. Food and Drug Administration. U.S. Food and Drug Administration. General and Plastic Surgery Devices Panel Meeting Transcript. Washington, D.C. March 1–3, 2000. Online. Available: http://www.fda.gov/cdrh/gpsdp.html#030100.

4. Hiebeler R, Kelly TT, Ketteman C: *Best practices: building your business with customer-focused solutions.* London: Simon and Schuster, 1998, pp 7–228.

5. Adams WP, Bengtson BP, Glicksman CA, Gryskiewicz JM, Jewell ML, McGrath MH, Reisman NR, Teitelbaum SA, Tebbetts JB, Tebbetts T: Decision and management algorithms to address patient and Food and Drug Administration concerns regarding breast augmentation and implants. *Plast Reconstr Surg* 114(5):1252–1257, 2004.

6. Tebbetts JB: An approach that integrates patient education and informed consent in breast augmentation. *Plast Reconstr Surg* 110(3):971–978, 2002.

7. Gorney M: Preventing litigation in breast augmentation. *Clin Plast Surg* 28(3):607–615, 2001.

8. Tebbetts JB: Patient acceptance of adequately filled breast implants using the tilt test. *Plast Reconstr Surg* 106(1):139–147, 2000.

9.   Tebbetts JB: Dual plane (DP) breast augmentation: optimizing implant–soft tissue relationships in a wide range of breast types. *Plast Reconstr Surg* 107:1255, 2001.

10.   Tebbetts JB: Achieving a predictable 24 hour return to normal activities after breast augmentation Part II: Patient preparation, refined surgical techniques and instrumentation. *Plast Reconstr Surg* 109:293–305, 2002.

11.   Tebbetts JB: Out points criteria for breast implant removal without replacement and criteria to minimize reoperations following breast augmentation. *Plast Reconstr Surg* 114(5):1258–1262, 2004.

12.   Tebbetts JB: Achieving a zero percent reoperation rate at 3 years in a 50 consecutive case augmentation mammaplasty PMA study. *Plast Reconstr Surg* 118(6):1453–1457, 2006.

Wound Healing, Capsular Contracture, and Tissue Stretch: Factors Surgeon and Patient Cannot Control

Surgeon decisions and technical execution largely determine patient outcomes in breast augmentation, but neither surgeons nor patients can control wound healing mechanisms and neither can predict or control tissue stretch following augmentation. Wound healing mechanisms and tissue stretch may seem unrelated, but these topics impact outcomes in two distinct ways: (1) wound healing mechanisms during capsule formation and contraction directly impact the degree of lower pole soft tissue stretch that occurs following augmentation, and (2) wound healing and tissue stretch mechanisms determine incidence of several causes of reoperations, including infection, capsular contracture, implant malposition or displacement, and lower pole stretch deformities.

■ THE ROLE OF PATIENT EDUCATION IN MANAGING POSTOPERATIVE CHALLENGES

Management of postoperative problems and complications begins preoperatively with patient education. When problems occur postoperatively and require reoperations, patients frequently question the causes of the problems and ask "Why me?" and "Whose fault is this?" When patients are thoroughly informed preoperatively of mechanisms and potential problems that neither surgeon nor patient can control, surgeons can address postoperative issues more effectively and efficiently. Patients are less prone to focus on unanswerable questions such as "Why me" and are less prone to assign blame for untoward events.

During the preoperative patient education process, surgeons should provide patients with written information that describes specific areas of wound healing and tissue stretch that are not controllable by surgeon or patient

During the preoperative patient education process, surgeons should provide patients with written information that describes specific areas of wound healing and tissue stretch that are not controllable by surgeon or patient. After reading the written information, patients should receive verbal reinforcement of key concepts and have an opportunity to ask questions about factors that surgeon and patient cannot control. Before surgery, patients should acknowledge their understanding and acceptance of factors that surgeon and patient cannot control, and acknowledge the problems, reoperations, costs, and risks that are associated with these uncontrollable mechanisms in clearly written informed consent documents.

■ EDUCATING THE PATIENT ABOUT FACTORS THE SURGEON CANNOT CONTROL

The following content is excerpted from a preoperative patient education DVD and accompanying document entitled "My Preferences and Information I Fully Understand and Accept" that are components from a staged, repetitive, and comprehensive system for augmentation patient education that is peer reviewed and published in the journal *Plastic and Reconstructive Surgery*.[1] As the DVD presents information in stages, the program pauses at intervals to allow the patient to read the accompanying printed document and document an understanding and acceptance of the information. Video content from the patient education program and the accompanying document are included in the Resources folder on the DVDs that accompany this book.

> *Video*: Hello, I am Dr. John Tebbetts. I appreciate your considering me to perform your breast augmentation, and assure you that I will do my best to take excellent care of you. At the same time, I want to be completely honest with you about certain areas that despite over two decades of surgical experience, I cannot predict or control. There are currently no tests I can perform to tell me how you will heal or exactly how your tissues will respond to your breast implants, and therefore I cannot control these factors before, during, or after your surgery. I have to work with what you bring me in terms of your specific tissue characteristics, and I cannot change your tissue characteristics. We can try to make good decisions to limit the potential negative effects of implants on your tissues, but even with the best decisions and surgery, there are factors that neither I nor you can control.
>
> Before I examine you, I want to discuss with you three specific areas that concern me the most, because they are areas that I cannot totally predict or control: (1) whether or not you will develop infection, (2) how much the capsule you form around your implants will tighten and how that capsule may affect the appearance, softness, or feeling in your

breasts, and (3) how much your tissues will stretch in response to your implants. Let's talk about each area separately, but first, *If you are at a computer equipped to interact with the DVD, please confirm your understanding of this information by placing your signature in the box onscreen. Next, on your paper informed consent document, carefully read and initial items 15 and 16. When you have completed this portion of the program, please click on the Next Topic button on the screen.

Document used by the patient while watching the video:

15. _____ From my reading of Dr. Tebbetts' book *The Best Breast*, and information provided me, I understand and accept that there are several factors related to my individual tissue characteristics, how I heal, and how my tissues respond to my breast implants that Dr. Tebbetts cannot predict by tests before surgery, and cannot control after surgery.

16. _____ I understand and accept that Dr. Tebbetts must work with what I bring him to work with, and that he cannot change the qualities of the tissues of my breasts that affect stretch following surgery or how I will heal. I also understand and accept that Dr. Tebbetts cannot perform tests before surgery, or in any other way predict (1) how my skin will stretch following my augmentation, and (2) how my body will heal or not heal following my augmentation.

Video: Infection can occur following any surgical procedure, despite all efforts to prevent it using the most state-of-the-art techniques and drugs.

Every woman's breasts contain bacteria that normally live on the skin and enter the breast through the nipple. In some women, the amounts or types of these bacteria may make them more likely to develop an infection following breast augmentation, but we currently have no tests to identify women who may be at increased risk.

We give every patient intravenous antibiotics immediately prior to starting surgery. These antibiotics are in the blood stream during surgery and in the tissues and tissue fluids following surgery. We do not routinely prescribe antibiotics following surgery because statistics show that they are unnecessary, and because of concern that antibiotics can kill many normal bacteria and encourage the overgrowth of other undesirable bacteria.

If you develop an infection following surgery, the safest and best treatment to avoid prolonged problems and possible permanent deformities is to remove the implants as soon as possible. My experience in trying to salvage infected breast implants is that in the vast majority of cases, the implants ultimately have to be removed, and the longer the delay, the greater the scarring and permanent deformities.

Once implants are removed, infection usually subsides with the help of antibiotics over a 1–3 week period, but the tissues of the breast require at least 3 months to soften and heal. The more aggressive the infection, the greater the risk of internal or external scarring that can leave permanent deformities.

Once the infection is treated, some surgeons attempt to replace implants after waiting 6 months to 1 year. Having tried this several times in patients referred to me with infection, I am convinced that when patients have had a previous infection in their breasts, at least half of them will develop another infection if we try to replace implants. Patients who can get by without recurrent infection, however, almost always develop severe capsular contractures that produce additional deformities and require additional surgery. The bottom line is that if you develop infection, you are at much less risk for future problems if you remove and do not replace your implants, despite your disappointment and mine.

Next, on your paper informed consent document, carefully read and initial item 17. When you have completed this portion of the program, please click on the Next Topic button on the screen.

Document:

17. _____ I fully understand and accept that if I develop an infection following my augmentation, Dr. Tebbetts will remove both of my breast implants, and will never replace either implant to minimize further reoperations, risks, and costs to me. I further understand and accept that, if implant removal is ever required for any reason, that deformities may result that may not be totally correctable.

Video: After we perform surgery and place implants in your breasts, your body healing mechanisms take over. These mechanisms can vary significantly from patient to patient, and despite our best efforts, we cannot precisely predict or control how you will heal.

When any medical device such as a breast implant is placed inside the body, the body forms a lining around that device. That lining is called a capsule, and it forms in the first few weeks to months following surgery. As the lining forms and matures, it usually tightens or contracts slightly, but in some patients it contracts or tightens excessively, putting pressure on the implant, causing it to feel too firm, or causing other deformities or discomfort.

Every patient who has an augmentation forms capsules around her implants. Unfortunately, there are no tests we can perform on you prior to surgery to predict whether the capsules you form will tighten excessively and cause deformities. If we could predict that you are likely to form an excessively tight capsule, we would advise you not to have an augmentation, but unfortunately we cannot predict or control how your body heals and how much your capsule will tighten.

Your capsules can tighten a small amount or a large amount, and they rarely tighten the same in both breasts. During the first 3–6 months, you may notice slight shape changes or severe shape changes, depending on how your capsule forms and tightens. If a capsule tightens a small amount in the lower portion of the breast, the capsule puts pressure on the lower implant, causing an upper bulge in the breast. If the capsule tightens at the outside of the pocket, it can push the implant inward, causing more bulging toward the middle of the breast. If the capsule tightens more toward the inside of the breast, it can displace the implant outward, widening the gap between your breasts. When the capsule displaces the implant, you may be able to feel or see implant edges.

If the entire capsule tightens excessively, your breasts will feel excessively firm. Some patients who form excessively tight capsules also form heavier scars where the incision is located, since both are part of the normal healing mechanism, and that mechanism seems to be overactive in some patients. If capsular tightening is severe, it can cause discomfort and a feeling of tightening, or in rare cases may cause pain. The tightening may interfere with sensation in any area of the breast, and other aspects of the healing mechanism may cause lymph node enlargement or the formation of small bands near the incision.

The risk of your developing an excessively tight capsule around your implants is at least 3%, or 3 chances in 100. In 1700 reported cases in our practice, capsules requiring reoperations occurred in less than 1% of patients with saline implants, but we think that it is prudent to consider at least a 3% capsule rate for purposes of decision making. Regardless of the rate you consider, if you develop an excessively tight capsule, and there is always that chance, the rate is 100% for you, so if you choose to have an augmentation, understand that problems with capsules are a very real consideration and risk, even though the percentage is relatively low.

Most patients who form excessively tight capsules will do so in the first 3–6 months following surgery. If you don't form a tight capsule within a year, at least 90% of your risk is over, but a small percentage of patients can form tight capsules at any time following augmentation.

If any of these problems caused by the capsule are mild to moderate, I may not recommend a reoperation. When the problems are mild, your body is sending us a message that your healing mechanisms tend to form tight capsules. If we reoperate, we are not changing your body's healing mechanisms, and you might form an even worse capsule with worse deformities than you already have. On the other hand, if the deformities are severe, and I have to be the judge of that, we may need to reoperate. Our experience has taught us that regardless of how rapidly a capsule tightens, we should not reoperate on that capsule until at least 6 months following the initial surgery. During that time, the capsule is forming and maturing, and if we interrupt that process, recurrence of the excessively tight capsule is almost certain.

When we reoperate on a capsule, we remove the implant, remove the capsule, and place a new implant into the pocket. Because we cannot control your healing mechanisms, and we already know that you are prone to form excessively tight capsules, our chances of correcting the problem are only about 60% successful, with a 40% chance that you will form another excessively tight capsule. Since the chance for correction is limited, we only recommend reoperations for severe capsular deformities, not mild to moderate ones. If you form another tight capsule after we reoperate one capsule, we will recommend that you live with the capsular tightening if it is mild or moderate, or if it is severe, remove and not replace your implants. What we will not do is continue to reoperate on you when your body has clearly shown that it tends to form recurrent tight capsules, because the risks of problems with additional surgeries far outweigh any chances of success.

Capsules can be very frustrating to you and to me, and it is important that you understand that we cannot control what the capsules do, the capsules will be different on the two sides, they may produce differences in appearance on the two sides, and capsular contractures cannot be controlled and may not be correctable by additional surgery.

Next, on your paper informed consent document, carefully read and initial items 18–24. When you have completed this portion of the program, please click on the Next Topic button on the screen.

Document:

18. _____ I understand and accept that Dr. Tebbetts has absolutely no control over how my body heals following my breast augmentation, and that he cannot predict (by tests prior to surgery) or control my individual healing characteristics.

19. _____ I understand and accept that my body will form a lining (capsule) around my breast implant following my augmentation, and that the capsule around the implant may contract (tighten) excessively, causing a variety of deformities that may require additional surgery and despite additional surgery, may be uncorrectable and require implant removal. The capsules that form and the amount that they tighten are never equal on both sides, so the effects of the capsule on each breast are usually different.

20. _____ I understand and accept that there are no tests or medical information that can accurately predict whether my capsules will tighten excessively, and that following my augmentation, Dr. Tebbetts has no control over how my body forms the capsule or how much the capsule will tighten or cause deformity.

21. _____ I understand and accept that any or all of the following deformities can result from how the capsule forms and tightens, and that Dr. Tebbetts cannot predict, prevent, or control the occurrence of any of these deformities:

    a. Closing of a portion of the lower implant pocket (can be mild or severe), causing slight or significant upward displacement of the implant, and raising the fold under the breast leaving the incision scar below the fold (if the incision was made under the breast).

    b. Closing of a portion of the outside of the implant pocket, causing flattening of areas of the outside contour of the breast and inward displacement of the implant.

    c. Excessive firmness of the implant or breast.

    d. Visible edges or bulging deformities in any area of the breast.

    e. The quality of the scar that I will form wherever my incision is located.

    f. The effects of my body healing and scarring in the area of the incision, adjacent areas to the incision or breast, or any area of the breast.

    g. Discomfort or pain in areas of the breast.

    h. Change in sensation or loss of sensation in any area of the breast or adjacent areas.

    i. Occurrence of lymph node enlargement or small bands near the incision caused by incision or obstruction of small lymph vessels (both of which usually subside without treatment in 3–6 weeks).

22. _____ I understand and accept that any or all of these deformities can occur in one or both breasts, and do not occur equally on the two sides. Although breasts never match exactly on the two sides, if any of these deformities occur, differences in the two breasts may be more noticeable and may not be correctable.

23. _____ I understand and accept that if any or all of the deformities caused by my healing characteristics or the characteristics of the capsule (lining) around my implants occur, even though the deformity may be visible, that Dr. Tebbetts alone will determine whether additional surgery is needed. Dr. Tebbetts will base this decision on whether he feels the potential benefits outweigh the potential risks of additional surgery and whether he feels I will get predictable improvement from additional surgery. I agree to abide by Dr. Tebbetts' decisions in all matters pertaining to whether or not additional surgery is performed.

24. _____ I understand and accept that if any of the deformities listed above occur following my augmentation, that additional surgery will not change the qualities of my tissues and healing characteristics that caused the deformity in the first place. As a result, additional surgery to correct these deformities (a) is unpredictable at best due to the limitations of my tissues and healing characteristics, (b) that surgery for any of the deformities listed above may not successfully correct the deformity, and (c) that any or all of these deformities can occur again after additional surgery because of my healing characteristics.

Video: When we place breast implants into your body, your tissues will stretch to accommodate the implants, and then will stretch additionally over time due to the additional weight of the implants in the breasts. The stretch characteristics of patients' tissues are built into the body genetically from birth, and may vary tremendously from one patient to another.

Obviously, the larger the breast implant we place into the breast, the more stretch and thinning of the overlying tissues we expect to see in the future as your tissues age and stretch under the weight of the implant. But occasionally, in rare instances, a patient's tissues may stretch excessively with even a small implant.

We cannot test you to predict how your tissues will stretch following augmentation, and we cannot control tissue stretch, except by limiting implant size and weight. If your tissues are thin and very stretchy on examination, you may be more prone to excessive stretching after surgery. This excessive stretching can occur rapidly, in the first 6–12 months following surgery, or it can occur more slowly, over several years. The important thing to remember is that we cannot predict or control it.

If excessive stretch occurs in the lower portion of the breasts, the implants will shift downward, the upper breast will lose fullness, and the nipple will point upward excessively. If excessive stretch occurs at the outside of the breasts, the implants will shift outward and widen the gap between the breasts. When tissues stretch, they become thinner, and you may be able to feel or see the edges or shell of your implant in any area of the breast. The weight of the implant pulling on the capsule and thin overlying tissues can produce visible traction rippling in any area of the breast. In patients who are prone to excess stretch, we are not aware of any bra or support device that will prevent it, regardless of how much it is worn.

If you develop a deformity from unpredictable or excessive stretch of your tissues, surgical correction of those stretch deformities is unpredictable at best, because we are operating on the same tissues that have already demonstrated that they will stretch excessively. We can change to a smaller implant to decrease weight, but the stitches placed internally to close off the excess pocket and reposition the implant may not hold in the thin tissues against the weight of even a smaller implant, and the stretch deformity may recur. If a stretch deformity recurs after a surgery to attempt to correct it, we will usually recommend implant removal without replacement to avoid even further stretch and thinning of your tissues that could cause permanent uncorrectable deformities.

Next, on your paper informed consent document, carefully read and initial items 25–28. When you have completed this portion of the program, please click on the Next Topic button on the screen.

Document:

25. _____ If my tissues stretch excessively in any area following my augmentation, deformities can result over which Dr. Tebbetts has no control. These deformities include the following:

   j. Excessive sagging or "bottoming out" of the breast with the implant too low and the nipple pointing excessively upwards

   k. Shift of the implants to the sides with widening of the gap between the breasts

   l. Thinning of tissues over the implant allowing the implant to become visible or palpable (able to be felt) in any area, and

   m. Visible rippling in any area that can result when the implant pulls on the overlying tissues.

26. _____ I understand and accept that any or all of these deformities can occur in one or both breasts, and do not occur equally on the two sides. I also understand and accept that the larger breast implant I choose or my breasts require for optimal aesthetic results, the greater the risk of these deformities occurring. Although breasts never match exactly on the two sides, if any of these deformities occur, differences in the two breasts may be more noticeable and may not be correctable.

27. _____ I understand and accept that if any or all of the deformities caused by tissue stretch listed above should occur, even though the deformity may be visible, that Dr. Tebbetts alone will determine whether additional surgery is needed. Dr. Tebbetts will base this decision on whether he feels the potential benefits outweigh the potential risks of additional surgery and whether he feels I will get predictable improvement from additional surgery. I agree to abide by Dr. Tebbetts' decisions in all matters pertaining to whether or not additional surgery is performed.

28. _____ I understand and accept that if my tissues stretch excessively for any reason following my augmentation, that additional surgery will not change the qualities of my tissues that allowed them to stretch in the first place. As a result, additional

surgery to correct stretch deformities is unpredictable at best due to the limitations my tissues impose, and that surgery for any of the stretch deformities listed above may not successfully correct the deformity, and that any or all of these deformities can occur again if my tissues stretch again. I understand and accept that if my tissues stretch excessively after surgery to correct a stretch deformity, Dr. Tebbetts will recommend that I remove and not replace my implants to avoid possible permanent, uncorrectable deformities.

Video: If problems occur due to your healing mechanisms that form a capsule or due to tissue stretch deformities following your augmentation, you may need additional surgery, and it is important that you understand and accept responsibility for the costs of that additional surgery.

Because we cannot predict which patients may develop problems as the result of their healing mechanisms or their tissue stretch characteristics, you are responsible for all costs for any reoperation that is necessary to attempt to correct a problem caused by the capsules or by tissue stretch. These costs include surgery fees, laboratory fees, surgical facility fees, anesthesia fees, costs of medications, costs of time away from work or other activities, mammogram fees, and electrocardiogram fees for patients over 40 years old.

We do not accept any payments from insurance companies or third parties for costs associated with any additional surgery following your augmentation. We will be happy to provide you with copies of your operative notes and medical records if you choose to pursue any third party payments, but you are responsible for all costs discussed previously, and these costs must be prepaid at least 2 weeks prior to any reoperation surgery.

If you have any type of problem that is not associated with capsules or tissue stretch, such as infection or bleeding, most surgeons do not charge a surgeon's fee for additional surgery to address those problems. In our practice, if any additional surgery is necessary for any problem whatever that is not associated with capsules or tissue stretch, we do not charge surgeon fees. In addition, for problems not related to capsules or tissue stretch, we will take care of all of the other expenses listed above, with the exception of medications and time off work or normal activities.

Next, on your paper informed consent document, carefully read and initial items 29–33. When you have completed this portion of the program, please click on the Next Topic button on the screen.

Document:

29. _____ Since Dr. Tebbetts cannot predict or control my tissue characteristics or healing characteristics and how they will affect my chances of developing any of the

deformities listed above related to tissue stretch and thinning or capsule or scar tissue formation following my augmentation, I understand and accept that should any of the deformities listed above (1–13) occur, if surgery is necessary to try to improve any of the following conditions, that *I will be personally responsible for all costs associated with any surgery that is performed (please initial beside each number indicating your complete understanding and acceptance of all costs associated with surgery for each deformity)*:

1. Excessive sagging or "bottoming out" of the breast with the implant too low and the nipple pointing excessively upwards

2. Shift of the implants to the sides with widening of the gap between the breasts

3. Thinning of tissues over the implant allowing the implant to become visible or palpable (able to be felt) in any area, and

4. Visible rippling in any area that can result when the implant pulls on the overlying tissues.

5. Closing of a portion of the lower implant pocket (can be mild or severe), causing slight or significant upward displacement of the implant, and raising the fold under the breast leaving the incision scar below the fold (if the incision was made under the breast).

6. Closing of a portion of the outside of the implant pocket, causing flattening of areas of the outside contour of the breast and inward displacement of the implant.

7. Excessive firmness of the implant or breast.

8. Visible edges or bulging deformities in any area of the breast.

9. Discomfort or pain in areas of the breast.

10. The effects of my body healing and scarring in the area of the incision, adjacent areas to the incision or breast, or any area of the breast.

11. Discomfort or pain in areas of the breast.

12. Change in sensation or loss of sensation in any area of the breast or adjacent areas.

13. Occurrence of lymph node enlargement or small bands near the incision caused by incision or obstruction of small lymph vessels (both of which usually subside without treatment in 3–6 weeks).

30. _____ I understand and accept that Dr. Tebbetts does not accept insurance or any third party reimbursement for any type of additional surgery that may be necessary

following my augmentation, and that I will be personally responsible for prepaying all costs of any additional surgery at least 2 weeks prior to the scheduled surgery. If I choose to pay by credit card, I understand and accept that I agree to sign additional documents authorizing full payment by my credit card company. Dr. Tebbetts will provide me with copies of my operative note from my surgery, but I assume all responsibility for any filing of insurance and understand that Dr. Tebbetts and his staff will not pursue payments from any third party.

31. _____ I understand and accept that costs of any additional surgery following my augmentation will likely exceed the costs of my original augmentation surgery, and that costs are determined by the complexity and length (time) of the surgery required. Fees for additional surgery will include laboratory fees, electrocardiogram fees if I am over 40 or have any heart condition, possible mammogram or magnetic resonance imaging fees, Dr. Tebbetts' surgeon fees, anesthesia fees, surgical facility fees, and costs of take home medications. I accept personal responsibility for all of these fees, and in addition, I understand and accept that I may have additional costs associated with time off work or normal activities.

32. _____ If following my breast augmentation, any additional surgery for the reasons listed above becomes necessary, and I later choose to dispute any of the items above for which I have indicated my full understanding and acceptance, I agree to pay any and all of Dr. Tebbetts' costs, including any attorney's fees, court costs, or any other costs associated with resolving the dispute.

33. _____ I have read all of Dr. [Surgeon's Name]' informational materials and have had an opportunity to visit with Dr. [Surgeon's Name]' patient educator _____. I have had an opportunity to ask questions and have had all of my questions answered to my satisfaction. I will have an additional opportunity to ask Dr. [Surgeon's Name] questions during our consultation.

■ SURGEON DISCUSSION OF WOUND HEALING AND TISSUE STRETCH FACTORS

During the surgeon consultation, a few minutes of the surgeon's time to explain the interactions of healing mechanisms and tissue stretch is invaluable. If uncontrollable mechanisms produce postoperative problems, the surgeon can remind the patient: "Remember, we discussed things we can't control and how those mechanisms can challenge us after surgery. Let's review our documents that we completed before surgery."

If uncontrollable mechanisms produce postoperative problems, the surgeon can remind the patient: "Remember, we discussed things we can't control and how those mechanisms can challenge us after surgery. Let's review our documents that we completed before surgery."

The following paraphrases the conversation that the author has with patients during the surgeon consultation:

I know that you've read and seen in the DVD that there are certain things that no surgeon and no patient can control after your augmentation. I'd like to spend a few minutes to be absolutely sure that you understand the things neither of us can control, and that you're willing to have your augmentation with the full understanding that we can't control every aspect of how your body heals and how your tissues stretch.

When we place implants in your body, we must create a space for the implant. We have developed techniques that allow us to do this with virtually no bleeding, and very little trauma to your tissues—most patients can go out to dinner the evening of surgery— but all surgery causes some tissue challenges that cause your body to start wound healing mechanisms, and neither you nor I can control those mechanisms. When we place a breast implant behind your breast, your body will form a lining around the implant. That lining is called a capsule. The capsule will form in the first few weeks after surgery, and it never forms the same in both breasts. The capsule lining tightens or contracts in every patient, and the capsules never tighten or contract the same on both sides.

On one side, the capsule will tighten more than the capsule on the other side. On the side where the capsule tightens more, the capsule will act as an internal bra and hold the implant in position more than the opposite side. On the opposite side, when the capsule tightens less, the implant pushes more on your tissues in the lower breast, and will cause more stretch in the lower breast. When the lower breast stretches more compared to the other side, you will lose some fill in the upper breast with the less tight capsule as the stretched tissue allows implant fill to shift to the lower breast.

The most important thing for you to understand is that your breasts will never match. Healing mechanisms will be different from one breast to the other, and we can't control those healing mechanisms. When the capsule lining tightens more around one implant, as it always does, that breast will always have more upper fill compared to the other breast in which less tightening of the capsule allows more of the fill to shift to the lower breast and cause more stretch in the lower breast. These mechanisms are very frustrating to both of us, because we would like to control them, but we can't. Breasts never match, and if you are expecting them to match, you shouldn't have a breast augmentation because no surgeon can make them match.

■ DISTINGUISHING INFERIOR POCKET CLOSURE FROM CAPSULAR CONTRACTURE

After every breast augmentation, some degree of dead space exists around the implant, regardless of the precision of pocket dissection. Small amounts of serous or

The most important thing for you to understand is that your breasts will never match. Healing mechanisms will be different from one breast to the other, and we can't control those healing mechanisms

After every breast augmentation, some degree of dead space exists around the implant, regardless of the precision of pocket dissection

serosanguinous fluid accumulate immediately postoperatively, even if a surgeon places drains which are unnecessary in primary augmentation. Wound healing mechanisms attempt to close dead space, but the amount and location of closure varies substantially from one case to another or from one breast to the other in the same patient.

The most common area of fluid accumulation is the inferior pocket sulcus along the inframammary fold. Small amounts of fluid accumulate in this area regardless of whether a surgeon uses a drain. Immediately postoperatively, a triangular dead space exists in the inferior-most portion of the pocket along the inframammary fold (Figure 18-1, *A*) because the implant does not completely fill the lower pocket due to pressure of overlying soft tissues. The larger or more projecting an implant, the larger the dead space along the inframammary fold, but some dead space exists in this area regardless of implant type, size, or pocket location (Figure 18-1, *B*).

Figure 18-1 A Dead space exists in the implant pocket inferior to the implant after every breast augmentation.
Figure 18-1 B The triangular dead space beneath the implant fills with serosanguinous fluid that the body reabsorbs in most cases.
Figure 18-1 C With more fluid or trauma stimulating inflammation, the dead space can undergo intense capsular thickening and tightening or fibrous replacement, causing inferior pocket closure and upward implant displacement (blue arrows).
Figure 18-1 D Black lines and red arrows indicate the degree of upward implant displacement that resulted from inferior pocket closure.

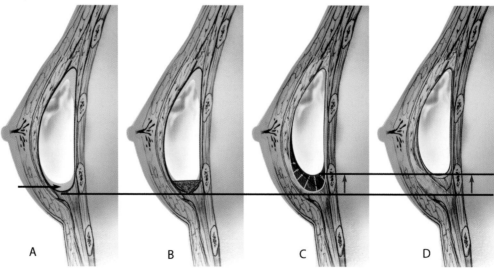

A   B   C   D

In most cases, the body's wound healing mechanisms attempt to close the inferior dead space, but inferior pole soft tissues rapidly stretch enough to allow the implant to settle inferiorly, contacting the anterior and posterior surfaces of the sulcus and filling the depth of the dead space to prevent pocket closure in this area. If greater accumulations of fluid or blood occur in the inframammary fold dead space, the inflammatory response increases and accumulations of fluid can undergo fibrous replacement that obliterates the inferior dead space and closes the inferior pocket (Figure 18-1, C), filling the space in the inferior pocket with fibrous tissue or thick capsule (Figure 18-1, D). Very small amounts of inferior pocket closure (as little as 1 cm) displace the implant superiorly and produce increased, often excessive fullness in the upper breast on the affected side. Patients frequently notice very small differences in upper pole fullness when comparing their breasts, and may request a revision procedure to achieve better symmetry of the upper poles.

Degrees of inferior pocket closure can vary widely, and despite patient wishes, revision procedures are not always indicated. Patients should be informed preoperatively and acknowledge in signed informed consent documents that inferior pocket closure always occurs to some degree, is unpredictable and uncontrollable by the surgeon, and is one of several factors that guarantee that the breasts will not match on the two sides. When inferior pocket closure occurs, the surgeon reminds the patient of wound healing factors that neither surgeon nor patient can control, and reviews the previously signed informed consent document with the patient.

■ DIAGNOSIS OF INFERIOR POCKET CLOSURE AND INDICATIONS FOR REVISION

Inferior pocket closure can occur as an isolated process that does not progress to clinically apparent (grades 2, 3, and 4) capsular contracture, but nevertheless causes enough superior implant displacement to create visually apparent differences in upper pole fill. If the affected breast is relatively soft (grade 1 or 2) and 1 cm or less inferior pocket closure occurs, surgeons should not diagnose capsular contracture. Instead, the condition should be diagnosed more appropriately as inferior pocket closure, because indications and methods of treatment of inferior pocket closure are different compared to clinically apparent capsular contracture (grades 3 and 4).

Indications for surgical revision of inferior pocket closure vary among surgeons and depend to some degree on the level of patient education and patient and surgeon

Inferior pocket closure can occur as an isolated process that does not progress to clinically apparent (grades 2, 3, and 4) capsular contracture, but nevertheless causes enough superior implant displacement to create visually apparent differences in upper pole fill

perceptions of likelihood of success of a surgical procedure weighed against its costs, risks, and tradeoffs. The author's indications for surgical correction of inferior pocket closure include any of the following:

- A 1.5 cm or greater closure of the inferior pocket, documented by an inframammary scar that is located 1.5 cm or more below the new, higher inframammary fold created by inferior pocket closure (in patients who had inframammary incision approach).

- A 1.5 cm or greater closure of the inferior pocket documented by measurement of nipple-to-inframammary fold (N:IMF) distance under maximal stretch and comparison to the known N:IMF distance that was set intraoperatively.

- A clearly visible stepoff in the upper breast on the affected side with the patient unclothed and standing upright.

- Grade 3 capsular contracture in conjunction with inferior pocket closure.

When none of these indications is present, regardless of the level of patient concern about differences in the upper poles of the breasts, a surgical procedure may temporarily improve the condition, but risks of recurrent inferior pocket closure or excessive correction with inferior implant displacement outweigh the potential benefits and predictability of surgical revision. Optimal preoperative education and detailed, signed informed consent documents are invaluable to assist with patient management when minor degrees of inferior pocket closure occur.

■ SURGICAL CORRECTION OF INFERIOR POCKET CLOSURE

Surgical correction of inferior pocket closure is technically more challenging than many surgeons realize. Correction requires reopening the inferior pocket to a precise, planned level and repositioning the implant to the desired new level inferiorly. Preoperative planning and measurement of $N:IMF_{max\ stretch}$ in the contralateral breast are critical to success. At the time of preoperative marking, the surgeon measures $N:IMF_{max\ stretch}$ on the unaffected breast and transfers this measurement to the affected side. If the patient had an inframammary approach, and if implant size and inframammary fold position were planned using the High Five™ System,[2] the position of the inframammary scar on the affected side is a good indicator for the level of the desired, new, lower inframammary fold and the desired inferior extent of pocket dissection. If the patient did not have an inframammary incision, but N:IMF was planned appropriately for the implant size selected preoperatively, the surgeon can accurately transfer the $N:IMF_{max\ stretch}$ measurement from the unaffected side to the affected side to mark the desired inferior extent of pocket dissection which is also the desired, new inframammary fold level.

With the desired inferior extent of the periprosthetic pocket determined objectively and marked preoperatively, the surgeon first performs an inferior capsulotomy across the entire inframammary fold, extending from the junction of the inframammary fold with the sternum medially to the 7 o'clock position of the pocket laterally using a handswitching needlepoint electrocautery pencil. While constantly visualizing the skin marking line inferiorly, the surgeon then dissects inferiorly to reopen the pocket in 0.5 cm increments, carefully avoiding inadvertent dissection below the optimal level, and carefully avoiding inadvertently enlarging the inferior pocket by excessive retractor force while exposing the lower sulcus. Keeping the fingers of the non-dominant hand on the line marked preoperatively while simultaneously holding the retractor provides the surgeon with a constant reference to avoid overdissection inferiorly.

After opening the inferior pocket to the desired level, the surgeon repositions the implant inferiorly and checks implant position and upper pole fill with the patient elevated to a sitting position on the operating table. While visual checking is helpful, it is not totally reliable due to the number of variables inherent to patient positioning sitting while under anesthesia. Precise measurements and preoperative planning are critical to optimizing predictability of correction of inferior pocket closure.

In most cases, the straightforward techniques for opening the inferior pocket described previously are adequate. Occasionally, the inferior edge of the anterior capsule has tightened transversely and produces banding across the lower pole of the breast superior to the new, lower inframammary fold. If banding of the anterior capsule produces a visible distortion of lower pole contour, the surgeon can either score the anterior capsule radially to release the banding, or perform a limited anterior capsulectomy to correct the banding.

If the patient did not have an inframammary incision *and* if implant size and $N:IMF$ were not objectively planned preoperatively, the surgeon must resort to alternative, less accurate methods. If the unaffected breast has optimal aesthetics, the surgeon can begin by transferring the $N:IMF_{max\ stretch}$ measurement from the unaffected side to the affected side. If the unaffected breast does not have optimal aesthetics, with either excessive or insufficient upper pole fill, the surgeon must mark an arbitrary estimate of where the new inframammary fold should be located, always erring on the conservative, short side. Intraoperatively, the surgeon should enlarge the inferior pocket in very small increments, reposition the implant inferiorly, and check upper pole fill with the patient in the sitting position on the operating table.

MANAGEMENT ALTERNATIVES FOR CAPSULAR CONTRACTURE

Chapter 17 includes a detailed decision and management flowchart that outlines management alternatives for clinically significant (grades 3 and 4) capsular contracture, with potential advantages, risks, and tradeoffs of each alternative. This algorithm is derived from the Breast Augmentation Surgeons for Patients Initiative (BASPI) recommendations that are peer reviewed and published in the journal *Plastic and Reconstructive Surgery*.[3] The flowchart is designed to enable surgeons to discuss alternatives for management with the patient and simultaneously document the patient's preference of alternatives to satisfy informed consent legal requirements. This document is available in the Resources folder on the DVDs that accompany this book.

> Chapter 17 includes a detailed decision and management flowchart that outlines management alternatives for clinically significant (grades 3 and 4) capsular contracture, with potential advantages, risks, and tradeoffs of each alternative

CURRENT RATES OF CAPSULAR CONTRACTURE

Over the past two decades, improvements in implant design and surgical techniques[4,5] have dramatically reduced the incidence of capsular contracture. In three peer reviewed and published studies by the author[4–6] of 1664 cases with up to 7 year followup, the overall average incidence of capsular contracture using saline implants was 0.7% compared to a 9% rate in the averaged McGhan and Mentor Food and Drug Administration (FDA) premarket approval (PMA) studies for saline implants. The majority of implants in the author's series were the McGhan Style 468 Biocell™ textured surface, anatomic implants. In the FDA PMA series of Mentor and McGhan, the majority of implants were smooth shell saline implants. Although these data are not scientifically comparable due to inability to equalize the preoperative variables in the cohorts, this 1260% difference in capsular contracture rates certainly suggests that the Style 468 implant combined with state-of-the-art surgical techniques that virtually eliminate bleeding, dramatically reduce tissue trauma, and allow 96% of patients to return to normal activities within 24 hours, also significantly reduces risks of capsular contracture.

> Comprehensive data for the entire PMA for the Style 410 have not been released by Allergan, but the author's personal series data again suggest that optimal proved processes and surgical techniques, combined with a state-of-the-art implant device, dramatically reduce risks of capsular contracture

In the FDA PMA study for the Allergan Style 410 form stable, cohesive gel, anatomic implant with Biocell™ textured surface, a consecutive series of 50 patients, reviewed by a CRO and peer reviewed and published in the journal *Plastic and Reconstructive Surgery*, had a zero percent incidence of capsular contracture at 3 year followup.[7] Comprehensive data for the entire PMA for the Style 410 have not been released by Allergan, but the author's personal series data again suggest that optimal proved processes and surgical techniques, combined with a state-of-the-art implant device, dramatically reduce risks of capsular contracture.

■ PERSONAL APPROACH TO MANAGEMENT OF CAPSULAR CONTRACTURE

The author's personal clinical approach to capsular contracture has evolved over three decades of clinical practice. Currently, when a patient presents with an excessively firm breast, with or without implant deformity or displacement, optimal management decisions require the following information:

1. When did the patient have her primary breast augmentation?
2. What implant device was implanted at the primary augmentation?
3. What subsequent reoperations has the patient had, and what devices were placed at each reoperation?
4. What was the pocket location for the primary augmentation, and if it has changed at a reoperation, what is the current pocket location?
5. If the patient has had more than one reoperation for capsular contracture, is she willing to remove and not replace her implants, understanding that this option minimizes risks of future reoperations and tissue compromises and understanding that repeated reoperations may result in uncorrectable tissue deformities?
6. What is the current measured pinch thickness of the *thinnest area of coverage* over any area of the patient's implants?
7. What are the patient's specific complaints regarding the condition of her breasts?
8. Is the patient willing and able to fund total costs associated with a reoperation and is she willing to confirm her ability and willingness to do so in written informed consent documents?
9. Does the patient clearly understand and accept in signed informed consent documents that additional reoperations do not assure correction of capsular contracture, might make the condition worse, and that the tradeoffs, costs, and risks of permanent tissue compromises or deformities increase with each reoperation?
10. What does the patient expect from a possible reoperation?

While the author basically follows the algorithm for management of capsular contracture that is presented in Chapter 17, personal criteria for reoperations and out points (implant removal without replacement) have become more stringent with increasing clinical experience.

The first practical question is: "What criteria would make me (the surgeon) decline to perform a reoperation for capsular contracture?" Table 18-1 lists criteria for declining to reoperate on capsular contracture conditions.

Surgeons and patients should remember that once a patient has developed inferior pocket closure or a capsular contracture grade 2 or greater, the patient is at significant risk of developing another capsular contracture due to her inherent body healing mechanisms, unless an isolated event such as a postoperative hematoma likely to cause capsular contracture occurred at the primary operation. No patient ever has matching breasts following any breast augmentation. The degree to which a patient notices differences in her breasts varies widely, and patients who are not thoroughly informed preoperatively

---

Table 18-1. Indications to decline reoperation for capsular contracture

If one or more of these criteria exist, the author declines to perform an additional operation (other than removing and not replacing the implants) for any sequelae of capsular contracture:

- A patient has a Grade 2 capsular contracture with less than 1 cm implant displacement due to isolated inferior pocket closure

- A patient has visual differences in the breasts that concern her, but a Grade 2 or less contracture and/or less than 1 cm implant displacement due to capsular pressure

- A history of more than one previous reoperation for capsular contracture (unless the patient has pre-1990 manufactured implants in place)

- Any area of coverage that has less than 0.5 cm pinch thickness over any area of the implant, unless a pocket change to subpectoral or dual plane is available and certain to provide adequate soft tissue coverage

- Patient is not willing to accept and document in informed consent written documents at least a 50% risk of recurrent capsular contracture, regardless of what operation is performed

- Patient is not willing to accept that her breasts will never match following surgery, that she will likely see and will certainly feel areas of her implants, and that visible traction rippling may occur in areas of thin tissue coverage postoperatively

- Patient is unwilling or unable to fund costs of a reoperation, or patient expects insurance to cover reoperation

- Patient is not willing to sign informed consent documents stating that if a recurrent capsular contracture occurs following an attempted reoperation, the surgeon will recommend removal of both implants without replacement and will not perform additional reoperations

and acknowledge their understanding in writing are much more likely to notice and complain about minor differences in the breasts postoperatively.

Many minor differences in the breasts postoperatively tempt surgeons to perform reoperations, because the "solution" seems so simple. An example is performing an isolated capsulotomy to open an area of the pocket that closed postoperatively. In the author's three decade clinical experience, when deformities or differences are less than those specified for a grade 3 capsular contracture (significant excessive firmness to palpation with distortion of breast shape), operating on minor differences or deformities often produces only a "different set of differences". In other words, while it is always possible to alter the appearance of a breast with capsular contracture, the surgeon should ask the following questions before proceeding:

1. What am I really trying to accomplish in this case?
2. What are the chances that I'll be successful?
3. What are the chances that after a reoperation I'll only be dealing with a different set of tradeoffs or compromises instead of a "cure"?
4. What are the chances that the patient will really be better served by a reoperation?

Patients who have silicone gel implants in place that were manufactured prior to 1990 and present with capsular contracture have a higher percentage risk of a ruptured implant, regardless of the findings on clinical examination. MRI may or may not suggest rupture, but in the presence of a grade 3 or 4 capsular contracture, exploration, treatment of the capsule (capsulectomy or capsulotomy), and replacement of both implants is well worth the patient's consideration. If the patient desires exploration and implant replacement, MRI adds nothing but preoperative expense, and is unnecessary. Grade 3 or 4 contracture alone is adequate indication for exploration and treatment of the capsule, and the older the silicone gel implant, the greater the indication.

SURGICAL TREATMENT OF GRADE 2 CAPSULAR CONTRACTURE

While grade 2 capsular contracture may produce minor increased firmness and visible differences in the breasts, surgical intervention for grade 2 capsular contracture rarely provides predictable outcomes that really outweigh risks, costs, and tradeoffs of the surgery. In most cases, treatment of grade 2 contractures may simply produce a different set of compromises or differences, so the author routinely tries to educate patients about these realities and avoid surgical intervention for grade 2 conditions.

Many minor differences in the breasts postoperatively tempt surgeons to perform reoperations, because the "solution" seems so simple

Patients who have silicone gel implants in place that were manufactured prior to 1990 and present with capsular contracture have a higher percentage risk of a ruptured implant, regardless of the findings on clinical examination

While grade 2 capsular contracture may produce minor increased firmness and visible differences in the breasts, surgical intervention for grade 2 capsular contracture rarely provides predictable outcomes that really outweigh risks, costs, and tradeoffs of the surgery

SURGICAL TREATMENT OF GRADES 3 AND 4 CAPSULAR CONTRACTURES

Table 18-2 lists indications for reoperation for capsular contracture.

Classical grading of capsular contractures is largely useless, because all of the criteria are subjective and non-standardized, so any data gleaned using those criteria cannot be validated scientifically for comparisons. Even the criteria listed above are subjective, and surgeons must individualize judgments according to clinical case presentation when deciding whether a reoperation is in a patient's best interests.

Pain or discomfort, while included in some classifications of capsular contracture, is a poor criterion to justify reoperation, because it is so subjective. Few patients experience true pain, even with severe contractures, with most patients with grade 4 contractures describing a feeling of "tightness" or "pulling" with body or arm movement. Occasional patients may experience true pain, presumably due to traction or compression on sensory nerves.

An important principle when addressing severe capsular contracture (grade 3 or 4, or any of the conditions listed previously to justify surgical intervention) is: *remove as much of the existing capsule as possible without causing additional tissue damage, severe bleeding, or leaving less than 5 mm thickness of tissue coverage in any area.*

When treating severe capsular contractures, surgeons should have one or more definitive reasons to NOT perform a total capsulectomy. Reasons to perform less than a complete capsulectomy may include:

- Inadequate surgical skills, instrumentation, or patience

- Excessive bleeding occurs while attempting to perform complete capsulectomy that the surgeon is unable to optimally control

> Pain or discomfort, while included in some classifications of capsular contracture, is a poor criterion to justify reoperation, because it is so subjective

> An important principle when addressing severe capsular contracture (grade 3 or 4, or any of the conditions listed previously to justify surgical intervention) is: remove as much of the existing capsule as possible without causing additional tissue damage, severe bleeding, or leaving less than 5 mm thickness of tissue coverage in any area

Table 18-2. Indications for reoperation for capsular contracture

· Breast firmness that is dramatically firmer (not slightly firmer) compared to a normal breast
· Substantial distortion of breast shape or implant displacement
· Breast shape distortion that is visible in normal clothing
· Capsular contracture in the presence of infection or suspected infection

- Removing the capsule will leave less than 5 mm soft tissue coverage over the implant.

Assuring adequate soft tissue coverage in all areas over an implant is the number one priority in breast augmentation. The safety of performing complete capsulectomy is directly related to the surgeon's technical skills, instrumentation, and patience. With electrocautery instrumentation and retractors available today, complete capsulectomy is straightforward, regardless of pocket location. The larger the implant size, the more surface area of capsule requires removal. If removing capsule will leave less than 5 mm of soft tissue coverage, surgeons should prioritize coverage and leave the capsule, accepting that residual capsule and attachments may compromise tissue redraping and breast shape.

Complete capsulectomy is preferable to partial capsulectomy for many reasons:

- With silicone gel implants, especially older generation gel implants, removal of the capsule enables the most complete removal of silicone that may have "bled" into the surrounding capsule or silicone adjacent to a disrupted implant.

- Complete removal of the capsule allows optimal redraping of breast parenchyma and soft tissues over a new implant.

- Removal of the capsule prevents potential fluid accumulation in the capsular space if the capsule is left behind and the implant simply relocated.

- Capsulotomy or partial capsulectomy may provide focal "release" in the area of capsulotomy or capsulectomy, but both techniques leave capsule and capsule attachments in other areas that usually compromise optimal tissue redraping and breast shape.

One of the most definitive studies evaluating treatment options for capsular contracture compared complete capsulectomy with replacement of implants with polyurethane covered implants to partial capsulectomy.[8] This study, performed independently by three investigators during the late 1980s and early 1990s, was interesting because of the degree of correlation between independent authors' findings, and the finding that capsulotomy and partial capsulectomy were extremely ineffective compared to complete capsulectomy in preventing recurrent capsular contracture.

Isolated capsulotomy and scoring of the capsule in various areas seems appealing and less difficult compared to complete capsulectomy, but these assumptions are not necessarily true. For example, when removing a capsule from the posterior surface of the pectoralis muscle (a procedure many surgeons feel is so difficult that it should be avoided), with optimal instrumentation, less bleeding occurs by precise electrocautery dissection in the proper plane compared to scoring the capsule and inadvertently cutting into the pectoralis and causing marked bleeding that is difficult to control.

Posterior Capsulectomy

Opinions vary regarding indications for posterior capsulectomy, particularly with a subpectoral implant location. If a silicone gel implant has been in place and the patient desires maximal removal of silicone that may have "bled" from an implant or escaped from a disrupted shell, the most complete removal requires posterior capsulectomy. If the surgeon plans to replace a textured surface device with a texturing that may develop adherence (the only one at present is the Biocell™ surfact of Allergan implants), posterior capsulectomy provides a virgin tissue surface to optimize the potential performance of the implant. In other clinical situations where a smooth shell saline device is present, posterior capsulectomy is less logical and less indicated.

Removing the posterior capsule following submammary or subfascial augmentation is very straightforward. Details of technique are presented later in this chapter. Removing a posterior capsule that is attached to the ribs and intercostal musculature following subpectoral augmentation is usually straightforward provided the surgeon establishes the correct plane and maintains traction on the capsule with claw retractors to define the plane of dissection. Keeping the electrocautery dissecting instrument parallel to the plane of the thoracic wall in all areas minimizes risks of inadvertent pneumothorax. In some cases, the posterior capsule is so adherent to ribs and intercostals, or is so thin that removal is technically impractical.

En Bloc Surgical Technique for Complete Capsulectomy

The en bloc approach to complete capsulectomy prioritizes leaving the implant in place within the capsule while performing extracapsular dissection. The logic of this principle is that tension on tissue planes defines visual planes for dissection. Retractors place tension on tissues external to the capsule to define the plane between capsule and adjacent tissues. Leaving the implant inside the capsule enables the implant to maintain tension on the capsule through internal pressure, keeping a constant curve to the capsule as extracapsular dissection proceeds.

The en bloc approach to complete capsulectomy prioritizes leaving the implant in place within the capsule while performing extracapsular dissection. The logic of this principle is that tension on tissue planes defines visual planes for dissection

Surgeons can perform en bloc complete capsulectomy through inframammary or periareolar approaches

Surgeons can perform en bloc complete capsulectomy through inframammary or periareolar approaches. While the periareolar approach is appealing from the perspective that all points of the circumference are equidistant from the incision, limitations of the size of the periareolar incision limit width of retractor blades, limit exposure, and limit capability to remove the implant within the capsule compared to the inframammary approach. The remainder of this discussion focuses on complete capsulectomy via the inframammary approach. Similar principles apply for the periareolar approach, but the optimal sequence of dissection differs for the periareolar approach.

Techniques for en bloc complete capsulectomy are included in the DVDs that accompany this book.

Through the inframammary approach, the surgeon dissects through subcutaneous tissue and breast tissue (if present) to the surface of the capsule using handswitching needlepoint electrocautery pencil dissection. Electrocautery settings differ from case to case, and require adjustment by the surgeon. If the surgeon can use pure coagulation current or blended cut and coagulation with substantial coagulation current, bleeding is minimal and extracapsular dissection can proceed rapidly.

Figure 18-2 illustrates the optimal sequence of dissection for en bloc complete capsulectomy. Leaving the implant in place and carefully avoiding incising the capsule, the surgeon places the shorter end of a double ended retractor to lift the soft tissues anteriorly and establishes the plane of dissection anterior to the capsule and posterior to overlying tissues. The surgeon should avoid any dissection posterior to the capsule initially, allowing the posterior capsular attachments to stabilize the encapsulated implant and facilitate anterior dissection. With the short blade of the double ended retractor lifting superiorly, the surgeon places counter retraction pressure on the capsule and implant using a spatula retractor. This counter pressure is

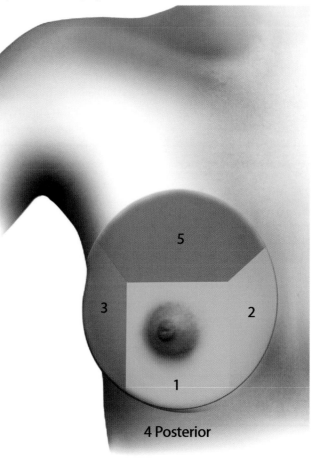

Figure 18-2. Zones of dissection for complete capsulectomy in numbered sequence for dissection. Zones 1–3 and 5 dissection separates the intact capsule from adjacent structures. Zone 4 frees the posterior capsule from underlying structures.

indispensable throughout the reminder of dissection in all zones of dissection to optimally define the plane of dissection. Sweeping the needlepoint dissector and retractor side to side, the surgeon separates the capsule from attached overlying tissues in Zone 1.

Changing to the longer end of the double ended retractor, the surgeon dissects medially into Zone 2 and laterally into Zone 3, separating the capsule from adjacent tissues in these areas. As dissection anterior to the capsule proceeds cephalad, the surgeon changes to an extended needle tip in the handswitching electrocautery pencil. When the surgeon has separated as much capsule as possible from adjacent tissues anteriorly, medially, and laterally, posterior dissection proceeds.

The surgeon places the short end of the double ended retractor between the posterior surface of the capsule containing the implant and the adjacent, adherent tissues posterior to the capsule. In submammary and subfascial cases, the retractor lifts the encapsulated implant off the underlying pectoralis major and serratus muscles. In subpectoral and dual plane augmentations, the retractor lifts the encapsulated implant off the underlying ribs, costal cartilages, and intercostal musculature.

In the plane posterior to the capsule, the surgeon dissects medially, laterally, and superiorly to free the capsule from adjacent tissues in the area of Zone 4. Similar to the anterior dissection in Zones 1–3, as dissection proceeds cephalad, the surgeon switches to the longer blade of the double ended retractor and the extended needle tip on the electrocautery pencil. At the conclusion of the posterior dissection, the only remaining attachments of the capsule to adjacent tissues are in Zone 5 superiorly. In some cases, usually with smaller implants in place, the surgeon can continue dissection in Zone 5 to completely free the capsule containing the implant from adjacent tissues and even remove the implant with the intact capsule surrounding it.

In many cases, especially with larger implants, the surgeon can facilitate Zone 5 dissection to complete capsule excision by first removing the implant from the capsule through an incision through the inferior border of the capsule. With the implant removed, the surgeon can easily expose Zone 5 by placing traction on the capsule directed inferiorly and exposing tissue attachments to the capsule superiorly in Zone 5 using the longer blade of the double ended retractor or a fiberoptic retractor with a longer blade.

Strip Surgical Technique for Complete Capsulectomy

In some cases, varying thicknesses of the capsule and dense adherence of the capsule to adjacent tissues can compromise the en bloc dissection techniques described previously. If the surgeon makes multiple entries into the capsule during initial attempts to perform an en bloc dissection, the surgeon can remove the implant and remove the capsule using strip capsulectomy techniques.

Techniques for strip removal complete capsulectomy are included in the DVDs that accompany this book.

After removing the implant from the capsule, the surgeon places the longer blade of the double ended retractor inside the capsule and uses the needlepoint electrocautery to score the capsule to create 3 cm wide strips anteriorly and posteriorly. Dividing the capsule into strips of this width greatly facilitates capsulectomy, because the surgeon can maintain a wider field of view inside the pocket during dissection and avoid having larger masses of mobilized capsule blocking the field of vision. Regardless of the pocket plane, when scoring the capsule to divide it into strips, the surgeon should use coagulation electrocautery current and very light strokes of the needle tip cautery to incise the capsule incrementally, stopping before entering adjacent tissues and producing bleeding that obscures the remainder of the dissection. If coagulation current does not cut adequately, the surgeon can blend cutting current with the coagulation current. Avoiding bleeding or immediately controlling all bleeding when performing any type of capsulectomy is essential to optimize visualization and avoid dissection into adjacent tissues that always causes even more bleeding. Controlled and accurate capsulectomy to separate a capsule from the anterior or posterior surface of the pectoralis major muscle requires general anesthesia and complete pectoralis relaxation with muscle relaxants.

> Avoiding bleeding or immediately controlling all bleeding when performing any type of capsulectomy is essential to optimize visualization and avoid dissection into adjacent tissues that always causes even more bleeding

The assistant then grasps each strip immediately adjacent to the inframammary incision using Lahey clamps and places inferior or side-to-side traction on each strip to create counter traction opposite to the direction of traction created by the retractor in the surgeon's non-dominant hand. Using the needlepoint electrocautery, the surgeon dissects immediately adjacent to the capsule to separate the individual strips of capsule from adjacent tissues. Maintaining optimal traction and counter traction, and optimizing exposure with optimal retractor instrumentation are essential to minimize trauma and bleeding in adjacent tissues. As dissection frees the capsular strips from adjacent tissues, frequent repositioning of the Lahey clamp and retractors optimizes traction and counter traction to define the plane of dissection.

Adjunctive Techniques and Care for Complete Capsulectomy

Complete hemostasis is essential to minimize risks of recurrent capsular contracture. Complete capsulectomy creates a large wound surface area, and even with excellent hemostasis, substantial transudation and serous fluid accumulation occurs postoperatively. Regardless of the degree of hemostasis, surgeons should place closed suction drains following complete capsulectomy, and leave the drains in place until drainage is less than 25 cc for a 24 hour period or for a maximum of 10 days. While drains are in place, the author keeps the patient on low dose oral cephalosporins.

Tight wraps or tight compressive dressings or bras, while theoretically beneficial in reducing transudation and drainage, can be very uncomfortable for patients. None of these devices has ever been shown to be beneficial in valid scientific studies. Precise surgical techniques, complete hemostasis, and closed drainage are far more important compared to special dressings, pressure devices, or special bras or garments.

> Regardless of the degree of hemostasis, surgeons should place closed suction drains following complete capsulectomy

■ TISSUE STRETCH DEFORMITIES—CAUSES AND PREVENTION

Tissue stretch problems that occur postoperatively are largely outside surgeons' control, but surgeons can minimize tissue stretch problems by selecting implant size to match patient tissue characteristics using the High Five System™ and by avoiding excessively projecting implants.

Problems caused by excessive tissue stretch postoperatively include lateral implant displacement, inferior implant displacement (ptosis and/or "bottoming"), visible implant edges medially, and visible traction rippling. Inferior and lateral implant displacement may be surgically correctable, but visible traction rippling and implant edges that occur after tissue thinning from excessive stretch and the result are largely uncorrectable.

> Tissue stretch problems that occur postoperatively are largely outside surgeons' control, but surgeons can minimize tissue stretch problems by selecting implant size to match patient tissue characteristics using the High Five System™ and by avoiding excessively projecting implants

Irreversible tissue changes that produce surgically uncorrectable stretch deformities are almost totally preventable. In 1664 reported cases with up to 7 year followup,[4-6] visible rippling or implant edges with the patient upright did not occur, and implant malposition required reoperation in only 0.1% of cases. Prioritizing soft tissue coverage during the preoperative decision making process and implementing proved processes of patient education and tissue based implant selection clearly impact occurrence of irreversible tissue deformities. A zero percent reoperation rate in a consecutive series in an FDA PMA study[7] further confirms the efficacy of these proved processes.

> Irreversible tissue changes that produce surgically uncorrectable stretch deformities are almost totally preventable

Prevention of uncorrectable deformities using proved processes is infinitely more effective compared to attempts at surgical correction after irreversible tissue changes

Prevention of uncorrectable deformities using proved processes is infinitely more effective compared to attempts at surgical correction after irreversible tissue changes.

Stretch deformities that may be surgically correctable include lateral implant displacement with widening of the intermammary distance and inferior implant displacement with "bottoming" or ptosis. Prevention of these deformities is much more effective compared to surgical correction. Lateral implant displacement that occurs after conventional subpectoral augmentation (leaving inferior pectoralis origins intact) increases muscle pressure on the implant that transmits inferolaterally to stretch the lateral pocket envelope. Dual plane augmentation divides inferior pectoralis origins across the inframammary fold and virtually eliminates occurrence of lateral implant displacement.[4-7] Dividing inferior pectoralis origins to create a dual plane pocket does not increase incidence of inferior implant displacement or bottoming deformities based on 7 year followup in 1664 reported cases.[4-6]

Dividing inferior pectoralis origins to create a dual plane pocket does not increase incidence of inferior implant displacement or bottoming deformities based on 7 year followup in 1664 reported cases[4-6]

Despite surgeons' best decisions and best technical efforts, some patients' tissues simply do not support the weight of an average size (less than 300 cc) breast implant. Unfortunately, no preoperative tests or physical examination findings accurately predict patients whose tissues will stretch excessively. Excessive lower pole stretch with appropriate size breast implants occurs rarely, but unfortunately bottoming or lower pole stretch deformities are not predictable or preventable using current tissue measurement and decision processes.

A detailed decision support and management algorithm flowchart for stretch deformities was presented in Chapter 17, and is one of the algorithms from the Breast Augmentation Surgeons for Patients Initiative (BASPI) to address patient and FDA concerns. This flowchart is included in the Resources folder on the DVDs that accompany this book.

■ SURGICAL CORRECTION OF LATERAL IMPLANT DISPLACEMENT

Lateral implant displacement usually occurs following overdissection of the lateral pocket at the time of augmentation. Surgeons can prevent overdissection of the lateral pocket by stopping dissection at the lateral border of the pectoralis major in submammary and subfascial augmentations, and stopping lateral dissection at the lateral border of the pectoralis minor in subpectoral and dual plane augmentations. After inserting the implant, if lateral pocket dissection is properly limited, the lateral breast contour will appear somewhat flattened. The surgeon can then insert a double ended retractor pulling laterally and a spatula retractor protecting the implant medially to expose the lateral pocket sulcus for enlargement in small, 0.5 cm increments with the electrocautery pencil or handswitching, monopolar, electrocautery forceps.

Correction of excessive lateral implant displacement requires surgical closure of the lateral pocket with a lateral capsulorrhaphy. Precise lateral capsulorrhaphy, leaving a smooth, optimal lateral breast contour, can be challenging. The thinner the tissues overlying the lateral pocket, the more likely sutures placed for the capsulorrhaphy will create visible dimpling externally, especially if the capsule is thin and achieving good suture purchase requires incorporating deep dermis into the sutures that close the lateral pocket. If the capsule is adequately thick and dense, the surgeon can approximate capsule to capsule with a reasonable expectation of success. In many cases, however, if the patient had a thick or dense capsule, lateral stretch would not have occurred, so a thin capsule is a common tissue finding that limits the efficacy of lateral capsulorrhaphy. Table 18-3 lists requirements for optimal capsulorrhaphy.

> Patient tissue quality does not improve with time, and unless patient and surgeon are willing to decrease forces that created the deformity initially, both should expect a high rate of recurrent stretch and deformity

When correcting stretch deformities, if initial pocket dissection was accurate, surgeons must acknowledge that implant and overlying soft tissue forces caused excessive stretch. Patient tissue quality does not improve with time, and unless patient and surgeon are willing to decrease forces that created the deformity initially, both should expect a high rate of recurrent stretch and deformity. Decreasing implant forces requires decreasing the mass, size, or weight of the implant. Surgeons can decrease soft tissue forces on the implant in three specific ways: (1) decrease implant size to decrease the effects of pressure from overlying tissues, (2) decrease implant projection to disperse soft tissue forces over a greater surface area of the implant, and (3) decrease soft tissue pressure on the implant by converting a traditional subpectoral pocket (with intact pectoralis origins across the inframammary fold) to a dual plane pocket (by dividing pectoralis origins across the inframammary fold, stopping where the inframammary fold joins the sternum). Controlling forces applied to the lateral tissues is far more important compared to any

> Decreasing implant forces requires decreasing the mass, size, or weight of the implant

Table 18-3. **Requirements for optimal capsulorrhaphy**
• Controlling and minimizing forces on the suture line by selection of appropriate implant type and size
• Controlling and minimizing tissue forces on the implant transmitted to the lateral envelope
• Accurate suture placement (position and depth) to provide long-term stability with minimal skin dimpling
• Optimal healing of opposing surfaces that allows scar formation to reinforce and strengthen the suture line

specific technique of lateral capsulorrhaphy, but surgeons frequently fail to address forces that created the deformity when planning correction.

A specific decision algorithm for planning correction of all stretch deformities reminds surgeons to prioritize reducing implant and tissue forces that contributed to the initial problem (Table 18-4).

■ PRINCIPLES OF CORRECTION OF INFERIOR IMPLANT DISPLACEMENT OR "BOTTOMING"

Excessive inferior pole stretch following breast augmentation usually produces deformities that differ from breast ptosis. As breasts become more ptotic, the entire breast envelope stretches and the nipple-areola complex moves inferiorly proportionate to the degree of overall envelope stretch, increasing the sternal notch-to-nipple distance as the nipple-to-inframammary fold distance increases. Inferior pole stretch differs from ptosis, because the nipple-to-inframammary fold distance increases disproportionately, while sternal notch-to-nipple

Excessive inferior pole stretch following breast augmentation usually produces deformities that differ from breast ptosis

Table 18-4. Optimizing surgical correction of stretch deformities following breast augmentation.

**Management alternatives are listed prioritizing alternatives most likely to reduce risks of additional operations, reduce additional risks and costs to the patient, and reduce risks of permanent, uncorrectable deformities.

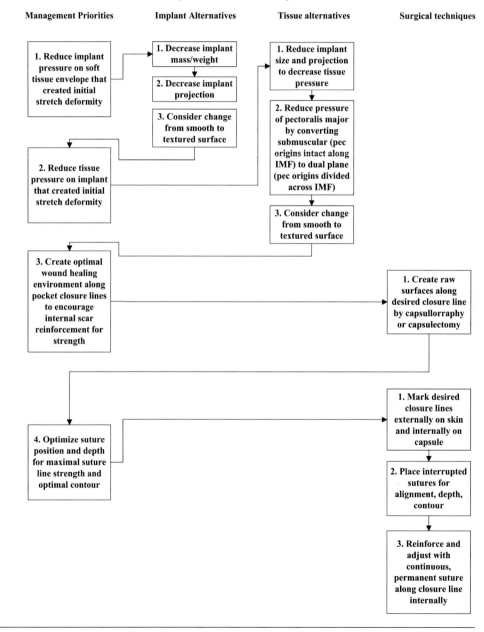

distance changes minimally. Excessive inferior pole stretch produces a deformity that many surgeons refer to as "bottoming" in which excessive lower pole breast envelope stretch allows the breast implant to move inferiorly, decreasing upper pole fill in the breast, while simultaneously causing excessive fill in the lower breast that causes upward displacement of the nipple-areola complex on the breast mound.

Nipple-to-inframammary fold distance can increase while the position of the inframammary fold remains constant. This type of stretch produces glandular ptosis, and may cause excessive upward nipple tilt. A more common and problematic inferior pole stretch deformity occurs when excessive N:IMF stretch combines with separation of the deep subcutaneous fascia from underlying tissues along the inframammary fold, enlarging the inferior pocket, relocating the inframammary fold inferior to its position at the time of surgery, and allowing a true inferior displacement of the implant into the enlarged pocket. The exact mechanism of this second, more severe type of bottoming deformity is undefined, but anatomically, pocket enlargement inferiorly following breast augmentation requires a separation of the deep subcutaneous fascia from the underlying anterior rectus sheath medially, and the serratus fascia more laterally.

> Nipple-to-inframammary fold distance can increase while the position of the inframammary fold remains constant

Principles of surgical correction for inferior implant displacement are similar to principles described previously for correction of lateral implant displacement. The decision algorithm in Table 18-4 applies equally to inferior implant displacement correction and lateral implant displacement correction.

If a patient had an inframammary incision approach for her primary augmentation, and significant excessive inferior pole stretch with enlargement of the inferior pocket occurs, the inframammary incision scar migrates superiorly on the breast mound. A 1–1.5 cm elevation of an inframammary scar can occur with isolated lower pole stretch (N:IMF elongation) *without* any significant enlargement of the lower pocket. This type and degree of stretch rarely require surgical correction.

When significant enlargement of the inferior pocket occurs, the inframammary fold-to-umbilicus distance shortens. Measuring and documenting the distance from the central umbilicus to the 6 o'clock position of the inframammary fold at the conclusion of a breast augmentation enables the surgeon to make a definitive diagnosis with exact quantitation of the degree of inferior pocket enlargement and inframammary fold descent. Measurements from the clavicle or sternal notch to the inframammary fold are far less accurate compared to umbilicus-to-fold measurements.

When correcting bottoming or inferior pole stretch deformities, surgeons frequently compromise corrections by attempting to place both inframammary folds at the same level on the torso. In most women, the levels of the inframammary folds on the torso differ on the two sides. The critical relationship to optimize breast aesthetics is the nipple-to-inframammary fold distance relative to breast width. If a surgeon does not set N:IMF to be equal on the two sides, and instead adjusts inframammary fold levels to match, N:IMF distances will differ on the two sides, causing nipple-areola malposition on the breast mound. When planning primary augmentations or planning correction of inferior pole stretch deformities, surgeons should set optimal N:IMF for breast width on both sides and ignore differences in the levels of the inframammary folds on the torso. Obviously, a balance between N:IMF symmetry and IMF level symmetry is desirable, but equalizing N:IMF on the two sides is always the priority if optimal aesthetics are the goal. Patients must be informed and aware preoperatively that the breasts do not develop at exactly the same level on the torso, and that differences in IMF level on the torso almost always differ from one side to the other.

■ SURGICAL CORRECTION OF INFERIOR IMPLANT DISPLACEMENT OR "BOTTOMING"

Surgical correction of bottoming deformities can be accomplished through inframammary or periareolar incision approaches. Limited incision or puncture incision approaches to correction of inferior pole stretch deformities are not as predictable, accurate, or controllable compared to inframammary or periareolar approaches to correction. This discussion will focus on correction through an inframammary approach. If the contralateral breast has good aesthetics and an appropriate N:IMF distance compared to the breast width, the surgeon can place dots at 1 cm intervals along the normal breast inframammary fold (IMF), measure N:IMF distances to each of these dots with the skin under maximal stretch, and transfer those measurements to the contralateral breast with the inferior pole stretch deformity to define the desired level of the IMF. Alternatively, or if both breasts are affected, the surgeon should measure base width (BW) of the breast, and consult Table 18-5, excerpted from the TEPID[TM,9] and High Five[TM,2] systems to determine an appropriate N:IMF to set under maximal stretch.

Table 18-5. Breast base width relationship to optimal nipple-to-inframammary fold distance

Base width (BW) in cm	10.5	11.0	11.5	12.0	12.5	13.0	13.5	14.0	14.5
Appropriate nipple to inframammary fold distance (N:IMF) measured under maximal stretch	7.0	7.0	7.5	8.0	8.0	8.0	8.5	9.0	9.5

These measurements provide surgeons a guideline for an appropriate N:IMF to set for any given BW. Objective measurements are always more accurate compared to "eyeballing" decisions intraoperatively where countless variables can detract from the accuracy of correction. Visual checks during preoperative marking and surgery are obviously logical, but the visual impressions are always more accurate if they reconcile with objective measurements.

The surgeon first determines an appropriate N:IMF measurement for correction by measuring the opposite breast N:IMF if opposite breast aesthetics are optimal, or by deriving an appropriate N:IMF from Table 18-5. The surgeon marks the desired, new N:IMF distance on the affected side, measuring downward from the nipple and placing a dot at the 6 o'clock position of the desired, new inframammary fold. The surgeon can then transfer radial measurements from an opposite, unaffected breast, or visually freehand draw a desired, new inframammary fold on the affected side. Using either method, the surgeon places dots at 1 cm intervals along the desired, new inframammary fold. If the patient had an inframammary incision placed at the appropriate level for breast width at the primary operation, the incision scar will be located within 0.5 cm of the desired new fold level.

The following technique for inferior and lateral capsulorrhaphy is based on the principles and decision processes discussed previously. If the contralateral breast has optimal contours, the surgeon can transfer radial measurements from the nipple to the 6 through 10 o'clock positions of the pocket to the contralateral affected side, making all measurements under maximal stretch (Figure 18-3). Connecting these dots creates an approximate, desired lateral pocket limit. If both breasts are affected, the surgeon displaces the implant medially with the spread fingers of the non-dominant hand to simulate the desired

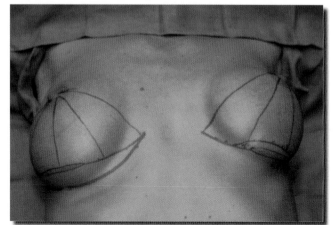

Figure 18-3. Radial measurements and markings from the patient's unaffected left breast are transferred to the right breast with stretched lower pole. Each radial is carefully measured under maximal stretch.

lateral limit of pocket closure, and marks similar points on the skin to define points along the desired lateral pocket limit.

Through an inframammary or periareolar incision approach, the surgeon removes the implant and then places a double ended retractor to expose the capsular surfaces of the lateral pocket. Using the tip of a handswitching needle tip electrocautery pencil, the surgeon presses the needle tip against the inner surface of the anterior capsule medially and laterally to identify points immediately beneath the points previously marked on the skin (Figure 18-4). When the needle tip of the electrocautery pencil is positioned exactly beneath the points marked on the skin, the surgeon momentarily touches the coagulation switch on the electrocautery pencil to mark a corresponding point internally on the capsule. This simple technique avoids the necessity of pushing needles through the skin from externally to mark exact corresponding points on the capsule, and is much more efficient. The surgeon repeats this process, creating a dotted line of pinpoint electrocautery marks on the anterior capsule along the desired line of closure.

To free the surgeon's hands, the surgeon then transfers the retractor to the assistant. Using the non-dominant hand, the surgeon presses against each point marked externally on the skin while visualizing the dotted marks on the capsule inside the pocket to make each of these points contact the opposite, posterior capsular surface. At the exact point where the marked point on the anterior capsule contacts the posterior capsule, the surgeon places an electrocautery "dot" on the posterior capsule by momentarily depressing the coagulation switch (Figure 18-5).

Using the needle tip or extended needle tip electrocautery, the surgeon

Figure 18-4. The surgeon uses the tip of the needle tip cautery to identify points on the anterior capsule inside the pocket that correspond exactly to marks on the skin for desired pocket borders. At these exact points, the surgeon activates the coagulation current for an instant to mark the point on the anterior capsule, and repeats this process across the inframammary fold and lateral pocket.

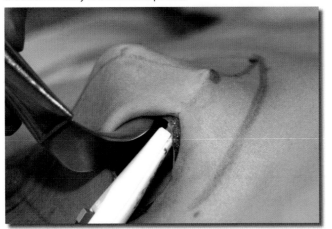

Figure 18-5. The surgeon presses at each point on the skin while viewing inside the pocket. At each point where the cautery mark on the anterior capsule contacts the posterior capsule, the surgeon places and electrocautery "dot" on the posterior capsule.

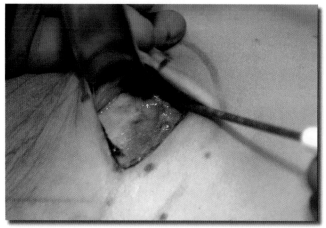

Figure 18-6.

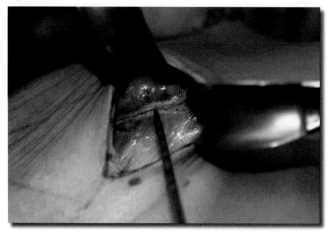

then connects the dots on the anterior and posterior capsules using a blended cut and coagulation current to create a continuous, precise, line anteriorly and posteriorly on the capsule that corresponds to desired suture line for pocket closure (Figure 18-6). Slight separation of the edges of the incised capsule creates a raw surface area for optimal wound healing and scar reinforcement, and simultaneously provides a distinct, precise capsular edge for precise suture placement. On the posterior capsule, the surgeon does not need to incise deeply and does not need to elevate the capsule edge for approximation to the anterior capsule. Creating a raw surface line with the electrocautery pencil is all that is required for accurate and effective approximation of the anterior to the posterior capsule.

Removal of anterior and posterior capsules inferior to the desired line of closure is unnecessary, because the increased raw surface will produce more transudate and the strength of the inferior closure is in the suture materials, not adherence of raw surfaces. Before beginning closure, the surgeon should assure at least a 3–4 mm gap between the edges of the capsular incisions anteriorly and posteriorly. Suture placement incorporates both edges of the anterior and posterior capsules for

Slight separation of the edges of the incised capsules creates a raw surface area for optimal wound healing and scar reinforcement, and simultaneously provides a distinct, precise capsular edge for precise suture placement

Removal of anterior and posterior capsule inferior to the desired line of closure is unnecessary

Figure 18-7. The continuous Prolene suture incorporates both edges of both the anterior and posterior capsule incision lines for optimal strength and to coapt the cut surfaces along the scoring lines.

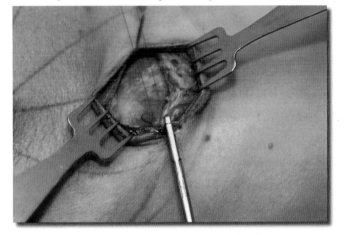

optimal suture strength in the best tissue, while coapting the narrow raw surfaces created by the anterior and posterior scoring incisions (Figure 18-7).

Initial approximation of the capsular scored edges anterior to posterior with interrupted, absorbable sutures at 1 cm increments along the desired line of closure allows the surgeon to check and adjust the position and depth of each suture to create the desired line of closure and minimize visible dimpling on the skin while trying to incorporate as dense tissue as possible in each suture. After placing several interrupted sutures, the surgeon can check lateral pocket contour by three alternative methods. The most efficient is to place two or three fingers into the incision, lift the soft tissues to allow the pocket to fill with air, then occlude the incision with the fingers and compress the overlying tissues to define the contour of the lateral pocket. Alternatively, the surgeon can place an inflatable implant or sizer into the pocket and inflate it with air or saline to check lateral pocket contour. A final alternative is to place the definitive implant, but this alternative is not optimal because it may require repeated insertion and removal of the device, subjecting it to more risks of shell damage or contamination. The surgeon should check contours with the patient supine and sitting on the operating table, marking areas of irregularity on the skin and replacing the interrupted sutures to achieve an optimal, smooth contour. This process can be very tedious and time consuming, but an accurate closure with minimal or no dimpling and smooth contour is essential to avoid patient complaints and recurrent deformities postoperatively.

When contours are optimal with the interrupted sutures, a few minor irregularities along the closure line may be visible on the skin. To reinforce the interrupted suture closure and make final, minor adjustments to optimize contour, the surgeon places two, continuous 3-0 polypropylene or nylon sutures for final approximation of the anterior capsular edge to the posterior capsular edge. *The surgeon starts one suture at the medial-most extent of the closure, and another suture at the lateral-most extent of the desired closure.* The lateral continuous suture stops at the lateral aspect of the inframammary incision, and the medial continuous suture approximates the deep fascial edge and capsule across the incision to join the point where the lateral suture stopped. The surgeon then loosens the medial suture adequately to permit implant insertion (Figure 18-8). *Placing both sutures before inserting the implant greatly simplifies the closure and provides optimal protection for the implant.* Performing total capsulectomy in the sulcus area lateral to the closure line is unnecessary using the techniques described, and only causes more tissue trauma, bleeding and fluid accumulation without increasing the efficacy or longevity of the correction. The surgeon ties the two continuous sutures at the lateral aspect of the inframammary incision, and assures that the knot is tucked as deeply as possible to minimize knot palpability postoperatively. In many patients with thinned tissues, knot palpability is unavoidable, and patients should be informed preoperatively and acknowledge this fact in signed informed consent documents. Figure 18-9 shows the completed capsulorrhaphy closure, and Figure 18-10 shows the patient before and 2 years after capsulorrhaphy.

Figure 18-8. With continuous medial and lateral Prolene sutures in place, the surgeon loosens the medial suture to permit implant insertion.

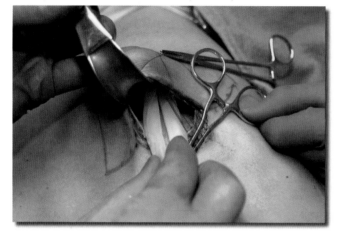

Figure 18-9. Completed capsulorrhaphy closure with elevation of the inframammary fold.

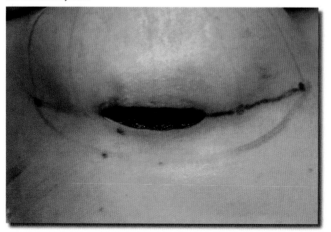

Figure 18-10. Top row: Patient with inferior pole stretch and "bottoming" right breast. Bottom row: Two years after capsulorrhaphy to elevate and reconstruct the right inframammary fold.

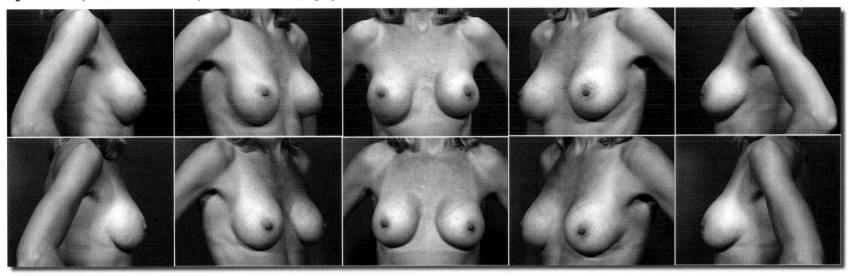

■ ADJUNCTIVE MEASURES FOLLOWING CAPSULORRHAPHY

Using the techniques described in this chapter minimizes the necessity of inferior capsulectomy, minimizes excessive wound surface area inside the pocket, minimizes transudation, and negates the necessity of drains in most cases. If significant bleeding occurs at any point of the dissection, a drain exiting an axillary puncture is a logical adjunct.

Although no scientifically valid studies prove any efficacy of compressive dressing or garments along the inframammary fold closure, a flexible foam tape dressing or elastic garment that provides support at the level of the inframammary fold repair is logical and may provide compression along the fold to minimize dead space and fluid accumulation in the inferior sulcus. Maintaining elastic garment support for 1–3 weeks postoperatively is logical, and is somewhat reassuring to the patient, even if the adjunct is unproved scientifically.

▓ REFERENCES

1. Tebbetts JB: An approach that integrates patient education and informed consent in breast augmentation. *Plast Reconstr Surg* 110(3):971–978, 2002.

2. Tebbetts JB, Adams WP: Five critical decisions in breast augmentation using 5 measurements in 5 minutes: the high five system. *Plast Reconstr Surg* 116(7):2005–2016, 2005.

3. Adams WP, Bengtson BP, Glicksman CA, Gryskiewicz JM, Jewell ML, McGrath MH, Reisman NR, Teitelbaum SA, Tebbetts JB, Tebbetts T: Decision and management algorithms to address patient and Food and Drug Administration concerns regarding breast augmentation and implants. *Plast Reconstr Surg* 114(5):1252–1257, 2004.

4. Tebbetts JB: Dual plane (DP) breast augmentation: optimizing implant–soft tissue relationships in a wide range of breast types. *Plast Reconstr Surg* 107:1255, 2001.

5. Tebbetts JB: Achieving a predictable 24 hour return to normal activities after breast augmentation Part II: Patient preparation, refined surgical techniques and instrumentation. *Plast Reconstr Surg* 109:293–305, 2002.

6. Tebbetts JB: Patient acceptance of adequately filled breast implants using the tilt test. *Plast Reconstr Surg* 106(1):139–147, 2000.

7. Tebbetts JB: Achieving a zero percent reoperation rate at 3 years in a 50 consecutive case augmentation mammaplasty PMA study. *Plast Reconstr Surg* 118(6):1453–1457, 2006.

8. Hester TR, Tebbetts JB, Maxwell GP: The polyurethane-covered mammary prosthesis: facts and fiction (II): a look back and a "peek" ahead. *Clin Plast Surg* 28(3):579–586, 2001.

9. Tebbetts JB: A system for breast implant selection based on patient tissue characteristics and implant–soft tissue dynamics. *Plast Reconstr Surg* 109(4):1396–1409, 2002.

Glandular Ptotic and Constricted Lower Pole Breasts

Achieving optimal augmentation results in breasts with glandular ptosis or a constricted lower pole requires that surgeons have a detailed knowledge of the anatomy and implant–soft tissue dynamics that are unique to these two breast types. Suboptimal outcomes occur frequently following augmentation of these breast types when surgeons apply routine augmentation principles to operative planning and implant and technique selection.

■ REQUIREMENTS FOR OPTIMAL CORRECTION IN GLANDULAR PTOTIC AND CONSTRICTED LOWER POLE BREASTS

Glandular ptotic breasts and constricted lower pole breasts have significant anatomic differences, but optimal correction of both deformities with augmentation has common requirements (Table 19-1): (1) surgical correction of the anatomic layer(s) that produce the deformity, (2) selection of implant type and size that allows the surgeon to control distribution of fill and pressure that the implant exerts on adjacent tissues, (3) redistribution or repositioning of tissue relative to the implant, (4) tissue layer interface control, (5) precise intraoperative control of implant pocket dimensions, and (6) precise positioning of the implant within the soft tissue pocket.

■ CATEGORIZING BREAST PTOSIS

The most commonly recognized classification of breast ptosis was first published in 1976 by Paula Regnault.[1] This classification and subsequent modifications of the classification, while useful for many years, share common deficiencies that confuse many surgeons and contribute to selection of suboptimal surgical techniques for correction.

Table 19-1. **Requirements for correction of glandular ptotic and constricted lower pole breasts**

Requirement for Correction	Reason(s) for the Requirement
1. Surgical correction of the anatomic layer(s) that produce the deformity	Glandular ptosis (GP): must *disrupt and convert the parenchyma–muscle interface* to a parenchyma–anterior capsule interface Constricted lower pole (CLP): Must *release constricting tissue layers* to allow subsequent stretch by implant forces
2. Selection of implant type and size that allows the surgeon to control distribution of fill and pressure that the implant exerts on adjacent tissues	GP: Requires full height, moderate projection implant selected using the High Five™ System in order to exert maximal pressure over the greatest surface area of the posterior parenchymal surface CLP: Same as GP; in addition, exert widest (not focal) pressure across the entire lower pole area of soft tissue constriction—all layers
3. Redistribution or repositioning of tissue relative to the implant	GP: Must redistribute parenchymal mass over the widest surface area to provide maximal opportunity for the posterior surface of the parenchyma to attach to the anterior capsule to provide support to minimize inferior descent CLP: Parenchyma, often constricted with minimal base width, needs to be redistributed more widely by radial and/or concentric scoring to redistribute the parenchymal mass over as wide an area of the implant as possible for coverage and for optimal aesthetics
4. Tissue layer interface control	GP: Disrupt existing parenchyma–muscle interface that allowed inferior migration of parenchyma; establish widest possible surface area for attachment of redistributed parenchyma to anterior capsule CLP: Release/disrupt attachments at the parenchyma–muscle interface to allow subsequent redistribution of narrow, constricted parenchymal mass; provide maximal surface area for implant to exert pressure on overlying constricted soft tissue layers to effect stretch to reform and reshape the lower pole
5. Precise intraoperative control of implant pocket dimensions	GP: Implant pocket dimensions control implant position; implant position is critical to exert pressure and provide controlled fill in specific areas CLP: Same as for GP
6. Precise positioning of the implant within the soft tissue pocket	GP: Implant position within the pocket is critical to exert pressure and provide controlled fill in specific areas for optimal correction. CLP: Same as for GP

All current classifications of breast ptosis that relate the position of the nipple to the level of the projected inframammary fold are extremely subjective, non-quantitative, and subject to a wide range of surgeon interpretations

All current classifications of breast ptosis that relate the position of the nipple to the level of the projected inframammary fold are extremely subjective, non-quantitative, and subject to a wide range of surgeon interpretations. Absent measurements to quantify the amount of skin in the lower pole of the breast (nipple-to-inframammary fold distance measured under maximal stretch[2,3]) surgeons make judgments and select techniques for correction by viewing the breast laterally in photographs or in the clinical setting, and subjectively assign a level of the nipple relative to the level of the projected inframammary fold anteriorly. This method, though widely used, is exceedingly inaccurate and subject to a wide range of variables. When surgeons use this method, and then select a surgical technique for correction of the deformity based on a subjective and relatively inaccurate and inconsistent visual estimation, it is not surprising that a large number of suboptimal corrections and subsequent revision or reoperation procedures occur.

Surgeons should recognize the critical importance of establishing quantitative guidelines to define degrees of breast ptosis that may be correctable by an implant alone versus degrees of ptosis that require mastopexy, with or without augmentation. *The single quantitative factor that best defines whether a breast implant alone may correct a ptosis deformity is nipple-to-inframammary fold distance measured under maximal stretch ($N{:}IMF_{max\ stretch}$). When N:IMF exceeds 9.5 cm and/or breast width exceeds 13 cm, surgeons should not attempt correction of the ptosis deformity with an implant alone.*[2,3] Figure 19-1 emphasizes the need to strongly consider mastopexy when N:IMF measured under maximal stretch exceeds 9.5–10 cm.

> When N:IMF exceeds 9.5 cm and/or breast width exceeds 13 cm, surgeons should not attempt correction of the ptosis deformity with an implant alone

The most accurate, reproducible, and scientifically valid method of classifying and quantifying the degree of ptosis is a single measurement: nipple-to-inframammary fold distance measured under maximal stretch. This measurement not only serves as a criterion for performing mastopexy in lieu of or in conjunction with augmentation as described previously, but it also provides an objective method of documenting degree of lower pole skin stretch preoperatively and at intervals postoperatively. Objectively documenting further stretch following augmentation or mastopexy provides surgeons with objective evidence to document positive or negative postoperative changes that may become issues to patients.

Figure 19-1. Criteria for mastopexy in lieu of augmentation in the glandular ptotic breast.

If N: IMF (max stretch) is > 9.5-10cm	**and/or**	Base width >13 cm and APSS > 4 cm

The degree to which an implant is likely to accomplish optimal correction of a sagging breast is determined by the amount of skin in the lower pole of the breast (N:IMF$_{max\ stretch}$) and the amount of filler material required to optimally and fully expand the lower pole

Using quantitative measurements to define limits for augmentation alone versus mastopexy (with or without an implant) eliminates the inherent inaccuracies of subjective judgments of nipple position relative to the inframammary fold

The degree to which an implant is likely to accomplish optimal correction of a sagging breast is determined by the amount of skin in the lower pole of the breast (N:IMF$_{max\ stretch}$) and the amount of filler material required to optimally and fully expand the lower pole. The *longer* the N:IMF measurement, the *wider* the breast, and the *less* parenchyma present preoperatively, the greater the implant volume required to optimally expand the skin envelope and create adequate projection to optimally correct the deformity.

The less parenchyma present in a patient's breast, the lower the nipple position may appear for any N:IMF measurement. Traditional classifications of ptosis that base technique selection on nipple position relative to the projected inframammary fold do not consider three critical factors that determine whether an implant alone may accomplish optimal correction: N:IMF$_{max\ stretch}$, base width (BW), and the amount of parenchyma present within the existing envelope.

Using quantitative measurements to define limits for augmentation alone versus mastopexy (with or without an implant) eliminates the inherent inaccuracies of subjective judgments of nipple position relative to the inframammary fold.[2,3] Ptosis deformities in which the nipple–areola complex is located 1–1.5 cm *below* the level of the projected inframammary fold, indicate formal mastopexy according to most systems that classify ptosis using nipple position relative to the projected inframammary fold. A subset of these cases, however, has a low nipple position relative to the inframammary fold, but may have a N:IMF of 8.0–9.0 cm or less, indicating that the deformity is likely correctable by implant alone, avoiding unnecessary tradeoffs and risks of mastopexy. In subjective terms, a patient can have an "empty" breast that appears "sagging", but if N:IMF is 9.5 cm or less and base width is 13 cm or less, the "emptiness" factor that is causing the sagging appearance can likely be corrected with an implant alone. When N:IMF and BW exceed the previously defined parameters, the volume of implant required to optimally expand the envelope for optimal correction becomes excessive, often exceeding 400–500 cc, and surgeons should counsel the patient regarding the tradeoffs of excessively large, low breasts compared to the tradeoffs of mastopexy.

■ THE GLANDULAR PTOTIC BREAST

The generic term "glandular ptotic" is inherently subjective and poorly defines one segment of a range of breast ptosis deformities. Three components must exist simultaneously to create a glandular ptotic or ptotic breast: (1) weakness or stretch of soft tissue attachments at the parenchyma–muscle interface, (2) a mobile mass of parenchyma, and (3) excess skin (by stretch) in the *lower pole* envelope to allow descent of the parenchymal mass. Descent of the nipple–areola complex is a separate component, and the extent to which the complex descends depends on the degree of stretch in the skin of the *upper* breast envelope.

In the glandular ptotic breast, the tissue interface between the pectoralis major muscle and the overlying breast parenchyma is extremely mobile, allowing the parenchyma to migrate inferiorly over time or following pregnancy. Stretched skin is present in the lower pole envelope that allows descent of the parenchymal mass. The degree to which the nipple-to-inframammary fold skin stretches to lengthen N:IMF and the quality of the soft tissue attachments at the parenchyma–muscle interface determine the degree to which the glandular mass migrates inferiorly.

> The degree to which the nipple-to-inframammary fold skin stretches to lengthen N:IMF and the quality of the soft tissue attachments at the parenchyma–muscle interface determine the degree to which the glandular mass migrates inferiorly

Criteria for Augmentation without Mastopexy for Correcting the Glandular Ptotic Breast

Theoretically, the nipple–areola complex (NAC) in the glandular ptotic breast is located at or above the level of the anteriorly projected inframammary fold (Figure 19-2). The position of the nipple with respect to the projected inframammary fold, as previously discussed, does not accurately define the variables that affect correction of this type of breast deformity. For example, the nipple can appear to be below the level of the projected inframammary fold, but N:IMF may be only 8–8.5 cm if minimal parenchyma is present. This degree of lower pole stretched envelope certainly does not require a mastopexy for optimal fill and aesthetic

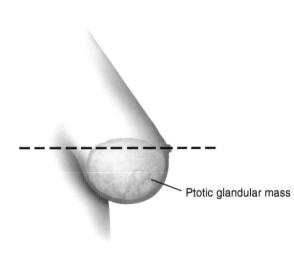

Figure 19-2. Nipple position at level of projected inframammary fold in the glandular ptotic breast.

Ptotic glandular mass

correction. A 300 cc breast implant in conjunction with a dual plane type 2 pocket dissection predictably corrects this deformity without subjecting the patient to all of the tradeoffs and risks of a mastopexy.

Analyzing this type of deformity using the High Five™ System[3] quickly identifies and quantifies indications for augmentation alone or mastopexy (Table 19-2).

According to the system, a 13 cm base width requires 325 cc volume for optimal fill. If anterior pull skin stretch (APSS) exceeds 3 cm, as it virtually always does with a stretched envelope (glandular ptotic) breast, the system recommends adding 30 cc to the starting volume for a total of 355 cc. If APSS exceeds 4 cm, an additional 30 cc or a 385 cc volume would be required. Finally, if N:IMF exceeds 9.5 cm, the system recommends adding another 30 cc for a total of 415 cc. While this size implant may adequately expand

Table 19-2. Applying the High Five™ System to determine the necessity of mastopexy or augmentation alone

Prioritized Decisions Based on Breast Measurements and Tissue Characteristics
The High Five™ System   Copyright 2005   John B. Tebbetts, M.D.

I. POCKET LOCATION SELECTED BASED ON THICKNESS OF TISSUE COVERAGE (Circle One)

			DP
STPTUP		If <2.0 cm, consider dual plane (DP) or partial retropectoral (PRP, pectoralis origins intact across IMF)	**PRP RM**
STPTIMF		If STPTIMF <0.5 cm, consider subpectoral pocket and leave pectoralis origins intact along IMF	

II. IMPLANT VOLUME/WEIGHT   BASED ON BREAST DIMENSIONS, TISSUE STRETCH, AND EXISTING PARENCHYMA, ALL IN CM.

Base Width	13	B.W. Parenchyma (cm)	10.5	11.0	11.5	12.0	12.5	13.0	13.5	14.0	14.5	15.0	325 cc
		Initial Volume (cc)	**200**	**250**	**275**	**300**	**300**	325	**350**	**375**	**375**	**400**	
APSS$_{MaxStr}$	4.4	[2]If APSS <2.0, −30 cc; If APSS >3.0, +30 cc; If APSS >4.0, +60 cc **Place appropriate number in blank at right**											+60 cc
N:IMF$_{MaxSt}$	9.8	**If N:IMF >9.5, +30 cc** Place appropriate number in blank at right											+30 cc
PCSEF %	30	**If PCSEF <20%, +30 cc; If PCSEF >80%, −30 cc** Place appropriate number in blank at right											cc
IDFDD cc		**If Inamed Style 468, −30 cc** Place appropriate number in blank at right											cc
Pt. request													cc

NET ESTIMATED VOLUME TO FILL ENVELOPE BASED ON PATIENT TISSUE CHARACTERISTICS	415 cc

III. IMPLANT TYPE   MFR: Allergan STYLE/MODEL: 410 Form Stable Gel, Full Height, Moderate Profile   VOLUME: cc

Volume: N:IMF Relationships	200	250	275	300	325	350	375	400	**PreN:IMF**
	7.0	7.0	7.5	8	8	8.5	9.0	9.5	**9.8 cm**

IV. NEW INFRAMAMMARY FOLD LEVEL	N:IMF$_{MaxSt}$ **to set with preoperative markings and intraoperatively**	9.8 cm

V. INCISION LOCATION (Circle One)   IM   AX   PA   UMB

the lower pole envelope and improve appearance, even this significant volume may not adequately fill the upper pole of the breast. Regardless, this weight implant in an envelope that has already proved it stretches excessively as a result of genetics, aging, or pregnancy, is unlikely to sustain a satisfactory aesthetic result at best, and at worst could quickly develop a "rock in a sock" appearance of a much larger breast that appears low on the torso. Rationale for implant type selection and level of the inframammary fold in this example are discussed later in this chapter.

No breast implant lifts a breast

No breast implant lifts a breast. When treating significant glandular ptosis with an implant alone, patients should be informed and acknowledge in written, informed consent documents that their result will be a substantially larger breast that remains low on the torso, likely with poor fill of the breast upper pole.

Informed Consent Considerations for Patients with Glandular Ptosis

Most patients with glandular ptosis, if presented with alternatives, prefer augmentation alone, avoiding the scars and other potential tradeoffs of mastopexy. In order to obtain valid, legal informed consent, however, patients who select augmentation and decline mastopexy should understand and acknowledge the following in written and signed informed consent documents:

1. The surgeon must place adequate volume (a large enough implant) to adequately fill the breast envelope, or the middle and upper breast will not be adequately filled, and the breast may have a "rock in a sock" appearance.

2. The very fact that the breast is sagging preoperatively proves that the genetic qualities of the skin were unable to support the weight of the breast alone without excessive stretching.

3. Adding weight, especially the weight of an implant large enough to fill an already stretched envelope, to a breast that has already proved it stretches excessively is at best a temporary improvement, and any correction achieved may be lost rapidly due to further stretch of the skin with the added weight of an implant.

4. No implant in this type breast, regardless of type or size, will predictably maintain fill in the upper breast. Mastopexy, with or without augmentation, will also not predictably maintain fill in the upper breast. Patients with skin that has already stretched excessively should be aware that despite some surgeons' claims, no implant or technique will ever change the genetic realities of the skin, and therefore the patient should never expect long-term upper breast fill.

No implant in this type breast, regardless of type or size, will predictably maintain fill in the upper breast. Mastopexy, with or without augmentation, will also not predictably maintain fill in the upper breast

5. No breast implant effectively lifts a breast. Filling the envelope may create an appearance of nipple lift, but any lifted appearance is more apparent than real. True lifting of the breast requires removal of excess stretched skin that allowed downward displacement of the breast tissue that created the ptosis.

6. Augmenting a breast with a stretched lower pole envelope can often result in a breast that appears "bottomed", fuller in the lower breast and emptier in the upper breast, with or without an excessively upward tilted or located nipple–areola complex.

7. Augmenting a glandular ptotic breast results in a larger breast that may continue to appear low on the torso. Augmentation in this type breast never produces a "perkier" appearing breast that appears higher on the torso.

8. Mastopexy may be required as a secondary procedure for any patient with a significant degree of glandular ptosis who is treated with augmentation alone.

Implant–Soft Tissue Dynamics in the Glandular Ptotic Breast

The key to success or failure in treating glandular ptotic breasts with augmentation alone is the posterior interface of the parenchyma with either the anterior capsule in submammary, subfascial, or dual plane[4] 2 augmentations, or the parenchyma–muscle interface if the surgeon places the implant subpectorally. Traditional subpectoral augmentation, leaving pectoralis origins intact along the inframammary fold, is almost predictably doomed to failure, because the surgeon has not addressed the weak attachments at the parenchyma–muscle interface that allowed the glandular tissue to slide inferiorly to create the preoperative deformity of glandular ptosis. A traditional subpectoral augmentation almost predictably results in the parenchyma sliding inferiorly off the pectoralis and underlying implant to create a "double bubble" deformity in the breast lower pole. Correction of the "double bubble" deformity requires either: (1) a conversion to a dual plane[4] 2 pocket with division of pectoralis origins along the inframammary fold and separation of parenchyma–muscle attachments to allow superomedial rotation of the lower pectoralis edge (this option optimizes soft tissue coverage medially and superiorly), or (2) conversion to a submammary or subfascial pocket which does not provide as good long-term soft tissue coverage medially and superiorly. With either conversion option, radial scoring of any palpable banding transversely at the level of the preoperative inframammary fold is often necessary for optimal release and correction.

Regardless of whether a surgeon chooses to augment the glandular ptotic patient using a submammary, subfascial, or dual plane[4] 2 pocket, the surgeon must realize and inform the patient that the glandular tissue may unavoidably slide downward off the anterior surface of the anterior capsule that forms around the implant. No type of implant, regardless of surface characteristics, shape, or profile/projection can predictably assure that glandular tissue will not continue to slide inferiorly off the capsule. If inferior descent of glandular tissue occurs despite a properly performed dual plane[4] 2 or 3 pocket, or following submammary or subfascial placement, correction will require formal mastopexy to remove skin from the lower envelope (excess skin envelope is present by definition if the parenchymal mass descends, and the excess is both vertical and horizontal). Surgeons should be especially cautious when attempting to correct this secondary deformity, and assure adequate removal of skin vertically in the breast lower pole. Mastopexy techniques that limit scars to periareolar and vertical usually fail to correct this secondary deformity because they fail to remove adequate skin from the breast lower pole, choosing to rotate excess skin upward to minimize scar length.

Regardless of whether a surgeon chooses to augment the glandular ptotic patient using a submammary, subfascial, or dual plane[4] 2 pocket, the surgeon must realize and inform the patient that the glandular tissue may unavoidably slide downward off the anterior surface of the anterior capsule that forms around the implant

Surgical Correction of the Glandular Ptotic Breast

Figure 19-3 is a flowchart that summarizes alternatives for surgical correction of the glandular ptotic breast.

Provided that N:IMF is 9.5 cm or less, and base width 13 cm or less, a dual plane type 2 pocket dissection and a full height, form stable, moderate profile implant selected according to the High Five™ system[3] provides excellent correction and optimal long-term outcomes in a majority of cases. Submammary and subfascial pocket locations are not best for the patient long-term, because neither provides maximal soft tissue coverage medially and superiorly for the patient's lifetime, risking reoperations or uncorrectable deformities such as visible implant edges and traction rippling medially or superiorly. A dual plane type 2 or 3 pocket provides optimal correction and optimal long-term soft tissue coverage for most areas of a glandular ptotic breast. Disrupting the parenchyma–muscle interface by using the dual plane[4] 2 technique is critically important to minimize risks of the parenchyma sliding inferiorly off the muscle. With the dual plane 2, the inferior cut edge of the pectoralis moves superiorly by superomedial rotation to the level of the nipple or lower border of the areola. Details of technique are included in Chapters 8 and 11.

Submammary and subfascial pocket locations are not best for the patient long-term, because neither provides maximal soft tissue coverage medially and superiorly for the patient's lifetime

A dual plane type 2 or 3 pocket provides optimal correction and optimal long-term soft tissue coverage for most areas of a glandular ptotic breast

Figure 19-3. Surgical correction of the glandular ptosis.

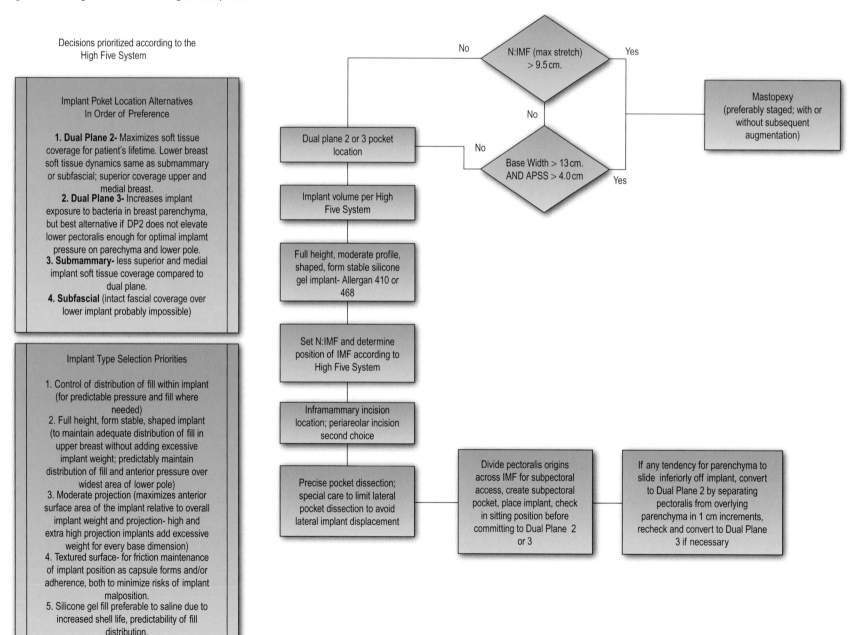

Decisions prioritized according to the
High Five System

**Implant Poket Location Alternatives
In Order of Preference**

1. Dual Plane 2- Maximizes soft tissue
coverage for patient's lifetime. Lower breast
soft tissue dynamics same as submammary
or subfascial; superior coverage upper and
medial breast.
2. Dual Plane 3- Increases implant
exposure to bacteria in breast parenchyma,
but best alternative if DP2 does not elevate
lower pectoralis enough for optimal implant
pressure on parechyma and lower pole.
3. Submammary- less superior and medial
implant soft tissue coverage compared to
dual plane.
4. Subfascial (intact fascial coverage over
lower implant probably impossible)

Implant Type Selection Priorities

1. Control of distribution of fill within implant
(for predictable pressure and fill where
needed)
2. Full height, form stable, shaped implant
(to maintain adequate distribution of fill in
upper breast without adding excessive
implant weight; predictably maintain
distribution of fill and anterior pressure over
widest area of lower pole)
3. Moderate projection (maximizes anterior
surface area of the implant relative to overall
implant weight and projection- high and
extra high projection implants add excessive
weight for every base dimension)
4. Textured surface- for friction maintenance
of implant position as capsule forms and/or
adherence, both to minimize risks of implant
malposition.
5. Silicone gel fill preferable to saline due to
increased shell life, predictability of fill
distribution.

N:IMF (max stretch)
> 9.5 cm.

No ——— No ——— Yes

Mastopexy
(preferably staged; with or
without subsequent
augmentation)

Dual plane 2 or 3 pocket
location

No

Base Width > 13 cm.
AND APSS > 4.0 cm

No

Yes

Implant volume per High
Five System

Full height, moderate profile,
shaped, form stable silicone
gel implant- Allergan 410 or
468

Set N:IMF and determine
position of IMF according to
High Five System

Inframammary incision
location; periareolar incision
second choice

Precise pocket dissection;
special care to limit lateral
pocket dissection to avoid
lateral implant displacement

Divide pectoralis origins
across IMF for subpectoral
access, create subpectoral
pocket, place implant, check
in sitting position before
committing to Dual Plane 2
or 3

If any tendency for parenchyma to
slide inferiorly off implant, convert
to Dual Plane 2 by separating
pectoralis from overlying
parenchyma in 1 cm increments,
recheck and convert to Dual Plane
3 if necessary

An inframammary incision approach provides the most exposure, control, and versatility for adjusting the position of the pectoralis for a dual plane[4] 2 or 3 pocket. A periareolar approach does not provide as much exposure, control, or versatility. A common error is committing initially to a dual plane 3 pocket, when often a dual plane 1 or 2 pocket preserves more soft tissue coverage without limiting anterior projection of the implant. Surgeons should plan to first divide inferior origins of the pectoralis across the inframammary fold and dissect a dual plane 1 pocket. By placing two fingers in the pocket and pulling anteriorly, the surgeon can determine whether the inferior border of the pectoralis is limiting full anterior displacement of the overlying parenchyma by an implant. If any limitation is present, the surgeon separates the pectoralis from overlying parenchyma in 1 cm increments, rechecks by pulling the envelope anteriorly, and limits separation of pectoralis from overlying parenchyma to the minimal amount that allows unrestricted anterior expansion of the soft tissue envelope.

When the surgeon has removed all limitations to full anterior expansion of the envelope, the surgeon inserts the implant and elevates the patient to a sitting position on the operating table. If the parenchyma tends to slide inferiorly off the anterior surface of the implant, or if nipple–areola position is not optimal, or if excess laxity remains in the central envelope around the nipple–areola, the surgeon should remove the implant and convert from a dual plane 2 to a dual plane 3 by additional separation of pectoralis from overlying parenchyma.

Pocket dissection must be precise to optimally control the position of the implant, because implant position is critical to provide fill and apply pressure to specific areas required for correction. To prevent the common error of excessive dissection of the lateral pocket, the surgeon should limit lateral pocket dissection, and stop dissection at the lateral border of the pectoralis minor. After placing the implant, if the posterior surface of the implant is compressed medially–laterally, the surgeon enlarges the lateral pocket in 0.5 cm increments until the base of the implant lies uncompressed on the chest wall. Keeping the implant centralized medially by precise pocket creation is essential to optimal correction. If the implant can displace laterally, it cannot transmit optimal pressure directly anterior, which is key to optimizing implant–soft tissue dynamics for optimal correction.

> An inframammary incision approach provides the most exposure, control, and versatility for adjusting the position of the pectoralis for a dual plane[4] 2 or 3 pocket

> Pocket dissection must be precise to optimally control the position of the implant, because implant position is critical to provide fill and apply pressure to specific areas required for correction

> Keeping the implant centralized medially by precise pocket creation is essential to optimal correction

If the parenchymal mass is globular or has a base width less than 11.5 cm, radial scoring of the parenchyma can help redistribute the parenchyma more widely, providing a greater surface area for pressure from the implant, and for potential attachments from parenchyma to the anterior capsule. When scoring parenchyma, most surgeons do not begin far enough superiorly. Radial scoring should begin well above the top of the areola, at the superior-most extent of the parenchyma. While scoring may increase the likelihood of better adherence of parenchyma to anterior capsule to decrease risks of parenchyma sliding inferiorly postoperatively, scoring also increases exposure of the implant to endogenous bacteria in the breast and may increase risks of capsular contracture. Scoring, therefore, should be performed only when absolutely necessary to effect optimal correction.

Implant Selection for the Glandular Ptotic Breast

High and extra high profile implants have often been promoted for augmenting glandular ptotic breasts, emphasizing the role of implant projection to the sagging parenchyma and skin of the lower pole of the breast anteriorly to "lift" the breast and "correct" the ptosis. High and extra high profile implants may contribute projection, but they are not the best choice for correction of glandular ptosis if surgeons carefully consider all of the factors of implant–soft tissue dynamics that contribute to optimal correction.

High and extra high profile implants are *not* the optimal choice for correction of glandular ptosis for the following reasons:

1. For any given base width implant, adding projection adds volume and weight. A ptotic or glandular ptotic breast has, by the occurrence of the deformity, proved that soft tissue support is compromised, so every increment of weight must be justified and offset by potential benefits.

2. High profile implants focus pressure in the worst location possible in a glandular ptotic breast—the central lower pole area. This is the area that is already thinned and stretched, the area that allowed the ptosis to occur. Worse yet, high profile devices focus the pressure over a smaller anterior surface area of the implant compared to an equal volume moderate profile implant.

3. Optimal correction of the glandular ptotic breast does not occur by simply adding projection to the implant. "Lift" produced by an implant is not true lift. Instead, the

High and extra high profile implants may contribute projection, but they are not the best choice for correction of glandular ptosis if surgeons carefully consider all of the factors of implant–soft tissue dynamics that contribute to optimal correction

appearance of lift occurs when the implant optimally expands the entire breast envelope, not only anteriorly, but also in a medial–lateral direction. If the base width of the implant is not adequate, medial–lateral expansion of the envelope is not optimal, and the medial–lateral laxity allows the central lower envelope to sag inferiorly. An optimal width implant, if high profile, always adds considerably more weight to the breast compared to a moderate profile implant.

4. All smooth shell, high profile implants currently manufactured, whether saline or silicone gel filled, are not form stable. When tilted upright, the upper shell collapses inferiorly. This characteristic is exactly what is not needed in glandular ptotic breasts where middle and upper breast fill are essential to aesthetically balance fill in the stretched lower pole. A high profile implant that fills the lower pole but does not adequately fill the upper pole produces a "rock in a sock" appearance.

5. Many currently available high profile implants have smooth shell surfaces. Smooth shell implants do not allow surgeons to control distribution of fill within the breast envelope, because the surgeon cannot control the position of any smooth shell implant. The implant falls to the bottom of the pocket, and does not allow predictable control of middle and upper breast fill.

6. A high profile implant of equivalent volume to a moderate profile implant is narrower than the moderate profile implant, with a smaller anterior surface area on the higher profile implant. The anterior surface area of the implant is critical in addressing the glandular ptotic breast. The greater the anterior surface area of the implant, the more even the pressure the implant transmits to the overlying parenchyma to splay the parenchyma and prevent parenchyma from concentrating medially where it exerts maximal stretch on the already stretched envelope and tends to slide inferiorly off the anterior surface of the implant, causing a double bubble deformity.

7. A moderate profile, full height, form stable (upper pole of implant does not collapse when implant is upright) implant provides adequate projection, less weight for any given base width compared to high or **extra** high profile implants, and predictable distribution of fill.

An optimal implant for correction of glandular ptosis should have the following characteristics:

1. Adequate base width for optimal medial–lateral expansion of the entire breast skin envelope.

2. Adequate projection to fill the envelope in an anterior–posterior direction.

3. For any given volume or weight, maximum anterior implant surface area to distribute pressure over the widest area of the posterior surface of the parenchyma.

4. Control of implant position in the pocket to control distribution of fill in the breast.

5. Control of distribution of fill within the implant to optimally control distribution of fill in the breast.

6. A shaped implant that puts projection where it is needed in the lower pole, but not at the expense of excess weight. The shaped implant must be form stable, with no collapse of the upper shell when the implant is upright.

7. A full height, form stable implant that offers the best opportunity to maintain upper breast fill as it provides dimensions and projection to optimally expand the lower pole envelope and apply pressure to the ptotic parenchyma to minimize its sliding inferiorly.

8. Surface texturing that provides friction immediately postoperatively as the capsule forms to: (a) maintain implant position, and (b) provide an opportunity for adherence to capsule and parenchyma to minimize risks of inferior migration of the parenchyma over the implant causing a double bubble deformity.

The optimal implant design for augmentation of the glandular ptotic breast, therefore, is a full height, moderate profile, shaped, textured, form stable saline or silicone gel filled implant. The Allergan Style 410 full height, form stable, silicone gel filled implant is the author's preferred implant for this application. If a patient prefers a saline filled implant, the Allergan Style 468 implant is the most form stable saline filled implant that meets these criteria.

No current implant, however, can totally assure prevention of glandular descent due to weak attachments to the anterior capsule after the implant is in place. When all measures described previously have been addressed pre- and intraoperatively, if the glandular mass markedly descends with the patient elevated to the sitting position on the operating table, the surgeon should consider performing mastopexy over the implant at the same time as

The optimal implant design for augmentation of the glandular ptotic breast, therefore, is a full height, moderate profile, shaped, textured, form stable saline or silicone gel filled implant

No current implant can totally assure prevention of glandular descent due to weak attachments to the anterior capsule after the implant is in place augmentation. To not do so virtually assures a reoperation to correct what could and should have been corrected at the primary procedure. This approach requires that patients be educated, informed, and accept in written documents that if their parenchymal mass is exceedingly mobile, simultaneous mastopexy may be required, and that the surgeon must be consented to make the decision intraoperatively. This is one of the very few indications for simultaneous augmentation-mastopexy in the author's opinion.

A common misconception is that a high or extra high projection round or shaped, form stable implant is the optimal implant to select for glandular ptotic breasts or breasts with more lax skin (APSS > 3cm.). The author learned this concept as a resident and intuitively applied the concept during the first 10 years of clinical practice. With additional clinical experience, long-term tissue measurement data instead of intuitive opinion strongly indicates that any potentially positive effect of current high and extra high profile implants in glandular ptotic breasts is outweighed by specific negatives. The additional weight of a high or extra high profile implant for any given base width imparts more negatives of additional parenchymal atrophy, lower pole skin stretch and thinning, and potential implant edge visibility or visible traction rippling. These negatives and the fact that some of these tissue consequences are irreversible and uncorrectable far outweigh any potential improvement in aesthetic outcomes of high and extra high profile implants compared to moderate profile implants. The case studies in this chapter and the author's peer reviewed and published clinical outcomes data clearly indicate that optimally sized, moderate profile implants provide excellent aesthetic correction of glandular ptosis, while reducing risk of reoperations uncorrectable tissue consequences.

Surgeons often have intuitive opinions, not necessarily based on peer reviewed and published data. Breast implant manufacturers' want to provide the widest possible range of implant projection to satisfy the surgeon market. As a result, surgeons should be aware that current implant selection systems of both breast implant manufacturers may recommend or tacitly endorse high or extra high profile implants for patients with glandular ptosis or more lax skin envelopes. Surgeons should evaluate subjective or non-data based implant selections critically to avoid irreversibly damaging or compromising patients' tissues or creating deformities based on implant selection systems that are intuitive, subjective and not based on valid scientific data. Scientifically valid implant selection systems are based on peer reviewed and published data in leading professional journals, and are not proprietary and product oriented.

Text continued on p. 482

Case Studies of Glandular Ptotic Breasts

CASE STUDY 19-1

Age 33
Gravida 3
Para 2
Bra **Band** Size: 34
Breast **Cup** Size (Pt. estimate)
Prior to pregnancy C
Largest with preg DD
Current Cup Size B
Desired Cup Size D
Previous Breast Disease: None
Breast Biopsies: No
Family Hx. Breast Cancer: No
Pertinent Medical or Breast
Imaging History: None
Breast Masses: None

TISSUE ASSESSMENT AND HIGH FIVE™ SYSTEM CRITICAL DECISIONS PROCESS

Prioritized Decisions Based on Breast Measurements and Tissue Characteristics
The High Five™ System   Copyright 2005   John B. Tebbetts, M.D.

I. POCKET LOCATION SELECTED BASED ON THICKNESS OF TISSUE COVERAGE (Circle One)

STPTUP	1.4	**If <2.0 cm., consider dual plane (DP) or partial retropectoral (PRP, pectoralis origins intact across IMF)**	**DP 2**
STPTIMF	0.8	**If STPTIMF <0.5 cm, consider subpectoral pocket and leave pectoralis origins intact along IMF**	**PRP RM**

II. IMPLANT VOLUME/WEIGHT BASED ON BREAST DIMENSIONS, TISSUE STRETCH, AND EXISTING PARENCHYMA

Base Width	13.0	**B.W. Parenchyma (cm)**	10.5	11.0	11.5	12.0	12.5	13.0	13.5	14.0	14.5	15.0	**325 cc**
		Initial Volume (cc)	200	250	275	300	300	325	350	375	375	400	
APSS$_{MaxStr}$	3.6	^{2}**If APSS <2.0, −30 cc; If APSS >3.0, +30 cc; If APSS >4.0, +60 cc Place appropriate number in blank at right**											**+30 cc**
N:IMF$_{MaxSt}$	9.5	**If N:IMF >9.5, +30 cc Place appropriate number in blank at right**											**+30 cc**
PCSEF %	30%	**If PCSEF <20%, +30 cc; If PCSEF >80%, −30 cc Place appropriate number in blank at right**											**cc**
IDFDD cc		**If Allergan Style 468 or other form stable saline implant, −30 cc Place appropriate number in blank at right**											**−30 cc**
Pt. request													**cc**

NET ESTIMATED VOLUME TO FILL ENVELOPE BASED ON PATIENT TISSUE CHARACTERISTICS	**355 cc**

III. IMPLANT TYPE MFR: Allergan STYLE/MODEL: Style 468 Anatomic Saline VOLUME: 350–370 cc									**370 cc**
Volume: N:IMF Relationships: Locate Final Selected Implant Volume at Right; Set N:IMF to the disstance shown in the cell beneath, or leave at preop N:IMF, whichever is longer.	200	250	275	300	325	350	375	400	**PreN:IMF**
	7.0	7.0	7.5	8	8	8.5	9.0	9.5	**9.5 cm**

IV. NEW INFRAMAMMARY FOLD LEVEL	**N:IMF**$_{MaxSt}$ **to set with preoperative markings and intraoperatively**	**9.5 cm**

V. INCISION LOCATION	**IM AX PA UMB**	

PREOPERATIVE ASSESSMENT AND OBSERVATIONS

WNBCS = Will not be corrected surgically
Breast size asymmetry- WNBCS
Breast level asymmetry- WNBCS
Nipple level asymmetry- WNBCS
Breast width asymmetry- WNBCS
Thin soft tissue coverage
Nipples located laterally on breast mound R > L- WNBCS
Downpointing nipples
Glandular ptosis

POSTOPERATIVE ASSESSMENT AND OBSERVATIONS

Pre- to Post- bra size change by patient questionnaire: B to D.
Breasts soft, mobile, compressible at 22 months followup.
Very good breast shape and fill
Good correction glandular ptosis
Maintenance of upper pole fill and shape at 22 months with full height, anatomic saline implant
All WNBCS items as predicted preoperatively.

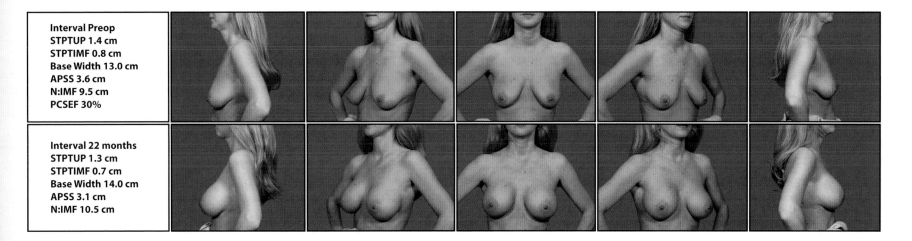

Interval Preop				
STPTUP 1.4 cm				
STPTIMF 0.8 cm				
Base Width 13.0 cm				
APSS 3.6 cm				
N:IMF 9.5 cm				
PCSEF 30%				

Interval 22 months				
STPTUP 1.3 cm				
STPTIMF 0.7 cm				
Base Width 14.0 cm				
APSS 3.1 cm				
N:IMF 10.5 cm				

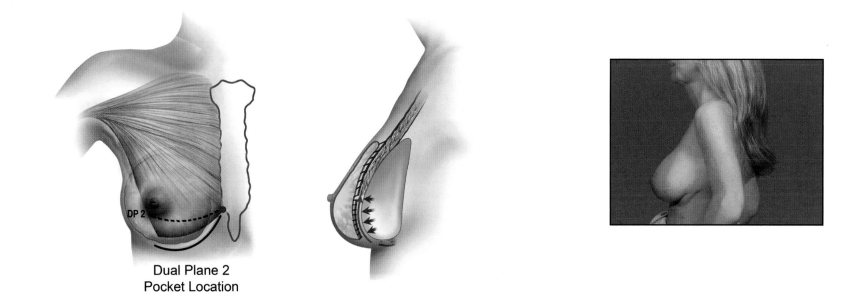

Dual Plane 2
Pocket Location

CASE STUDY 19-2

HISTORY

Age 31
Gravida 3
Para 3
Bra **Band** Size: 36
Breast **Cup** Size (Pt. estimate)
Prior to pregnancy B
Largest with preg C
Current Cup Size B
Desired Cup Size C/D
Previous Breast Disease: None
Breast Biopsies: No
Family Hx. Breast Cancer: No
Pertinent Medical or Breast
Imaging History: None
Breast Masses: None

TISSUE ASSESSMENT AND HIGH FIVE™ SYSTEM CRITICAL DECISIONS PROCESS

Prioritized Decisions Based on Breast Measurements and Tissue Characteristics
The High Five™ System   Copyright 2005   John B. Tebbetts, M.D.

I. POCKET LOCATION SELECTED BASED ON THICKNESS OF TISSUE COVERAGE (Circle One)

STPTUP	1.5	**If <2.0 cm., consider dual plane (DP) or partial retropectoral (PRP, pectoralis origins intact across IMF)**	**DP 2**
STPTIMF	0.9	**If STPTIMF <0.5 cm, consider subpectoral pocket and leave pectoralis origins intact along IMF**	**PRP RM**

II. IMPLANT VOLUME/WEIGHT BASED ON BREAST DIMENSIONS, TISSUE STRETCH, AND EXISTING PARENCHYMA

Base Width	13.5	**B.W. Parenchyma (cm)**	10.5	11.0	11.5	12.0	12.5	13.0	13.5	14.0	14.5	15.0	350 cc
		Initial Volume (cc)	200	250	275	300	300	325	350	375	375	400	
APSS$_{MaxStr}$	3.4	**If APSS <2.0, −30 cc; If APSS >3.0, +30 cc; If APSS >4.0, +60 cc Place appropriate number in blank at right**											+30 cc
N:IMF$_{MaxSt}$	9.0	**If N:IMF >9.5, +30 cc Place appropriate number in blank at right**											**cc**
PCSEF %	40%	**If PCSEF <20%, +30 cc; If PCSEF >80%, −30 cc Place appropriate number in blank at right**											**cc**
IDFDD cc	*	**If Allergan Style 468 or other form stable saline implant, −30 cc Place appropriate number in blank at right**											−30 cc
Pt. request														**cc**

NET ESTIMATED VOLUME TO FILL ENVELOPE BASED ON PATIENT TISSUE CHARACTERISTICS — 350 cc

III. IMPLANT TYPE MFR: Allergan STYLE/MODEL: Style 468 Anatomic Saline   VOLUME: 350 cc — 350 cc

Volume: N:IMF Relationships: Locate Final Selected Implant Volume at Right; Set N:IMF to the disstance shown in the cell beneath, or leave at preop N:IMF, whichever is longer.	200	250	275	300	325	350	375	400	**PreN:IMF**
	7.0	7.0	7.5	8	8	8.5	9.0	9.5	**9.0 cm**

IV. NEW INFRAMAMMARY FOLD LEVEL	N:IMF$_{MaxSt}$ to set with preoperative markings and intraoperatively	9.0 cm
V. INCISION LOCATION	IM AX PA UMB	

PREOPERATIVE ASSESSMENT AND OBSERVATIONS

WNBCS = Will not be corrected surgically
Breast size asymmetry- WNBCS
Breast level asymmetry- WNBCS
Nipple level asymmetry- WNBCS
Breast width asymmetry- WNBCS
Thin soft tissue coverage
Glandular ptosis

POSTOPERATIVE ASSESSMENT AND OBSERVATIONS

Pre- to Post- bra size change by patient questionnaire: B to D.
Breasts soft, mobile, compressible at 50 months followup.
Excellent breast shape and fill
Very slight loss of upper pole fill and shape over 4 years postoperatively
Very natural appearing upper pole with full height anatomic, saline implant
All WNBCS items as predicted preoperatively.

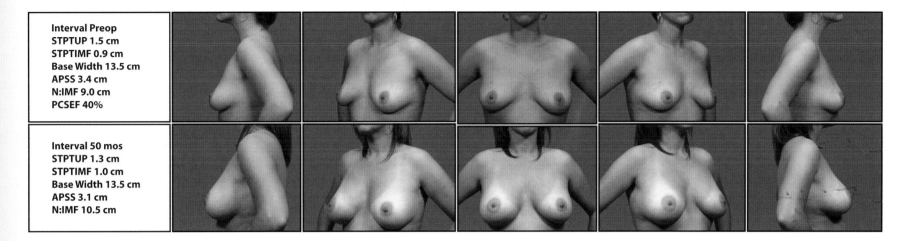

Interval Preop				
STPTUP 1.5 cm				
STPTIMF 0.9 cm				
Base Width 13.5 cm				
APSS 3.4 cm				
N:IMF 9.0 cm				
PCSEF 40%				

Interval 50 mos				
STPTUP 1.3 cm				
STPTIMF 1.0 cm				
Base Width 13.5 cm				
APSS 3.1 cm				
N:IMF 10.5 cm				

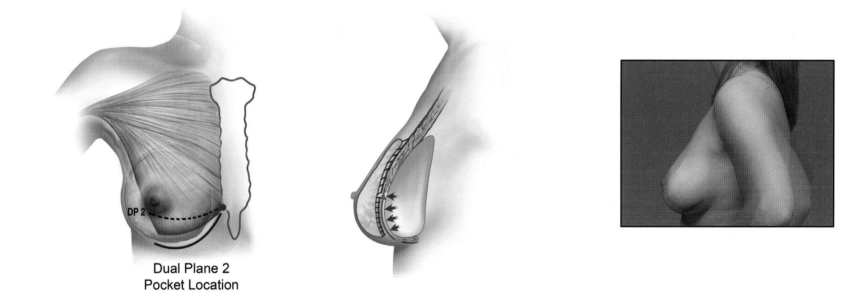

DP 2

Dual Plane 2
Pocket Location

CASE STUDY 19-3

HISTORY

Age 31
Gravida 1
Para 1
Bra **Band** Size: 34
Breast **Cup** Size (Pt. estimate)
Prior to pregnancy B
Largest with preg C
Current Cup Size B
Desired Cup Size D
Previous Breast Disease: None
Breast Biopsies: No
Family Hx. Breast Cancer: No
Pertinent Medical or Breast
Imaging History: None
Breast Masses: None

TISSUE ASSESSMENT AND HIGH FIVE™ SYSTEM CRITICAL DECISIONS PROCESS

Prioritized Decisions Based on Breast Measurements and Tissue Characteristics		
The High Five™ System Copyright 2005 John B. Tebbetts, M.D.		

I. POCKET LOCATION SELECTED BASED ON THICKNESS OF TISSUE COVERAGE (Circle One)

STPTUP	1.7	**If <2.0 cm., consider dual plane (DP) or partial retropectoral (PRP, pectoralis origins intact across IMF)**	DP 2
STPTIMF	1.0	**If STPTIMF <0.5 cm, consider subpectoral pocket and leave pectoralis origins intact along IMF**	PRP RM

II. IMPLANT VOLUME/WEIGHT BASED ON BREAST DIMENSIONS, TISSUE STRETCH, AND EXISTING PARENCHYMA

Base Width	12.5	B.W. Parenchyma (cm)	10.5	11.0	11.5	12.0	12.5	13.0	13.5	14.0	14.5	15.0	300 cc
		Initial Volume (cc)	200	250	275	300	300	325	350	375	375	400	
$APSS_{MaxStr}$	2.6	[2]**If APSS <2.0, −30 cc; If APSS >3.0, +30 cc; If APSS >4.0, +60 cc Place appropriate number in blank at right**											cc
$N:IMF_{MaxSt}$	8.0	**If N:IMF >9.5, +30 cc Place appropriate number in blank at right**											cc
PCSEF %	50%	**If PCSEF <20%, +30 cc; If PCSEF >80%, −30 cc Place appropriate number in blank at right**											cc
IDFDD cc	NA	**If Allergan Style 468 or other form stable saline implant, −30 cc Place appropriate number in blank at right**											NA
Pt. request													cc

NET ESTIMATED VOLUME TO FILL ENVELOPE BASED ON PATIENT TISSUE CHARACTERISTICS	300 cc
III. IMPLANT TYPE MFR: Allergan STYLE/MODEL: Style 410FM Full Height Mod Profile Form Stable Anatomic Gel VOLUME: 310 gm	**310 gm**

Volume: N:IMF Relationships: Locate Final Selected Implant Volume at Right; Set N:IMF to the disstance shown in the cell beneath, or leave at preop N:IMF, whichever is longer.	200	250	275	300	325	350	375	400	PreN:IMF 8 cm
	7.0	7.0	7.5	8	8	8.5	9.0	9.5	

IV. NEW INFRAMAMMARY FOLD LEVEL	$N:IMF_{MaxSt}$ **to set with preoperative markings and intraoperatively**	8 cm
V. INCISION LOCATION	IM AX PA UMB	

PREOPERATIVE ASSESSMENT AND OBSERVATIONS

WNBCS = Will not be corrected surgically
Breast size asymmetry- WNBCS
Breast level asymmetry- WNBCS
Nipple level asymmetry- WNBCS
Nipple tilt asymmetry- WNBCS
Thin soft tissue coverage
Nipples located laterally on breast mound- WNBCS
Glandular ptosis
Narrow base width breast

POSTOPERATIVE ASSESSMENT AND OBSERVATIONS

Pre- to Post- bra size change by patient questionnaire: B to D.
Breasts soft, mobile, compressible at 17 months followup.
Very good breast shape and fill
Maintenance of upper pole fill and shape over 17 months postoperatively
Slight excess fullness right upper pole secondary to slight inferior pocket closure right
All WNBCS items as predicted preoperatively.

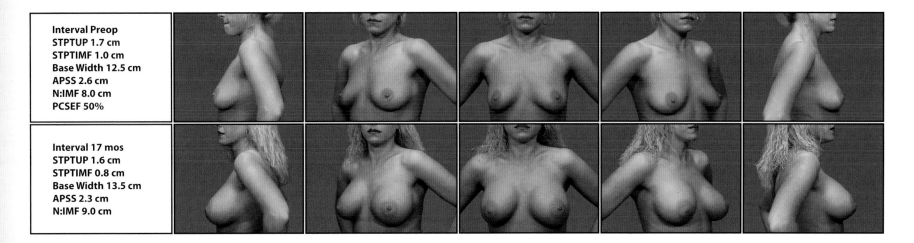

Interval Preop	Interval 17 mos
STPTUP 1.7 cm	STPTUP 1.6 cm
STPTIMF 1.0 cm	STPTIMF 0.8 cm
Base Width 12.5 cm	Base Width 13.5 cm
APSS 2.6 cm	APSS 2.3 cm
N:IMF 8.0 cm	N:IMF 9.0 cm
PCSEF 50%	

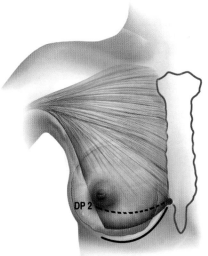

DP 2

Dual Plane 2
Pocket Location

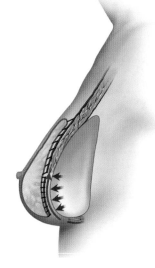

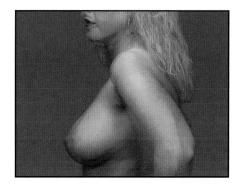

CASE STUDY 19-4

HISTORY

Age 27
Gravida 2
Para 2
Bra **Band** Size: 32
Breast **Cup** Size (Pt. estimate)
Prior to pregnancy B
Largest with preg C
Current Cup Size A
Desired Cup Size C
Previous Breast Disease: None
Breast Biopsies: No
Family Hx. Breast Cancer: No
Pertinent Medical or Breast
Imaging History: None
Breast Masses: None

TISSUE ASSESSMENT AND HIGH FIVE™ SYSTEM CRITICAL DECISIONS PROCESS

Prioritized Decisions Based on Breast Measurements and Tissue Characteristics
The High Five™ System   Copyright 2005   John B. Tebbetts, M.D.

I. POCKET LOCATION SELECTED BASED ON THICKNESS OF TISSUE COVERAGE (Circle One)

STPTUP	1.2	**If <2.0 cm., consider dual plane (DP) or partial retropectoral (PRP, pectoralis origins intact across IMF)**	DP 2
STPTIMF	0.8	**If STPTIMF <0.5 cm, consider subpectoral pocket and leave pectoralis origins intact along IMF**	PRP RM

II. IMPLANT VOLUME/WEIGHT BASED ON BREAST DIMENSIONS, TISSUE STRETCH, AND EXISTING PARENCHYMA

Base Width	11.0	B.W. Parenchyma (cm)	10.5	11.0	11.5	12.0	12.5	13.0	13.5	14.0	14.5	15.0	250 cc
		Initial Volume (cc)	200	250	275	300	300	325	350	375	375	400	
$APSS_{MaxStr}$	3.2	[2]**If APSS <2.0, −30 cc; If APSS >3.0, +30 cc; If APSS >4.0, +60 cc Place appropriate number in blank at right**											+30 cc
$N{:}IMF_{MaxSt}$	6.5	**If N:IMF >9.5, +30 cc Place appropriate number in blank at right**											cc
PCSEF %	30%	**If PCSEF <20%, +30 cc; If PCSEF >80%, −30 cc Place appropriate number in blank at right**											cc
IDFDD cc	*	**If Allergan Style 468 or other form stable saline implant, −30 cc Place appropriate number in blank at right**											−30 cc
Pt. request													cc

NET ESTIMATED VOLUME TO FILL ENVELOPE BASED ON PATIENT TISSUE CHARACTERISTICS	250 cc

III. IMPLANT TYPE MFR: Allergan STYLE/MODEL: Style 468 Anatomic Saline VOLUME: 230–240 cc		240 cc

Volume: N:IMF Relationships: Locate Final Selected Implant Volume at Right; Set N:IMF to the disstance shown in the cell beneath, or leave at preop N:IMF, whichever is longer.	200	250	275	300	325	350	375	400	PreN:IMF 6.5 cm
	7.0	7.0	7.5	8	8	8.5	9.0	9.5	

IV. NEW INFRAMAMMARY FOLD LEVEL	$N{:}IMF_{MaxSt}$ **to set with preoperative markings and intraoperatively**	7.0 cm
V. INCISION LOCATION	IM AX PA UMB	

PREOPERATIVE ASSESSMENT AND OBSERVATIONS

WNBCS = Will not be corrected surgically

Breast size asymmetry- WNBCS

Breast level asymmetry- WNBCS

Nipple level asymmetry- WNBCS

Thin soft tissue coverage

Nipples located laterally on breast mound L > R- WNBCS

Wide intermammary distance- WNBCS

Glandular ptosis

Narrow base width breast

POSTOPERATIVE ASSESSMENT AND OBSERVATIONS

Pre- to Post- bra size change by patient questionnaire: 32 A to 32 C.

Breasts soft, mobile, compressible at 26 months followup.

Very good breast shape and fill

Maintenance of upper pole fill and shape at 26 months postoperatively

Upper breast transition to chest wall slightly angular, even with a full height, anatomic saline implant that does not experience upper pole collapse when upright at manufacturer's recommended fill.

All WNBCS items as predicted preoperatively.

Interval Preop STPTUP 1.2 cm STPTIMF 0.8 cm Base Width 11.0 cm APSS 3.2 cm N:IMF 6.5 cm PCSEF 30%	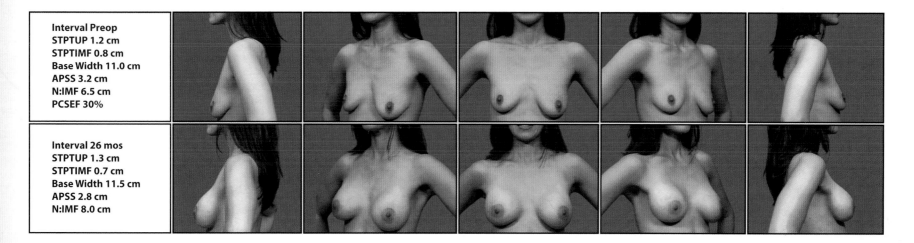
Interval 26 mos STPTUP 1.3 cm STPTIMF 0.7 cm Base Width 11.5 cm APSS 2.8 cm N:IMF 8.0 cm	

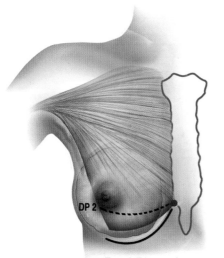

Dual Plane 2
Pocket Location

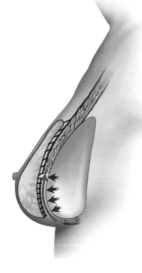

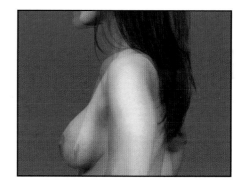

CASE STUDY 19-5

<table>
<tr><th colspan="2" align="center">HISTORY</th><th colspan="15" align="center">TISSUE ASSESSMENT AND HIGH FIVE™ SYSTEM CRITICAL DECISIONS PROCESS</th></tr>
</table>

HISTORY
Age 36
Gravida 3
Para 3
Bra **Band** Size: 34
Breast **Cup** Size (Pt. estimate)
Prior to pregnancy D
Largest with preg G
Current Cup Size B
Desired Cup Size C/D
Previous Breast Disease: None
Breast Biopsies: No
Family Hx. Breast Cancer: No
Pertinent Medical or Breast Imaging History: None
Breast Masses: Previous biopsy of left breast mass 5 years ago, reportedly benign.

TISSUE ASSESSMENT AND HIGH FIVE™ SYSTEM CRITICAL DECISIONS PROCESS

Prioritized Decisions Based on Breast Measurements and Tissue Characteristics
The High Five™ System   Copyright 2005   John B. Tebbetts, M.D.

I. **POCKET LOCATION** SELECTED BASED ON THICKNESS OF TISSUE COVERAGE (Circle One)			
STPTUP	1.1	**If <2.0 cm., consider dual plane (DP) or partial retropectoral (PRP, pectoralis origins intact across IMF)**	DP2
STPTIMF	0.6	**If STPTIMF <0.5 cm, consider subpectoral pocket and leave pectoralis origins intact along IMF**	PRP RM

II. IMPLANT VOLUME/WEIGHT BASED ON BREAST DIMENSIONS, TISSUE STRETCH, AND EXISTING PARENCHYMA

Base Width	12.5	B.W. Parenchyma (cm)	10.5	11.0	11.5	12.0	12.5	13.0	13.5	14.0	14.5	15.0	300 cc
		Initial Volume (cc)	200	250	275	300	300	325	350	375	375	400	
APSS$_{MaxStr}$	3.5	[2]**If APSS <2.0, −30 cc; If APSS >3.0, +30 cc; If APSS >4.0, +60 cc Place appropriate number in blank at right**											+30 cc
N:IMF$_{MaxSt}$	8.5	**If N:IMF >9.5, +30 cc Place appropriate number in blank at right**											cc
PCSEF %	20%	**If PCSEF <20%, +30 cc; If PCSEF >80%, −30 cc Place appropriate number in blank at right**											+30 cc
IDFDD cc	*	**If Allergan Style 468 or other form stable saline implant, −30 cc Place appropriate number in blank at right**											−30 cc
Pt. request													cc

NET ESTIMATED VOLUME TO FILL ENVELOPE BASED ON PATIENT TISSUE CHARACTERISTICS	330 cc
III. **IMPLANT TYPE** MFR: Allergan STYLE/MODEL: Style 468 Anatomic Saline VOLUME: 300–315 cc	315 cc

Volume: N:IMF Relationships: Locate Final Selected Implant Volume at Right; Set N:IMF to the disstance shown in the cell beneath, or leave at preop N:IMF, whichever is longer.	200	250	275	300	325	350	375	400	PreN:IMF
	7.0	7.0	7.5	8	8	8.5	9.0	9.5	8.5 cm

IV. **NEW INFRAMAMMARY FOLD LEVEL**	N:IMF$_{MaxSt}$ to set with preoperative markings and intraoperatively	8.5 cm
V. **INCISION LOCATION**	IM AX PA UMB	

PREOPERATIVE ASSESSMENT AND OBSERVATIONS

WNBCS = Will not be corrected surgically
Breast size asymmetry- WNBCS
Breast level asymmetry- WNBCS
Nipple level asymmetry- WNBCS
Thin soft tissue coverage
Glandular ptosis

POSTOPERATIVE ASSESSMENT AND OBSERVATIONS

Pre- to Post- bra size change by patient questionnaire: 34 B to 34 D.
Breasts soft, mobile, compressible at 75 months followup.
Excellent breast shape and fill
Maintenance of upper pole fill and shape over 6 years postoperatively with a full height, textured anatomic saline implant
All WNBCS items as predicted preoperatively.

Interval Preop				
STPTUP 1.1 cm **STPTIMF 0.6 cm** **Base Width 12.5 cm** **APSS 3.5 cm** **N:IMF 8.5 cm** **PCSEF 20%**				

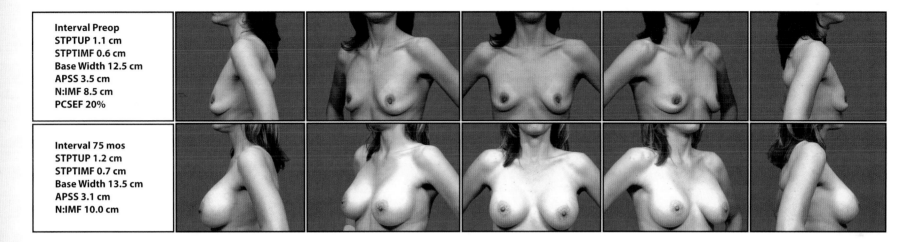

Interval 75 mos				
STPTUP 1.2 cm **STPTIMF 0.7 cm** **Base Width 13.5 cm** **APSS 3.1 cm** **N:IMF 10.0 cm**				

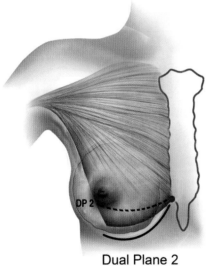

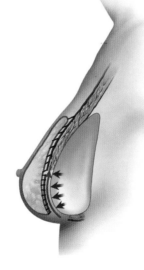

Dual Plane 2
Pocket Location

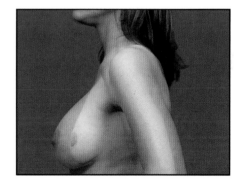

◼ CONSTRICTED LOWER POLE BREASTS

For the past three or more decades, variations of constricted lower pole breasts have been labeled with different terms (tuberous breast, tubular breast, etc.), when all of these terms actually represent variations of a common set of characteristics that can occur singly or in combination to produce a range of deformities.

Table 19-3 lists characteristics that are common to constricted lower pole breasts with modes of correction.

Table 19-3. **Characteristics of constricted lower pole breasts**

Characteristic/Deformity	Modes of Correction
1. Narrow base width, especially in lower pole (narrow base of parenchyma)	Radial and/or concentric scoring of parenchyma at incremental, progressive depth from deep to superficial until complete release and parenchymal redistribution is achieved
2. Maldistribution of breast parenchyma, constricted, narrow transversely, sometimes tight and globular	Same as #1; once released, implant selection becomes critical to help maintain redistribution of parenchyma and apply controlled pressure to areas of lower envelope that need to be stretched
3. Inframammary fold (IMF) is "tight" (more fixed to deeper structures compared to normal)	Thorough release of all tight or banding soft tissue attachments at the preoperative fold that extend deep to the fold and attach to deeper structures. Also, vertical cuts across fold area internally to interrupt continuity of any transverse banding or dense fascial structures at the preoperative IMF
4. Existing IMF is short transversely (due to misdistribution of parenchyma and focal fixation of fold over short distance transversely)	After release of all fold attachments, create new fold, usually at lower level by selecting optimal base width and projection implant to apply pressure across entire lower pole, resulting in lower pole skin stretch and passive formation of wider new IMF
5. Inadequate expansion of breast lower pole skin over the entire width of an average breast	Create pocket dimensions to accommodate implant of desired new breast base width, release any constricting layers overlying implant, use textured surface implant to optimally control implant position, and select implant projection (moderate, not high) to spread stretch forces optimally across entire lower pole
6. Excessive expansion of narrow, focal area of skin in central lower pole of the breast, creating pseudoptosis or "tubular" configuration where narrow base width parenchyma has stretched only a narrow portion of lower pole skin	Same as (5) above
7. Downpointing nipple–areola complex (when lower pole is constricted and upper pole parenchyma continues to develop)	Assess nipple position intraoperatively with patient sitting after optimal release and placement of implant. If nipple remains downpointing, especially if overlying mobile parenchyma, reposition NAC with periareolar + vertical (not periareolar alone) technique
8. Pseudoherniation of subareolar tissue, creating areolar deformities and asymmetries	Obtain informed consent for possible nipple sensory loss and/or loss of ability to nurse; leaving NAC based opposite area of most pseudoherniation, excise at least a 2 cm thick wedge of the herniated parenchyma for most predictable correction
9. Nipple–areola complex malposition on breast mound	Reposition NAC with periareolar + vertical (not periareolar alone) technique. Isolated periareolar or "doughnut" designs are more prone to excessive postoperative stretch or areolar asymmetries because all tension is periareolar
10. Thickened deep subcutaneous fascia with or without thickening of pectoralis fascia deep to lower pole parenchyma	Radial and, if necessary, concentric scoring from NAC inferiorly to level of new inframammary fold to completely release all constricting fascia. Perform in increments, scoring to subdermis if necessary to obtain optimal, complete release. Assess at intervals by inserting fingers and pulling anteriorly on lower pole tissues to identify areas of remaining restriction

These characteristics can occur singly or in various combinations, so constricted lower pole (CLP) breasts represent a wide range of deformities. While some surgeons attempt to classify CLP deformities as mild, moderate, or severe, this type of classification is inaccurate and imprecise, because it does not specify the tissue conditions or deformities that must be surgically addressed for successful correction of the deformity. Each of the 10 characteristics listed in Table 19-3 should be assessed individually in each case, and the operative plan should include specific modes of correction to individually address each characteristic that is present.

Informed Consent Considerations for Patients with Constricted Lower Pole Breasts

To achieve optimal correction of constricted lower pole (CLP) breasts, especially with the more severe forms of the deformity, the surgeon must have the patient's informed consent to perform surgical maneuvers that have significant tradeoffs. Without this permission, predictable correction is impossible. Although many of the key surgical maneuvers to correct CLP breasts can and should be performed incrementally, optimal correction nevertheless requires that a surgeon be able to continue scoring deeply or to a greater extent in more different directions to effectively release areas of constriction and to effectively redistribute breast parenchyma.

In order to give valid informed consent, patients must understand and accept each of the following potential risks and tradeoffs that are essential to optimal correction:

1. *Potential loss of nipple sensation*: risk increases with necessity of excising subareolar tissue if pseudoherniation is present, and increases with increasing extent and depth of parenchymal scoring

2. *Potential loss of ability to nurse*: for all of the same reasons listed in #1 above.

3. *Possible striae over areas of the breast, especially the lower breast*: risks of striae increase as depth of scoring increases and nears the dermis, a maneuver that is often necessary in more severe deformities.

4. *Increased risk of capsular contracture*: risk increases as the extent and depth of parenchymal scoring increases, exposing the implant to endogenous bacteria in the breast parenchyma.

5. *Very narrow base width CPL breasts*: in order to widen the base of very narrow (<10.5 cm base width) CLP breasts, an implant with a base width wider than the

While some surgeons attempt to classify CLP deformities as mild, moderate, or severe, this type of classification is inaccurate and imprecise, because it does not specify the tissue conditions or deformities that must be surgically addressed for successful correction of the deformity

In order to give valid informed consent, patients must understand and accept each of the potential risks and tradeoffs that are essential to optimal correction

base width of the existing breast tissue may be necessary. When the width of the implant is greater than the width of the existing breast tissue, risks of implant edge visibility, palpability, and visible traction rippling from the implant pulling downward on thin overlying tissue may occur. These problems may be uncorrectable.

6. *Incomplete correction of the deformities* (*residual deformity, double bubble or persistent preoperative inframammary fold*): despite all surgical maneuvers applied to the greatest extent possible, and despite selection and placement of an optimal breast implant, complete correction may not occur as tissues may not stretch adequately.

Each of these items should be thoroughly explained to the patient preoperatively, and the patient should acknowledge her understanding of the information and acceptance of the risks and tradeoffs in detailed, signed informed consent documents.

Surgical Correction of the Constricted Lower Pole Breast

Optimal surgical correction of the constricted lower pole breast requires an incremental, sequenced surgical approach that incorporates the six principles listed in Table 19-1. Figure 19-4 is a flowchart that outlines the planning and surgical approach to constricted lower pole breasts.

> Approaching the decision making process optimally requires that the surgeon prioritize soft tissue coverage over the implant as the highest priority, and sequence decisions according to the High Five™ System

Approaching the decision making process optimally requires that the surgeon prioritize soft tissue coverage over the implant as the highest priority, and sequence decisions according to the High Five™ System.[3] The first decision is implant pocket location, because that decision determines soft tissue coverage for the patient's entire lifetime. A narrow base, constricted lower pole breast is one of the few exceptions to the High Five™ System[3] rule that the base width of the implant should not exceed the base width of the patient's existing parenchyma for optimal, long-term soft tissue coverage.

Pocket Location for Correction of Constricted Lower Pole Breasts

Prior to the development of dual plane pocket techniques, optimal correction of CLP breasts required a submammary pocket to allow access for adequate scoring of parenchyma and to assure direct contact of the implant with scored parenchyma and skin envelope for optimal stretching of the constricted areas and redistribution of parenchyma. The tradeoff of submammary placement, however, is that it does not provide as optimal long-term coverage compared to dual plane techniques that assure more than 1 cm of

Figure 19-4. Surgical correction of constricted lower pole breasts.

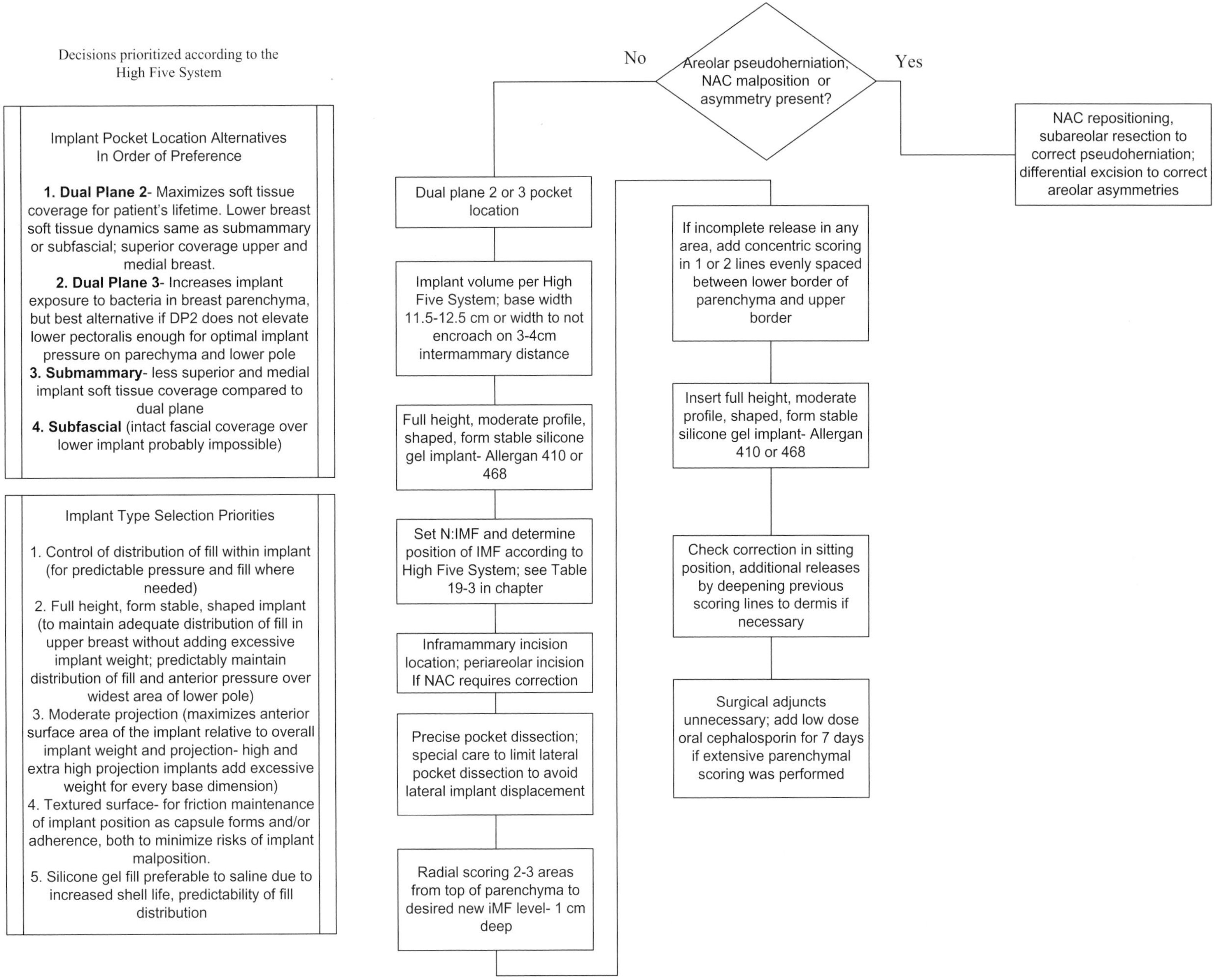

Decisions prioritized according to the
High Five System

```
                                          ┌──────────────────┐
                                          │ Areolar          │
                                   No     │ pseudoherniation;│   Yes
                                          │ NAC malposition  │
                                          │ or asymmetry     │
                                          │ present?         │
                                          └──────────────────┘
```

Areolar pseudoherniation; NAC malposition or asymmetry present? — No / Yes

Implant Pocket Location Alternatives In Order of Preference

1. Dual Plane 2- Maximizes soft tissue coverage for patient's lifetime. Lower breast soft tissue dynamics same as submammary or subfascial; superior coverage upper and medial breast.

2. Dual Plane 3- Increases implant exposure to bacteria in breast parenchyma, but best alternative if DP2 does not elevate lower pectoralis enough for optimal implant pressure on parechyma and lower pole

3. Submammary- less superior and medial implant soft tissue coverage compared to dual plane

4. Subfascial (intact fascial coverage over lower implant probably impossible)

Implant Type Selection Priorities

1. Control of distribution of fill within implant (for predictable pressure and fill where needed)

2. Full height, form stable, shaped implant (to maintain adequate distribution of fill in upper breast without adding excessive implant weight; predictably maintain distribution of fill and anterior pressure over widest area of lower pole)

3. Moderate projection (maximizes anterior surface area of the implant relative to overall implant weight and projection- high and extra high projection implants add excessive weight for every base dimension)

4. Textured surface- for friction maintenance of implant position as capsule forms and/or adherence, both to minimize risks of implant malposition.

5. Silicone gel fill preferable to saline due to increased shell life, predictability of fill distribution

---

Flowchart (No branch):

Dual plane 2 or 3 pocket location

↓

Implant volume per High Five System; base width 11.5-12.5 cm or width to not encroach on 3-4cm intermammary distance

↓

Full height, moderate profile, shaped, form stable silicone gel implant- Allergan 410 or 468

↓

Set N:IMF and determine position of IMF according to High Five System; see Table 19-3 in chapter

↓

Inframammary incision location; periareolar incision If NAC requires correction

↓

Precise pocket dissection; special care to limit lateral pocket dissection to avoid lateral implant displacement

↓

Radial scoring 2-3 areas from top of parenchyma to desired new iMF level- 1 cm deep

Flowchart (middle column):

If incomplete release in any area, add concentric scoring in 1 or 2 lines evenly spaced between lower border of parenchyma and upper border

↓

Insert full height, moderate profile, shaped, form stable silicone gel implant- Allergan 410 or 468

↓

Check correction in sitting position, additional releases by deepening previous scoring lines to dermis if necessary

↓

Surgical adjuncts unnecessary; add low dose oral cephalosporin for 7 days if extensive parenchymal scoring was performed

Flowchart (Yes branch):

NAC repositioning, subareolar resection to correct pseudoherniation; differential excision to correct areolar asymmetries

The dual plane pocket provides the best of both worlds by incorporating all of the benefits of the same exposure and scoring potential in the lower breast, while maximizing soft tissue coverage long-term in the medial and upper breast

pectoralis coverage medially along the sternum and over the superior pole of the breast. The dual plane pocket provides the best of both worlds by incorporating all of the benefits of the same exposure and scoring potential in the lower breast, while maximizing soft tissue coverage long-term in the medial and upper breast. To provide optimal access for scoring, redistribution of parenchyma, and implant pressure for inferior pole expansion, a dual plane 2 or 3 pocket is indicated to assure that the inferior border of the pectoralis major is optimally positioned superior enough to allow full access to the lower parenchyma.

Implant Volume and Dimensions Selection for the Constricted Lower Pole Breast

The second highest priority decision in the High Five[TM] System[3] is implant volume and base width. If the base width of the CLP breast is less than 10.5 cm, the base width of the implant will almost certainly need to be wider than the parenchyma for optimal correction (this is one of only two exceptions to the High Five[3] principle that implant base width should not exceed base width of existing parenchyma). Patients must be informed and accept in signed documents that placing an implant wider than the base width of the existing parenchyma increases risks of implant edge visibility, palpability, and visible traction rippling that may be uncorrectable in the future. If a patient is unwilling to accept these risks and tradeoffs, surgeons should not proceed with attempted correction, because limiting the range of necessary surgical maneuvers limits the predictability and extent of correction.

In most cases, an implant with base dimension of 11.5–12.5 cm is a good choice, because it substantially widens the base of the CLP breast without encroaching excessively into the medial area where soft tissue coverage over the sternum is minimal

To determine optimal base width for the implant, the surgeon should outline a 3–4 cm intermammary distance using dots on either side of a row of sternal notch to xiphoid dots and never, under any circumstances, dissect medial to the lateral row of dots on each side. In most cases, an implant with base dimension of 11.5–12.5 cm is a good choice, because it substantially widens the base of the CLP breast without encroaching excessively into the medial area where soft tissue coverage over the sternum is minimal. The more laterally the NAC is located preoperatively, the narrower the base width of the implant should be to prevent even more lateralization of the NAC over a wider base implant placed centrally on the chest wall. If NAC repositioning is planned, the base width of the implant selected should be positioned beneath the new nipple location, assuring that the medial portion of the implant does not encroach into the minimal 3 cm intermammary distance previously outlined.

Selection of implant type follows principles similar to those described previously in this chapter for implants to correct glandular ptosis. An optimal implant for correction of constricted lower pole breasts should have the following characteristics:

1. Adequate base width and dimensions to widen the base of the preoperative breast if necessary, and adequate base width to deliver a N:IMF distance for optimal aesthetic proportion to the base width.

2. Adequate projection to apply pressure to parenchyma and overlying soft tissues in the lower breast to correct the constriction and fully expand the lower envelope.

3. For any given volume or weight, maximum anterior implant surface area to distribute pressure over the widest area of the posterior surface of the parenchyma to prevent focal parenchymal atrophy in the central breast while optimally maintaining redistribution of scored parenchyma over the widest possible area of the lower pole.

4. Control of implant position in the pocket to control distribution of fill in the breast and thereby control distribution of pressure applied to the constricted lower tissues of the breast.

5. Control of distribution of fill within the implant to optimally control distribution of fill in the breast.

6. A shaped implant that puts projection where it is needed in the lower pole, but not at the expense of excess weight (caused by a high profile, round implant). The shaped implant must be form stable, with no collapse of the upper shell when the implant is upright.

7. A full height, form stable implant that offers the best opportunity to maintain upper breast fill as it provides dimensions and projection to optimally expand the lower pole envelope and apply pressure to the lower pole tissues for optimal expansion while providing control over middle and upper pole fill.

8. Surface texturing that provides friction immediately postoperatively as the capsule forms to: (a) maintain implant position, and (b) provide an opportunity for adherence to capsule and parenchyma to optimize maintenance of position of the scored, redistributed parenchyma in the lower pole.

The optimal implant design for augmentation of the constricted lower pole breast, therefore, is a full height, moderate profile, shaped, textured, form stable saline or silicone gel filled implant. The Allergan Style 410 full height, form stable, silicone gel filled implant is the author's preferred implant for this application. If a patient prefers a

The optimal implant design for augmentation of the constricted lower pole breast is a full height, moderate profile, shaped, textured, form stable saline or silicone gel filled implant

saline filled implant, the Allergan Style 468 implant is the most form stable saline filled implant that meets these criteria. Lower height implants, regardless of type, do not assure as predictable upper pole fill long-term. Regardless of where a breast is located on the torso, even if high on the torso with a short sternal notch-to-nipple distance of less than 18 cm, optimal aesthetics requires optimal, long-term fill of the upper breast. Reduced height implants do not predictably deliver this requirement as effectively as full height, form stable implants.

Location of the New Inframammary Fold in Constricted Lower Pole Breasts

Knowing where to locate the new inframammary fold and predictably executing surgical techniques to accurately place the new fold are essential to optimal correction of constricted lower pole breasts. Subjective, "artistic" or "eyeballing" methods of determining new fold position are outmoded and substandard, because proved processes now exist[3] that provide surgeons quantifiable tools to make these decisions objectively instead of subjectively.

Knowing where to locate the new inframammary fold and predictably executing surgical techniques to accurately place the new fold are essential to optimal correction of constricted lower pole breasts

From a practical standpoint, the base width of the implant selected for correction of the CLP breast effectively determines the base width of the result, since the base width of existing parenchyma is usually much narrower compared to the base width of the implant. Optimal N:IMF distance is directly related to the base width of the result.[3] If the N:IMF is too short for the base width, the breast appears "boxy", and if N:IMF is too long in relation to base width, the breast appears "bottom heavy or bottomed".

Table 19-4 is excerpted from the High Five™ System.[3] To determine optimal N:IMF for each base width, the surgeon locates the base width in the top row, and the optimal N:IMF for that width is located in the cell directly beneath that base width. If the preoperative base width is longer than the base width recommended in Table 19-4, the surgeon accepts the longer preoperative distance and places the incision in the existing inframammary fold.

Table 19-4. **Appropriate nipple-to-fold distance for the base width of the breast when augmenting constricted lower pole breasts**

Selected implant base width (cm)	10.5	11.0	11.5	12.0	12.5	13.0	13.5	14.0
Set N:IMF to: (cm)	7.0	7.0	7.5	8	8	8.5	9.0	9.5

During preoperative marking, the surgeon first outlines the existing inframammary fold. Placing the tip of a flexible tape measure exactly opposite the nipple (or new nipple position if a change is planned), the surgeon lifts directly superiorly to place the lower pole skin under maximal stretch, and then places a dot at the 6 o'clock position of the inframammary fold at the High Five™ recommended N:IMF distance. Using that dot as the level of the new fold, the surgeon outlines the desired new inframammary fold contour from medial to lateral for optimal aesthetics.

Incision Location for Correction of Constricted Lower Pole Breasts

If nipple–areola complex (NAC) deformities are present that require correction (such as subareolar pseudoherniation, asymmetries, or NAC malposition), a periareolar incision approach is logical. If nipple–areola complex deformities are not significant, an inframammary approach provides better exposure, more control, and more versatility in adjusting the position of the pectoralis with dual plane techniques compared to the periareolar approach. In some cases, the author has combined periareolar and inframammary incision approaches to optimally address the deformities present while assuring optimal control over every aspect of the operation.

Surgical Techniques for Correction of Constricted Lower Pole Breasts

Table 19-1 lists modes of correction for each of the specific deformities that may occur in CLP breasts.

During preoperative marking, the surgeon should place a midline row of dots between the sternal notch and xiphoid, and then place dots 1.5–2.0 cm lateral to each of the midline dots to outline a 3–4 cm intermammary distance. The surgeon should outline the existing and desired new inframammary folds as described previously in this chapter. For an inframammary approach, the surgeon should drop a perpendicular line from the medial border of the proposed postoperative nipple position down to cross the new, lowered inframammary fold, and mark one-third of the incision medial to the point of crossing, and two-thirds lateral to the point of crossing.

After making the inframammary incision, the surgeon angles dissection superiorly to minimize risks of excessively lowering the inframammary fold, and continues electrocautery dissection through the pectoralis fascia. Lifting with a double ended retractor, if the muscle visualized tents upward with traction, the muscle is pectoralis major. If it does not tent, it is likely serratus or intercostals. If the muscle tents upward

If nipple–areola complex deformities are not significant, an inframammary approach provides better exposure, more control, and more versatility in adjusting the position of the pectoralis with dual plane techniques compared to the periareolar approach

Lifting with a double ended retractor, if the muscle visualized tents upward with traction, the muscle is pectoralis major

with traction, the surgeon proceeds incrementally through the muscle with monopolar electrocautery dissecting forceps to create a dual plane 1 pocket as detailed in Chapters 8 and 11. When lowering the fold, frequently the inframammary incision lies inferior to the origins of the pectoralis major along the inframammary fold, and the surgeon should carefully dissect superficial to the intercostals and serratus (if visible) to identify the pectoralis (which tents under anterior traction) before dissecting through the muscle.

When performing any dual plane pocket dissection, surgeons should always dissect the entire subpectoral pocket *before performing any dissection in the submammary plane or before separating the pectoralis from overlying parenchyma*. If surgeons perform submammary dissection *before* dissecting the entire *subpectoral* pocket, they sacrifice optimal control of the inferior border of the pectoralis and risk excessive elevation of the muscle with loss of coverage and potential banding or window shading of the pectoralis.

> When performing any dual plane pocket dissection, surgeons should always dissect the entire subpectoral pocket before performing any dissection in the submammary plane or before separating the pectoralis from overlying parenchyma

Pocket dissection must be precise to optimally control the position of the implant when correcting CLP breasts, because controlling distribution of fill by position of the implant and fill distribution within the implant are the factors that control the amount and location of pressure that the implant applies to correct the deformities. To prevent the common error of excessive dissection of the lateral pocket, the surgeon should limit lateral pocket dissection, and stop dissection at the lateral border of the pectoralis minor. After placing the implant, if the posterior surface of the implant is compressed medially–laterally, the surgeon enlarges the lateral pocket in 0.5 cm increments until the base of the implant lies uncompressed on the chest wall. Keeping the implant centralized medially by precise pocket creation is essential to optimal correction. If the implant can displace laterally, it cannot transmit optimal pressure directly anterior, which is key to optimizing implant–soft tissue dynamics for optimal correction.

> To prevent the common error of excessive dissection of the lateral pocket, the surgeon should limit lateral pocket dissection, and stop dissection at the lateral border of the pectoralis minor

After dissecting a dual plane[4] 1 pocket, the surgeon inserts two fingers in the pocket and by pulling anteriorly, the surgeon can determine whether the inferior border of the pectoralis is limiting full anterior displacement of the overlying parenchyma by an implant. If any limitation is present, the surgeon separates the pectoralis from overlying parenchyma in 1 cm increments, rechecks by pulling the envelope anteriorly, and limits separation of pectoralis from overlying parenchyma to the minimal amount that allows unrestricted access to the posterior surface of the parenchyma.

Surgeons must address five specific tissue problems in CLP breasts: (1) excessively narrow base width, (2) tight, fixed, and usually short transverse inframammary fold,

> Surgeons must address five specific tissue problems in CLP breasts

(3) centralized, globular, maldistributed parenchyma, (4) internal fascial thickenings and bands that may exist, and (5) non-expanded, tight skin inferior, medial, and lateral that must be recruited into the lower pole breast envelope and stretched adequately to expand and obliterate the preexisting inframammary fold. Areolar pseudoherniation and NAC abnormalities may also require correction.

The narrow base width is corrected by selecting an optimal base width implant and dissecting a very accurate pocket to fit the implant. The tight, fixed, short inframammary fold is passively corrected by maneuvers that release constriction and redistribute the parenchyma. Figure 19-5 illustrates the staged, incremental steps in surgical correction that follow initial creating of a dual plane[4] 2 or 3 pocket. Release of constrictions and redistribution of parenchyma begin with two or three radial scoring cuts with needlepoint electrocautery, *beginning at the cephalad-most extent of the parenchyma and continuing to the level of the desired, new inframammary fold, approximately 1 cm deep* to enable medial–lateral expansion of the parenchyma (Figure 19-5, *A*). A common error is not starting these radial cuts far enough cephalad, at the most cephalad border of parenchyma, which is often cephalad to the cephalad border of the areola. Starting these scoring cuts excessively low precludes optimal medial–lateral expansion and redistribution of parenchyma.

After completing the first series of scoring cuts, the surgeon inserts fingers and pulls anteriorly while sweeping right to left to assess the degree of release and redistribution of parenchyma, and to identify any residual areas of palpable banding or restriction in the overlying soft tissues. In the process, the surgeon assesses the superior–inferior distribution of parenchyma, a step that is often omitted when correcting CLP breasts.

If vertical expansion (in a superior–inferior direction) of parenchyma is not optimal, or if constrictions persist within the parenchymal segments, the surgeon then adds concentric scoring cuts (Figure 19-5, *B*) of the same 1 cm depth at two levels spaced equally between the superior and inferior borders of the parenchymal mass (or through specific areas that palpation has identified with residual bands or constriction).

The surgeon should then deepen the scoring cuts as necessary in 0.5–1.0 cm increments (Figure 19-5, *C*), all the way to dermis if necessary, to minimize or eliminate all areas of palpable banding or constriction and to optimally redistribute the parenchyma over the widest possible area. Deep scoring to dermis should be limited to a maximum of three

Figure 19-5. (*A–C*) Surgical correction of the constricted lower pole breast.

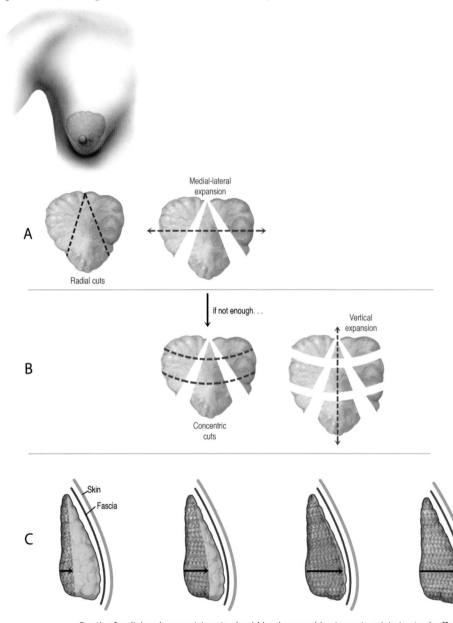

Depth of radial and concentric cuts should be deepened in stages to minimize tradeoffs, but should proceed through subcutaneous fascia if necessary to correct the deformity.

radial and/or concentric cuts to minimize risks of vascular compromise. Vigilance and attention to detail is essential with deep scoring to avoid inadvertent injury to dermis or skin.

Implant Placement and Positioning

With pocket dissection, soft tissue releases, and parenchymal redistribution complete, the surgeon inserts the implant and elevates the patient to a sitting position on the operating table to assess the degree of expansion of the lower pole and the position of the implant. *It is critically important when using full height, form stable implants to accurately position the inferior border of the implant exactly at the level of the new, desired inframammary fold.* A common error is leaving the lower border of the implant one or more centimeters too cephalad, precluding optimal fold position, lower pole expansion, and increasing risk of excessive upper pole fullness. The surgeon can assure correct implant positioning by visualizing the breast in direct lateral view, and then grasp the medial corner of the inframammary incision and displace it directly posteriorly to identify the point at which it touches the chest wall. This point is the precise level at which the surgeon should position the lower border of the implant. After incision closure, if the implant is in proper position, the incision line will appear to have pulled upward onto the breast at least 1 cm. In reality, a triangular dead space exists inferior to the implant that allows the incision line to tent upward and produce this appearance. This dead space closes within 48 hours postoperatively, and a check at that interval will demonstrate that the incision is located precisely in the desired, new inframammary fold line.

> It is critically important when using full height, form stable implants to accurately position the inferior border of the implant exactly at the level of the new, desired inframammary fold

Postoperative Adjuncts

The author does not use any postoperative adjuncts such as drains, straps, special bandages, special bras, positioning devices, pain pumps, or narcotic pain medications postoperatively for patients with either glandular ptotic or constricted lower pole breasts. These patients are treated exactly as routine primary augmentation patients, and 85% are out to dinner the evening of their augmentation, with 96% resuming full, normal activities within 24 hours. The only medication difference is the addition of a low dose, oral cephalosporin for 1 week postoperatively if deep parenchymal scoring has been performed in the breast.

Text continued on p. 500

Case Studies of Constricted Lower Pole Breasts

CASE STUDY 19-6

HISTORY

Age 23
Gravida 0
Para 0
Bra **Band** Size: 34
Breast **Cup** Size (Pt. estimate)
Prior to pregnancy A
Largest with preg NA
Current Cup Size A
Desired Cup Size C
Previous Breast Disease: None
Breast Biopsies: No
Family Hx. Breast Cancer: No
Pertinent Medical or Breast
    Imaging History: None
Breast Masses: None

TISSUE ASSESSMENT AND HIGH FIVE™ SYSTEM CRITICAL DECISIONS PROCESS

Prioritized Decisions Based on Breast Measurements and Tissue Characteristics												
The High Five™ System Copyright 2005 John B. Tebbetts, M.D.												

I. POCKET LOCATION SELECTED BASED ON THICKNESS OF TISSUE COVERAGE (Circle One)

STPTUP	1.6	**If <2.0 cm., consider dual plane (DP) or partial retropectoral (PRP, pectoralis origins intact across IMF)**		DP 3
STPTIMF	1.2	**If STPTIMF <0.5 cm, consider subpectoral pocket and leave pectoralis origins intact along IMF**		PRP RM

II. IMPLANT DIMENSIONS **In constricted lower pole breasts with narrow base width, select implant width to achieve 3.0 cm intermammary distance

Base Width	10.5	B.W. Parenchyma (cm)	10.5	11.0	11.5	12.0	12.5	13.0	13.5	14.0	14.5	15.0	300 cc
		Initial Volume (cc)	200	250	275	300	300	325	350	375	375	400	
APSS$_{MaxStr}$	2.1	[2]**If APSS <2.0, −30 cc; If APSS >3.0, +30 cc; If APSS >4.0, +60 cc Place appropriate number in blank at right**											cc
N:IMF$_{MaxSt}$	5.5	**If N:IMF >9.5, +30 cc Place appropriate number in blank at right**											cc
PCSEF %	70%	**If PCSEF <20%, +30 cc; If PCSEF >80%, −30 cc Place appropriate number in blank at right**											cc
IDFDD cc	NA	**If Allergan Style 468 or other form stable saline implant, −30 cc Place appropriate number in blank at right**											NA
Pt. request	*	****Patient specifically request ed a round, smooth saline implant**											cc

NET ESTIMATED VOLUME TO FILL ENVELOPE BASED ON PATIENT TISSUE CHARACTERISTICS — cc

III. IMPLANT TYPE MFR: Allergan   STYLE/MODEL: Style 68 Round Smooth Saline   VOLUME: 300 + 30 cc — **330 cc**

Volume: N:IMF Relationships: Locate Final Selected Implant Volume at Right; Set N:IMF to the disstance shown in the cell beneath, or leave at preop N:IMF, whichever is longer.	200	250	275	300	325	350	375	400	PreN:IMF
	7.0	7.0	7.5	8	8	8.5	9.0	9.5	5.5 cm

IV. NEW INFRAMAMMARY FOLD LEVEL	N:IMF$_{MaxSt}$ to set with preoperative markings and intraoperatively	8.0 cm
V. INCISION LOCATION	IM AX PA UMB	

PREOPERATIVE ASSESSMENT AND OBSERVATIONS

WNBCS = Will not be corrected surgically
Breast size asymmetry- WNBCS
Breast level asymmetry- WNBCS
Nipple level asymmetry- WNBCS
Tight skin envelope
Breasts high on torso (short SN:N)- WNBCS
Wide intermammary distance- WNBCS
Relative constriction or inadequate expansion of breast lower pole
Narrow base width breast
When selecting implant base width/desired breast width for a narrow base, constricted lower pole breast, draw a 3 cm wide intermammary distance and then measure laterally to determine the optimal width for the postoperative breast. Then select a base width implant approximately 0.5–1.0 cm. less than the desired base width. A full height, moderate profile anatomic implant is most ideal long-term, because it achieves excellent lower pole expansion while avoiding the parenchymal atrophy caused by high profile implants.

POSTOPERATIVE ASSESSMENT AND OBSERVATIONS

Pre- to Post- bra size change by patient questionnaire: A to C.
Breasts remain somewhat tight, no capsular contracture, at 16 months followup.
Very good breast shape and fill
Very good expansion breast lower pole
All WNBCS items as predicted preoperatively.

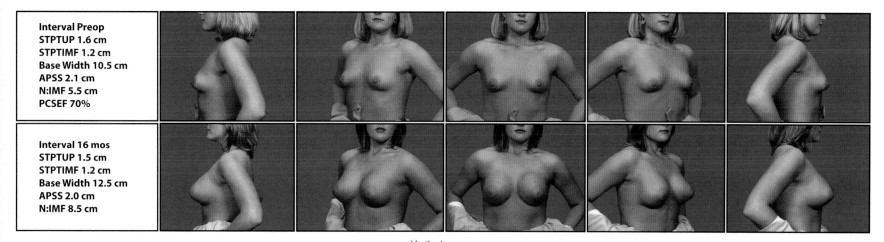

Interval Preop					
STPTUP 1.6 cm					
STPTIMF 1.2 cm					
Base Width 10.5 cm					
APSS 2.1 cm					
N:IMF 5.5 cm					
PCSEF 70%					

Interval 16 mos					
STPTUP 1.5 cm					
STPTIMF 1.2 cm					
Base Width 12.5 cm					
APSS 2.0 cm					
N:IMF 8.5 cm					

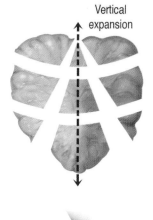

Concentric cuts

Vertical expansion

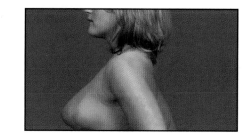

CASE STUDY 19-7

HISTORY

Age 31
Gravida 1
Para 1
Bra **Band** Size: 34
Breast **Cup** Size (Pt. estimate)
Prior to pregnancy B
Largest with preg B/C
Current Cup Size B
Desired Cup Size C
Previous Breast Disease: None
Breast Biopsies: No
Family Hx. Breast Cancer: No
Pertinent Medical or Breast
Imaging History: None
Breast Masses: None

TISSUE ASSESSMENT AND HIGH FIVE™ SYSTEM CRITICAL DECISIONS PROCESS

Prioritized Decisions Based on Breast Measurements and Tissue Characteristics
The High Five™ System   Copyright 2005   John B. Tebbetts, M.D.

I. POCKET LOCATION SELECTED BASED ON THICKNESS OF TISSUE COVERAGE (Circle One)

STPTUP	1.6	If <2.0 cm., consider dual plane (DP) or partial retropectoral (PRP, pectoralis origins intact across IMF)	**DP 3**
STPTIMF	1.2	If STPTIMF <0.5 cm, consider subpectoral pocket and leave pectoralis origins intact along IMF	**PRP RM**

II. IMPLANT DIMENSIONS **In constricted lower pole breasts with narrow base width, select implant width to achieve 3.0 cm intermammary distance

Base Width	11.5	B.W. Parenchyma (cm)	10.5	11.0	11.5	12.0	12.5	13.0	13.5	14.0	14.5	15.0	275 cc
		Initial Volume (cc)	200	250	275	300	300	325	350	375	375	400	

APSS$_{MaxStr}$	2.5	[2]If APSS <2.0, −30 cc; If APSS >3.0, +30 cc; If APSS >4.0, +60 cc Place appropriate number in blank at right	cc
N:IMF$_{MaxSt}$	7.0	If N:IMF >9.5, +30 cc Place appropriate number in blank at right	cc
PCSEF %	80%	If PCSEF <20%, +30 cc; If PCSEF >80%, −30 cc Place appropriate number in blank at right	−30 cc
IDFDD cc	NA	If Allergan Style 468 or other form stable saline implant, −30 cc Place appropriate number in blank at right	NA
Pt. request			cc

NET ESTIMATED VOLUME TO FILL ENVELOPE BASED ON PATIENT TISSUE CHARACTERISTICS	245 cc
III. IMPLANT TYPE MFR: Allergan STYLE/MODEL: Style 410FM Full Height Mod Profile Form Stable Anatomic Gel VOLUME: 235 gm gm	235 gm

Volume: N:IMF Relationships: Locate Final Selected Implant Volume at Right; Set N:IMF to the disstance shown in the cell beneath, or leave at preop N:IMF, whichever is longer.	200	250	275	300	325	350	375	400	**PreN:IMF**
	7.0	7.0	7.5	8	8	8.5	9.0	9.5	**7.0 cm**

IV. NEW INFRAMAMMARY FOLD LEVEL	N:IMF$_{MaxSt}$ to set with preoperative markings and intraoperatively	7.5 cm
V. INCISION LOCATION	IM AX PA UMB	

PREOPERATIVE ASSESSMENT AND OBSERVATIONS

WNBCS = Will not be corrected surgically
Breast size asymmetry- WNBCS
Breast level asymmetry- WNBCS
Nipple level asymmetry- WNBCS
Breast width asymmetry- WNBCS
Tight skin envelope
Thin soft tissue coverage
Nipples located laterally on breast mound- WNBCS
Relative constriction or inadequate expansion of breast lower pole
Downpointing nipples

POSTOPERATIVE ASSESSMENT AND OBSERVATIONS

Pre- to Post- bra size change by patient questionnaire: 34 A to 34 C.
Breasts remain somewhat tight, no capsular contracture, at 24 months followup.
Very good breast shape and fill
Very good expansion breast lower pole
All WNBCS items as predicted preoperatively.
Lowering this IMF an additional 0.5 cm. and adding concentric scoring similar to Case Study 19–6 would likely have improved nipple position and nipple tilt, though further stretching of the lower pole is likely.

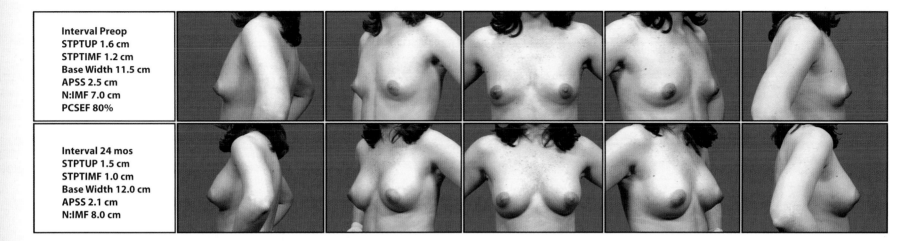

Interval Preop				
STPTUP 1.6 cm				
STPTIMF 1.2 cm				
Base Width 11.5 cm				
APSS 2.5 cm				
N:IMF 7.0 cm				
PCSEF 80%				

Interval 24 mos				
STPTUP 1.5 cm				
STPTIMF 1.0 cm				
Base Width 12.0 cm				
APSS 2.1 cm				
N:IMF 8.0 cm				

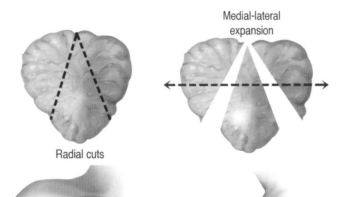

Radial cuts

Medial-lateral expansion

DP 3

Dual Plane 3
Pocket Location

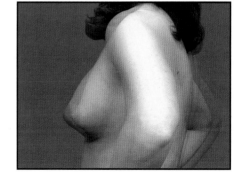

CASE STUDY 19-8

HISTORY

Age 25
Gravida 1
Para 1
Bra **Band** Size: 36
Breast **Cup** Size (Pt. estimate)
Prior to pregnancy A
Largest with preg B/C
Current Cup Size A
Desired Cup Size C/D
Previous Breast Disease: None
Breast Biopsies: No
Family Hx. Breast Cancer: No
Pertinent Medical or Breast
Imaging History: None
Breast Masses: None

TISSUE ASSESSMENT AND HIGH FIVE™ SYSTEM CRITICAL DECISIONS PROCESS

Prioritized Decisions Based on Breast Measurements and Tissue Characteristics
The High Five™ System   Copyright 2005   John B. Tebbetts, M.D.

I. POCKET LOCATION SELECTED BASED ON THICKNESS OF TISSUE COVERAGE (Circle One)

STPTUP	2.2	If <2.0 cm., consider dual plane (DP) or partial retropectoral (PRP, pectoralis origins intact across IMF)	DP 3
STPTIMF	1.6	If STPTIMF <0.5 cm, consider subpectoral pocket and leave pectoralis origins intact along IMF	PRP RM

II. IMPLANT DIMENSIONS **In constricted lower pole breasts with narrow base width, select implant width to achieve 3.0 cm intermammary distance

Base Width	11.0	B.W. Parenchyma (cm)	10.5	11.0	11.5	12.0	12.5	13.0	13.5	14.0	14.5	15.0	350 cc
		Initial Volume (cc)	200	250	275	300	300	325	350	375	375	400	

APSS$_{MaxStr}$	2.1	[2]If APSS <2.0, −30 cc; If APSS >3.0, +30 cc; If APSS >4.0, +60 cc Place appropriate number in blank at right	cc
N:IMF$_{MaxSt}$	5.5	If N:IMF >9.5, +30 cc Place appropriate number in blank at right	cc
PCSEF %	70%	If PCSEF <20%, +30 cc; If PCSEF >80%, −30 cc Place appropriate number in blank at right	cc
IDFDD cc	NA	If Allergan Style 468 or other form stable saline implant, −30 cc Place appropriate number in blank at right	NA
Pt. request			cc

NET ESTIMATED VOLUME TO FILL ENVELOPE BASED ON PATIENT TISSUE CHARACTERISTICS — cc

III. IMPLANT TYPE MFR: Allergan   STYLE/MODEL: Style 410FM Full Height Mod Profile Form Stable Anatomic Gel   VOLUME: 350 gm — **350 gm**

Volume: N:IMF Relationships: Locate Final Selected Implant Volume at Right; Set N:IMF to the disstance shown in the cell beneath, or leave at preop N:IMF, whichever is longer.	200	250	275	300	325	350	375	400	PreN:IMF
	7.0	7.0	7.5	8	8	8.5	9.0	9.5	5.5 cm

IV. NEW INFRAMAMMARY FOLD LEVEL — N:IMF$_{MaxSt}$ to set with preoperative markings and intraoperatively — **8.5 cm**

V. INCISION LOCATION — IM   AX   PA   UMB

PREOPERATIVE ASSESSMENT AND OBSERVATIONS

WNBCS = Will not be corrected surgically
Breast size asymmetry- WNBCS
Breast level asymmetry- WNBCS
Nipple level asymmetry- WNBCS
Tight skin envelope
Breasts high on torso (short SN:N)- WNBCS
Wide intermammary distance- WNBCS
Relative constriction or inadequate expansion of breast lower pole
Downpointing nipples
When selecting implant base width/desired breast width for a narrow base, constricted lower pole breast, draw a 3 cm wide intermammary distance and then measure laterally to determine the optimal width for the postoperative breast. Then select a base width implant approximately 0.5–1.0 cm. less than the desired base width (in this case, a 12.5 cm. wide implant 350 gm. A full height, moderate profile anatomic implant is most ideal long-term, because it achieves excellent lower pole expansion while avoiding the parenchymal atrophy caused by high profile implants.

POSTOPERATIVE ASSESSMENT AND OBSERVATIONS

Pre- to Post- bra size change by patient questionnaire: A to C.
Breasts remain somewhat tight, no capsular contracture, at 27 months followup.
Very good breast shape and fill
Very good expansion breast lower pole
All WNBCS items as predicted preoperatively.

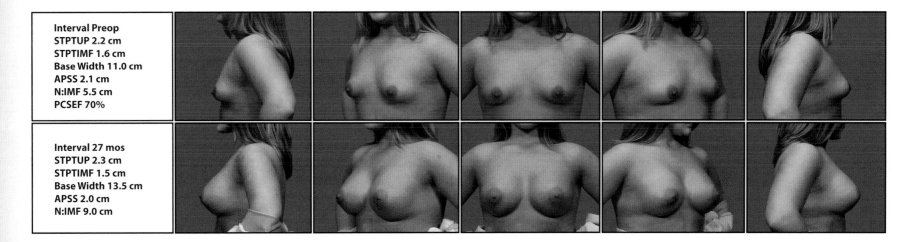

Interval Preop				
STPTUP 2.2 cm				
STPTIMF 1.6 cm				
Base Width 11.0 cm				
APSS 2.1 cm				
N:IMF 5.5 cm				
PCSEF 70%				

Interval 27 mos				
STPTUP 2.3 cm				
STPTIMF 1.5 cm				
Base Width 13.5 cm				
APSS 2.0 cm				
N:IMF 9.0 cm				

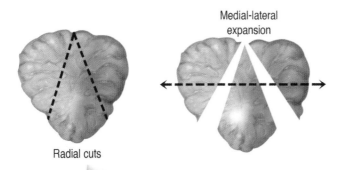

Medial-lateral expansion

Radial cuts

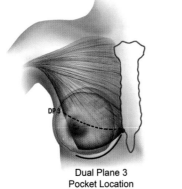

DP 3

Dual Plane 3
Pocket Location

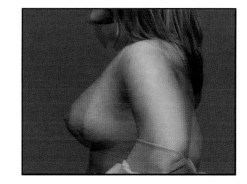

▥ REFERENCES

1. Regnault P: Breast ptosis. Definition and treatment. *Clin Plast Surg* 3(2):193–203, 1976.

2. Tebbetts JB: A system for breast implant selection based on patient tissue characteristics and implant–soft tissue dynamics. *Plast Reconstr Surg* 109(4):1396–1409, 2002.

3. Tebbetts JB, Adams WP: Five critical decisions in breast augmentation using 5 measurements in 5 minutes: the high five system. *Plast Reconstr Surg* 116(7):2005–2016, 2005.

4. Tebbetts JB: Dual plane (DP) breast augmentation: optimizing implant–soft tissue relationships in a wide range of breast types. *Plast Reconstr Surg* 107:1255, 2001.

Augmentation Mastopexy

The world we have made as a result of the level of thinking we have done thus far creates problems we cannot solve at the same level of thinking at which we created them.

Albert Einstein

■ INTRODUCTION

Breast augmentation and mastopexy are two distinctly different surgical procedures, performed for distinctly different reasons. The objectives or goals of mastopexy and breast augmentation are quite different. Nipple-areola repositioning or reshaping that repositions the nipple areola 2 cm or less is not a mastopexy. A true mastopexy that removes significant skin is an illogical procedure to perform simultaneously with a breast augmentation. Surgeons and patients sometimes choose to combine these two operations at a single surgical setting termed augmentation mastopexy or mastopexy augmentation. For practical purposes, surgeons use the terms augmentation mastopexy and mastopexy augmentation interchangeably to describe a single stage combination of the two procedures.

The challenges of the decision making process and surgical execution of augmentation mastopexy are evidenced by the fact that this combination of operations at a single stage has resulted in the highest rate of medical malpractice claims of any operation in aesthetic surgery. Despite large numbers of peer reviewed and published articles, and countless presentations in surgeon education venues over the past three decades, predictable and optimal outcomes and valid scientific data that prove the safety and efficacy of augmentation mastopexy remain elusive. Anecdotal studies of series of augmentation mastopexy that report good results with minimal complications all suffer from the same deficiency. No peer reviewed and published study currently exists that (1) quantifies the preoperative parameters that define indications for surgery, and (2) define quantified parameters that distinguish a true mastopexy or breast lift from a plethora of minor skin excisions or areola manipulations that surgeons also term "mastopexy". Without these quantified definitions, scientific analysis and definition of decision processes to optimize outcomes and minimize disasters cannot occur.

Persistent challenges require fresh approaches to critically and logically examine the processes and decisions that produce current results. The track record of single stage mastopexy augmentation is clear—three decades of high complication rates, suboptimal patient outcomes, and high rates of malpractice claims. This track record strongly suggests that if patient safety and optimal outcomes are priorities, surgeons and surgeon professional organizations that control surgeon education should critically reexamine the logic, decision processes, and surgical techniques of single stage mastopexy augmentation. Despite isolated anecdotal series published in peer reviewed literature, complication rates with simultaneous mastopexy-augmentation are well known to most experienced surgeons.

■ BREAST PTOSIS—CAUSES AND CLASSIFICATIONS

Breast ptosis occurs when the parenchymal mass of the breast exerts stretch forces on the breast soft tissue envelope, causing stretch of breast skin that allows descent of the parenchymal mass and changes in the shape and position of the nipple–areola complex. The weight of the parenchymal mass, genetic and hormonal factors, and a patient's pregnancy and nursing history determine the occurrence and degree of ptosis in individual patients.

Patients seek surgical improvement for a wide range of ptosis related complaints, ranging from minor degrees of stretch or breast shape change to major displacement and distortion of the breast. *When any patient presents with significant ptosis, the skin of the breast, by definition, failed to support the weight of the parenchymal mass.* This fact is true regardless of the underlying causes of the ptosis. *Performing any type of surgical procedure does not positively improve or alter the tissue characteristics that allowed the deformity to occur.*

When any patient presents with significant ptosis, the skin of the breast, by definition, failed to support the weight of the parenchymal mass

In 1976, Paula Regnault published a classification of breast ptosis that continues to be a predominant, common of classifying ptosis three decades later.[1,2] Although variations of this classification exist, key elements from Regnault's classification predominate when surgeons discuss and describe degrees of breast ptosis:

- Grade 1: Mild ptosis—Nipple just below inframammary fold but still above lower pole of breast
- Grade 2: Moderate ptosis—Nipple further below inframammary fold but still with some lower pole tissue below nipple

- Grade 3: Severe ptosis—Nipple well below inframammary fold and no lower pole tissue below nipple

- Pseudoptosis—Inferior pole ptosis with nipple at or above inframammary fold.

This classification and virtually all classifications of breast ptosis in common use today are based on a surgeon's subjective, visual assessment of the breast in lateral view. The degree of subjectivity and variability with this classification is enormous, and no scientific study has ever documented reproducibility with single surgeon or multiple surgeon use of this classification.

Lack of an objective, quantifiable classification for breast ptosis is a major contributor to persisting problems with mastopexy and mastopexy augmentation. When problems or suboptimal outcomes occur postoperatively, absent objective data, surgeons cannot objectively and scientifically assess and define the root causes of the problem. Was the assessment suboptimal? Was the decision process flawed? Was the surgical technique less than appropriate? Decision processes based on subjective impressions are often flawed when compared to the same processes based on objective, reproducible, scientifically verified data.

> Lack of an objective, quantifiable classification for breast ptosis is a major contributor to persisting problems with mastopexy and mastopexy augmentation

Outcomes and complications with mastopexy augmentation relate directly to the preoperative condition of the patient's tissues, the extent of the preoperative deformities, and the decision processes for surgical technique and implant. Absent objective, quantifiable, scientifically verified criteria for surgical indications to perform mastopexy or mastopexy augmentation, surgeons rely on subjective opinion and personal preferences in the decision process to perform the surgery and select the surgical technique and implant. The wide range of variations in indications and techniques for mastopexy augmentation, and the track record of high complication and reoperation rates suggest that subjectivity has not produced predictably optimal outcomes for patients. Objectivity and science based methodologies are needed.

■ DEFINING MASTOPEXY

The Medline Plus® Medical Dictionary defines mastopexy as "breast lift: plastic surgery to elevate and often reshape a sagging breast".[2] Other definitions in the medical literature include the following in the definition of mastopexy:

1. removal of excess skin from the breast
2. relocation of the breast mound upward (relocating the breast parenchymal mass)
3. reshaping of the breast parenchymal tissue
4. repositioning of the nipple–areola complex, and
5. reshaping the areola.

Current definitions of mastopexy are unscientifically broad and misleading for patients and surgeons. Excision of an ellipse of skin less than 1 cm wide around the areola is currently termed a "crescent mastopexy". Circumferentially extended around the areola, a 1 mm skin excision can be termed a "concentric or doughnut mastopexy". A "periareolar mastopexy" can be anything from excision of 1 mm of skin around the areola to a very large periareolar skin excision with extensive breast parenchyma modifications. Current terminology for "mastopexy" is subjective, poorly defined, and often misleading. Minor skin excisions for nipple–areola modification are orders of magnitude less risky and unpredictable for patients compared to major excisions of lower pole skin and major repositioning of the parenchymal mass and nipple–areola complex. Current terminology for mastopexy does not objectively distinguish amounts of skin excision, modifications and movement of breast parenchyma, and degree of nipple–areola repositioning.

Until surgeons more precisely define quantitative parameters that in turn define the degree of each of the five surgical areas of mastopexy listed in the previous paragraph, confusion will continue. When is a mastopexy really a mastopexy, and when is a so-called mastopexy nothing more than a minor areolar reshaping or minor nipple repositioning? At present, the term mastopexy applies to both, but the degree of technical difficulty, degree of potential devascularization and denervation, and the potential for wound healing problems and permanent, often uncorrectable tissue compromises are dramatically different. A breast augmentation combined with minor nipple repositioning or nipple–areola repositioning in a narrow breast in a young patient is distinctly less risky and unpredictable compared to an augmentation in an older patient that involves greater degrees of skin excision, skin undermining, parenchymal modification, and greater implant size.

When does a mastopexy become a mastopexy? For the past decade, the author has used the following criteria to define a mastopexy and distinguish mastopexy from much more minor nipple repositioning or minor skin excisions in the breast:

[margin notes]

Current definitions of mastopexy are unscientifically broad and misleading for patients and surgeons

Current terminology for mastopexy does not objectively distinguish amounts of skin excision, modifications and movement of breast parenchyma, and degree of nipple–areola repositioning.

When does a mastopexy become a mastopexy?

---

1. Nipple–areola repositioning of at least 2 cm.

2. Horizontal skin excision (vertical incision) of at least 2 cm width.

3. Vertical skin excision (horizontal incision along inframammary fold) only when vertical skin excess (VSE) exceeds 2 cm. Vertical skin excess is defined as the distance from the defined postoperative nipple position to the inframammary fold, minus 10 cm (VSE = N_{post} : IMF − 10 cm).

4. Parenchymal mass repositioning, with or without parenchymal modifications.

■ QUANTIFYING CRITICAL PARAMETERS IN MASTOPEXY AND MASTOPEXY AUGMENTATION

Currently, no objective, quantifiable criteria exist to provide objective data for scientific assessment of augmentation mastopexy. As a result, scientifically valid outcomes studies for mastopexy augmentation that identify risk factors are non-existent and will remain scientifically invalid until surgeons quantify key parameters that are now totally subjective. Objective, quantifiable tissue parameters that optimize outcomes and minimize reoperation rates dramatically for *breast augmentation* patients have been peer reviewed and published in the most respected journal in plastic surgery for more than 5 years.[3–11] The same simple, easy to perform measurements from these studies[4,5] generate quantified information and prioritized, defined decision processes that can provide surgeons the tools to improve outcomes in mastopexy augmentation just as they have done for breast augmentation patients.

The following basic parameters should be measured and documented preoperatively for every mastopexy augmentation patient. Detailed descriptions for the first five measurements are included in Chapter 7.[4,5]

- Soft tissue pinch thickness of the upper pole (STPTUP)

- Base width of the breast (BW)

- Anterior pull skin stretch (APSS)

- Nipple-to-inframammary fold distance, measured under maximal stretch (N : $IMF_{maxstretch}$)

- Sternal notch-to-nipple distance (SN : N)

- Nipple-to-midline distance (N : ML)

- Desired new nipple position (N_{post})

- Vertical skin excess (VSE)—a calculation (VSE = N_{post} : $IMF_{max\ stretch}$ − 10 cm) where N_{post} is the desired, marked postoperative nipple position

- Horizontal skin excess (HSE)—measured width of vertical skin excision at widest point

These basic measurements and calculations provide quantified data which surgeons can use for scientifically valid study design in augmentation mastopexy. Comparing these and other variables pre- and postoperatively enables valid scientific outcomes data to define best practices and proved processes to optimize patient outcomes. If quantified data are available, surgeons can define and prioritize scientifically valid decision processes that can dramatically change the current track record of mastopexy augmentation. Objectivity and science are required to substantively improve the dismal track record of subjectivity and opinion in mastopexy augmentation.

> Objectivity and science are required to substantively improve the dismal track record of subjectivity and opinion in mastopexy augmentation

■ PATIENTS AND PATIENT REQUESTS—IMPLANT ONLY OR MASTOPEXY AUGMENTATION?

Many patients schedule a consultation for breast augmentation, and on examination, their skin is stretched to an extent that, combined with breast width, requires an exceedingly large implant (>400 cc) to adequately fill the envelope for optimal results. Some of these patients like the idea of a large implant, until they understand that regardless of implant size, absent a mastopexy, their result will be a much larger breast that continues to appear low on the torso. Educating patients to this fact changes some patients' minds, and they elect a mastopexy or mastopexy augmentation instead, because they do not want a very large breast that hangs low on the torso.

In the same wide, ptotic breast patient group, some patients will simply ask the surgeon to place a specific, smaller than ideal size implant in the ptotic breast to avoid excessive size. With a wide (<13 cm base width breast) with substantial skin stretch (N : IMF > 10.0 cm and/or APSS > 3.5), placing an implant volume that is inadequate to completely fill the envelope will result in a full, larger lower breast with a still empty upper breast that creates a "rock in a sock" appearance. When patients hear the term "rock in a sock" and "empty upper breast", virtually no patient wants either of these aesthetic outcomes.

> A basic principle that every patient must understand during the education process is that an optimal aesthetic result requires that the surgeon place adequate volume in the breast

A basic principle that every patient must understand during the education process is that an optimal aesthetic result requires that the surgeon place adequate volume in the breast.

The wider the breast, the greater the skin stretch, and the longer the nipple to inframammary fold distance under maximal stretch, the greater the volume required to fill the envelope. Inadequate fill produces a full lower or middle breast, but leaves an empty upper breast. Once the ideal volume is in place, additional volume produces a more bulging upper pole, often with a stepoff. Every patient with a ptotic breast should clearly understand and acknowledge that despite any amount of implant volume a surgeon places in order to create upper breast fullness, additional lower pole stretch over time will result in loss of upper breast fullness. Hence *the premise that placing any implant in conjunction with a mastopexy will maintain upper breast fullness is patently false, unless the patient develops a capsular contracture.*

Understanding these principles, patients with significant ptosis and wide breasts have two realistic choices: (1) place adequate volume to fill the wide, stretched, ptotic envelope and live with the consequences of the appearance and adding significant additional weight in a breast that has already proved it stretches and doesn't support weight well, or (2) reduce the skin envelope to allow less volume to provide optimal fill (mastopexy).

■ MASTOPEXY WITHOUT OR WITH AN IMPLANT—PATIENT REQUESTS AND SURGEON RESPONSIBILITIES

Mastopexy can significantly improve the relationships between the inframammary fold, breast parenchymal mass, and nipple–areola complex. No current mastopexy or mastopexy augmentation surgical technique can predictably and consistently maintain upper fill in the post mastopexy breast. Despite publication of numerous techniques that purport to maintain upper fill in the breast, if surgeons examine the publications carefully, they will find that most publications contain the following: short-term results; pictured results rarely show five views of the breast; many of the best results are clearly in younger patients under the age of 40; no independently monitored, consecutive series of patients with long-term mastopexy or mastopexy augmentation results exists in the medical literature; and regardless of surgical technique, the quality of moderate to long-term (3–5 year) results relates more to the age and tissue qualities of the patient compared to one surgical technique or another.

The prevalence of mastopexy augmentation is due in part to the inability of mastopexy to maintain fill in the upper breast, and the misconception among surgeons and patients that a breast implant can predictably create and maintain upper fill. Recognizing that patients want upper fill and that mastopexy, regardless of technique, does not predictably

The premise that placing any implant in conjunction with a mastopexy will maintain upper breast fullness is patently false, unless the patient develops a capsular contracture

No current mastopexy surgical technique can predictably and consistently maintain upper fill in the post mastopexy breast

The prevalence of mastopexy augmentation is due in part to the inability of mastopexy to maintain fill in the upper breast, and the misconception among surgeons and patients that a breast implant can predictably create and maintain upper fill

deliver it, for decades surgeons have advised patients that a breast implant is necessary to produce upper fill with a mastopexy. In addition, a subset of patients wants their breasts both lifted and larger.

Patient desires generate powerful economic incentives for aesthetic surgeons to perform medically unnecessary procedures. The degree to which those procedures are logically justified depends on many factors, the most important of which is the safety of the patient and the safety of the patient's tissues long-term. Few patients consider the long-term implications of mastopexy augmentation before consulting a surgeon; hence the surgeon is responsible for assuring that patients are accurately and comprehensively informed of all potential short- and long-term consequences of performing the surgery.

The FDA and breast implant manufacturers also introduced significant financial incentives to surgeons. During the multi-year adjunct study of older generation silicone gel implants, surgeons were able to provide silicone gel implants to patients who needed or had a concurrent "mastopexy". By performing a minor periareolar skin ellipse excision or similar minor procedure and terming it a "mastopexy", surgeons who were willing to "stretch" the system could offer silicone gel implants to patients who requested them long before the implants were approved for the general public. This topic is seldom discussed in surgeon venues, and breast implant manufacturers and the FDA have never released segmented data on mastopexy augmentation patients from any FDA study. Whether these economic factors have affected the popularity of mastopexy augmentation remains a mystery from a scientific data perspective.

The quality of patient education and informed consent documentation determines the patient's knowledge base and the validity of her decisions that define informed consent. The demands on the surgeon to deliver the required information regarding mastopexy augmentation are immense, and the track record of malpractice claim rates with this operation suggests that deficiencies exist in patient education and informed consent for mastopexy augmentation.

Every mastopexy or mastopexy augmentation patient should learn and acknowledge the following in signed informed consent documents:

- Surgeons cannot consistently predict or change the quality of any patient's tissue.

- No surgical technique can predictably change and improve the quality of any patient's tissues.

- No surgical technique for mastopexy can predictably assure long-term fill of the upper breast.

- Placement of a breast implant may *create* upper fill in the breast, with or without mastopexy, but in either case, absent capsular contracture, no mastopexy technique or implant can predictably *maintain* upper breast fill.

- As a single operation, mastopexy has a set of tradeoffs, risks, and consequences.

- As a single operation, breast augmentation has a set of tradeoffs, risks, and consequences.

- When mastopexy and breast augmentation are performed at a single surgical stage, the tradeoffs, risks, and potential negative consequences are much more than additive for the two procedures.

■ FACTORS THAT DETERMINE OUTCOMES IN MASTOPEXY AUGMENTATION

Outcomes and consequences of mastopexy and augmentation relate directly to patient knowledge base, preoperative tissue parameters, the decision processes preceding the surgery, the level of technical execution during surgery, and the characteristics of any prosthetic device implanted during the surgery. Decision processes derive directly from the level of education and knowledge base of the patient and the surgeon.

Preoperative decisions based on subjective assessment have not established an optimal track record of patient outcomes in mastopexy augmentation. Patient and surgeon education determine the content of the patient and surgeon knowledge base used to make decisions. Decisions determine outcomes before any surgical technique occurs. Few, if any, surgical techniques can compensate for suboptimal preoperative assessment and decisions.

Mastopexy augmentation outcomes continue to be challenged by the following:

1. *Suboptimal patient and surgeon education* that poorly defines the consequences of prioritizing scar length or any aspect of breast aesthetics above optimal safety for the patient's tissues, optimal outcomes, and minimal negative short- or long-term consequences.

2. *Subjective preoperative tissue assessment* and subjectively based decisions—lack of defined, scientifically verified, quantifiable methods to define tissue parameters

Outcomes and consequences of mastopexy and augmentation relate directly to patient knowledge base, preoperative tissue parameters, the decision processes preceding the surgery, the level of technical execution during surgery, and the characteristics of any prosthetic device implanted during the surgery

Few, if any, surgical techniques can compensate for suboptimal preoperative assessment and decisions and characterize the preoperative tissue conditions that predispose to untoward outcomes.

3. *Lack of defined and prioritized decision processes* that are based on scientifically valid methodologies and techniques.

4. *Selection of surgical techniques* based on surgeon preference, scar length, marketing considerations, and other parameters that do not relate directly to patient tissue condition, optimal patient outcomes, patient safety, and low risks of problems and complications.

5. Prioritizing wishes above tissues—what the patient *wants* above what is *safest and best* for the patient. The classic example is the patient request for a lifted breast that is a specific size with a specific amount of upper pole fullness and the shortest possible scar.

■ REEXAMINING THE CHALLENGES OF MASTOPEXY AUGMENTATION FROM NEW PERSPECTIVES

Improving the unenviable track record of mastopexy augmentation requires that surgeons reexamine the most basic factors and logic that impact patient outcomes. Defining surgeons' area of focus is straightforward by examining any program from any surgeon education venue. Mastopexy augmentation presentations and discussions routinely focus on scar length and surgical techniques, and rarely focus on the level of objectivity in decision making or the basic, underlying factors that determine the level of patient outcome and the track record.

This chapter is not about techniques for breast augmentation or mastopexy. Instead, this chapter focuses on two levels of reexamining the logic and processes that ultimately define decisions that determine outcomes. The first level is a simple comparison of the goals of mastopexy and augmentation as separate operations to identify areas where each operation's goals contradict the other operation's goals. The second level is a detailed reexamination of the factors that affect outcomes using methodologies from business reliability engineering and process engineering to identify factors that cause untoward events, and to use these analyses to define improved processes. Each of these approaches provides a different perspective of the factors and processes that define outcomes in mastopexy augmentation.

> Improving the unenviable track record of mastopexy augmentation requires that surgeons reexamine the most basic factors and logic that impact patient outcomes

■ CONTRADICTORY OBJECTIVES IN MASTOPEXY AUGMENTATION

A fundamental problem with mastopexy augmentation is that the goals and objectives of each operation contradict the goals and objectives of the other

A fundamental problem with mastopexy augmentation is that the goals and objectives of each operation contradict the goals and objectives of the other. Regardless of surgical specialty or procedure, surgeons rarely combine operations with contradictory goals and objectives. Even when medical necessity dictates combining surgical procedures with potentially conflicting goals, surgeons are usually exceedingly cautious and concerned about their ability to deliver optimal outcomes with minimal tradeoffs and complications. For some reason, in the author's 30 year clinical experience, augmentation mastopexy, a medically unnecessary operation, somehow continues to defy logic in the decision processes of performing both operations in a single stage.

Table 20-1A lists the goals of mastopexy, and for each goal, the corresponding, contradictory effect of placing a breast implant in the breast. Table 20-1B lists the goals of breast augmentation, and for each goal, the corresponding, contradictory objective of mastopexy.

Table 20-1A. Goals of mastopexy and contradictory effects of breast augmentation

Mastopexy goals	Contradictory effects of augmentation
1. Long-term repositioning and reshaping of the breast	1. Additional weight, additional skin stretch, more rapid skin stretch, sagging, bottoming
2. Maximize innervation and vascularity	2. Pocket creation denervates and devascularizes in direct proportion to the size of the pocket and surgical techniques*
3. Scars of minimal width, optimal quality, and optimal predictability	3. Implant creates additional tension directly proportionate to implant dimensions and size; encourages scar widening; may necessitate pursestring sutures that potentially increase morbidity by palpability or failure with areolar distortion and stretch*
4. Optimal wound healing from an operation that inherently devascularizes tissues to varying degrees	4. Implant adds pressure in the breast envelope that impedes venous drainage and potentially impedes arterial inflow depending on implant size and dimensions and surgical techniques.*
5. Minimize risk of reoperations	5. Presence of a breast implant inherently increases risks of reoperations; implant device failure, wound healing problems, scar revisions, capsular contracture, and other reoperations
6. Predictable outcome for the patient	6. By adding risks, augmentation inherently makes the outcome less predictable*
7. Minimize risks of uncorrectable tissue compromises or deformities	7. Implant potential effects on wound healing, implant exposure, infection, wound dehiscence, and tissue stretch/thinning increase risks of permanent tissue compromises or deformities*
8. Optimize patient outcome while minimizing surgeon malpractice risk	8. Track record of suboptimal patient outcome and increased malpractice risk increases when mastopexy is simultaneously combined with breast augmentation*

*Risks or untoward occurrence factors that can be substantially reduced or eliminated by performing a mastopexy and staging the breast augmentation 6 months later.

Table 20-1B. **Goals of mastopexy and contradictory effects of breast augmentation**

Breast augmentation goals	Contradicting factors regarding mastopexy
1. Enlarge the breast	1. The larger the breast, the greater the risk of recurrent stretching and ptosis. Mastopexy is more predictable and safe in a smaller breast
2. Create predictable improvement in breast shape	2. Adding weight to a breast with mastopexy makes control of shape less predictable
3. Minimize risks of capsular contracture	3. Manipulation of breast parenchyma during mastopexy increases exposure of the implant to endogenous bacteria in the breast*
4. Preserve breast sensation	4. Mastopexy inherently increases denervation*
5. Minimize scar variables and maximize scar quality	5. Mastopexy with skin excision, skin undermining and parenchymal movement or modification inherently increases scar variables; tension of mastopexy closures inherently introduces factors that often compromise scar quality*
6. Minimize risks of interference with nursing	6. Manipulation or movement of the nipple–areola complex and manipulation or rearrangement of breast parenchyma in mastopexy inherently increase risks of interference with nursing
7. Minimize stretching, shape distortion, and scarring of the areola	7. Mastopexy inherently increases risks of areolar stretch, shape distortion, and unpredictability of periareolar scarring*
8. Optimize patient outcome while minimizing surgeon malpractice risk	8. Malpractice risk inherently increases when combining mastopexy with augmentation

*Risks or untoward occurrence factors that can be substantially reduced or eliminated by performing a mastopexy and staging the breast augmentation 6 months later.

Even the most cursory review of Tables 20-1A and 20-1B leaves any objective observer questioning the logic of combining mastopexy and breast augmentation at a single surgical setting. *Of the total 16 contradictory objectives of mastopexy augmentation, 10 of the 16 factors (62%) can be substantially reduced or eliminated by performing a mastopexy and staging the breast augmentation 6 months later. Patients should consider a potential 62% reduction in risk factors when considering economic factors of a one versus a two stage mastopexy augmentation.* While surgeons could legitimately argue that this number is not supported by peer reviewed and published, valid scientific data, few surgeons could legitimately dispute the simple logic presented in Tables 20-1A and 20-1B.

The potentially negative impacts of performing a breast augmentation simultaneously with a mastopexy depend on a myriad of factors that are more clearly defined later in this chapter. A minor nipple–areola repositioning that does not require skin undermining or

> Patients should consider a potential 62% reduction in risk factors when considering economic factors of a one versus a two stage mastopexy augmentation

parenchymal repositioning certainly involves fewer risks compared to a major skin excision, parenchymal shape modification and repositioning, and extensive skin undermining. Until quantified parameters exist to distinguish the level of tissue manipulation at which patient risks increase, to optimize outcomes surgeons must analyze the combined operation from the perspective of a legitimate mastopexy augmentation instead of a minor areolar or skin excision.

■ MASTOPEXY AND AUGMENTATION RISKS—MORE THAN ADDITIVE

Table 20-2 lists recognized risks for mastopexy and breast augmentation when surgeons perform the operations separately.

When surgeons perform mastopexy or breast augmentation separately, patients incur risks 1–8 with either operation. However, when surgeons combine the operations at one stage, augmentation separately increases the inherent risks of mastopexy by increasing risks when adding augmentation risks 3, 4, 5, 6, 8, 10, 11, 12, 13, 14, and 15 in the right column of Table 20-2. Placement of any breast implant inevitably increases the risk of

Table 20-2. Risks and costs of mastopexy and breast augmentation

Risks of mastopexy	Risks of breast augmentation
1. Asymmetry	1. Asymmetry
2. Hematoma/seroma	2. Hematoma/seroma
3. Infection	3. Infection
4. Delayed wound healing	4. Delayed wound healing
5. Poor quality scars	5. Poor quality scars
6. Nipple sensory loss	6. Nipple sensory loss
7. Unsatisfactory aesthetic result	7. Unsatisfactory aesthetic result
8. Interference with breast feeding	8. Interference with breast feeding
9. Recurrent deformity, ptosis, bottoming	9. Implant size issues
10. Nipple–areola loss	10. Skin stretch
11. Skin necrosis	11. Skin, subcutaneous, and parenchymal atrophy, thinning
12. Fat necrosis	12. Capsular contracture
13. Costs of mastopexy	13. Interference with breast imaging
	14. Costs of breast augmentation
	15. Device failure reoperation risk

delayed wound healing, skin or fat necrosis, scar widening or poor quality scars, nipple–areola loss or asymmetry, and by increasing those risks, also increases the risk of the patient perceiving an unsatisfactory cosmetic result.

Breast augmentation at the time of mastopexy not only increases the risks already inherent to mastopexy (risks 1–8 in Table 20-2), but adds significant risks and costs: additional weight that increases risk of recurrent deformity after mastopexy, additional pressure that risks skin, subcutaneous tissue and parenchymal atrophy or thinning, capsular contracture risk, increased reoperation risk due to implant device failure, interference with breast imaging, and the additional costs of the breast augmentation portion of the procedure. One perspective could argue that breast augmentation only adds risks 9–15 in Table 20-2, but even that perspective means that patients could avoid *seven additional risks and cost* by not adding augmentation to mastopexy.

A more accurate perspective recognizes that a comparison of complication rates for mastopexy and augmentation performed separately is dramatically less for each operation compared to similar rates for a one stage mastopexy augmentation. Experienced surgeons recognize this fact and have warned colleagues in peer reviewed studies in the most respected journal in plastic surgery.[12,13] Despite anecdotal studies in the literature that suggest that a one stage mastopexy augmentation is as safe as either operation performed separately, no prospective, independently monitored study of consecutive cases is published. In FDA premarket approval (PMA) studies where independent clinical review organization monitoring is required, breast implant manufacturers and the FDA have never released breakdown data on complication rates of mastopexy augmentation compared to augmentation performed separately. The medical malpractice claims rate for mastopexy augmentation clearly indicates the increased risks associated with combining the operations.

In addition to the lack of quantified data and objective, data based decision processes, the sheer number of variables associated with either operation, much less the two combined, makes structuring a scientifically valid clinical study exceedingly difficult. Until scientifically valid studies are available, surgeons can do three things to improve mastopexy outcomes for patients: (1) reexamine currently held tenets and beliefs using new methodologies, (2) adjust current processes and define new process algorithms using business process engineering principles, and (3) implement objective measurements and collect objective, quantified data to produce valid scientific studies.

> A more accurate perspective recognizes that a comparison of complication rates for mastopexy and augmentation performed separately is dramatically less for each operation compared to similar rates for a one stage mastopexy augmentation

The effects of mastopexy on patients' tissues are often not apparent for many years following surgery. Each operation performed individually without the other has long-term potentially negative effects on patient's tissues. Mastopexy devascularizes and denervates areas of the breast, may interfere with nursing, and leave scars. Breast augmentation, especially with excessively large or excessively projecting implants, can cause skin stretch and thinning, subcutaneous tissue atrophy, breast parenchyma atrophy, and chest wall deformities. Ranges of breast implant size and projection that optimize patient outcomes are beginning to be defined in the literature.[4–10] But no prospective, non-anecdotal, independently monitored study exists to define safe practices and best processes to assure optimal outcomes in mastopexy augmentation.

Rarely does a patient who has marked breast ptosis ask the surgeon who may be performing a breast lift with placement of a breast implant, "How does my having this combination of procedures now affect my risks and outcomes should I need another lifting operation in the future?" Most patients at the initial consultation for ptosis want (1) their breasts to look as they did at age 20 or 25, or before pregnancy, (2) a perpetually full upper breast, and (3) minimal costs and risks. Even more rarely does a surgeon focus on the long-term implications of potential choices that ultimately determine a patient's outcome.

One of the most disturbing perspectives of the potential negatives of the effects of augmentation and mastopexy is documented in a paper that cautions surgeons performing mastopexy on previously augmented patients.[13] The challenges of performing mastopexy on previously augmented breasts are the focus of the paper, but the message is more ominous. Augmentation mammaplasty clearly makes future mastopexy (with or without implant replacement) much riskier and less predictable for patients. If augmentation alone presents these challenges, any astute surgeon recognizes that a mastopexy combined with a primary augmentation would leave tissues in a much more compromised situation. The "what ifs" in the event that additional surgery is required in the future are not a common topic of surgeon discussion, but this topic is critically important to long-term patient outcomes. Every surgeon that performs simultaneous augmentation mastopexy should read this paper and consider the implications should their patient ever require a reoperation in the future.

▪ BUSINESS RELIABILITY ENGINEERING AND TOTAL QUALITY MANAGEMENT ANALYSES OF MASTOPEXY AUGMENTATION

Why should surgeons apply business reliability engineering principles and methodologies to analyze current practices and define improved processes? Analysis of breast

Many of the world's most successful businesses use a structured approach of Total Quality Management (TQM) to constantly seek improvements in processes to deliver constantly improved products and services to customers

augmentation processes using principles of process engineering and motion and time studies has been shown to dramatically improve patient recovery and outcomes.[6,9,10] Many of the world's most successful businesses use a structured approach of Total Quality Management (TQM) to constantly seek improvements in processes to deliver constantly improved products and services to customers. TQM emphasizes management and process refinement from the customer's point of view, emphasizing customer satisfaction. The goal of TQM is to discard flawed processes and seek improved processes. Surgeons can adapt many of the methodologies of TQM and process engineering to refine decision and surgical processes and deliver improved outcomes (the product) to patients.

The goal of TQM is to discard flawed processes and seek improved processes

TQM methodologies address four sequential categories: plan, do, check, and act (the PDCA cycle)

TQM methodologies address four sequential categories: plan, do, check, and act (the PDCA cycle). In the first of these categories, *planning*, the goal is to define the problem to be addressed, collect relevant data, and use the data to identify root causes of the problem. In the *doing* phase, personnel define, develop, and implement a "solution" and define measurements to judge its effectiveness. During the *checking* phase, personnel collect comparison data before and after the "solution" is implemented to assess results, and in the *acting* phase, personnel document refined processes and disseminate those processes to others.

A modified PDCA cycle enables surgeons to use valuable information to benefit patients while implementing scientifically valid clinical studies that ultimately define optimal processes. Table 20-3 illustrates the classic PDCA cycle, and a modified PDCA cycle with specific subprocesses that allow surgeons to improve processes while awaiting definitive scientific studies.

Surgeons tend to think linearly using a "solution for problem" algorithm

Surgeons tend to think linearly using a "solution for problem" algorithm. Given a problem or clinical situation, a board examiner expects a surgeon to produce a "solution' answer. The problem–solution, linear approach to thinking has not improved outcomes for augmentation mastopexy patients in valid scientific studies and has not reduced malpractice claims for mastopexy augmentation. Analysis from a different, non-linear perspective is logical. The first step in the PDCA "plan" process is to identify potential problem areas in mastopexy augmentation. Table 20-4 presents typical problem areas that occur following augmentation mastopexy.

For each potential problem area, brainstorming encourages non-linear thinking

For each potential problem area, brainstorming encourages non-linear thinking. Instead of attempting to establish cause and effect relationships, surgeons should simply throw

Table 20-3. Applying the TQM PDCA cycle to analysis of mastopexy augmentation processes.

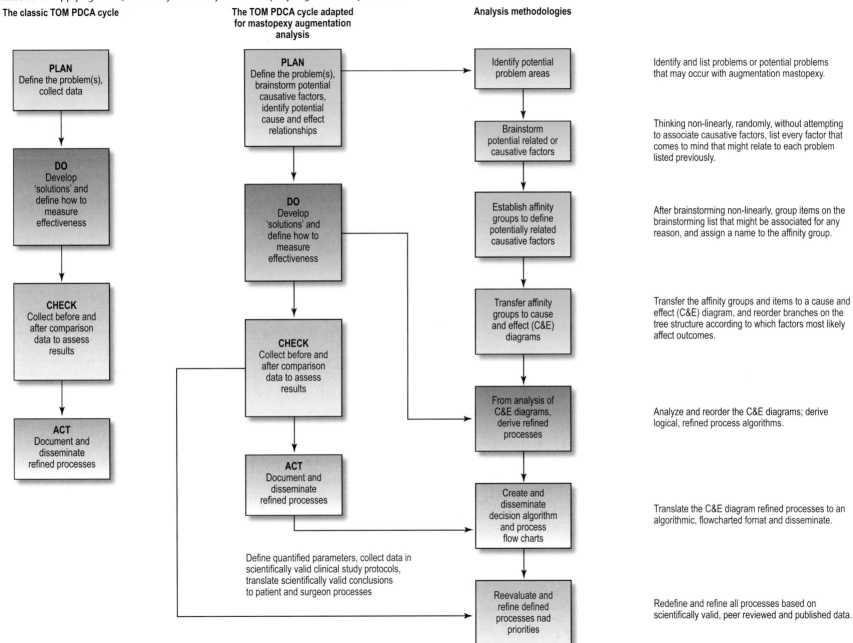

The classic TOM PDCA cycle

PLAN
Define the problem(s), collect data

DO
Develop 'solutions' and define how to measure effectiveness

CHECK
Collect before and after comparison data to assess results

ACT
Document and disseminate refined processes

The TOM PDCA cycle adapted for mastopexy augmentation analysis

PLAN
Define the problem(s), brainstorm potential causative factors, identify potential cause and effect relationships

DO
Develop 'solutions' and define how to measure effectiveness

CHECK
Collect before and after comparison data to assess results

ACT
Document and disseminate refined processes

Define quantified parameters, collect data in scientifically valid clinical study protocols, translate scientifically valid conclusions to patient and surgeon processes

Analysis methodologies

Identify potential problem areas

Brainstorm potential related or causative factors

Establish affinity groups to define potentially related causative factors

Transfer affinity groups to cause and effect (C&E) diagrams

From analysis of C&E diagrams, derive refined processes

Create and disseminate decision algorithm and process flow charts

Reevaluate and refine defined processes nad priorities

Identify and list problems or potential problems that may occur with augmentation mastopexy.

Thinking non-linearly, randomly, without attempting to associate causative factors, list every factor that comes to mind that might relate to each problem listed previously.

After brainstorming non-linearly, group items on the brainstorming list that might be associated for any reason, and assign a name to the affinity group.

Transfer the affinity groups and items to a cause and effect (C&E) diagram, and reorder branches on the tree structure according to which factors most likely affect outcomes.

Analyze and reorder the C&E diagrams; derive logical, refined process algorithms.

Translate the C&E diagram refined processes to an algorithmic, flowcharted fornat and disseminate.

Redefine and refine all processes based on scientifically valid, peer reviewed and published data.

Table 20-4. **Problems following augmentation mastopexy**
1. Scar widening
2. Scar puckering or contour irregularities
3. Nipple–areola shape or position irregularities
4. Recurrent ptosis, bottoming, and inferior pole stretch deformities
5. Scar malposition
6. Wound problems occurring postoperatively including dehiscence and delayed healing
7. Sensory problems postoperatively

out and list any factor that comes to mind when presented with the listed problem. It is not about solutions or techniques; instead, it is all about anything that comes to mind that might be associated in any way with the listed problem. This list is a brainstorming list, and does not attempt to associate anything with anything else. Instead, brainstorming encourages those involved to introduce any and all factors that may come to mind when thinking about a problem area. This process is challenging for many surgeons, because surgical education is built on linear, problem–solution thought processes.

Identifying Key Problems

Table 20-4 identifies potential factors that may contribute to problems in mastopexy or mastopexy augmentation. For each of the seven categories listed in Table 20-4, surgeons should ask a specific question and brainstorm that question. For example, "What are tissue characteristics that might contribute to problems in mastopexy augmentation?" When creating the brainstorming list, a surgeon or group of surgeons should list any and all factors that come to mind for any reason, avoiding trying to establish cause and effect relationships, substituting lateral for linear thinking, and simply listing everything that comes to mind. A summary brainstorming list is included in Table 20-5.

Creating Affinity Sets or Affinity Groups

The affinity group concept was developed by Kawakita Jiro (the KJ method) to *discover meaningful groups of ideas within a raw list.* While the method is designed to let the groupings or affinity sets emerge naturally instead of using preordained categories. In the first cycle through this entire process 5 years ago to look at mastopexy augmentation from a different perspective, the author used the classic method. In this chapter, for expediency, the affinity lists are presented already named.

Table 20-5. Summary brainstorming list for potential problems in mastopexy augmentation

Tissue characteristics problems

Genetic tissue characteristics

Age

Previous pregnancies

Width of breast preoperatively

Previous surgery

Previous implant (size)

Smoking history

Weight problems

Amount of parenchyma preoperatively

Amount of parenchyma left intraoperatively

Size of breast implant preoperatively if placed

Size of breast implant intraoperatively if placed

Patient education factors

Inadequate patient education

Unrealistic expectations regarding result or longevity

Failure to sign detailed informed consent documents detailing limitations and risks, documenting patient acceptance

Failure to review preoperative pictures and specify limitations and risks

Failure to specify inevitability of relapse

Failure to specify increased rate of relapse with any increase in weight factors

Failure to inform patient of scar widening risk

Failure to inform patient of potential of scar contour irregularities with scar length limiting techniques

Failure to advise patient preoperatively of possible nipple–areolar shape irregularities

Failure to advise patient preoperatively of possible scar malposition occurring postoperatively

Failure to advise patient preoperatively of possible postoperative wound problems

Failure to advise patient preoperatively of possible sensory compromise or loss postoperatively

Patient physical factors

Excess breast size, weight requested or present preoperatively

Inadequate extrinsic breast support

Request for implant placed at time of mastopexy

Request for implant at any time associated with mastopexy

Table 20-5. Summary brainstorming list for potential problems in mastopexy augmentation—cont'd

Surgeon preoperative factors

Failure to document breast and tissue measurements preoperatively

Failure to plan incision lengths and location related to breast width and distance of nipple movement

Prioritizing scar length over scar contour and adequate skin removal

Prioritizing scar length over optimal redistribution of skin left intraoperatively

Planning excessive skin removal

Planning inadequate skin removal

Planning excessively high nipple–areola position

Failure to plan specific N:IMF distance preoperatively

Planning techniques that leave excessively large discrepancies between sides of incision closures, necessitating gathering

Planning inadequate incision length leaving standing cones or excess skin

Planning placement of breast implant at time of mastopexy when tissues are mobilized

Planning placement of implant when soft tissue coverage is inadequate

Planning excessive mobilization and potential devascularization

Planning transposition of parenchymal flaps

Planning techniques that leave dead space in the breast

Planning excessive central skin excision that flattens the breast

Planning excessively long N:IMF relative to breast width or leaving excess skin and rotating superiorly to shorten scar

Planning excessively short N:IMF distance relative to breast width

Failure to assure optimal instrumentation

Planning technique that excises skin at areolar position prior to closure of skin envelope

Failure to plan technique to assure adequate venous and arterial supply to nipple–areola

Failure to plan technique that spares sensory innervation

Suboptimal or inaccurate preoperative marking

Preoperative marking with patient in any position other than standing

Failure to measure nipple to midline during preoperative marking

Planning transposition or relocation of parenchymal flaps

Planning inadequate movement distance of any component

Failure to plan incision lengths and location related to breast width and distance of nipple movement

Setting nipple position relative only to projected IMF

Setting nipple position only relative to sternal notch to nipple distance

Setting nipple position relative to any single anatomic landmark

Table 20-5. Summary brainstorming list for potential problems in mastopexy augmentation—cont'd

Surgeon intraoperative factors

Committing to excision of skin at areola site with initial skin excisions

Failure to achieve adequate hemostasis

Failure to establish drainage as needed relative to tissue trauma

Gathering skin in any area to achieve wound closure

Leaving discrepant lengths on two sides of any incision closures

Excessive skin excision, creating tension

Failure to remove adequate parenchyma when indicated

Adding a breast implant at time of mastopexy

Adding a breast implant at any time after mastopexy

Adding an excessively large implant at any time

One layer closure any area

Placing excessive tension on any remaining parenchymal components

Placing excessive pressure on residual parenchymal components by excessively tight closure

Increasing weight of the breast with a breast implant

Increasing pressure on envelope and parenchyma with breast implant

Creating potential strangulation of pedicles with pull through techniques

Adding alloplastic mesh or other supporting material internally

Using any technique that increases tissue trauma

Using any technique that traumatizes more normal anatomic components

Creating excessively short N:IMF distance for breast width

Creating excessively long N:IMF for breast width

Incorporating questionable assumptions

Absorbable sutures effectively suspend or hold weight long-term

Permanent sutures effectively suspend or hold weight long-term

Adding an implant adds upper fullness to the breast long-term

Alloplastic material slings or suspension decrease rate of recurrent lower pole stretch or ptosis

Breast shaping using parenchymal flaps outweighs potential risks of vascular compromise or fat necrosis

Breast implants are preferably placed at the time of mastopexy

The tighter the inferior pole closure, the greater the longevity of the result

Rotating relative skin excesses superiorly to obviate a horizontal scar does not increase risks of future bottoming or excessive N:IMF lengths

Gathering relative skin excesses along discrepant incision length lines is preferable to longer incisions

Table 20-5. **Summary brainstorming list for potential problems in mastopexy augmentation—cont'd**
Skin closures with visible gathering due to discrepant incision lengths results in acceptable revision rates or residual deformities
Optimal sutures and closure techniques can overcome scar widening due to excess tension
Optimal sutures and closure techniques can overcome scar widening due to excess weight in the skin envelope
Scars crossing the inframammary fold are preferable to scars placed medially and/or laterally in the IMF
Leaving excess skin or standing cone centrally in or around the IMF is preferable to a longer scar placed in the IMF
Breast implant factors
Implant costs
Increased implant weight added to breast
Increased pressure on adjacent parenchyma and skin envelope caused by implant
Potential reoperation risks and costs when implant added
Capsular contracture
Skin stretch caused by implant
Skin thinning caused by implant
Parenchymal atrophy caused by implant long-term
Increased rate of recurrent ptosis or bottoming implant related
Hematoma
Seroma
Periprosthetic infection
Sensory compromise from additional surgical trauma associated with creating implant pocket
Sensory compromise from additional stretch on residual innervation from implant
Implant shell failure necessitating replacement
Implant interference with mammography
Implant exposure
Implant extrusion
Optimal implant width limitations due to excess pressure and tension created by implant of optimal width
Visible traction rippling from additional weight under thin soft tissue cover

An affinity group or affinity set is a sorted and named brainstorming list

An affinity group or affinity set is a sorted and named brainstorming list. To create an affinity set, the surgeon simply takes an item from the brainstorming list, places it at the top of an unnamed affinity set list, and then moves down the brainstorming list, and for each item asks, "Could this item in any way be related to the item I already moved to the affinity set list?" If the surgeon feels that it is related in any way, without any thought of cause and effect or other linear thinking, the surgeon copies the item to the affinity set list.

The affinity set list or diagram is particularly effective to reexamine or refine preexisting ideas, processes, or paradigms

The affinity set list or diagram is particularly effective to reexamine or refine preexisting ideas, processes, or paradigms. By continually regrouping items within the affinity set before naming them, surgeons gain a different perspective of basic tenets and paradigms they learned in residency and often identify parameters that may be important, but have been overlooked in traditional training. That different perspective can translate into refined processes that the surgeon uses every day.

Having transferred all pertinent items from the brainstorming list to the affinity set list, the surgeon sorts the affinity set into groups of seemingly related ideas and repeats this process until clearly related groups occur. Only then should the surgeon name the affinity set. During this process, users should:

1. Rapidly group ideas that seem to belong together without overanalyzing why they belong together.
2. Refine and clarify any ideas in question.
3. Copy an idea into more than one affinity set if appropriate.
4. When small sets emerge, ask if they really belong in a larger set.
5. Do large sets need to be broken down more precisely?
6. When most of the ideas have been sorted, the surgeon can begin to name each set.

Several software programs facilitate all of these processes. The program used for this chapter is PathMaker™, distributed by SkyMark Corporation, 7300 Penn Avenue, Pittsburg, PA 15208, telephone 412.371.0630 or on the Web at www.skymark.com. This program greatly simplifies the process by an interface design that places the brainstorming list on the left and the affinity group list on the right, allowing surgeons to drag items from the brainstorming list onto the affinity set list. This company's website has excellent content that summarizes most of the basic concepts and tools used in process engineering and TQM.

Initially, some business process analysis methodologies are strange and cumbersome to surgeons, because the processes stimulate lateral thinking rather than linear thinking, and because they force users to "think out of the box". The power of the TQM methodologies is their ability to encourage surgeons or users to think more openly about problems or processes that are ingrained and taken for granted. The processes are extremely stimulating and reward the surgeon user with ideas and perspectives that might otherwise remain obscure.

Table 20-6 lists affinity sets that are derived from the brainstorming list in Table 20-5, with each list titled with a potential cause of a mastopexy augmentation problem. Affinity sets include the following:

1. Scar widening
2. Scar puckering or contour irregularities
3. Nipple–areola shape or position irregularities
4. Recurrent ptosis, bottoming, and inferior pole stretch deformities
5. Scar malposition
6. Wound problems occurring postoperatively
7. Sensory problems postoperatively.

Within each affinity set subcategory, surgeons should prioritize the items in order of likely importance for later transfer to a cause and effect diagram. This process, depending on the affinity set and items, can be very enlightening and assist surgeons in reevaluating current concepts from a different perspective.

Text continued on p. 537

> Initially, some business process analysis methodologies are strange and cumbersome to surgeons, because the processes stimulate lateral thinking rather than linear thinking, and because they force users to "think out of the box"

Table 20-6. Affinity sets for effects or problems associated with mastopexy augmentation

Scar widening affinities

Tissue characteristics problems

Genetic tissue characteristics

Age

Previous pregnancies

Preoperative breast size

Previous surgery

Previous implant (size)

Weight problems

Amount of parenchyma left intraoperatively

Size of breast implant preoperatively if placed

Size of breast implant intraoperatively if placed

Inadequate patient education

Patient education factors

Failure to inform patient of scar widening risk

Patient physical factors

Request for implant placed at time of mastopexy

Request for implant at any time associated with mastopexy

Surgeon preoperative factors

Planning excessive skin removal

Planning techniques that leave excessively large discrepancies between sides of incision closures, necessitating gathering

Planning placement of breast implant at time of mastopexy when tissues are mobilized

Planning excessive central skin excision that flattens the breast

Failure to plan technique to assure adequate venous and arterial supply to nipple–areola

Planning excessively short N:IMF distance relative to breast width

Planning technique that excises skin at areolar position prior to closure of skin envelope

Failure to document breast and tissue measurements preoperatively

Surgeon intraoperative factors

Planning excessive skin removal

Committing to excision of skin at areola site with initial skin excisions

Excessive skin excision, creating tension

Adding a breast implant at time of mastopexy

Adding an excessively large implant at any time

One layer closure any area

Table 20-6. Affinity sets for effects or problems associated with mastopexy augmentation—cont'd

Increasing weight of the breast with a breast implant

Using any technique that increases tissue trauma

Creating excessively short N:IMF distance for breast width

Incorporating questionable assumptions

Absorbable sutures effectively suspend or hold weight long-term

Permanent sutures effectively suspend or hold weight long-term

Alloplastic material slings or suspension decrease rate of recurrent lower pole stretch or ptosis

Breast implants are preferably placed at the time of mastopexy

The tighter the inferior pole closure, the greater the longevity of the result

Optimal sutures and closure techniques can overcome scar widening due to excess tension

Optimal sutures and closure techniques can overcome scar widening due to excess weight in the skin envelope

Breast implant factors

Increased implant weight added to breast

Increased pressure on adjacent parenchyma and skin envelope caused by implant

Skin stretch caused by implant

Skin thinning caused by implant

Hematoma

Seroma

Periprosthetic infection

Implant exposure

Implant extrusion

Skin puckering or contour irregularities affinities

Tissue characteristics problems

Genetic tissue characteristics

Age

Previous pregnancies

Preoperative breast size

Width of breast preoperatively

Patient education factors

Inadequate patient education

Failure to sign detailed informed consent documents detailing limitations and risks, documenting patient acceptance

Failure to review preoperative pictures and specify limitations and risks

Failure to inform patient of potential of scar contour irregularities with scar length limiting techniques

Table 20-6. Affinity sets for effects or problems associated with mastopexy augmentation—cont'd

Surgeon preoperative factors

Failure to plan incision lengths and location related to breast width and distance of nipple movement

Prioritizing scar length over scar contour and adequate skin removal

Prioritizing scar length over optimal redistribution of skin left intraoperatively

Planning excessive skin removal

Planning inadequate skin removal

Planning techniques that leave excessively large discrepancies between sides of incision closures, necessitating gathering

Planning inadequate incision length leaving standing cones or excess skin

Planning excessively long N:IMF relative to breast width or leaving excess skin and rotating superiorly to shorten scar

Suboptimal or inaccurate preoperative marking

Preoperative marking with patient in any position other than standing

Failure to document breast and tissue measurements preoperatively

Failure to plan incision lengths and location related to breast width and distance of nipple movement

Nipple–areola shape and position irregularities affinities

Tissue characteristics problems

Genetic tissue characteristics

Age

Width of breast preoperatively

Weight problems

Amount of parenchyma preoperatively

Amount of parenchyma left intraoperatively

Size of breast implant preoperatively if placed

Size of breast implant intraoperatively if placed

Patient education factors

Inadequate patient education

Unrealistic expectations regarding result or longevity

Failure to sign detailed informed consent documents detailing limitations and risks, documenting patient acceptance

Failure to advise patient preoperatively of possible nipple–areolar shape irregularities

Patient physical factors

Request for implant placed at time of mastopexy

Request for implant at any time associated with mastopexy

Table 20-6. Affinity sets for effects or problems associated with mastopexy augmentation—cont'd

Surgeon preoperative factors

Failure to document breast and tissue measurements preoperatively

Failure to plan incision lengths and location related to breast width and distance of nipple movement

Prioritizing scar length over scar contour and adequate skin removal

Prioritizing scar length over optimal redistribution of skin left intraoperatively

Planning excessive skin removal

Planning inadequate skin removal

Planning excessively high nipple–areola position

Planning techniques that leave excessively large discrepancies between sides of incision closures, necessitating gathering

Planning excessive central skin excision that flattens the breast

Planning excessively long N:IMF relative to breast width or leaving excess skin and rotating superiorly to shorten scar

Planning technique that excises skin at areolar position prior to closure of skin envelope

Suboptimal or inaccurate preoperative marking

Failure to measure nipple to midline during preoperative marking

Preoperative marking with patient in any position other than standing

Surgeon intraoperative factors

Committing to excision of skin at areola site with initial skin excisions

Gathering skin in any area to achieve wound closure

Leaving discrepant lengths on two sides of any incision closures

Excessive skin excision, creating tension

Adding a breast implant at time of mastopexy

Adding a breast implant at any time after mastopexy

Adding an excessively large implant at any time

One layer closure any area

Increasing weight of the breast with a breast implant

Increasing pressure on envelope and parenchyma with breast implant

Creating excessively short N:IMF distance for breast width

Creating excessively long N:IMF for breast width

Incorporating questionable assumptions

Absorbable sutures effectively suspend or hold weight long-term

Permanent sutures effectively suspend or hold weight long-term

Breast implants are preferably placed at the time of mastopexy

The tighter the inferior pole closure, the greater the longevity of the result

Table 20-6. Affinity sets for effects or problems associated with mastopexy augmentation—cont'd

Rotating relative skin excesses superiorly to obviate a horizontal scar does not increase risks of future bottoming or excessive N:IMF lengths

Gathering relative skin excesses along discrepant incision length lines is preferable to longer incisions

Optimal sutures and closure techniques can overcome scar widening due to excess tension

Optimal sutures and closure techniques can overcome scar widening due to excess weight in the skin envelope

Breast implant factors

Increased implant weight added to breast

Increased pressure on adjacent parenchyma and skin envelope caused by implant

Skin stretch caused by implant

Skin thinning caused by implant

Recurrent ptosis, bottoming, inferior pole stretch deformities affinities

Tissue characteristics problems

Genetic tissue characteristics

Age

Previous pregnancies

Preoperative breast size

Width of breast preoperatively

Previous surgery

Previous implant (size)

Weight problems

Amount of parenchyma preoperatively

Amount of parenchyma left intraoperatively

Size of breast implant preoperatively if placed

Size of breast implant intraoperatively if placed

Patient education factors

Inadequate patient education

Unrealistic expectations regarding result or longevity

Failure to sign detailed informed consent documents detailing limitations and risks, documenting patient acceptance

Failure to review preoperative pictures and specify limitations and risks

Failure to specify inevitability of relapse

Failure to specify increased rate of relapse with any increase in weight factors

Failure to inform patient of scar widening risk

Failure to inform patient of potential of scar contour irregularities with scar length limiting techniques

Table 20-6. Affinity sets for effects or problems associated with mastopexy augmentation—cont'd

Patient physical factors

Excess breast size, weight requested or present preoperatively

Inadequate extrinsic breast support

Request for implant placed at time of mastopexy

Request for implant at any time associated with mastopexy

Surgeon preoperative factors

Failure to document breast and tissue measurements preoperatively

Failure to plan incision lengths and location related to breast width and distance of nipple movement

Prioritizing scar length over scar contour and adequate skin removal

Prioritizing scar length over optimal redistribution of skin left intraoperatively

Planning excessive skin removal

Planning inadequate skin removal

Planning excessively high nipple–areola position

Failure to plan specific N:IMF distance preoperatively

Planning techniques that leave excessively large discrepancies between sides of incision closures, necessitating gathering

Planning inadequate incision length leaving standing cones or excess skin

Planning placement of breast implant at time of mastopexy when tissues are mobilized

Planning placement of implant when soft tissue coverage is inadequate

Planning excessive central skin excision that flattens the breast

Planning excessively long N:IMF relative to breast width or leaving excess skin and rotating superiorly to shorten scar

Planning excessively short N:IMF distance relative to breast width

Planning technique that excises skin at areolar position prior to closure of skin envelope

Suboptimal or inaccurate preoperative marking

Preoperative marking with patient in any position other than standing

Failure to document breast and tissue measurements preoperatively

Failure to plan incision lengths and location related to breast width and distance of nipple movement

Setting nipple position relative only to projected IMF

Setting nipple position only relative to sternal notch to nipple distance

Setting nipple position relative to any single anatomic landmark

Surgeon intraoperative factors

Committing to excision of skin at areola site with initial skin excisions

Gathering skin in any area to achieve wound closure

Leaving discrepant lengths on two sides of any incision closures

Table 20-6. Affinity sets for effects or problems associated with mastopexy augmentation—cont'd

Excessive skin excision, creating tension

Failure to remove adequate parenchyma when indicated

Adding a breast implant at time of mastopexy

Adding a breast implant at any time after mastopexy

Adding an excessively large implant at any time

One layer closure any area

Placing excessive pressure on residual parenchymal components by excessively tight closure

Increasing weight of the breast with a breast implant

Increasing pressure on envelope and parenchyma with breast implant

Creating excessively short N:IMF distance for breast width

Creating excessively long N:IMF for breast width

Incorporating questionable assumptions

Absorbable sutures effectively suspend or hold weight long-term

Permanent sutures effectively suspend or hold weight long-term

Adding an implant adds upper fullness to the breast long-term

Alloplastic material slings or suspension decrease rate of recurrent lower pole stretch or ptosis

Breast implants are preferably placed at the time of mastopexy

The tighter the inferior pole closure, the greater the longevity of the result

Rotating relative skin excesses superiorly to obviate a horizontal scar does not increase risks of future bottoming or excessive N:IMF lengths

Gathering relative skin excesses along discrepant incision length lines is preferable to longer incisions

Optimal sutures and closure techniques can overcome scar widening due to excess weight in the skin envelope

Leaving excess skin or standing cone centrally in or around the IMF is preferable to a longer scar placed in the IMF

Breast implant factors

Increased implant weight added to breast

Increased pressure on adjacent parenchyma and skin envelope caused by implant

Potential reoperation risks and costs when implant added

Skin stretch caused by implant

Skin thinning caused by implant

Parenchymal atrophy caused by implant long-term

Increased rate of recurrent ptosis or bottoming implant related

Visible traction rippling from additional weight under thin soft tissue cover

Table 20-6. Affinity sets for effects or problems associated with mastopexy augmentation—cont'd

Scar malposition affinities

Tissue characteristics problems

Width of breast preoperatively

Weight problems

Size of breast implant preoperatively if placed

Size of breast implant intraoperatively if placed

Patient education factors

Inadequate patient education

Failure to review preoperative pictures and specify limitations and risks

Failure to specify inevitability of relapse

Failure to specify increased rate of relapse with any increase in weight factors

Failure to advise patient preoperatively of possible scar malposition occurring postoperatively

Patient physical factors

Request for implant placed at time of mastopexy

Request for implant at any time associated with mastopexy

Surgeon preoperative factors

Failure to document breast and tissue measurements preoperatively

Failure to plan incision lengths and location related to breast width and distance of nipple movement

Planning excessive skin removal

Planning excessively high nipple–areola position

Failure to plan specific N:IMF distance preoperatively

Planning techniques that leave excessively large discrepancies between sides of incision closures, necessitating gathering

Planning excessive central skin excision that flattens the breast

Planning excessively short N:IMF distance relative to breast width

Planning technique that excises skin at areolar position prior to closure of skin envelope

Suboptimal or inaccurate preoperative marking

Preoperative marking with patient in any position other than standing

Failure to plan incision lengths and location related to breast width and distance of nipple movement

Setting nipple position only relative to sternal notch to nipple distance

Setting nipple position relative to any single anatomic landmark

Surgeon intraoperative factors

Committing to excision of skin at areola site with initial skin excisions

Failure to remove adequate parenchyma when indicated

Table 20-6. Affinity sets for effects or problems associated with mastopexy augmentation—cont'd

Adding a breast implant at time of mastopexy

Adding a breast implant at any time after mastopexy

Placing excessive tension on any remaining parenchymal components

Increasing weight of the breast with a breast implant

Increasing pressure on envelope and parenchyma with breast implant

Creating excessively short N:IMF distance for breast width

Creating excessively long N:IMF for breast width

Incorporating questionable assumptions

Absorbable sutures effectively suspend or hold weight long-term

Permanent sutures effectively suspend or hold weight long-term

Breast implants are preferably placed at the time of mastopexy

The tighter the inferior pole closure, the greater the longevity of the result

Scars crossing the inframammary fold are preferable to scars placed medially and/or laterally in the IMF

Breast implant factors

Increased implant weight added to breast

Increased pressure on adjacent parenchyma and skin envelope caused by implant

Skin stretch caused by implant

Wound problems postoperatively affinities

Tissue characteristics problems

Genetic tissue characteristics

Age

Preoperative breast size

Width of breast preoperatively

Previous surgery

Previous implant (size)

Smoking history

Weight problems

Amount of parenchyma preoperatively

Amount of parenchyma left intraoperatively

Size of breast implant preoperatively if placed

Size of breast implant intraoperatively if placed

Patient education factors

Inadequate patient education

Failure to sign detailed informed consent documents detailing limitations and risks, documenting patient acceptance

Failure to advise patient preoperatively of possible postoperative wound problems

Table 20-6. Affinity sets for effects or problems associated with mastopexy augmentation—cont'd

Patient physical factors

Excess breast size, weight requested or present preoperatively

Request for implant placed at time of mastopexy

Surgeon preoperative factors

Failure to document breast and tissue measurements preoperatively

Planning excessive skin removal

Planning excessively high nipple–areola position

Failure to plan specific N:IMF distance preoperatively

Planning techniques that leave excessively large discrepancies between sides of incision closures, necessitating gathering

Planning placement of breast implant at time of mastopexy when tissues are mobilized

Planning placement of implant when soft tissue coverage is inadequate

Planning transposition of parenchymal flaps

Planning techniques that leave dead space in the breast

Planning excessively short N:IMF distance relative to breast width

Planning technique that excises skin at areolar position prior to closure of skin envelope

Suboptimal or inaccurate preoperative marking

Preoperative marking with patient in any position other than standing

Planning transposition or relocation of parenchymal flaps

Failure to plan incision lengths and location related to breast width and distance of nipple movement

Surgeon intraoperative factors

Committing to excision of skin at areola site with initial skin excisions

Excessive skin excision, creating tension

Failure to remove adequate parenchyma when indicated

Adding a breast implant at time of mastopexy

Adding a breast implant at any time after mastopexy

Adding an excessively large implant at any time

One layer closure any area

Placing excessive tension on any remaining parenchymal components

Placing excessive pressure on residual parenchymal components by excessively tight closure

Increasing weight of the breast with a breast implant

Increasing pressure on envelope and parenchyma with breast implant

Creating potential strangulation of pedicles with pull through techniques

Using any technique that increases tissue trauma

Creating excessively short N:IMF distance for breast width

Table 20-6. Affinity sets for effects or problems associated with mastopexy augmentation—cont'd

Incorporating questionable assumptions

Absorbable sutures effectively suspend or hold weight long-term

Adding an implant adds upper fullness to the breast long-term

Breast implants are preferably placed at the time of mastopexy

The tighter the inferior pole closure, the greater the longevity of the result

Optimal sutures and closure techniques can overcome scar widening due to excess tension

Optimal sutures and closure techniques can overcome scar widening due to excess weight in the skin envelope

Breast implant factors

Increased implant weight added to breast

Increased pressure on adjacent parenchyma and skin envelope caused by implant

Skin stretch caused by implant

Skin thinning caused by implant

Hematoma

Seroma

Periprosthetic infection

Implant exposure

Implant extrusion

Sensory problems post mastopexy affinities

Tissue characteristics problems

Preoperative breast size

Width of breast preoperatively

Previous surgery

Previous implant (size)

Weight problems

Amount of parenchyma preoperatively

Amount of parenchyma left intraoperatively

Size of breast implant preoperatively if placed

Size of breast implant intraoperatively if placed

Patient education factors

Inadequate patient education

Failure to sign detailed informed consent documents detailing limitations and risks, documenting patient acceptance

Failure to advise patient preoperatively of possible sensory compromise or loss postoperatively

Table 20-6. Affinity sets for effects or problems associated with mastopexy augmentation—cont'd

Patient physical factors

Excess breast size, weight requested or present preoperatively

Request for implant placed at time of mastopexy

Request for implant at any time associated with mastopexy

Surgeon preoperative factors

Planning placement of breast implant at time of mastopexy when tissues are mobilized

Planning excessive mobilization and potential devascularization

Planning transposition of parenchymal flaps

Failure to plan technique that spares sensory innervation

Planning transposition or relocation of parenchymal flaps

Surgeon intraoperative factors

Adding a breast implant at time of mastopexy

Adding a breast implant at any time after mastopexy

Adding an excessively large implant at any time

Increasing weight of the breast with a breast implant

Increasing pressure on envelope and parenchyma with breast implant

Using any technique that traumatizes more normal anatomic components

Incorporating questionable assumptions

Adding an implant adds upper fullness to the breast long term

Breast shaping using parenchymal flaps outweighs potential risks of vascular compromise or fat necrosis

Breast implants are preferably placed at the time of mastopexy

Breast implant factors

Increased implant weight added to breast

Increased pressure on adjacent parenchyma and skin envelope caused by implant

Periprosthetic infection

Sensory compromise from additional surgical trauma associated with creating implant pocket

Sensory compromise from additional stretch on residual innervation from implant

Transferring Affinity Sets to Cause and Effect Diagrams

The cause and effect (C&E or "fishbone') diagram is a tool that is used to explore all the potential or real causes (inputs) that result in a single effect (output)

The cause and effect (C&E or "fishbone') diagram (Figure 20-1) is a tool that is used to explore all the potential or real causes (inputs) that result in a single effect (output). Designed by Kaoru Ishikawa, a process engineering pioneer who introduced these processes in the Kawasaki shipyards, C&E diagrams are used to:

- arrange factors or causes according to their level of importance

- produce a graphic depiction of relationships between factors and causes

- depict a hierarchy of events that lead to an effect or output.

Figure 20.1. Basic cause and effect (C&E) diagram. The term "effect" refers to any untoward event or undesired result from a process; hence the Effect diagrammed to the right in the diagram could be any unplanned or undesired event that could occur following augmentation mastopexy. Causes in the diagram are derived by prioritizing a brainstorming list of factors that might produce an untoward outcome into an affinity group, and then naming the affinity group, with the affinity group name used as a Cause. Subcauses or factors contributing to each Cause are connected by arrows. Throughout the diagram, the more important factors contributing to each Cause or to the Effect are placed to the right, with progressively less important factors placed in sequence to the left.

One of the most effective methods for surgeons to examine existing processes is to create the branches of the cause and effect tree from the titles of the affinity set. Initially, each title of an affinity set is listed in the box at the top of each branch as a "cause" or factor associated with producing an effect. Each item in each affinity set becomes a sub branch attached to the main branch. The sub branches are arranged according to their relationship to other causes and the main cause. The main branches and all sub branches attached to a main branched are arranged in a hierarchy of

One of the most effective methods for surgeons to examine existing processes is to create the branches of the cause and effect tree from the titles of the affinity set

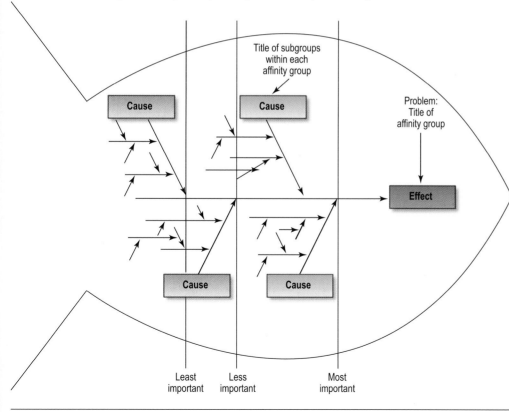

importance with the most likely important cause branch placed closest to the effect (in these illustrations, to the right), and each less important causal branch placed sequentially further from the effect.

Another and often more effective method of illustrating the C&E diagram is to draw the diagram as a tree diagram, with the tree lying on its side and its trunk to the right (Figure 20-2). As the classic fishbone diagram becomes more cluttered, it is difficult to locate and compare items and accurately judge their distance from the effect (hence their level of importance to the effect). With the tree structure, all items on the same causal level are aligned vertically.

Another and often more effective method of illustrating the C&E diagram is to draw the diagram as a tree diagram, with the tree lying on its side and its trunk to the right

Figure 20.2. Hierarchy of branches on a cause and effect diagram depicted as a tree diagram. Transposing a classic C&E diagram to a tree diagram depicted as a tree lying on its side with its trunk to the right more clearly depicts the hierarchy and relationships of causes or factors that contribute to the effect. Causes (blue) that are of equal importance to the Effect (red), are aligned vertically, with other Causes or subcauses (purple, pink) aligned sequentially to the left along the trunk with the least important farthest left.

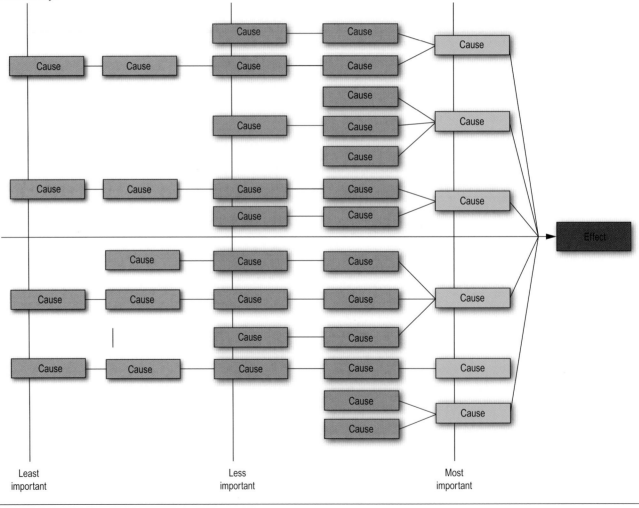

Space limitations preclude including all of the various C&E diagrams for each untoward effect that can occur in mastopexy augmentation. The following C&E diagrams depict cause and effect relationships for scar perceptibility (Figure 20-3) and for nipple–areola deformities (Figure 20-4).

Surgeons who are interested in refining their processes in augmentation mastopexy can transfer the other five affinity groups listed previously in Table 20-6 and transfer them to a C&E diagram, and then derive "solutions" in the form of flowcharted algorithms for each group.

Fault Tree Analysis

Fault tree analysis (FTA) is another method of assessing potential causes of a problem for reliability and safety analysis.[14,15] Developed by Bell Laboratories for the US Air Force Minuteman Project, FTA analysis and similar reliability block diagrams (RBDs) are large block diagrams that graphically depict factors in a system that could lead to failure of the system or occurrence of a single untoward event that represents a failure in the system. Surgeons can access an excellent summary of the principles of reliability analysis and fault tree analysis at http://www.weibull.com/basics/fault-tree/index.htm.[15]

Figure 20-5 is a fault tree analysis diagram that graphically displays factors that contribute to scar widening, scar puckering, or wound dehiscence in mastopexy augmentation. The basic events in this analysis are derived directly from the previously created affinity sets for this topic. Due to space limitations in this book, surgeons who are interested in further analysis can create FTAs for the other six named affinity groups.

> Fault tree analysis provides similar information as a cause and effect diagram, but often provides a different perspective of combinations of factors that cause an untoward event

Fault tree analysis provides similar information as a cause and effect diagram, but often provides a different perspective of combinations of factors that cause an untoward event. By rearranging and prioritizing basic events and using gates to delineate combinations of basic events that are likely to cause the main negative event, surgeons gain a wider perspective of factors that are likely to lead to compromised outcomes. Further, surgeons can graphically see the bigger picture combinations of items that challenge the logic of single stage mastopexy augmentation.

Deriving Flowchart Algorithms for Process Refinement

The next step in the PDCA cycle is *doing*, in which surgeons should define, develop, and implement a "solution" and define measurements to judge its effectiveness. One of the

> One of the most effective methodologies to define and refine a "solution" is to depict the process and all its subprocesses in an algorithmic flowchart

Figure 20.3. Cause and effect diagram for excessive scar perceptibility using affinity set names for primary branches. Hierarchy and prioritization of causes and subcauses to an effect are subjective, and are ideally derived from a workgroup setting in which multiple group members share input.

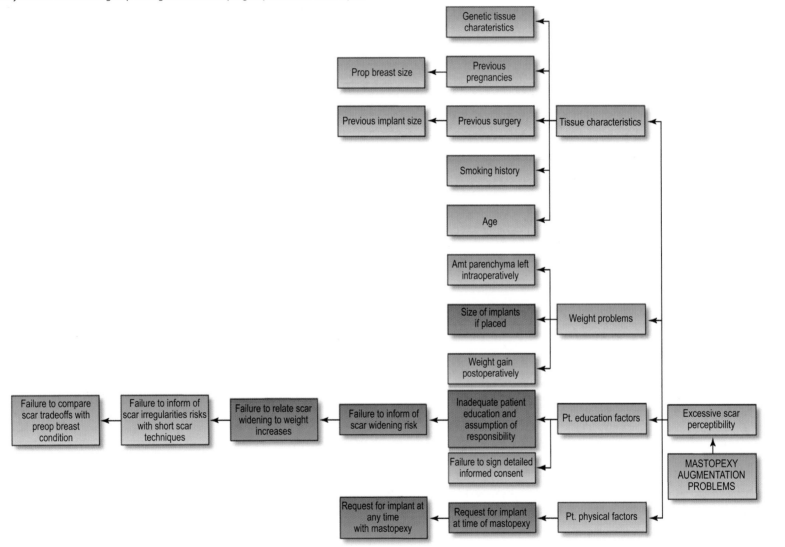

Figure 20.3. *Continued.*

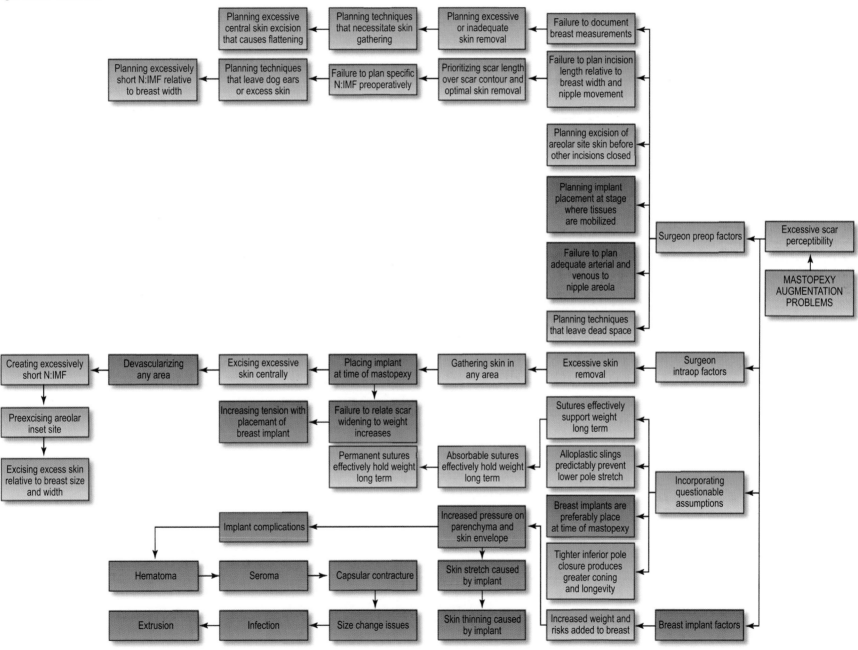

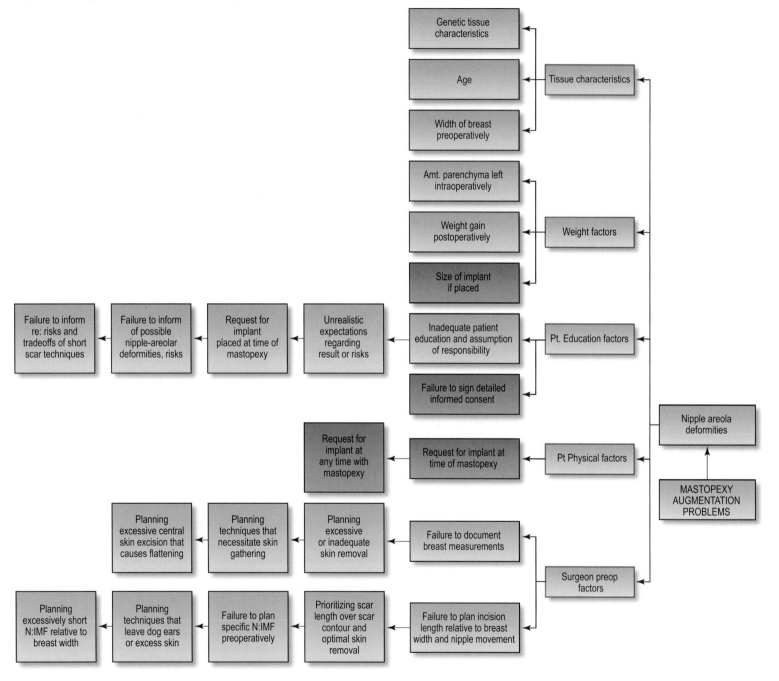

Figure 20.4. Cause and effect diagram for nipple–areola deformities in mastopexy augmentation. The desired effect of this or any other C&E diagram is to stimulate lateral thinking and develop a diagram through brainstorming and discussion from which the group can derive or formulate a solution or solutions to prevent the undesired effect.

Figure 20.4. *Continued.*

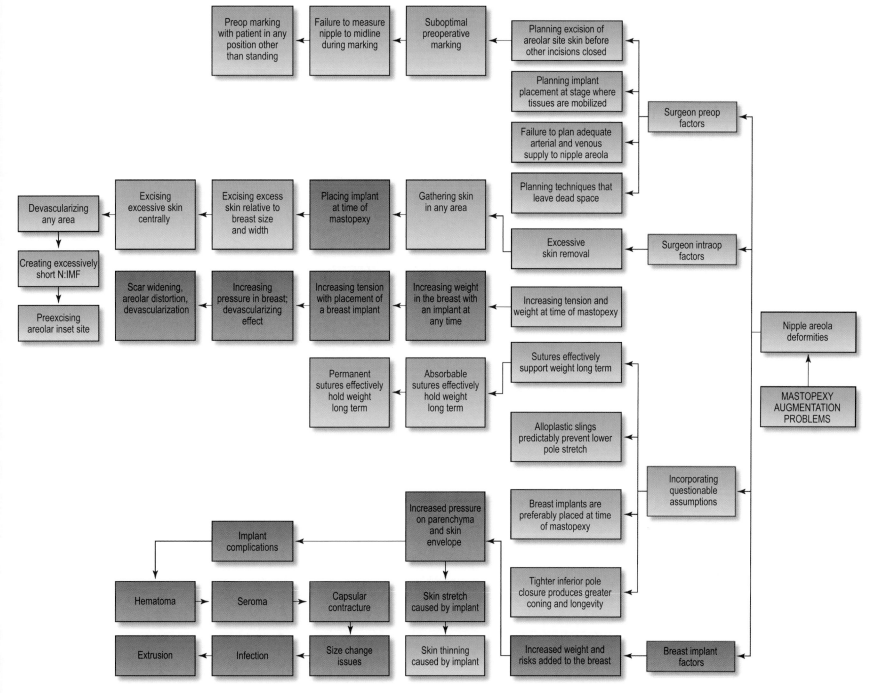

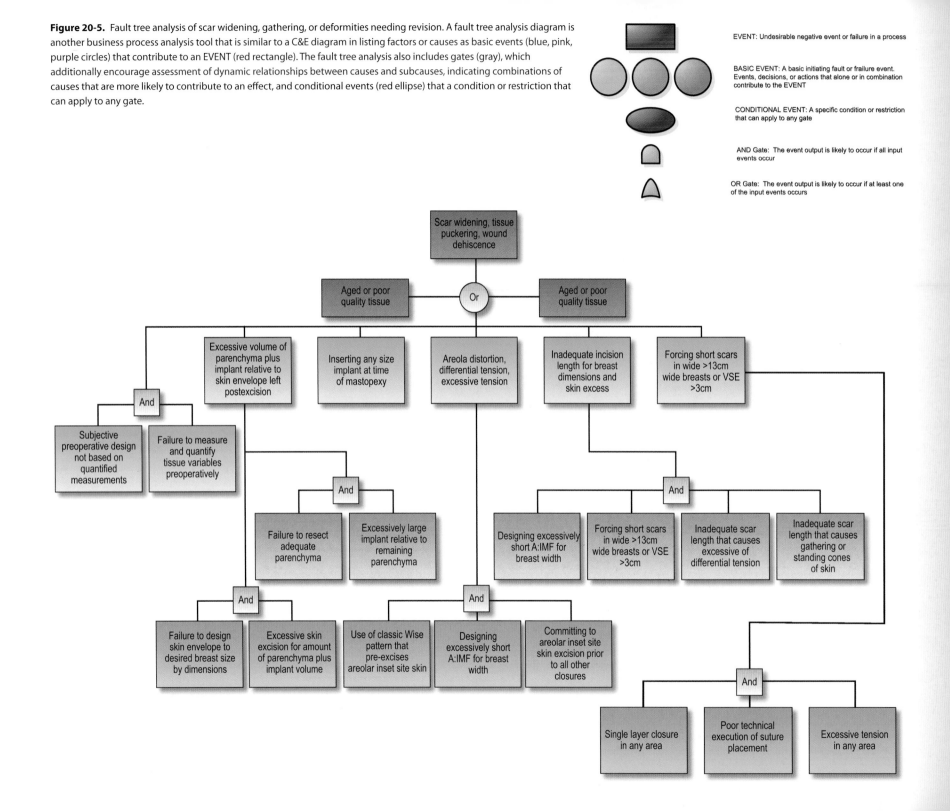

Figure 20-5. Fault tree analysis of scar widening, gathering, or deformities needing revision. A fault tree analysis diagram is another business process analysis tool that is similar to a C&E diagram in listing factors or causes as basic events (blue, pink, purple circles) that contribute to an EVENT (red rectangle). The fault tree analysis also includes gates (gray), which additionally encourage assessment of dynamic relationships between causes and subcauses, indicating combinations of causes that are more likely to contribute to an effect, and conditional events (red ellipse) that a condition or restriction that can apply to any gate.

EVENT: Undesirable negative event or failure in a process

BASIC EVENT: A basic initiating fault or frailure event. Events, decisions, or actions that alone or in combination contribute to the EVENT

CONDITIONAL EVENT: A specific condition or restriction that can apply to any gate

AND Gate: The event output is likely to occur if all input events occur

OR Gate: The event output is likely to occur if at least one of the input events occurs

most effective methodologies to define and refine a "solution" is to depict the process and all its subprocesses in an algorithmic flowchart. Figure 20-6 is an algorithm flowchart derived from the C&E diagrams for excessive scar perceptibility (Figure 20-3) that presents solutions for the most prominent factors in the TQM PDCA analysis that are most likely to positively affect patient outcomes with mastopexy or mastopexy augmentation.

Process analysis tools used in business management and manufacturing are powerful and useful in the surgical environment. Surgical outcomes derive from decision processes and surgical execution. Most surgeons learn decision making processes passively during apprenticeship residency training. Few opportunities currently exist in surgical education venues that focus primarily on process analysis and decision making. As a result, most surgeons make decisions on two basic levels: (1) using a few of the most basic parameters that define indications for an operation, and (2) selecting from a virtual checklist of available surgical techniques.

Rethinking categories of surgical procedures using process analysis tools encourages lateral thinking and new, improved processes to improve patient outcomes, compared to linear thinking and a basic problem–technique process that has not substantially changed patient outcomes in augmentation mastopexy for almost three decades.

■ THE REALITIES OF MASTOPEXY AUGMENTATION

Simultaneous mastopexy and augmentation of the breast is an illogical combination of surgical procedures.

Multiple peer reviewed and published, retrospective, anecdotal series of mastopexy augmentation suggest that one technique or another makes mastopexy augmentation logical and safe. The fact that mastopexy augmentation is responsible for more medical malpractice claims than any other operation in aesthetic surgery proves otherwise, and suggests that the level of predictability and safety with this combination of operations is inversely proportional to the procedure's complication and reoperation rates. Not a single prospective, consecutive series study of mastopexy augmentation exists in the plastic surgery literature that has been supervised by an independent clinical review organization (CRO). Data from FDA PMA studies that include mastopexy augmentation

Simultaneous mastopexy and augmentation of the breast is an illogical combination of surgical procedures

Figure 20-6. Solutions to decrease problems in mastopexy augmentation: an algorithmic flowchart. In a total quality management (TQM) analysis "plan, do, check, act" (PDCA) cycle, having completed C&E analyses, the group then formulates a "solution" derived from the analysis. The solution is translated graphically to an algorithmic flowchart to be disseminated and implemented. In the surgical environment, the C in PDCA for "check" represents scientific studies that test the hypotheses of the solution, and A for "act" are modifications to the process or processes for product (outcome) improvement to the customer (patient).

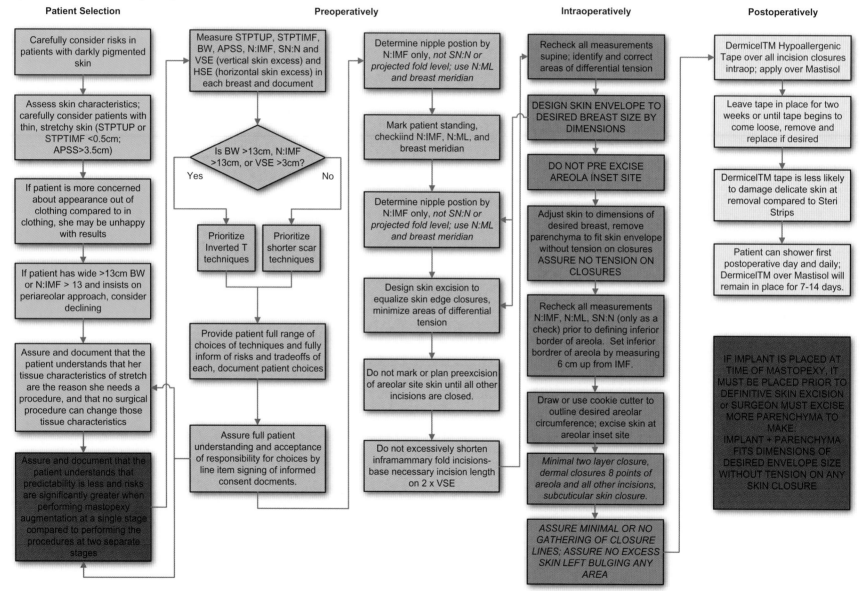

Patient Selection

- Carefully consider risks in patients with darkly pigmented skin
- Assess skin characteristics; carefully consider patients with thin, stretchy skin (STPTUP or STPTIMF <0.5cm; APSS>3.5cm)
- If patient is more concerned about appearance out of clothing compared to in clothing, she may be unhappy with results
- If patient has wide >13cm BW or N:IMF > 13 and insists on periareolar approach, consider declining
- Assure and document that the patient understands that her tissue characteristics of stretch are the reason she needs a procedure, and that no surgical procedure can change those tissue characteristics
- Assure and document that the patient understands that predictability is less and risks are significantly greater when performing mastopexy augmentation at a single stage compared to performing the procedures at two separate stages

Preoperatively

- Measure STPTUP, STPTIMF, BW, APSS, N:IMF, SN:N and VSE (vertical skin excess) and HSE (horizontal skin excess) in each breast and document
- Is BW >13cm, N:IMF >13cm, or VSE >3cm?
  - Yes → Prioritize Inverted T techniques
  - No → Prioritize shorter scar techniques
- Provide patient full range of choices of techniques and fully inform of risks and tradeoffs of each, document patient choices
- Assure full patient understanding and acceptance of responsibility for choices by line item signing of informed consent docments.

- Determine nipple postion by N:IMF only, *not SN:N or projected fold level; use N:ML and breast meridian*
- Mark patient standing, checkiind N:IMF, N:ML, and breast meridian
- Determine nipple postion by N:IMF only, *not SN:N or projected fold level; use N:ML and breast meridian*
- Design skin excision to equalize skin edge closures, minimize areas of differential tension
- Do not mark or plan preexcision of areolar site skin until all other incisions are closed.
- Do not excessively shorten inframammary fold incisions- base necessary incision length on 2 x VSE

Intraoperatively

- Recheck all measurements supine; identify and correct areas of differential tension
- DESIGN SKIN ENVELOPE TO DESIRED BREAST SIZE BY DIMENSIONS
- DO NOT PRE EXCISE AREOLA INSET SITE
- Adjust skin to dimensions of desired breast, remove parenchyma to fit skin envelope without tension on closures ASSURE NO TENSION ON CLOSURES
- Recheck all measurements N:IMF, N:ML, SN:N (only as a check) prior to defining inferior border of areola. Set inferior bordrer of areola by measuring 6 cm up from IMF.
- Draw or use cookie cutter to outline desired areolar circumference; excise skin at areolar inset site
- *Minimal two layer closure, dermal closures 8 points of areola and all other incisions, subcuticular skin closure.*
- *ASSURE MINIMAL OR NO GATHERING OF CLOSURE LINES; ASSURE NO EXCESS SKIN LEFT BULGING ANY AREA*

Postoperatively

- DermicelTM Hypoallergenic Tape over all incision closures intraop; apply over Mastisol
- Leave tape in place for two weeks or until tape begins to come loose, remove and replace if desired
- DermicelTM tape is less likely to damage delicate skin at removal compared to Steri Strips
- Patient can shower first postoperative day and daily; DermicelTM over Mastisol will remain in place for 7-14 days.

- IF IMPLANT IS PLACED AT TIME OF MASTOPEXY, IT MUST BE PLACED PRIOR TO DEFINITIVE SKIN EXCISION or SURGEON MUST EXCISE MORE PARENCHYMA TO MAKE: IMPLANT + PARENCHYMA FITS DIMENSIONS OF DESIRED ENVELOPE SIZE WITHOUT TENSION ON ANY SKIN CLOSURE

have never been published with the mastopexy augmentation data filtered and presented separately from augmentation data alone.

Despite the numerous publications and podium time committed to augmentation mastopexy in professional venues, an unbiased observer might logically question the following:

1. In the history of plastic surgery, why have surgeons apparently never learned to perform this combination of operations with a high degree of safety and predictability?

2. Is the combination of operations inherently safe, but the majority of surgeons simply cannot deliver predictable results with low complication rates?

3. Are low predictability and high complication and reoperation rates with mastopexy augmentation the result of surgeons' and patients' priorities and decision processes promoting an illogical combination of operations in a single stage procedure?

While facts strongly and directly challenge the safety and predictability of mastopexy augmentation for patients, surgeons continue to perform the operations simultaneously in record numbers. The obvious question is why and the obvious answers are economic. The answers are simple and straightforward. Patient demand exists for lifting and filling ptotic breasts. No patient wants two surgical procedures with increased costs if they believe they can safely achieve the same results with one operation. Surgeons who refuse to perform mastopexy and augmentation simultaneously will unquestionably lose patients and revenues to surgeons who are willing to perform the operations simultaneously. Demand, supply, and patient and surgeon priorities have kept mastopexy augmentation alive and well, despite all the evidence that alternatives might be safer and better for the patient.

> While facts strongly and directly challenge the safety and predictability of mastopexy augmentation for patients, surgeons continue to perform the operations simultaneously in record numbers. The obvious question is why and the obvious answers are economic

■ COMPARING A TWO STAGE TO A ONE STAGE MASTOPEXY AND AUGMENTATION

The following are logical and factual observations. With a two stage procedure, performing mastopexy first, and breast augmentation 6 months later:

1. The surgeon does not perform simultaneous operations with directly contradictory objectives.

2. The surgeon isolates the risks of mastopexy and breast augmentation for the patient instead of exponentially combining the risks.

3. Risks of wound complications are minimized by avoiding placement of a breast implant that inevitably increases pressure and tension on all incision lines.

4. Risks of compromised scar results are minimized by not placing a breast implant that inevitably increases pressure and tension on all incision lines. The patient is allowed to assess what the best possible scar results can be with mastopexy alone without the tension and pressure factors inherent to a simultaneous breast augmentation.

5. The surgeon minimizes risks of denervation by minimizing the extent of tissue dissection at the same time as inevitably devascularizing and denervating tissues to accomplish parenchymal mass repositioning and nipple–areola repositioning with mastopexy.

6. The surgeon allows incision lines to heal optimally without tension, minimizing scar widening and wound dehiscence risks.

7. The surgeon minimizes areas of devascularization at a single procedure, allowing revascularization following mastopexy before introducing the pocket dissection and tension devascularizing effects of a breast implant.

8. The surgeon allows tissues to heal and stretch following mastopexy alone, allowing (a) objective measurement assessment of the degree to which the tissues restretch following mastopexy without addition of weight and pressure to the breast, and (b) allows the patient to assess the benefits of mastopexy alone without the additional risks and tradeoffs of a breast implant.

9. The surgeon does not assume unnecessary risks of a patient not understanding and accepting responsibility for the potential consequences of a simultaneous mastopexy and breast augmentation. If tissues stretch excessively (N:IMF increase >20%) within 6 months following mastopexy, the surgeon has the opportunity to further inform the patient of additional risks of augmentation and decline operating on patients who ask the surgeon to assume illogical risks.

10. A staged augmentation, especially inframammary or dual plane or retropectoral, allows the surgeon to isolate areas of breast dissection to those that are exactly required to accommodate the implant, eliminating unnecessary devascularization and denervation, and minimizing exposure of the implant to bacteria in the breast.

11. At the time of breast augmentation 6 months following mastopexy, surgeons can adjust the many factors associated with mastopexy design or healing that leave a less than optimal result, improving the final outcome.

12. The surgeon makes a logical case to the patient, based on known risk factors and logical analyses of a combined versus staged procedures.

The bottom line is clear. Facts demonstrate a 12 to 1 logical case for staged mastopexy and augmentation, with the 1 being the economic benefit to the patient of a single stage procedure. Surgeons and patients can choose, but surgeons are ultimately responsible for educating patients and for assuring that patients assume responsibility for their choices.

> Facts demonstrate a 12 to 1 logical case for staged mastopexy and augmentation, with the 1 being the economic benefit to the patient of a single stage procedure

■ CONCLUDING THOUGHTS AND RECOMMENDATIONS

Figure 20-6 summarizes the factors that challenge the logic of single stage mastopexy augmentation.

The combination of mastopexy and augmentation at a single stage procedure is illogical from a scientific or process engineering analysis perspective. Mastopexy and breast augmentation have directly contradictory goals and objectives that no surgical procedure can change.

Excluding minor nipple or areola procedures and minor skin excisions that surgeons continue to term "mastopexy", combining a true mastopexy (criteria outlined earlier in this chapter) with a breast augmentation is not in the patient's best interests, if outcomes and minimal complications are priorities. Patient requests and economic incentives for surgeons have established an unenviable track record for mastopexy augmentation for decades.

To prioritize the patient and optimize patient outcomes, surgeons must assure the most thorough patient education and informed consent. Patients must be aware and acknowledge preoperatively in informed consent documents that if economic or other considerations prompt them or their surgeon to combine mastopexy and augmentation, they are choosing to inevitably increase risks that can produce irreversible tissue compromises and uncorrectable deformities.

> The combination of mastopexy and augmentation at a single stage procedure is illogical from a scientific or process engineering analysis perspective

Mastopexy at a single stage eliminates at least seven major categories of tradeoffs and risks associated with breast augmentation. Additionally, staged mastopexy eliminates an increase in 11 other mastopexy risks caused by simultaneous breast augmentation. Staging the operations isolates risk factors to those routinely associated with either procedure performed as a primary operation.

The immediate solution to decreasing risks, improving patient outcomes in mastopexy augmentation, and decreasing malpractice liability is straightforward: stage the mastopexy and augmentation, always performing the mastopexy first, with an interim delay of 6 months. Measure and document nipple-to-inframammary fold distance measured under maximal stretch at the time of surgery. Six months later, perform the same measurement again. If $N:IMF_{max\ stretch}$ has increased 20% or more in the first 6 months postoperatively, *do not place an implant in a breast that has unequivocally proved that its tissues do not support even the weight of the existing parenchyma.*

> The immediate solution to decreasing risks, improving patient outcomes in mastopexy augmentation, and decreasing malpractice liability is straightforward: stage the mastopexy and augmentation, always performing the mastopexy first, with an interim delay of 6 months

The decrease in risks and potential long-term costs more than offsets any additional incremental costs to the patient of staging mastopexy and augmentation. Staged mastopexy and augmentation are unquestionably more predictable and safer for patients compared to simultaneous mastopexy augmentation.

> The decrease in risks and potential long-term costs more than offsets any additional incremental costs to the patient of staging mastopexy and augmentation

Mastopexy augmentation at one stage is an illogical combination of operations that is not in the best interests of patients. In this context, mastopexy is defined as an operation that removes more than 3 cm of vertical and horizontal skin excess, and repositions the nipple more than 2 cm. When untoward outcomes occur following single stage mastopexy augmentation, the burden of proof to justify compromised outcomes to patients and plaintiff attorneys rests with the surgeon.

■ REFERENCES

1. Regnault P: Breast ptosis. Definition and treatment. *Clin Plast Surg* 3(2):193–203, 1976.

2. Pub Med abstract: http://www.ncbi.nlm.nih.gov/sites/entrez?db=pubmed&uid=1261176&cmd=showdetailview&indexed=google.

3. Medline Plus Medical Dictionary. http://www2.merriam-webster.com/cgi-bin/mwmednlm?book=Medical&va=breast+lift.

4. Tebbetts JB: A system for breast implant selection based on patient tissue characteristics and implant–soft tissue dynamics. Plast Reconstr Surg 109(4):1396–1409, 2002.

5. Tebbetts JB, Adams WP: Five critical decisions in breast augmentation using 5 measurements in 5 minutes: the high five system. *Plast Reconstr Surg* 116(7):2005–2016, 2005.

6. Tebbetts JB: Achieving a zero percent reoperation rate at 3 years in a 50 consecutive case augmentation mammaplasty PMA study. *Plast Reconstr Surg* 118(6):1453–1457, 2006.

7. Tebbetts JB: Patient acceptance of adequately filled breast implants using the tilt test. *Plast Reconstr Surg* 106(1):139–147, 2000.

8. Tebbetts JB: Dual plane (DP) breast augmentation: optimizing implant–soft tissue relationships in a wide range of breast types. *Plast Reconstr Surg* 107:1255, 2001.

9. Tebbetts JB: Achieving a predictable 24-hour return to normal activities after breast augmentation Part I: Refining practices using motion and time study principles. *Plast Reconstr Surg* 109:273–290, 2002.

10. Tebbetts JB: Achieving a predictable 24-hour return to normal activities after breast augmentation Part II: Patient preparation, refined surgical techniques and instrumentation *Plast Reconstr Surg* 109:293–305, 2002.

11. Spear SL, Giese SY: Simultaneous breast augmentation and mastopexy. *Aesthetic Surg J* 20:155, 2002.

12. Spear SL: Augmentation/mastopexy: surgeon beware. *Plast Reconstr Surg* 112:905, 2003.

13. Handel N: Secondary mastopexy in the augmented patient: a recipe for disaster. *Plast Reconstr Surg* 118(7S):52S–163S, 2006.

14. US Nuclear Regulatory Commission. Fault tree handbook. US Nuclear Regulatory Commission, Washington, DC, 1981. Online. Available: http://www.nrc.gov/reading-rm/doc-collections/nuregs/staff/sr0492/sr0492.pdf.

15. Weibull.com. Fault trees and reliability block diagrams. Weibull.com Team, Tucson, AZ. Online. Available: http://www.weibull.com/basics/fault-tree/index.htm.

Applying Proved Processes: Clinical Case Studies

■ INTRODUCTION AND BACKGROUND

Patient outcomes and the patient experience ultimately determine the quality, efficacy, and safety of all surgical processes. Historically, most peer reviewed and published articles, book chapters and books on breast augmentation have focused on surgical techniques. Validation usually consists of a small number of short-term, selected case results photographs, with even further selected views of each patient. Surgeon education and professional presentations have allowed and promoted similar practices that encourage subjectivity and opinion over quantifiable data and scientifically valid conclusions. The result for patients has been an unenviable track record over the past three decades according to FDA premarket approval (PMA) data from independently supervised studies. Reoperation rates of 15–20% or more in just 3 years following augmentation remain unchanged over three decades according to data from the latest PMA studies,[1] and a majority of breast augmentation patients continue to experience unnecessarily prolonged recovery times.

History indicates that improvement in patient recovery, the patient experience, reoperation rates, and long-term patient outcomes do not result from surgeons' viewing and discussing case results photographs. As the case studies in this chapter demonstrate, visual assessment of images can be very misleading without accompanying objective clinical measurements. Photographs are not the best measure of quality of surgery that determines the patient experience and patient outcomes. The best quality photographs do not provide objective data that are critical to scientifically evaluate the processes that determine patient outcomes. Photographs invariably encourage surgeon subjectivity and opinion based premises in lieu of objective, science based conclusions. Surgeons cannot evaluate critical processes in surgeon education, informed consent, tissue assessment, implant selection, and decision processes from any photograph.

If photographs have any scientific validity, the photographs must be directly linked to objective data from prospectively designed studies in consecutive case series.

Photographic views must be standardized and show at least five views of the patient. Ideally, the objective data and data collection from prospective, consecutive series studies should be supervised by an independent clinical review organization (CRO). If these criteria are satisfied, surgeons can begin to scientifically interpret photographic documentation of results instead of continuing to promote subjective opinions.

No professional journal or book has ever published a large number of cases from a consecutive series of breast augmentation photographic results from a study that was independently supervised and monitored by a CRO. More importantly, no publication has ever offered surgeons the opportunity to correlate photographic results with sequential, objective tissue measurements. In the December 2006 issue of *Plastic and Reconstructive Surgery Journal*, the author published a prospective, consecutive series of his first 50 cases from the FDA PMA study for the Allergan Style 410 anatomic, form stable, cohesive silicone gel implant.[2] This study focused on the processes that enabled a zero percent reoperation rate at 3 years' followup in the series.

The photographs of case results that follow in this chapter are cases from this unique series of 50 consecutive patients with up to 7 year followup. At each followup interval, measurements are listed that correlate with the critical tissue assessment measurements from the TEPID[TM,3] and High Five[TM,4] systems. Followup intervals vary by patient, and are listed with each series of images. Five views of each patient at each followup interval are presented to preclude any selection bias. Squeeze and supine views of patients were taken at 1 year followup.

Surgeons are familiar with various categories of breast types that are in common use, including, for example, "tight envelope", "loose envelope", glandular ptotic, pseudoptotic, constricted lower pole, and other categories. Each of these categories has been traditionally based on subjective or visual parameters instead of objective, quantifiable measurements. This series of cases, combined with future studies that collect objective tissue measurement data, provide surgeons with a unique opportunity to more accurately and scientifically categorize breast types and correlate process outcomes with quantifiable tissue characteristics.

■ PRINCIPLES AND GROUND RULES APPLIED IN CASE STUDIES

Readers can use the case studies in this chapter in many different ways. The most superficial and least productive use of these case studies is a cursory pictorial review of results accompanied by a completely subjective assessment of the visual results. A more constructive, educational, and productive process is to study each case individually and in depth after reading Chapters 2–8.

Every patient in these case studies was a participant in the Allergan FDA PMA study for the Allergan Style 410, textured, anatomic, form stable, cohesive silicone gel filled implant. Each patient received comprehensive information on all available implant types with accompanying manufacturer and scientific data about each type, following the patient educational processes detailed in our earlier publications.[2-4]

The following principles are applied to the cases presented in this chapter:

1. All patient case studies are from a 50 consecutive case series with a zero percent reoperation rate at 3 years' followup in an FDA PMA study supervised by an independent CRO.

2. No patient in the case studies or in the series developed a Class 3 or 4 capsular contracture at 3 years' followup.

3. No patient in the series had a failed implant device or any other device related sequelae that required reoperation.

4. All patients in the series completed all records for the PMA study during their period of followup, and completed additional breast measurements and patient satisfaction studies developed by the author.

5. All 50 patients resumed full normal activity within 24 hours postoperatively. More than 80% of patients were able to go out to dinner the evening of surgery.

6. Interval High Five™ measurements are located to the left of five view photographs at each indicated followup interval.

7. Visual impressions from preoperative and intraoperative photographs are subjective and relatively meaningless unless and until the visual observations are confirmed by and correlated with objective, quantifiable, clinical measurements.

8. As explained in detail in Chapter 7 and again in this chapter, no surgeon can ever make breasts exactly symmetrical. Attempting to place more volume in the smaller breast to make sizes similar is a common error. The smaller breast has a smaller skin envelope. When the smaller envelope is full, it is full, and attempting to put more volume in that breast must result in more bulging superiorly and/or laterally. This creates a shape difference in most patients that is much more apparent compared to a size difference that every woman already has and that the eye is accustomed to seeing. The author required more than 15 years to learn and follow this concept.

9. Prioritizing soft tissue coverage using the High Five™ System criteria for pocket location and the form stable Allergan Style 410 FM implant, no patient at any duration of followup up to 7 years developed any visible rippling or visible implant edges in any location.

10. Surgeons and patients categorically cannot accurately judge breast implant size in a patient from any photograph or combinations of photographs. Photographs, therefore, are not an accurate or valid tool for preoperatively choosing breast implant size, and should never be used for this purpose without the patient receiving the above information and signing appropriate informed consent documents and disclaimers.

11. Full height, form stable, silicone gel implants offer more control of appropriate upper breast fill. For this reason, upper pole shape is maintained longer and more predictably in these long term results and in many cases, maintenance of appropriate upper fill makes the breast appear larger with smaller form stable Style 410 implants compared to implants that collapse in the upper pole.

12. The longer the preoperative N:IMF, the more percent stretch is likely to occur in the lower pole skin in most patients, because implant weight is acting on a much larger surface area of lower pole envelope.

13. Only criteria and data pertinent to the most critical decisions in breast augmentation defined by the High Five™ processes are included.

14. Preoperative measurements are presented on the case description and planning page for each case. Each pertinent measurement is recorded in the appropriate cell of the High Five™ decision and operative planning form.

15. Patient height and weight are not included because all decisions are tissue based and breast size and shape are determined by the quantified measurements that indicate the amount and characteristics of the patient's tissues that define requirements and limits for optimal aesthetic results[3,4] and unparalleled patient outcomes and reoperation rates.[2] Regardless of a patient's height, torso width, or weight, the existing dimensions and characteristics of the breast skin envelope parenchyma define safe limits of breast augmentation without irreversible compromises, and define parameters for an optimal aesthetic result.

16. When the patient's *wishes* exceed the limits of the patient's *tissues* (defined by peer reviewed and published data for the lowest complication and reoperation rates[2-8]), surgeons must reconcile the two in the "patient request" line of the High Five™ form, and assure that patients are completely informed of possible irreversible tissue compromises that can result from excessively large or

excessively projecting implants. Further, the surgeon is responsible for documenting the patient's accepting responsibility for her requests or choices in written and signed informed consent documents.

17. All preoperative and postoperative measurements of nipple-to-inframammary fold distance (N:IMF) are *always measured with the skin under maximal stretch.*

18. Every breast has an "ideal" height that is relative to breast width, for optimal aesthetic results. The full height, moderate projection Style 410 FM is designed with a height that is proportionate to each width of the implant.

19. The concept that the vertical height of an implant should be shorter for patients with shorter sternal notch to nipple measurements, regardless of the arbitrary numbers associated with SN:N, is a faulty concept. More than a decade ago, the author subscribed to using reduced height implants when SN:N was less than 18 cm. Patients with reduced height implants ultimately lose upper breast fill more rapidly compared to patients with full, height, form stable implants, *provided the full height implant volume is determined by the High Five™ System, and provided the surgeon appropriately sets the nipple-to-inframammary fold distance intraoperatively according to the High Five™ System.*

20. A reduced height implant is any implant that is not taller than it is wide, whether a form stable implant designed with those parameters or any type of saline or silicone filled, conventional implant that collapses vertically due to inadequate fill relative to mandrel volume (fails to pass the tilt test outside the body).

21. Breasts never match in any woman, and no surgeon can ever make them match. Symmetry does not exist, and every patient in this series was thoroughly informed of conditions in each case that surgery would not correct (see Chapters 3 and 5, and review the informed consent document entitled "Patient Images Analysis" that patient and surgeon complete while looking at an AP image of the patient's breasts).

22. Although surgeons can implant the Style 410 implant through inframammary, periareolar, and axillary incisions, all patients in this series selected the inframammary incision approach. No patient in the series had any complaint regarding scar quality or visibility, no patient had any scar revision procedure, and hypoallergenic tape over the incision line for 2 weeks postoperatively was the only treatment of any incision line.

23. Supine views of patients taken at approximately 1 year postoperatively demonstrate compressibility, softness of breasts, and natural mobility and appearance supine, dispelling misconceptions that this form stable implant is too firm and does not move normally.

Legend for Case Studies Abbreviations

When measurements vary on the two sides they are listed as XX (right)/XX (left)

NA—Not applicable

WNBCS—will not be corrected surgically

Categories of Breast Conditions included in Case Studies

Breast size asymmetry: WNBCS

Breast level asymmetry: WNBCS

Nipple level asymmetry: WNBCS

Breast width asymmetry: WNBCS

Tight skin envelope

Thin soft tissue coverage

Breasts high on torso (short SN:N): WNBCS

Nipples located laterally on breast mound: WNBCS

Wide intermammary distance: WNBCS

Breasts low on torso: WNBCS

Breasts high on torso: WNBCS

Relative constriction or inadequate expansion of breast lower pole

Downpointing nipples

Glandular ptosis

Narrow base width breast

▥ SUMMARY OF OBSERVATIONS FROM CASE STUDIES

- Following the proved, scientifically verified processes in the High Five™ System resulted in a zero percent reoperation rate at 3 years in an FDA PMA study for the first time in history.

- All patients experienced return to full, normal activities within 24 hours of their augmentation, and 80% were able to go out to dinner the evening of their surgery.

- The aesthetic results in this series viewed in five views for up to 7 years demonstrates a consistency of results and maintenance of shape and upper pole fill that has never been demonstrated in a comparable series in the literature or in any plastic surgery book.

- The Allergan Style 410, textured anatomic, form stable, cohesive silicone gel implant, especially the Style 410 FM, demonstrates that a single, optimal implant design delivers the most long-term consistency in breast shape and control of fill published to date.

- The squeeze, displacement, and supine views of results at 1 year followup demonstrate that this form stable implant is highly compressible, displaces and moves normally, and has as normal appearance with the patient supine as any breast implant product, provided surgeons apply the processes and guidelines of the High Five™ System when using the device.

- The consistency of aesthetic results demonstrated in this patient series is currently unparalleled in plastic surgery professional publications. This series demonstrates that proved processes that produce optimal patient outcomes and low reoperation rates also produce the most consistent, predictable, and long-term aesthetic results.

■ REFERENCES

1. U.S. Food and Drug Administration. Product labeling data for Mentor and Allergan/Inamed core studies of saline implants. Online. Available: http://www.fda.gov/cdrh/breastimplants/labeling/mentor_patient_labeling_5900.html.

2. Tebbetts JB: Achieving a zero percent reoperation rate at 3 years in a 50 consecutive case augmentation mammaplasty PMA study. *Plast Reconstr Surg* 118(6):1453–1457, 2006.

3. Tebbetts JB: A system for breast implant selection based on patient tissue characteristics and implant–soft tissue dynamics. *Plast Reconstr Surg* 109(4):1396–1409, 2002.

4. Tebbetts JB, Adams WP: Five critical decisions in breast augmentation using 5 measurements in 5 minutes: the high five system. *Plast Reconstr Surg* 116(7):2005–2016, 2005.

5. Tebbetts JB: Patient acceptance of adequately filled breast implants using the tilt test. *Plast Reconstr Surg* 106(1):139–147, 2000.

6. Tebbetts JB: Dual plane (DP) breast augmentation: optimizing implant–soft tissue relationships in a wide range of breast types. *Plast Reconstr Surg* 107:1255, 2001.

7. Tebbetts JB: Achieving a predictable 24-hour return to normal activities after breast augmentation Part I: Refining practices using motion and time study principles. *Plast Reconstr Surg* 109:273–290, 2002.

8. Tebbetts JB: Achieving a predictable 24-hour return to normal activities after breast augmentation Part II: Patient preparation, refined surgical techniques and instrumentation *Plast Reconstr Surg* 109:293–305, 2002.

CASE STUDY 21-1

HISTORY

Age: 45
Gravida: 1
Para: 1
Bra **Band** Size: 32
Breast **Cup** Size (Pt. estimate.)
  Prior to pregnancy: A
  Largest with preg: B/C
  Current Cup Size: A
  Desired Cup Size: B/C
Previous Breast Disease: None
Breast Biopsies: None
Family Hx. Breast Cancer: Yes
  (Maternal grandmother,
  postmenopausal)
Pertinent Medical or Breast
  Imaging History: None
Breast Masses: **None**

TISSUE ASSESSMENT AND HIGH FIVE™ SYSTEM CRITICAL DECISIONS PROCESS

Prioritized Decisions Based on Breast Measurements and Tissue Characteristics
The High Five™ System   Copyright 2005   John B. Tebbetts, M.D.

I. POCKET LOCATION SELECTED BASED ON THICKNESS OF TISSUE COVERAGE (Circle One)			
STPTUP	0.8	If <2.0 cm, consider dual plane (DP) or partial retropectoral (PRP, pectoralis origins intact across IMF)	DP 1
STPTIMF	0.6	If STPTIMF <0.5 cm, consider subpectoral pocket and leave pectoralis origins intact along IMF	PRP RM

II. IMPLANT VOLUME/WEIGHT BASED ON BREAST DIMENSIONS, TISSUE STRETCH, AND EXISTING PARENCHYMA

Base Width	11.0	B.W. Parenchyma (cm)	10.5	11.0	11.5	12.0	12.5	13.0	13.5	14.0	14.5	15.0	
		Initial Volume (cc)	200	250	275	300	300	325	350	375	375	400	250 cc
APSS$_{MaxStr}$	2.2	[2]If APSS <2.0, −30 cc; If APSS >3.0, +30 cc; If APSS >4.0, +60 cc Place appropriate number in blank at right											NA
N:IMF$_{MaxSt}$	5.5	If N:IMF >9.5, +30 cc Place appropriate number in blank at right											NA
PCSEF %	70	If PCSEF <20%, +30 cc; If PCSEF >80%, −30 cc Place appropriate number in blank at right											NA
IDFDD cc	NA	If Allergan Style 468, or other form stable saline implant, −30 cc Place appropriate number in blank at right											NA
Pt. request													NA

NET ESTIMATED VOLUME TO FILL ENVELOPE BASED ON PATIENT TISSUE CHARACTERISTICS			250 cc
III. IMPLANT TYPE MFR: Allergan	STYLE/MODEL: Style 410 FM	VOLUME: 235 gm	235 gm

Volume: N:IMF Relationships: Locate final selected implant volume at right; Set N:IMF to the distance shown in the cell beneath, or leave at preop N:IMF, whichever is longer.	200	250	275	300	325	350	375	400	PreN:IMF 5.5 cm
	7.0	7.0	7.5	8	8	8.5	9.0	9.5	

IV. NEW INFRAMAMMARY FOLD LEVEL	N:IMF$_{MaxSt}$ to set with preoperative markings and intraoperatively	7.0 cm
V. INCISION LOCATION	IM AX PA UMB	

PREOPERATIVE ASSESSMENT AND OBSERVATIONS

Breast level asymmetry: Breasts at different levels on torso; left breast and
  nipple higher on torso, WNBCS
Nipple level asymmetry: WNBCS
Breast width asymmetry: Left breast narrower, WNBCS
Tight skin envelope: APSS 2.2
Envelope filled by parenchyma preoperatively: PCSEF 70%
Thin soft tissue coverage: STPTUP 0.8 cm; STPTIMF 0.6 cm

POSTOPERATIVE ASSESSMENT AND OBSERVATIONS

Pre- to post- bra size change by patient questionnaire: 34A to 36C

Slight excess volume fill (excessively large implant for tissue characteristics) for envelope size and stretch at 1 year, persisting to more than 2 years, slight excessive upper pole fullness

Upper pole fill and shape maintained to 6 years

Breast and nipple level asymmetry: WNBCS as predicted

IMF scar redness present at 7 months followup; resolved

Breasts soft, mobile, compressible at 7 months followup

Interval: Preop STPTUP 0.8 cm STPTIMF 0.6 cm Base Width 11 cm APSS 2.2 cm N:IMF 5.5 cm PCSEF 70%				
Interval: 1 yr STPTUP 1.6 cm STPTIMF 1.2 cm Base Width 12.5 cm APSS 1.9 cm N:IMF 8.5 cm				
Interval: 2 yr STPTUP 1.7 cm STPTIMF 1.4 cm Base Width 12.5 cm APSS 2.0 cm N:IMF 8.5 cm				
Interval: 5 yr STPTUP 1.6 cm STPTIMF 1.3 cm Base Width 12 .5 cm APSS 2.0 cm N:IMF 8.5 cm				
Interval: 6 yr STPTUP 1.7 cm STPTIMF 1.2 cm Base Width 12.5 cm APSS 2.4 cm N:IMF 8.5 cm				
Interval: 1 yr STPTUP 1.6 cm STPTIMF 1.2 cm Base Width 12.5 cm APSS 1.9 cm N:IMF 8.5 cm				

CASE STUDY 21-2

HISTORY

Age: 38
Gravida: 1
Para: 0
Bra **Band** Size: 36
Breast **Cup** Size (Pt. estimate)
  Prior to pregnancy: B
  Largest with preg: C
  Current Cup Size: B
  Desired Cup Size: C
Previous Breast Disease: None
Breast Biopsies: No
Family Hx. Breast Cancer: No
Pertinent Medical or Breast
  Imaging History: None
Breast Masses: **None**

TISSUE ASSESSMENT AND HIGH FIVE™ SYSTEM CRITICAL DECISIONS PROCESS

Prioritized Decisions Based on Breast Measurements and Tissue Characteristics
The High Five™ System   Copyright 2005   John B. Tebbetts, M.D.

I. POCKET LOCATION SELECTED BASED ON THICKNESS OF TISSUE COVERAGE (Circle One)			
STPTUP	1.3	If <2.0 cm, consider dual plane (DP) or partial retropectoral (PRP, pectoralis origins intact across IMF)	DP 1
STPTIMF	1.0	If STPTIMF <0.5 cm, consider subpectoral pocket and leave pectoralis origins intact along IMF	PRP RM

II. IMPLANT VOLUME/WEIGHT BASED ON BREAST DIMENSIONS, TISSUE STRETCH, AND EXISTING PARENCHYMA

Base Width	12.5	B.W. Parenchyma (cm)	10.5	11.0	11.5	12.0	12.5	13.0	13.5	14.0	14.5	15.0	
		Initial Volume (cc)	200	250	275	300	300	325	350	375	375	400	
APSS$_{MaxStr}$	3.0	[2]If APSS <2.0, −30 cc; If APSS >3.0, +30 cc; If APSS >4.0, +60 cc Place appropriate number in blank at right											300 cc
N:IMF$_{MaxSt}$	7.0	If N:IMF >9.5, +30 cc Place appropriate number in blank at right											+30 cc
PCSEF %	70	If PCSEF <20%, +30 cc; If PCSEF >80%, −30 cc Place appropriate number in blank at right											NA
IDFDD cc	NA	If Allergan Style 468 or other form stable saline implant, −30 cc Place appropriate number in blank at right											NA
Pt. request	NA												NA

NET ESTIMATED VOLUME TO FILL ENVELOPE BASED ON PATIENT TISSUE CHARACTERISTICS	330 cc
III. IMPLANT TYPE MFR: Allergan STYLE/MODEL: Style 410 FM VOLUME: 310 gm	310 gm

Volume: N:IMF Relationships: Locate final selected implant volume at right; Set N:IMF to the distance shown in the cell beneath, or leave at preop N:IMF, whichever is longer.	200	250	275	300	325	350	375	400	PreN:IMF 7.0 cm
	7.0	7.0	7.5	8	8	8.5	9.0	9.5	

IV. NEW INFRAMAMMARY FOLD LEVEL	N:IMF$_{MaxSt}$ to set with preoperative markings and intraoperatively	8.0 cm
V. INCISION LOCATION	IM AX PA UMB	

PREOPERATIVE ASSESSMENT AND OBSERVATIONS

Breasts low on torso
Nipple level asymmetry: WNBCS
Nipples located laterally on breast mound: WNBCS
Moderately wide intermammary distance with visible rib protrusions medially
  upper breast area preoperatively

POSTOPERATIVE ASSESSMENT AND OBSERVATIONS

Pre- to post- bra size change by patient questionnaire: 36B to 36C
Excellent upper and lower breast fill and contour
Upper breast fill and shape maintained for over 6 years
Breasts soft, mobile, compressible at 13 months followup
Nipple level asymmetry: WNBCS as predicted
When breasts are low on torso, any type of implant other than a form stable, full height device will leave the breasts looking even lower on the torso. This full height implant shortens the distance from the top of the breast to the clavicle and improves aesthetics
Nipples located laterally on breast mound: WNBCS as predicted
Intermammary distance decreased while preserving all attachments of pectoralis major medially with a dual plane 1 pocket
Less visible rib protrusions medially upper breast area compared to preoperatively
Apparent increased lower pole stretch at 3 and 5 years confirmed by measurements

Interval: Preop STPTUP 1.3 cm STPTIMF 1.0 cm Base Width 12.5 cm APSS 3.0 cm N:IMF 7.0 cm PCSEF 70%					
Interval: 6 mo STPTUP 1.7 cm STPTIMF 1.0 cm Base Width 13.5 cm APSS 1.7 cm N:IMF 9.0 cm					
Interval: 1 yr STPTUP 1.6 cm STPTIMF 1.1 cm Base Width 13.5 cm APSS 2.0 cm N:IMF 9.0 cm					
Interval: 3 yr STPTUP 1.6 cm STPTIMF 1.4 cm Base Width 13.5 cm APSS 2.0 cm N:IMF 11.0 cm					
Interval: 5 yr STPTUP 1.5 cm STPTIMF 1.4 cm Base Width 13.5 cm APSS 1.9 cm N:IMF 11.0 cm					
Interval: 1 yr STPTUP 1.6 cm STPTIMF 1.1 cm Base Width 13.5 cm APSS 2.0 cm N:IMF 9.0 cm					

CASE STUDY 21-3

HISTORY

Age: 60 (oldest patient in series)
Gravida: 2
Para: 2
Bra **Band** Size: 34
Breast **Cup** Size (Pt. estimate)
   Prior to pregnancy: A
   Largest with preg: C
   Current Cup Size: B
   Desired Cup Size: C/D
Previous Breast Disease: None
Breast Biopsies: No
Family Hx. Breast Cancer: No
   (Mother Grandmother Aunt)
Pertinent Medical or Breast
   Imaging History: None
Breast Masses: **None**

TISSUE ASSESSMENT AND HIGH FIVE™ SYSTEM CRITICAL DECISIONS PROCESS

Prioritized Decisions Based on Breast Measurements and Tissue Characteristics
The High Five™ System Copyright 2005 John B. Tebbetts, M.D.

I. POCKET LOCATION SELECTED BASED ON THICKNESS OF TISSUE COVERAGE (Circle One)

STPTU	1.3	If <2.0 cm, consider dual plane (DP) or partial retropectoral (PRP, pectoralis origins intact across IMF)	DP2
STPTIMF	0.8	If STPTIMF <0.5 cm, consider subpectoral pocket and leave pectoralis origins intact along IMF	PRP RM

II. IMPLANT VOLUME/WEIGHT BASED ON BREAST DIMENSIONS, TISSUE STRETCH, AND EXISTING PARENCHYMA

Base Width	12.0	B.W. Parenchyma (cm)	10.5	11.0	11.5	12.0	12.5	13.0	13.5	14.0	14.5	15.0	
		Initial Volume (cc)	200	250	275	300	300	325	350	375	375	400	300 cc
APSS$_{MaxStr}$	3.0	²If APSS <2.0, −30 cc; If APSS >3.0, +30 cc; If APSS >4.0, +60 cc Place appropriate number in blank at right											+30 cc
N:IMF$_{MaxSt}$	5L/7R	If N:IMF >9.5, +30 cc Place appropriate number in blank at right											NA
PCSEF %	60	If PCSEF <20%, +30 cc; If PCSEF >80%, −30 cc Place appropriate number in blank at right											NA
IDFDD cc	NA	If Allergan Style 468 or other form stable saline implant, −30 cc Place appropriate number in blank at right											NA
Pt. request													NA

NET ESTIMATED VOLUME TO FILL ENVELOPE BASED ON PATIENT TISSUE CHARACTERISTICS	330 cc

III. IMPLANT TYPE MFR: Allergan	STYLE/MODEL: Style 410 FM	VOLUME: 310 gm	310 gm

Volume: N:IMF Relationships: Locate final selected implant volume at right; Set N:IMF to the distance shown in the cell beneath, or leave at preop N:IMF, whichever is longer.	200	250	275	300	325	350	375	400	PreN:IMF
	7.0	7.0	7.5	8	8	8.5	9.0	9.5	5L/7R cm

IV. NEW INFRAMAMMARY FOLD LEVEL	N:IMF$_{MaxSt}$ to set with preoperative markings and intraoperatively	8.0 cm
V. INCISION LOCATION	IM AX PA UMB	

PREOPERATIVE ASSESSMENT AND OBSERVATIONS

Relative constriction or inadequate expansion of breast lower pole: N:IMF$_{MaxSt}$
   left 5.0 cm, right 7.0 cm preoperatively, set to N:IMF of 8 cm bilaterally
   intraoperatively.
Downpointing nipples: Plan IMF repositioning, DP2, but advise all patients
   with downpointing nipples to not expect complete correction, because
   regardless of surgical techniques and implant type, correction is not
   totally predictable.
Despite chronologic age, this patient is very active and athletic, and tissue
   "quality" good. Her APSS of 3.0 is typical of a parous patient of any age
   and comparable breast width.

POSTOPERATIVE ASSESSMENT AND OBSERVATIONS

Pre- to post- bra size change by patient questionnaire: 34A to 34D
Breasts soft, mobile, compressible at 9 months followup
Upper breast fill and shape maintained for over 5 years
Repositioning of inframammary folds inferiorly and DP2 improved, but did not totally correct downpointing nipples
   in lateral view
Despite planning according to High Five™, excess implant volume relative to limited lower pole expansion resulted in
   persistent mild excess upper pole fill at up to 5 years, that while appealing to the patient, did not correlate with
   the surgical plan
Breast shape and fill very consistent at up to 5 years in this older patient
In this case, with the oldest tissues in the series, lower pole expansion did not increase at up to 5 years followup,
   atypical of many patients over age 40

Interval: Preop STPTUP 1.3 cm STPTIMF 0.8 cm Base Width 12.0 cm APSS 3.0 cm N:IMF R: 5 cm L: 7 cm PCSEF 60%				
Interval: 1 yr STPTUP 1.8 cm STPTIMF 0.8 cm Base Width 13.5 cm APSS 1.8 cm N:IMF 9.0 cm				
Interval: 2 yr STPTUP 2.0 cm STPTIMF 1.0 cm Base Width 13.5 cm APSS 1.9 cm N:IMF 9.0 cm				
Interval: 3 yr STPTUP 2.1 cm STPTIMF 1.0 cm Base Width 13.5 cm APSS 1.8 cm N:IMF 9.0 cm				
Interval: 5 yr STPTUP 2.0 cm STPTIMF 0.9 cm Base Width 13.5 cm APSS 1.8 cm N:IMF 9.0 cm				
Interval: 1 yr STPTUP 1.8 cm STPTIMF 0.8 cm Base Width 13.5 cm APSS 1.8 cm N:IMF 9.0 cm				

CASE STUDY 21-4

HISTORY

Age: 44
Gravida: 1
Para: 1
Bra **Band** Size: 36
Breast **Cup** Size (Pt. estimate)
  Prior to pregnancy: A
  Largest with preg: B/C
  Current Cup Size: 34B
  Desired Cup Size: C
Previous Breast Disease: None
Breast Biopsies: No
Family Hx. Breast Cancer: No
Pertinent Medical or Breast
  Imaging History: None
$1/2$ pack/day smoker
Takes Zithromax, Macrobin, BCPs
Breast Masses: **None**

TISSUE ASSESSMENT AND HIGH FIVE™ SYSTEM CRITICAL DECISIONS PROCESS

Prioritized Decisions Based on Breast Measurements and Tissue Characteristics
The High Five™ System   Copyright 2005   John B. Tebbetts, M.D.

I. POCKET LOCATION SELECTED BASED ON THICKNESS OF TISSUE COVERAGE (Circle One)				
STPTUP	1.2	If <2.0 cm, consider dual plane (DP) or partial retropectoral (PRP, pectoralis origins intact across IMF)		DP1
STPTIMF	0.8	If STPTIMF <0.5 cm, consider subpectoral pocket and leave pectoralis origins intact along IMF		PRP RM

II. IMPLANT VOLUME/WEIGHT BASED ON BREAST DIMENSIONS, TISSUE STRETCH, AND EXISTING PARENCHYMA

Base Width	12.5	B.W. Parenchyma (cm)	10.5	11.0	11.5	12.0	12.5	13.0	13.5	14.0	14.5	15.0	
		Initial Volume (cc)	200	250	275	300	300	325	350	375	375	400	300 cc
APSS$_{MaxStr}$	3.3	[2]If APSS <2.0, −30 cc; If APSS >3.0, +30 cc; If APSS >4.0, +60 cc Place appropriate number in blank at right											+30 cc
N:IMF$_{MaxSt}$	8	If N:IMF >9.5, +30 cc Place appropriate number in blank at right											NA
PCSEF %	60	If PCSEF <20%, +30 cc; If PCSEF >80%, −30 cc Place appropriate number in blank at right											NA
IDFDD cc	NA	If Allergan Style 468 or other form stable saline implant, −30 cc Place appropriate number in blank at right											NA
Pt. request													NA

NET ESTIMATED VOLUME TO FILL ENVELOPE BASED ON PATIENT TISSUE CHARACTERISTICS	330 cc

III. IMPLANT TYPE MFR: Allergan STYLE/MODEL: Style 410 FM VOLUME: 310 gm	310 gm

Volume: N:IMF Relationships: Locate final selected implant volume at right; Set N:IMF to the distance shown in the cell beneath, or leave at preop N:IMF, whichever is longer.	200	250	275	300	325	350	375	400	PreN:IMF 8.0 cm
	7.0	7.0	7.5	8	8	8.5	9.0	9.5	

IV. NEW INFRAMAMMARY FOLD LEVEL	N:IMF$_{MaxSt}$ to set with preoperative markings and intraoperatively	8.0 cm

V. INCISION LOCATION	IM AX PA UMB

PREOPERATIVE ASSESSMENT AND OBSERVATIONS

Breasts low on torso: WNBCCS
Breast level asymmetry: WNBCS
Breast width asymmetry: WNBCS
Nipple level asymmetry: WNBCS
Nipples located laterally on breast mound: WNBCS
Moderately wide IMD
Marked chest wall protrusion left medial breast area on supine view

POSTOPERATIVE ASSESSMENT AND OBSERVATIONS

Pre- to post- bra size change by patient questionnaire: 34B to 36C
Breasts soft, mobile, compressible at 14 months followup
Upper breast fill and shape maintained for over 5 years
Chest wall protrusion hidden well by implant but causes slightly more apparent fill this area
Excellent breast fill and shape
Breasts remain low on torso as predicted preop; augmentation does not move the breast on the torso
IMD width remains unchanged as planned to preserve all medial pectoralis coverage medially for long-term coverage; eliminate risks of visible edges, traction rippling
Asymmetry and nipple position items listed preop WNBCS as predicted
When breasts are low on torso, any type of implant other than a form stable, full height device will leave the breasts looking even lower on the torso. This full height implant shortens the distance from the top of the breast to the clavicle and improves aesthetics

Interval: Preop STPTUP 1.2 cm STPTIMF 0.8 cm Base Width 12.5 cm APSS 3.3 cm N:IMF 8.0 cm PCSEF 60%					
Interval: 1 yr STPTUP 1.4 cm STPTIMF 0.9 cm Base Width 13.5 cm APSS 2.0 cm N:IMF 9.5 cm					
Interval: 2 yr STPTUP 1.8 cm STPTIMF 1.2 cm Base Width 13.5 cm APSS 2.1 cm N:IMF 9.5 cm					
Interval: 4 yr STPTUP 1.4 cm STPTIMF 1.4 cm Base Width 13.5 cm APSS 2.3 cm N:IMF 10.0 cm					
Interval: 5 yr STPTUP 1.3 cm STPTIMF 1.2 cm Base Width 13.5 cm APSS 2.3 cm N:IMF 10.0 cm					
Interval: 1 yr STPTUP 1.4 cm STPTIMF 0.9 cm Base Width 13.5 cm APSS 2.0 cm N:IMF 9.5 cm					

CASE STUDY 21-5

HISTORY

Age: 31
Gravida: 3
Para: 3
Bra **Band** Size: 36
Breast **Cup** Size (Pt. estimate)
   Prior to pregnancy: B
   Largest with preg: C
   Current Cup Size: A/B
   Desired Cup Size: C/D
Previous Breast Disease: None
Breast Biopsies: No
Family Hx. Breast Cancer: No
Pertinent Medical or Breast
   Imaging History: None
Breast Masses: **None**

TISSUE ASSESSMENT AND HIGH FIVE™ SYSTEM CRITICAL DECISIONS PROCESS

Prioritized Decisions Based on Breast Measurements and Tissue Characteristics
The High Five™ System   Copyright 2005   John B. Tebbetts, M.D.

I. POCKET LOCATION SELECTED BASED ON THICKNESS OF TISSUE COVERAGE (Circle One)			
STPTUP	1.5	**If <2.0 cm, consider dual plane (DP) or partial retropectoral (PRP, pectoralis origins intact across IMF)**	DP2
STPTIMF	0.9	**If STPTIMF <0.5 cm, consider subpectoral pocket and leave pectoralis origins intact along IMF**	PRP RM

II. IMPLANT VOLUME/WEIGHT BASED ON BREAST DIMENSIONS, TISSUE STRETCH, AND EXISTING PARENCHYMA

Base Width	13.5	B.W. Parenchyma (cm)	10.5	11.0	11.5	12.0	12.5	13.0	13.5	14.0	14.5	15.0	
		Initial Volume (cc)	200	250	275	300	300	325	350	375	375	400	350 cc
APSSMaxStr	3.0	²**If APSS <2.0, −30 cc; If APSS >3.0, +30 cc; If APSS >4.0, +60 cc Place appropriate number in blank at right**	+30 cc
N:IMF MaxSt	9.0	**If N:IMF >9.5, +30 cc Place appropriate number in blank at right**	NA
PCSEF %	60	**If PCSEF <20%, +30 cc; If PCSEF >80%, −30 cc Place appropriate number in blank at right**	NA
IDFDD cc	NA	**If Allergan Style 468 or other form stable saline implant, −30 cc Place appropriate number in blank at right**	NA
Pt. request		**One and one-half cup size increase—requests not to be a full D or larger breast**	−60 cc

NET ESTIMATED VOLUME TO FILL ENVELOPE BASED ON PATIENT TISSUE CHARACTERISTICS	320 cc

III. IMPLANT TYPE MFR: Allergan STYLE/MODEL: Style 410 FM VOLUME: 310 gm	310 gm

Volume: N:IMF Relationships: Locate final selected implant volume at right; **Set N:IMF to the distance shown in the cell beneath, or leave at preop N:IMF, whichever is longer.**	200	250	275	300	325	350	375	400	PreN:IMF 9.0 cm
	7.0	7.0	7.5	8	8	8.5	9.0	9.5	

IV. NEW INFRAMAMMARY FOLD LEVEL	**N:IMF**MaxSt **to set with preoperative markings and intraoperatively**	9.0 cm
V. INCISION LOCATION	IM AX PA UMB	

PREOPERATIVE ASSESSMENT AND OBSERVATIONS

Breast size asymmetry: WNBCS
Breast level asymmetry: WNBCS
Nipple level asymmetry: WNBCS
Breast size asymmetry: WNBCS

POSTOPERATIVE ASSESSMENT AND OBSERVATIONS

Pre- to post- bra size change by patient questionnaire: 36A/B to 36C
Breasts soft, mobile, compressible at 13 months followup
Excellent breast shape and fill
Upper fill and contour maintained for more than 4 years
All WNBCS items as predicted preoperatively
Patient had significant weight gain between 1 and 2 year followup
N:IMF had early predictable stretch from 9.0 to 9.5 cm, but stretched further to 11.5 cm at 2 years and 12 cm at 3 years, presumably related to the weight gain

Interval: Preop					
STPTUP 1.5 cm					
STPTIMF 0.9 cm					
Base Width 13.5 cm					
APSS 3.0 cm					
N:IMF 9.0 cm					
PCSEF 60%					

Interval: 6 mo
STPTUP 1.5 cm
STPTIMF 1.2 cm
Base Width 14.0 cm
APSS 2.7 cm
N:IMF 10.0 cm

Interval: 1 yr
STPTUP 1.6 cm
STPTIMF 1.2 cm
Base Width 14.0 cm
APSS 2.5 cm
N:IMF 10.5 cm

Interval: 2 yr
STPTUP 1.7 cm
STPTIMF 2.0 cm
Base Width 16.0 cm
APSS 2.5 cm
N:IMF 11.5 cm

Interval: 4 yr
STPTUP 1.7 cm
STPTIMF 1.3 cm
Base Width 16.0 cm
APSS 2.4 cm
N:IMF 12.0 cm

Interval: 1 yr
STPTUP 1.6 cm
STPTIMF 1.2 cm
Base Width 14.0 cm
APSS 2.5 cm
N:IMF 10.5 cm

CASE STUDY 21-6

HISTORY

Age: 37
Gravida: 2
Para: 2
Bra **Band** Size: 34
Breast **Cup** Size (Pt. estimate)
　Prior to pregnancy: B
　Largest with preg: C
　Current Cup Size: A/B
　Desired Cup Size: C
Previous Breast Disease: None
Breast Biopsies: No
Family Hx. Breast Cancer: Yes
　(Maternal grandmother,
　postmenopausal)
Pertinent Medical or Breast
　Imaging History: None
Breast Masses: **None**

TISSUE ASSESSMENT AND HIGH FIVE™ SYSTEM CRITICAL DECISIONS PROCESS

Prioritized Decisions Based on Breast Measurements and Tissue Characteristics
The High Five™ System　Copyright 2005　John B. Tebbetts, M.D.

I. POCKET LOCATION SELECTED BASED ON THICKNESS OF TISSUE COVERAGE (Circle One)			
STPTUP	1.9	If <2.0 cm, consider dual plane (DP) or partial retropectoral (PRP, pectoralis origins intact across IMF)	DP
STPTIMF	1.2	If STPTIMF <0.5 cm, consider subpectoral pocket and leave pectoralis origins intact along IMF	PRP RM

II. IMPLANT VOLUME/WEIGHT BASED ON BREAST DIMENSIONS, TISSUE STRETCH, AND EXISTING PARENCHYMA

Base Width	12.5	B.W. Parenchyma (cm)	10.5	11.0	11.5	12.0	12.5	13.0	13.5	14.0	14.5	15.0	
		Initial Volume (cc)	200	250	275	300	300	325	350	375	375	400	300 cc
APSS_{MaxStr}	2.0	²**If APSS <2.0, −30 cc; If APSS >3.0, +30 cc; If APSS >4.0, +60 cc Place appropriate number in blank at right**											−30 cc
N:IMF_{MaxSt}	8/7.5	**If N:IMF >9.5, +30 cc Place appropriate number in blank at right**											NA
PCSEF %	60	**If PCSEF <20%, +30 cc; If PCSEF >80%, −30 cc Place appropriate number in blank at right**											NA
IDFDD cc		**If Allergan Style 468 or other form stable saline implant, −30 cc Place appropriate number in blank at right**											NA
Pt. request													NA

NET ESTIMATED VOLUME TO FILL ENVELOPE BASED ON PATIENT TISSUE CHARACTERISTICS			270 cc

III. IMPLANT TYPE MFR: Allergan	STYLE/MODEL: Style 410 FM	VOLUME: 270 gm	270 gm

Volume: N:IMF Relationships: Locate final selected implant volume at right; Set N:IMF to the distance shown in the cell beneath, or leave at preop N:IMF, whichever is longer.	200	250	275	300	325	350	375	400	PreN:IMF 8R/7.5L cm
	7.0	7.0	7.5	8	8	8.5	9.0	9.5	

IV. NEW INFRAMAMMARY FOLD LEVEL	N:IMF_{MaxSt} to set with preoperative markings and intraoperatively	8.0 cm

V. INCISION LOCATION	IM　　AX　　PA　　UMB	

PREOPERATIVE ASSESSMENT AND OBSERVATIONS

Breast size asymmetry: WNBCS
Breast level asymmetry: WNBCS
Breast IMF level asymmetry
Tight skin envelope

POSTOPERATIVE ASSESSMENT AND OBSERVATIONS

Pre- to post- bra size change by patient questionnaire: 34A/B to 34C
Breasts soft, mobile, compressible at 13 months followup
Excellent breast shape and fill
All WNBCS items as predicted preoperatively
Breast IMF level asymmetry corrected by lowering left IMF to level of right by establishing equivalent N:IMF distances
　bilaterally
Upper fill and contour maintained to 6 years

Interval: Preop STPTUP 1.9 cm STPTIMF 1.2 cm Base Width 12.5 cm APSS 2.0 cm N:IMF R: 8 cm L: 7.5 cm PCSEF 60%					
Interval: 1 yr STPTUP 1.4 cm STPTIMF 1.7 cm Base Width 13.0 cm APSS 1.2 cm N:IMF R: 9 cm L: 8 cm					
Interval: 2 yr STPTUP 1.9 cm STPTIMF 1.0 cm Base Width 13.0 cm APSS 1.3 cm N:IMF R: 9 cm L: 8 cm					
Interval: 4 yr STPTUP 2.0 cm STPTIMF 1.3 cm Base Width 13.0 cm APSS 1.4 cm N:IMF R: 10 cm L: 9 cm					
Interval: 6 yr STPTUP 1.9 cm STPTIMF 1.4 cm Base Width 13.0 cm APSS 2.2 cm N:IMF R: 10 cm L: 9 cm					
Interval: 1 yr STPTUP 1.4 cm STPTIMF 1.7 cm Base Width 13.0 cm APSS 1.2 cm N:IMF R: 9 cm L: 8 cm					

CASE STUDY 21-7

HISTORY

Age: 27
Gravida: 0
Para: 0
Bra **Band** Size: 32
Breast **Cup** Size (Pt. estimate)
    Prior to pregnancy: NA
    Largest with preg: NA
    Current Cup Size: A
    Desired Cup Size: B/C
Previous Breast Disease: None
Breast Biopsies: No
Family Hx. Breast Cancer: No
Pertinent Medical or Breast
    Imaging History: MVP,
    asymptomatic, no meds
Breast Masses: **None**

TISSUE ASSESSMENT AND HIGH FIVE™ SYSTEM CRITICAL DECISIONS PROCESS

Prioritized Decisions Based on Breast Measurements and Tissue Characteristics
The High Five™ System   Copyright 2005   John B. Tebbetts, M.D.

I. POCKET LOCATION SELECTED BASED ON THICKNESS OF TISSUE COVERAGE (Circle One)

			DP 1
STPTUP	0.9	If <2.0 cm, consider dual plane (DP) or partial retropectoral (PRP, pectoralis origins intact across IMF)	
STPTIMF	0.6	If STPTIMF <0.5 cm, consider subpectoral pocket and leave pectoralis origins intact along IMF	PRP RM

II. IMPLANT VOLUME/WEIGHT BASED ON BREAST DIMENSIONS, TISSUE STRETCH, AND EXISTING PARENCHYMA

Base Width	10.5	B.W. Parenchyma (cm)	10.5	11.0	11.5	12.0	12.5	13.0	13.5	14.0	14.5	15.0	
		Initial Volume (cc)	200	250	275	300	300	325	350	375	375	400	200 cc
APSS~MaxStr~	2.0	[2]**If APSS <2.0, −30 cc; If APSS >3.0, +30 cc; If APSS >4.0, +60 cc Place appropriate number in blank at right**											NA
N:IMF~MaxSt~	8	**If N:IMF >9.5, +30 cc Place appropriate number in blank at right**											NA
PCSEF %	80	**If PCSEF <20%, +30 cc; If PCSEF >80%, −30 cc Place appropriate number in blank at right**											NA
IDFDD cc		**If Allergan Style 468 or other form stable saline implant, −30 cc Place appropriate number in blank at right**											NA
Pt. request													NA

NET ESTIMATED VOLUME TO FILL ENVELOPE BASED ON PATIENT TISSUE CHARACTERISTICS	200 cc

III. IMPLANT TYPE MFR: Allergan   STYLE/MODEL: Style 410 FM   VOLUME: 195 gm | **195 gm**

Volume: N:IMF Relationships: Locate final selected implant volume at right; Set N:IMF to the distance shown in the cell beneath, or leave at preop N:IMF, whichever is longer.	200	250	275	300	325	350	375	400	PreN:IMF
	7.0	7.0	7.5	8	8	8.5	9.0	9.5	8.0 cm

IV. NEW INFRAMAMMARY FOLD LEVEL	N:IMF~MaxSt~ to set with preoperative markings and intraoperatively	8.0 cm

V. INCISION LOCATION	IM AX PA UMB

PREOPERATIVE ASSESSMENT AND OBSERVATIONS

Breast size asymmetry: WNBCS
Tight skin envelope
Narrow base width breast
Thin soft tissue coverage
Left nipple located more laterally on breast mound: WNBCS
PCSEF of 80% indicates that for the dimensions and stretch capacity of the envelope, the envelope is already full of breast parenchyma (see lateral views) with little space for a breast implant (see upper pole of oblique views).

POSTOPERATIVE ASSESSMENT AND OBSERVATIONS

Pre- to post- bra size change by patient questionnaire: 32A to 32B
With APSS of 2.0 and PCSEF of 80% preoperatively, both were borderline for subtracting more volume in the High Five™ planning and implant selection process
Breasts soft, mobile, compressible at 13 months followup
Excellent breast shape and fill
Excellent upper breast shape and fill
All WNBCS items as predicted preoperatively
This case illustrates that it is impossible to accurately judge breast width preoperatively from a picture
2 months, 8 months and 1 year interval photographs show typical, rapid resolution to final breast shape, usually within 6 months
For up to a 200 cc implant, the High Five™ system recommends a N:IMF of 7.0, but the patient's preoperative N:IMF was 8.0, so that level was left unchanged intraoperatively

Interval: Preop STPTUP 0.9 cm STPTIMF 0.6 cm Base Width 10.5 cm APSS 2.0 cm N:IMF 8.0 cm PCSEF 80%					
Interval: 2 mo STPTUP 1.2 cm STPTIMF 0.7 cm Base Width 11.0 cm APSS 1.6 cm N:IMF 8.5 cm					
Interval: 6 mo STPTUP 1.0 cm STPTIMF 0.8 cm Base Width 11.0 cm APSS 2.0 cm N:IMF 9.0 cm					
Interval: 1 yr STPTUP 1.2 cm STPTIMF 0.8 cm Base Width 11.0 cm APSS 2.0 cm N:IMF 9.0 cm					
Interval: 2 yr STPTUP 1.1 cm STPTIMF 0.7 cm Base Width 11.0 cm APSS 2.2 cm N:IMF 9.5 cm					
Interval: 1 yr STPTUP 1.2 cm STPTIMF 0.8 cm Base Width 11.0 cm APSS 2.0 cm N:IMF 9.0 cm					

CASE STUDY 21-8

HISTORY

Age: 37
Gravida: 3
Para: 2
Bra **Band** Size: 34
Breast **Cup** Size (Pt. estimate)
  Prior to pregnancy: B
  Largest with preg: C/D
  Current Cup Size: B
  Desired Cup Size: C/D
Previous Breast Disease: None
Breast Biopsies: No
Family Hx. Breast Cancer: No
Pertinent Medical or Breast
  Imaging History: Negative
  needle biopsy L breast
  12 yrs ago
Breast Masses: **None**

TISSUE ASSESSMENT AND HIGH FIVE™ SYSTEM CRITICAL DECISIONS PROCESS

Prioritized Decisions Based on Breast Measurements and Tissue Characteristics
The High Five™ System   Copyright 2005   John B. Tebbetts, M.D.

I. POCKET LOCATION SELECTED BASED ON THICKNESS OF TISSUE COVERAGE (Circle One)

STPTUP	1.3	**If <2.0 cm, consider dual plane (DP) or partial retropectoral (PRP, pectoralis origins intact across IMF)**	**DP 1**
STPTIMF	0.9	**If STPTIMF <0.5 cm, consider subpectoral pocket and leave pectoralis origins intact along IMF**	**PRP RM**

II. IMPLANT VOLUME/WEIGHT BASED ON BREAST DIMENSIONS, TISSUE STRETCH, AND EXISTING PARENCHYMA

Base Width	12.0	B.W. Parenchyma (cm)	10.5	11.0	11.5	12.0	12.5	13.0	13.5	14.0	14.5	15.0	
		Initial Volume (cc)	200	250	275	300	300	325	350	375	375	400	300 cc
APSS~MaxStr~	3.2	²**If APSS <2.0, −30 cc; If APSS >3.0, +30 cc; If APSS >4.0, +60 cc Place appropriate number in blank at right**											**+30 cc**
N:IMF~MaxSt~	7.5	**If N:IMF >9.5, +30 cc Place appropriate number in blank at right**											**NA**
PCSEF %	60	**If PCSEF <20%, +30 cc; If PCSEF >80%, −30 cc Place appropriate number in blank at right**											**NA**
IDFDD cc		**If Allergan Style 468 or other form stable saline implant, −30 cc Place appropriate number in blank at right**											**NA**
Pt. request													**NA**

NET ESTIMATED VOLUME TO FILL ENVELOPE BASED ON PATIENT TISSUE CHARACTERISTICS	330 cc

III. IMPLANT TYPE MFR: Allergan   STYLE/MODEL: Style 410 FM   VOLUME: 315 gm | **315 gm**

Volume: N:IMF Relationships: Locate final selected implant volume at right; Set N:IMF to the distance shown in the cell beneath, or leave at preop N:IMF, whichever is longer.	200	250	275	300	325	350	375	400	PreN:IMF
	7.0	7.0	7.5	8	8	8.5	9.0	9.5	7.5 cm

IV. NEW INFRAMAMMARY FOLD LEVEL	**N:IMF**~MaxSt~ **to set with preoperative markings and intraoperatively**	8.0 cm

V. INCISION LOCATION	IM AX PA UMB	

PREOPERATIVE ASSESSMENT AND OBSERVATIONS

Breast size asymmetry: WNBCS
Breast level asymmetry: WNBCS
Nipple level asymmetry: WNBCS

POSTOPERATIVE ASSESSMENT AND OBSERVATIONS

Pre- to post- bra size change by patient questionnaire: 34B to 34D
Breast and nipple level asymmetries improved, but not totally corrected
Breasts soft, mobile, compressible at 13 months followup
Excellent breast shape and fill
Maintenance of upper pole fill and shape over 5 years postoperatively

Interval: Preop STPTUP 1.3 cm STPTIMF 0.9 cm Base Width 12.0 cm APSS 3.2 cm N:IMF 7.5 cm PCSEF 60%				
Interval: 1 yr STPTUP 1.5 cm STPTIMF 0.9 cm Base Width 13.5 cm APSS 2.6 cm N:IMF 9.0 cm				
Interval: 2 yr STPTUP 1.2 cm STPTIMF 1.0 cm Base Width 13.5 cm APSS 2.7 cm N:IMF 9.0 cm				
Interval: 3 yr STPTUP 1.4 cm STPTIMF 0.9 cm Base Width 13.5 cm APSS 2.6 cm N:IMF 9.0 cm				
Interval: 5 yr STPTUP 1.5 cm STPTIMF 1.1 cm Base Width 13.5 cm APSS 2.7 cm N:IMF 9.5 cm				
Interval: 1 yr STPTUP 1.5 cm STPTIMF 0.9 cm Base Width 13.5 cm APSS 2.6 cm N:IMF 9.0 cm				

CASE STUDY 21-9

HISTORY

Age: 24
Gravida: 0
Para: 0
Bra **Band** Size: 34
Breast **Cup** Size (Pt. estimate)
  Prior to pregnancy: NA
  Largest with preg: NA
  Current Cup Size: A/B
  Desired Cup Size: C
Previous Breast Disease: None
Breast Biopsies: No
Family Hx. Breast Cancer: No
Pertinent Medical or Breast
  Imaging History: None
Breast Masses: **None**

TISSUE ASSESSMENT AND HIGH FIVE™ SYSTEM CRITICAL DECISIONS PROCESS

Prioritized Decisions Based on Breast Measurements and Tissue Characteristics
The High Five™ System   Copyright 2005   John B. Tebbetts, M.D.

I. POCKET LOCATION SELECTED BASED ON THICKNESS OF TISSUE COVERAGE (Circle One)				DP 1
STPTUP	1.7	**If <2.0 cm, consider dual plane (DP) or partial retropectoral (PRP, pectoralis origins intact across IMF)**		
STPTIMF	0.7	**If STPTIMF <0.5 cm, consider subpectoral pocket and leave pectoralis origins intact along IMF**		**PRP RM**

II. IMPLANT VOLUME/WEIGHT BASED ON BREAST DIMENSIONS, TISSUE STRETCH, AND EXISTING PARENCHYMA

Base Width	12.0	B.W. Parenchyma (cm)	**10.5**	**11.0**	**11.5**	12.0	**12.5**	**13.0**	**13.5**	**14.0**	**14.5**	**15.0**	
		Initial Volume (cc)	**200**	**250**	**275**	300	**300**	**325**	**350**	**375**	**375**	**400**	**300 cc**
APSS_{MaxStr}	1.7	^{2}**If APSS <2.0, −30 cc; If APSS >3.0, +30 cc; If APSS >4.0, +60 cc Place appropriate number in blank at right**											**−30 cc**
N:IMF_{MaxSt}	7.5	**If N:IMF >9.5, +30 cc Place appropriate number in blank at right**											**NA**
PCSEF %	70	**If PCSEF <20%, +30 cc; If PCSEF >80%, −30 cc Place appropriate number in blank at right**											**NA**
IDFDD cc		**If Allergan Style 468 or other form stable saline implant, −30 cc Place appropriate number in blank at right**											**NA**
Pt. request													**NA**

NET ESTIMATED VOLUME TO FILL ENVELOPE BASED ON PATIENT TISSUE CHARACTERISTICS	**270 cc**
III. IMPLANT TYPE MFR: Allergan STYLE/MODEL: Style 410 FM VOLUME: 270 gm	**270 gm**

Volume: N:IMF Relationships: Locate final selected implant volume at right; Set N:IMF to the distance shown in the cell beneath, or leave at preop N:IMF, whichever is longer.	**200**	**250**	275	**300**	**325**	**350**	**375**	**400**	**PreN:IMF**
	7.0	**7.0**	7.5	**8**	**8**	**8.5**	**9.0**	**9.5**	**7.5 cm**

IV. NEW INFRAMAMMARY FOLD LEVEL	N:IMF_{MaxSt} to set with preoperative markings and intraoperatively	7.5 cm
V. INCISION LOCATION	IM AX PA UMB	

PREOPERATIVE ASSESSMENT AND OBSERVATIONS

Breast size asymmetry: WNBCS
Breasts high on torso (short SN:N): WNBCS
Nipple level asymmetry: WNBCS (left nipple lower)
Tight skin envelope
Breast level asymmetry: WNBCS
Wide intermammary distance: WNBCS

POSTOPERATIVE ASSESSMENT AND OBSERVATIONS

Pre- to post- bra size change by patient questionnaire: 34A to 34C
Breasts soft, mobile, compressible at 15 months followup
Excellent breast shape and fill
Maintenance of upper pole fill and shape over 5 years postoperatively
All WNBCS items as predicted preoperatively
IMD width remains unchanged as planned to preserve all medial pectoralis coverage medially for long-term coverage; eliminate risks of visible edges, traction rippling; however it appears visually narrower

Interval: Preop **STPTUP 1.7 cm** **STPTIMF 0.7 cm** **Base Width 12.0 cm** **APSS 1.7 cm** **N:IMF 7.5 cm** **PCSEF 70%**				
Interval: 6 mo **STPTUP 1.7 cm** **STPTIMF 1.0 cm** **Base Width 12.5 cm** **APSS 2.0 cm** **N:IMF 9.0 cm**				
Interval: 1 yr **STPTUP 1.9 cm** **STPTIMF 1.0 cm** **Base Width 12.5 cm** **APSS 2.2 cm** **N:IMF 10.0 cm**				
Interval: 3 yr **STPTUP 1.6 cm** **STPTIMF 1.2 cm** **Base Width 12.5 cm** **APSS 2.2 cm** **N:IMF 10.0 cm**				
Interval: 5 yr **STPTUP 1.7 cm** **STPTIMF 1.1 cm** **Base Width 12.5 cm** **APSS 2.6 cm** **N:IMF 10.5 cm**				
Interval: 1 yr **STPTUP 1.9 cm** **STPTIMF 1.0 cm** **Base Width 12.5 cm** **APSS 2.2 cm** **N:IMF 10.0 cm**				

CASE STUDY 21-10

HISTORY

Age: 20
GravidaL 0
Para: 0
Bra **Band** Size: 34
Breast **Cup** Size (Pt. estimate)
　Prior to pregnancy: NA
　Largest with preg: NA
　Current Cup Size: A/B
　Desired Cup Size: C
Previous Breast Disease: None
Breast Biopsies: No
Family Hx. Breast Cancer: No
Pertinent Medical or Breast
　Imaging History: None
Breast Masses: **None**

TISSUE ASSESSMENT AND HIGH FIVE™ SYSTEM CRITICAL DECISIONS PROCESS

Prioritized Decisions Based on Breast Measurements and Tissue Characteristics
The High Five™ System　Copyright 2005　John B. Tebbetts, M.D.

I. POCKET LOCATION SELECTED BASED ON THICKNESS OF TISSUE COVERAGE (Circle One)				DP 1
STPTUP	1.0	**If <2.0 cm, consider dual plane (DP) or partial retropectoral (PRP, pectoralis origins intact across IMF)**		**PRP RM**
STPTIMF	0.7	**If STPTIMF <0.5 cm, consider subpectoral pocket and leave pectoralis origins intact along IMF**		

II. IMPLANT VOLUME/WEIGHT BASED ON BREAST DIMENSIONS, TISSUE STRETCH, AND EXISTING PARENCHYMA

Base Width	11.5	B.W. Parenchyma (cm)	**10.5**	**11.0**	**11.5**	**12.0**	**12.5**	**13.0**	**13.5**	**14.0**	**14.5**	**15.0**	
		Initial Volume (cc)	**200**	**250**	**275**	**300**	**300**	**325**	**350**	**375**	**375**	**400**	**275 cc**
APSS_{MaxStr}	3.0	²**If APSS <2.0, −30 cc; If APSS >3.0, +30 cc; If APSS >4.0, +60 cc Place appropriate number in blank at right**											NA
N:IMF_{MaxSt}	6/7.5	**If N:IMF >9.5, +30 cc Place appropriate number in blank at right**											**NA**
PCSEF %	60	**If PCSEF <20%, +30 cc; If PCSEF >80%, −30 cc Place appropriate number in blank at right**											**NA**
IDFDD cc		**If Allergan Style 468 or other form stable saline implant, −30 cc Place appropriate number in blank at right**											**NA**
Pt. request													**NA**

NET ESTIMATED VOLUME TO FILL ENVELOPE BASED ON PATIENT TISSUE CHARACTERISTICS			**275 cc**
III. IMPLANT TYPE MFR: Allergan	STYLE/MODEL: Style 410 FM	VOLUME: 270 gm	**270 gm**

Volume: N:IMF Relationships: Locate final selected implant volume at right; Set N:IMF to the distance shown in the cell beneath, or leave at preop N:IMF, whichever is longer.	**200**	**250**	**275**	**300**	**325**	**350**	**375**	**400**	PreN:IMF 6/7.5 cm
	7.0	**7.0**	**7.5**	**8**	**8**	**8.5**	**9.0**	**9.5**	

IV. NEW INFRAMAMMARY FOLD LEVEL	N:IMF_{MaxSt} **to set with preoperative markings and intraoperatively**				7.5/7.5 cm
V. INCISION LOCATION		IM	AX	PA	UMB

PREOPERATIVE ASSESSMENT AND OBSERVATIONS

Breast size asymmetry: WNBCS
Wide intermammary distance: WNBCS
Nipples located laterally on breast mound: WNBCS
Breasts low on torso: WNBCS

POSTOPERATIVE ASSESSMENT AND OBSERVATIONS

Pre- to post- bra size change by patient questionnaire: 34A/B to 36C
Breasts soft, mobile, compressible at 13 months followup
Excellent breast shape and fill
Maintenance of upper pole fill and shape over 5 years postoperatively
The apparent size of the postoperative breasts with only a 270 gram implant demonstrates that it is impossible for surgeons or patients to accurately judge implant size in any picture. Further, the result demonstrates the excellent distribution of fill with a full height, form stable implant that makes the breast appear larger than it is
All WNBCS items as predicted preoperatively
IMD width remains unchanged as planned to preserve all medial pectoralis coverage medially for long-term coverage; eliminate risks of visible edges, traction rippling

Interval: Preop **STPTUP 1.0 cm** **STPTIMF 0.7 cm** **Base Width 11.5 cm** **APSS 3.0 cm** **N:IMF R: 6 cm L: 7.5 cm** **PCSEF 60%**				
Interval: 1 yr **STPTUP 1.4 cm** **STPTIMF 0.6 cm** **Base Width 12.0 cm** **APSS 2.8 cm** **N:IMF 10.0 cm**				
Interval: 2 yr **STPTUP 1.5 cm** **STPTIMF 0.7 cm** **Base Width 12.5 cm** **APSS 3.0 cm** **N:IMF 11.0 cm**				
Interval: 3 yr **STPTUP 1.8 cm** **STPTIMF 0.9 cm** **Base Width 12.5 cm** **APSS 2.8 cm** **N:IMF 11.0 cm**				
Interval: 5 yr **STPTUP 1.6 cm** **STPTIMF 0.7 cm** **Base Width 12.5 cm** **APSS 3.2 cm** **N:IMF 11.0 cm**				
Interval: 1 yr **STPTUP 1.4 cm** **STPTIMF 0.6 cm** **Base Width 12.0 cm** **APSS 2.8 cm** **N:IMF 10.0 cm**				

CASE STUDY 21-11

HISTORY

Age: 31
Gravida: 1
Para: 2
Bra **Band** Size: 32
Breast **Cup** Size (Pt. estimate)
   Prior to pregnancy: B
   Largest with preg: C
   Current Cup Size: A
   Desired Cup Size: C
Previous Breast Disease: None
Breast Biopsies: No
Family Hx. Breast Cancer: No
Pertinent Medical or Breast
   Imaging History: None
Breast Masses: **None**

TISSUE ASSESSMENT AND HIGH FIVE™ SYSTEM CRITICAL DECISIONS PROCESS

Prioritized Decisions Based on Breast Measurements and Tissue Characteristics
The High Five™ System   Copyright 2005   John B. Tebbetts, M.D.

I. POCKET LOCATION SELECTED BASED ON THICKNESS OF TISSUE COVERAGE (Circle One)			
STPTUP	1.3	**If <2.0 cm, consider dual plane (DP) or partial retropectoral (PRP, pectoralis origins intact across IMF)**	**DP 1** **PRP RM**
STPTIMF	0.6	**If STPTIMF <0.5 cm, consider subpectoral pocket and leave pectoralis origins intact along IMF**	

II. IMPLANT VOLUME/WEIGHT BASED ON BREAST DIMENSIONS, TISSUE STRETCH, AND EXISTING PARENCHYMA

Base Width	10.5	B.W. Parenchyma (cm)	10.5	11.0	11.5	12.0	12.5	13.0	13.5	14.0	14.5	15.0	
		Initial Volume (cc)	200	250	275	300	300	325	350	375	375	400	200 cc
APSS$_{MaxStr}$	3.2	[2]**If APSS <2.0, −30 cc; If APSS >3.0, +30 cc; If APSS >4.0, +60 cc Place appropriate number in blank at right**											+30 cc
N:IMF$_{MaxSt}$	7	**If N:IMF >9.5, +30 cc Place appropriate number in blank at right**											NA
PCSEF %	60	**If PCSEF <20%, +30 cc; If PCSEF >80%, −30 cc Place appropriate number in blank at right**											NA
IDFDD cc		**If Allergan Style 468 or other form stable saline implant, −30 cc Place appropriate number in blank at right**											NA
Pt. request													NA

NET ESTIMATED VOLUME TO FILL ENVELOPE BASED ON PATIENT TISSUE CHARACTERISTICS	230 cc
III. IMPLANT TYPE MFR: Allergan STYLE/MODEL: Style 410 FM VOLUME: 235 gm	235 gm

Volume: N:IMF Relationships: Locate final selected implant volume at right; Set N:IMF to the distance shown in the cell beneath, or leave at preop N:IMF, whichever is longer.	200	250	275	300	325	350	375	400	PreN:IMF
	7.0	7.0	7.5	8	8	8.5	9.0	9.5	7 cm

IV. NEW INFRAMAMMARY FOLD LEVEL	N:IMF$_{MaxSt}$ **to set with preoperative markings and intraoperatively**	7 cm

V. INCISION LOCATION	IM AX PA UMB

PREOPERATIVE ASSESSMENT AND OBSERVATIONS

Breast size asymmetry: WNBCS
Nipple level asymmetry: WNBCS
Breast level asymmetry: WNBCS
Wide intermammary distance: WNBCS
Thin soft tissue coverage
Narrow base width breast
Prominent upper chest rib visibility

POSTOPERATIVE ASSESSMENT AND OBSERVATIONS

Pre- to post- bra size change by patient questionnaire: 32A to 32C
Breasts soft, mobile, compressible at 13 months followup
Excellent breast shape and fill
Maintenance of upper pole fill and shape over 4 years postoperatively
Prominent upper chest rib visibility significantly improved postoperatively
All WNBCS items as predicted preoperatively
IMD width remains unchanged as planned to preserve all medial pectoralis coverage medially for long-term coverage; eliminate risks of visible edges, traction rippling

Interval: Preop STPTUP 1.2 cm STPTIMF 0.6 cm Base Width 10.5 cm APSS 3.2 cm N:IMF 7.0 cm PCSEF 60%				
Interval: 1 yr STPTUP 1.2 cm STPTIMF 0.6 cm Base Width 11.5 cm APSS 2.6 cm N:IMF R: 9 cm L: 8.5 cm				
Interval: 2 yr STPTUP 1.6 cm STPTIMF 0.6 cm Base Width 11.5 cm APSS 2.4 cm N:IMF R: 9 cm L: 8.5 cm				
Interval: 3 yr STPTUP 1.2 cm STPTIMF 0.6 cm Base Width 11.5 cm APSS 2.6 cm N:IMF R: 9 cm L: 8.5 cm				
Interval: 4 yr STPTUP 1.4 cm STPTIMF 0.7 cm Base Width 11.5 cm APSS 2.6 cm N:IMF R: 9 cm L: 8.5 cm				
Interval: 1 yr STPTUP 1.2 cm STPTIMF 0.6 cm Base Width 11.5 cm APSS 2.6 cm N:IMF R: 9 cm L: 8.5 cm				

CASE STUDY 21-12

HISTORY

Age: 36
Gravida: 2
Para: 2
Bra **Band** Size: 36
Breast **Cup** Size (Pt. estimate)
   Prior to pregnancy: A
   Largest with preg: C
   Current Cup Size: A
   Desired Cup Size: C
Previous Breast Disease: None
Breast Biopsies: No
Family Hx. Breast Cancer: No
Pertinent Medical or Breast
   Imaging History: None
Breast Masses: **None**

TISSUE ASSESSMENT AND HIGH FIVE™ SYSTEM CRITICAL DECISIONS PROCESS

Prioritized Decisions Based on Breast Measurements and Tissue Characteristics
The High Five™ System   Copyright 2005   John B. Tebbetts, M.D.

I. POCKET LOCATION SELECTED BASED ON THICKNESS OF TISSUE COVERAGE (Circle One)			
STPTUP	1.2	If <2.0 cm, consider dual plane (DP) or partial retropectoral (PRP, pectoralis origins intact across IMF)	DP 1
STPTIMF	0.9	If STPTIMF <0.5 cm, consider subpectoral pocket and leave pectoralis origins intact along IMF	**PRP RM**

II. IMPLANT VOLUME/WEIGHT BASED ON BREAST DIMENSIONS, TISSUE STRETCH, AND EXISTING PARENCHYMA													
Base Width	12.0	B.W. Parenchyma (cm)	10.5	11.0	11.5	12.0	12.5	13.0	13.5	14.0	14.5	15.0	**300 cc**
		Initial Volume (cc)	200	250	275	300	300	325	350	375	375	400	
APSS$_{MaxStr}$	2.5	^{2}If APSS <2.0, −30 cc; If APSS >3.0, +30 cc; If APSS >4.0, +60 cc Place appropriate number in blank at right											NA
N:IMF$_{MaxSt}$	6.5	If N:IMF >9.5, +30 cc Place appropriate number in blank at right											**NA**
PCSEF %	70	If PCSEF <20%, +30 cc; If PCSEF >80%, −30 cc Place appropriate number in blank at right											**NA**
IDFDD cc		If Allergan Style 468 or other form stable saline implant, −30 cc Place appropriate number in blank at right											**NA**
Pt. request													NA
NET ESTIMATED VOLUME TO FILL ENVELOPE BASED ON PATIENT TISSUE CHARACTERISTICS													**300 cc**
III. IMPLANT TYPE MFR: Allergan			STYLE/MODEL: Style 410 FM					VOLUME: 310 gm					**310 gm**

Volume: N:IMF Relationships: Locate final selected implant volume at right; Set N:IMF to the distance shown in the cell beneath, or leave at preop N:IMF, whichever is longer.	200	250	275	300	325	350	375	400	PreN:IMF
	7.0	7.0	7.5	8	8	8.5	9.0	9.5	6.5 cm

IV. NEW INFRAMAMMARY FOLD LEVEL	N:IMF$_{MaxSt}$ to set with preoperative markings and intraoperatively	8.0 cm
V. INCISION LOCATION	IM AX PA UMB	

PREOPERATIVE ASSESSMENT AND OBSERVATIONS

Breast size asymmetry: WNBCS
Breast level asymmetry: WNBCS
Nipple level and orientation asymmetry: WNBCS
Wide intermammary distance: WNBCS
Minimal breast parenchyma

POSTOPERATIVE ASSESSMENT AND OBSERVATIONS

Pre- to post- bra size change by patient questionnaire: 36A to 36C
Breasts soft, mobile, compressible at 14 months followup
Excellent breast shape and fill
Maintenance of upper pole fill and shape over 4 years postoperatively
IMD width remains unchanged as planned to preserve all medial pectoralis coverage medially for long-term coverage; eliminate risks of visible edges, traction rippling
All WNBCS items as predicted preoperatively

Interval: Preop					
STPTUP 1.2 cm					
STPTIMF 0.9 cm					
Base Width 12.0 cm					
APSS 2.5 cm					
N:IMF xx cm					
PCSEF 70%					

Interval: 6 mo					
STPTUP 1.3 cm					
STPTIMF 1.1 cm					
Base Width 13.5 cm					
APSS 3.0 cm					
N:IMF 9.5 cm					

Interval: 1 yr					
STPTUP 1.6 cm					
STPTIMF 1.0 cm					
Base Width 13.5 cm					
APSS 3.2 cm					
N:IMF 9.5 cm					

Interval: 2 yr					
STPTUP 1.4 cm					
STPTIMF 1.1 cm					
Base Width 13.5 cm					
APSS 3.1 cm					
N:IMF 9.5 cm					

Interval: 4 yr					
STPTUP 1.5 cm					
STPTIMF 1.0 cm					
Base Width 13.0 cm					
APSS 3.4 cm					
N:IMF R: 11 cm L: 10 cm					

Interval: 1 yr					
STPTUP 1.6 cm					
STPTIMF 1.0 cm					
Base Width 13.5 cm					
APSS 3.2 cm					
N:IMF 9.5 cm					

CASE STUDY 21-13

Age: 30
Gravida: 0
Para: 0
Bra **Band** Size: 34
Breast **Cup** Size (Pt. estimate)
  Prior to pregnancy: NA
  Largest with preg: NA
  Current Cup Size: A
  Desired Cup Size: C
Previous Breast Disease: None
Breast Biopsies: No
Family Hx. Breast Cancer: No
Pertinent Medical or Breast
  Imaging History: None
Breast Masses: **None**

TISSUE ASSESSMENT AND HIGH FIVE™ SYSTEM CRITICAL DECISIONS PROCESS

Prioritized Decisions Based on Breast Measurements and Tissue Characteristics
The High Five™ System   Copyright 2005   John B. Tebbetts, M.D.

I. POCKET LOCATION SELECTED BASED ON THICKNESS OF TISSUE COVERAGE (Circle One)				
STPTUP	2.2	**If <2.0 cm, consider dual plane (DP) or partial retropectoral (PRP, pectoralis origins intact across IMF)**	**DP 1**	
STPTIMF	1.3	**If STPTIMF <0.5 cm, consider subpectoral pocket and leave pectoralis origins intact along IMF**	**PRP RM**	

II. IMPLANT VOLUME/WEIGHT BASED ON BREAST DIMENSIONS, TISSUE STRETCH, AND EXISTING PARENCHYMA

Base Width	12.5	B.W. Parenchyma (cm)	**10.5**	**11.0**	**11.5**	**12.0**	**12.5**	**13.0**	**13.5**	**14.0**	**14.5**	**15.0**	
		Initial Volume (cc)	200	250	275	300	300	325	350	375	375	400	**300 cc**
APSS$_{MaxStr}$	1.8	[2]**If APSS <2.0, −30 cc; If APSS >3.0, +30 cc; If APSS >4.0, +60 cc Place appropriate number in blank at right**											**−30 cc**
N:IMF$_{MaxSt}$	9	**If N:IMF >9.5, +30 cc Place appropriate number in blank at right**											**NA**
PCSEF %	85	**If PCSEF <20%, +30 cc; If PCSEF >80%, −30 cc Place appropriate number in blank at right**											**−30 cc**
IDFDD cc		**If Allergan Style 468 or other form stable saline implant, −30 cc Place appropriate number in blank at right**											**NA**
Pt. request		Two cup size increase if possible with skin limitations											**+30 cc**

III. NET ESTIMATED VOLUME TO FILL ENVELOPE BASED ON PATIENT TISSUE CHARACTERISTICS			**270 cc**

III. IMPLANT TYPE MFR: Allergan	STYLE/MODEL: Style 410 FM	VOLUME: 270 gm	**270 gm**

Volume: N:IMF Relationships: Locate final selected implant volume at right; Set N:IMF to the disstance shown in the cell beneath, or leave at preop N:IMF, whichever is longer.	200	250	275	300	325	350	375	400	**PreN:IMF**
	7.0	7.0	7.5	8	8	8.5	9.0	9.5	**9 cm**

IV. NEW INFRAMAMMARY FOLD LEVEL	N:IMF$_{MaxSt}$ to set with preoperative markings and intraoperatively	**9 cm**

V. INCISION LOCATION		IM AX PA UMB	

PREOPERATIVE ASSESSMENT AND OBSERVATIONS

Breast size asymmetry: WNBCS
Breast level asymmetry: WNBCS
Nipple level asymmetry: WNBCS
Tight skin envelope: APSS 1.8 cm
Full skin envelope preoperatively: PCSEF 85%
Patient had adequate soft tissue thickness for a submammary pocket (STPTUP 2.2), but to minimize implant exposure to parenchymal flora and optimize imaging, a dual plane 1 pocket was selected.

POSTOPERATIVE ASSESSMENT AND OBSERVATIONS

Pre- to post- bra size change by patient questionnaire: 34A to 34C
Breasts soft, mobile, compressible at 13 months followup
Excellent breast shape and fill
Maintenance of upper pole fill and shape over 5 years postoperatively
Patient began significant weight gain between years 2 and 4 postoperatively, reflected in lower pole stretch measurements that increased disproportionately during that time
All WNBCS items as predicted preoperatively

| Interval: Preop |
| STPTUP 1.8 cm |
| STPTIMF 2.2 cm |
| Base Width 12.5 cm |
| APSS 1.8 cm |
| N:IMF 9.0 cm |
| PCSEF 70% |

| Interval: 1 yr |
| STPTUP 1.4 cm |
| STPTIMF 2.0 cm |
| Base Width 15.0 cm |
| APSS 1.4 cm |
| N:IMF 11.0 cm |

| Interval: 2 yr |
| STPTUP 1.8 cm |
| STPTIMF 2.1 cm |
| Base Width 15.0 cm |
| APSS 1.8 cm |
| N:IMF 12.0 cm |

| Interval: 4 yr |
| STPTUP 2.3 cm |
| STPTIMF 2.4 cm |
| Base Width 15.0 cm |
| APSS 2.3 cm |
| N:IMF 12.5 cm |

| Interval: 6 yr |
| STPTUP 2.4 cm |
| STPTIMF 2.3 cm |
| Base Width 16.0 cm |
| APSS 2.4 cm |
| N:IMF 12.5 cm |

| Interval: 1 yr |
| STPTUP 1.4 cm |
| STPTIMF 2.0 cm |
| Base Width 15.0 cm |
| APSS 1.4 cm |
| N:IMF 11.0 cm |

CASE STUDY 21-14

Age: 33
Gravida: 2
Para: 2
Bra **Band** Size: 34
Breast **Cup** Size (Pt. estimate)
  Prior to pregnancy: A
  Largest with preg: B
  Current Cup Size: A
  Desired Cup Size: B/C
Previous Breast Disease: None
Breast Biopsies: No
Family Hx. Breast Cancer: No
Pertinent Medical or Breast
  Imaging History: None
Breast Masses: **None**

TISSUE ASSESSMENT AND HIGH FIVE™ SYSTEM CRITICAL DECISIONS PROCESS

Prioritized Decisions Based on Breast Measurements and Tissue Characteristics
The High Five™ System   Copyright 2005   John B. Tebbetts, M.D.

I. POCKET LOCATION SELECTED BASED ON THICKNESS OF TISSUE COVERAGE (Circle One)			
STPTUP	0.9	**If <2.0 cm, consider dual plane (DP) or partial retropectoral (PRP, pectoralis origins intact across IMF)**	**DP**
STPTIMF	0.5	**If STPTIMF <0.5 cm, consider subpectoral pocket and leave pectoralis origins intact along IMF**	**PRP RM**

II. IMPLANT VOLUME/WEIGHT BASED ON BREAST DIMENSIONS, TISSUE STRETCH, AND EXISTING PARENCHYMA

Base Width	11.5	B.W. Parenchyma (cm)	**10.5**	**11.0**	**11.5**	**12.0**	**12.5**	**13.0**	**13.5**	**14.0**	**14.5**	**15.0**	
		Initial Volume (cc)	200	250	275	300	300	325	350	375	375	400	**275 cc**
APSS_{MaxStr}	3.5	²**If APSS <2.0, −30 cc; If APSS >3.0, +30 cc; If APSS >4.0, +60 cc Place appropriate number in blank at right**											**+30 cc**
N:IMF_{MaxSt}	7.0	**If N:IMF >9.5, +30 cc Place appropriate number in blank at right**											**NA**
PCSEF %	60	**If PCSEF <20%, +30 cc; If PCSEF >80%, −30 cc Place appropriate number in blank at right**											**NA**
IDFDD cc		**If Allergan Style 468 or other form stable saline implant, −30 cc Place appropriate number in blank at right**											**NA**
Pt. request													**NA**

NET ESTIMATED VOLUME TO FILL ENVELOPE BASED ON PATIENT TISSUE CHARACTERISTICS		**305 cc**

III. IMPLANT TYPE MFR: Allergan	STYLE/MODEL: Style 410 FM	VOLUME: 310 gm	**310 gm**

Volume: N:IMF Relationships: Locate final selected implant volume at right; **Set N:IMF to the disstance shown in the cell beneath, or leave at preop N:IMF, whichever is longer.**		**200**	**250**	**275**	**300**	**325**	**350**	**375**	**400**	**PreN:IMF**
		7.0	7.0	7.5	8	8	8.5	9.0	9.5	**7.0 cm**

IV. NEW INFRAMAMMARY FOLD LEVEL	**N:IMF**_{MaxSt} **to set with preoperative markings and intraoperatively**	**8.0 cm**

V. INCISION LOCATION	IM AX PA UMB	

PREOPERATIVE ASSESSMENT AND OBSERVATIONS

Breast size asymmetry: WNBCS
Breast level asymmetry: WNBCS
Nipple level asymmetry: WNBCS
Nipples located laterally on breast mound: WNBCS—R > L
Wide intermammary distance: WNBCS

POSTOPERATIVE ASSESSMENT AND OBSERVATIONS

Pre- to post- bra size change by patient questionnaire: 34A to 34C
Breasts soft, mobile, compressible at 12 months followup
Excellent breast shape and fill
Maintenance of upper pole fill and shape over 5 years postoperatively
IMD width remains unchanged as planned to preserve all medial pectoralis coverage medially for long-term
  coverage; eliminate risks of visible edges, traction rippling
All WNBCS items as predicted preoperatively
The base width of this implant was 12.0 cm, 0.5 cm wider than the patient's base parenchyma measurement. The
  11.5 cm measurement is always made very conservatively, hence soft tissue coverage remains optimal to 5 years

Interval: Preop STPTUP 0.9 cm STPTIMF 0.5 cm Base Width 11.5 cm APSS 3.5 cm N:IMF 7.0 cm PCSEF 60%					
Interval: 1 yr STPTUP 1.1 cm STPTIMF 0.7 cm Base Width 12.0 cm APSS 2.8 cm N:IMF 8 .5 cm					
Interval: 2 yr STPTUP 1.1 cm STPTIMF 0.7 cm Base Width 12.0 cm APSS 2.8 cm N:IMF 8.5 cm					
Interval: 3 yr STPTUP 1.1 cm STPTIMF 0.7 cm Base Width 12.0 cm APSS 2.6 cm N:IMF 8.5 cm					
Interval: 5 yr STPTUP 1.2 cm STPTIMF 0.8 cm Base Width 12.0 cm APSS 2.8 cm N:IMF 9.0 cm					
Interval: 1 yr STPTUP 1.1 cm STPTIMF 0.7 cm Base Width 12.0 cm APSS 2.8 cm N:IMF 8.5 cm					

587

CASE STUDY 21-15

HISTORY

Age: 19
Gravida: 0
Para: 0
Bra **Band** Size: 34
Breast **Cup** Size (Pt. estimate)
  Prior to pregnancy: NA
  Largest with preg: NA
  Current Cup Sizel A
  Desired Cup Size: B/C
Previous Breast Disease: None
Breast Biopsies: No
Family Hx. Breast Cancer: No
Pertinent Medical or Breast
  Imaging History: None
Breast Masses: **None**

TISSUE ASSESSMENT AND HIGH FIVE™ SYSTEM CRITICAL DECISIONS PROCESS

Prioritized Decisions Based on Breast Measurements and Tissue Characteristics
The High Five™ System   Copyright 2005   John B. Tebbetts, M.D.

I. POCKET LOCATION SELECTED BASED ON THICKNESS OF TISSUE COVERAGE (Circle One)			
STPTUP	1.2	**If <2.0 cm, consider dual plane (DP) or partial retropectoral (PRP, pectoralis origins intact across IMF)**	DP 1
STPTIMF	1.0	**If STPTIMF <0.5 cm, consider subpectoral pocket and leave pectoralis origins intact along IMF**	PRP RM

II. IMPLANT VOLUME/WEIGHT BASED ON BREAST DIMENSIONS, TISSUE STRETCH, AND EXISTING PARENCHYMA

Base Width	12.5	B.W. Parenchyma (cm)	**10.5**	**11.0**	**11.5**	**12.0**	**12.5**	**13.0**	**13.5**	**14.0**	**14.5**	**15.0**	
		Initial Volume (cc)	200	250	275	300	300	325	350	375	375	400	300 cc
APSSₘₐₓStr	1.8	²**If APSS <2.0, −30 cc; If APSS >3.0, +30 cc; If APSS >4.0, +60 cc Place appropriate number in blank at right**											−30 cc
N:IMFₘₐₓSt	9	**If N:IMF >9.5, +30 cc Place appropriate number in blank at right**											**NA**
PCSEF %	70	**If PCSEF <20%, +30 cc; If PCSEF >80%, −30 cc Place appropriate number in blank at right**											**NA**
IDFDD cc		**If Allergan Style 468 or other form stable saline implant, −30 cc Place appropriate number in blank at right**											**NA**
Pt. request													**NA**

NET ESTIMATED VOLUME TO FILL ENVELOPE BASED ON PATIENT TISSUE CHARACTERISTICS	270 cc
III. IMPLANT TYPE MFR: Allergan STYLE/MODEL: Style 410 FM VOLUME: 270 gm	270 gm

Volume: N:IMF Relationships: Locate final selected implant volume at right; Set N:IMF to the distance shown in the cell beneath, or leave at preop N:IMF, whichever is longer.	200	250	275	300	325	350	375	400	PreN:IMF
	7.0	7.0	7.5	8	8	8.5	9.0	9.5	9 cm

IV. NEW INFRAMAMMARY FOLD LEVEL	N:IMFₘₐₓSt to set with preoperative markings and intraoperatively	9 cm
V. INCISION LOCATION	IM AX PA UMB	

PREOPERATIVE ASSESSMENT AND OBSERVATIONS

Breast size asymmetry: WNBCS
Breast level asymmetry: WNBCS
Nipple level asymmetry: WNBCS
Tight skin envelope: APSS 2.0 cm
Nipples located laterally on breast mound: WNBCS

POSTOPERATIVE ASSESSMENT AND OBSERVATIONS

Pre- to post- bra size change by patient questionnaire: 34A to 34C
Breasts soft, mobile, compressible at 12 months followup
Excellent breast shape and fill
Maintenance of upper pole fill and shape over 5 years postoperatively
All WNBCS items as predicted preoperatively

Interval: Preop **STPTUP 1.2 cm** **STPTIMF 1.2 cm** **Base Width 12.0 cm** **APSS 1.8 cm** **N:IMF 9.0 cm** **PCSEF 70%**				
Interval: 6 mo **STPTUP 1.4 cm** **STPTIMF 1.2 cm** **Base Width 14.0 cm** **APSS 2.1 cm** **N:IMF 11.5 cm**				
Interval: 1 yr **STPTUP 1.6 cm** **STPTIMF 1.2 cm** **Base Width 14 cm** **APSS 2.4 cm** **N:IMF 11.5 cm**				
Interval: 2 yr **STPTUP 1.6 cm** **STPTIMF 1.2 cm** **Base Width 14 cm** **APSS 2.3 cm** **N:IMF 12.0 cm**				
Interval: 5 yr **STPTUP 1.8 cm** **STPTIMF 1.2 cm** **Base Width 14.0 cm** **APSS 2.3 cm** **N:IMF 12.0 cm**				
Interval: 1 yr **STPTUP 1.6 cm** **STPTIMF 1.2 cm** **Base Width 14 cm** **APSS 2.4 cm** **N:IMF 11.5 cm**				

INDEX

Please note that page references relating to non-textual content such as Figures or Tables are in *italic* print. Numbers, such as 24, are spelled out in words.